Continued on back

HYPERACTIVITY

HYPERACTIVITY

CURRENT ISSUES, RESEARCH, AND THEORY

SECOND EDITION

DOROTHEA M. ROSS
University of California
San Francisco, California

SHEILA A. ROSS
Research Institute
Palo Alto Medical Foundation for Health Care,
Research, and Education
Palo Alto, California

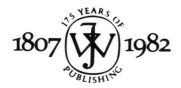

A Wiley-Interscience Publication
JOHN WILEY & SONS
New York • Chichester • Brisbane • Toronto • Singapore

Library of Congress Cataloging in Publication Data

Ross, Dorothea.
  Hyperactivity: Current issues, research, and theory.

  (Wiley series on personality processes, ISSN 0195-4008)
  "A Wiley-Interscience publication."
  Bibliography: p.
  Includes indexes.
  1. Hyperactive children   I. Ross, Sheila A.
II. Title. III. Series.
RJ506.H9R67 1982   618.92′8589   81-19780
ISBN 0-471-06331-2   AACR2

Printed in the United States of America

10 9 8 7 6 5 4 3 2 1

The world of the hyperactive child as described in taped quotes from therapy sessions by David, age nine:

... The very first day Mrs. K. (teacher) says, "Oh, *you're* David J.," and right in front of *everyone* she says when do I take my pills.

... then the new girl says, "Is your brother MR?" and Sal (sister) says that I got minimal brain dysfunction and the other girl says, "That's MR."

Chrissie Wilson had her Reckless Robert Robot in science class and it got started and wouldn't stop and Randy said, "Man, that robot's hyper like Davey! Give it a pill, Davey," and everyone laughed.

The doctor says I'll be OK when I'm 14. Well, I'm only *nine*. He acts like 14 is next week.

... and Gran said, "You get that child in Boys' Rec, Elmer," ... and Dad started telling the Rec Leader about me and he just laughed and says, "No problem, Mr. J., I was too and so was Tom Edison and two of my buddies who are in think tanks now" ... and when he told who were the new ones that day all he said was, "Glad to have you, Dave, I know your brother" ... just like I'm like the other kids.

... when it's special like a party I have to go to the sitter's. ... I heard my Mom say, "If *only* we could send him away to school."

... and then she (mother) gives Dad one of those looks and he like reads it and then he says, "Maybe just Sal and Peter (brother) should go this time." They think I'm really stupid. *I* know I *never* get picked to go. ... *Every* time is *this* time.

.... Sal has to take me places like I'm a dog and when we go to the Safeway where all the boys are Sal goes like, "Mom, do I *have* to take Davey?" and she's practically crying. So when we get to the park I say, "Sal, can I swing?" and she gets me on the way back.

I don't get them (pills) weekends so I can grow and it's scary because I'm one of the smallest in my class now and how can I catch up on only growing two days a week?

... medications is like in a big thick space suit with ear muffs and things get real fuzzy like far off.

I got no friends cos I don't play good and when they call me Dope Freak and David Dopey I cry, I just can't help it.

... in my best one (daydream) I pretend I'm Richard Dean and it's the city playoff the next day and Mr. Simpson (P.E. teacher) looks at me and says, "We *really* need *you* tomorrow, Rich."

Series Preface

This series of books is addressed to behavioral scientists interested in the nature of human personality. Its scope should prove pertinent to personality theorists and researchers as well as to clinicians concerned with applying an understanding of personality processes to the amelioration of emotional difficulties in living. To this end, the series provides a scholarly integration of theoretical formulations, empirical data, and practical recommendations.

Six major aspects of studying and learning about human personality can be designated: personality theory, personality structure and dynamics, personality development, personality assessment, personality change, and personality adjustment. In exploring these aspects of personality, the books in the series discuss a number of distinct but related subject areas: the nature and implications of various theories of personality; personality characteristics that account for consistencies and variations in human behavior; the emergence of personality processes in children and adolescents; the use of interviewing and testing procedures to evaluate individual differences in personality; efforts to modify personality styles through psychotherapy, counseling, behavior therapy, and other methods of influence; and patterns of abnormal personality functioning that impair individual competence.

IRVING B. WEINER

University of Denver
Denver, Colorado

Preface

In the space of less than a quarter century hyperactivity has become one of the most researched and easily the best known of the childhood behavior disorders, the single most common complaint presented to child psychiatrists, a ubiquitous and perplexing management task for pediatricians, and a significant problem for the elementary school system. Estimates of the prevalence of this disorder vary as a function of the social defining systems used, but the general consensus is that there is at least one and often two hyperactive children in most elementary school classrooms in this country. As recently as the early 1970s, hyperactivity was viewed as a time-limited disorder that disappeared early in the adolescent years and could be effectively controlled in the interim with stimulant medication. This erroneous view resulted in a certain complacency in the clinical domain and relative disinterest in the research ranks. The emergence of evidence in the mid-1970s that hyperactivity could persist into adolescence and early adulthood, with serious social and psychiatric sequelae, coupled with the finding that the central nervous stimulants were not in any sense a panacea, acted as a catalyst on the field.

The six years since the first edition have been the most exciting and productive years in the field of hyperactivity. There has been an exponential increase in productive collaboration such as high-level symposia, and in the quality and diversity of clusters of research. Significant changes have occurred in the approach to intervention, locale of research investigations, willingness to cross over into other fields, and particularly in the way of viewing the hyperactive child and awareness of the spread of effect of childhood hyperactivity. The face of hyperactivity has been drastically changed. These changes, along with their research bases, have justified a second edition with a wealth of new material.

This book is intended for researchers in hyperactivity, professionals in the medical, psychological, and educational domains who work with hyperactive children and their families, and students in graduate and undergraduate courses in the behavioral and medical sciences and in education. Because our text is addressed to this interdisciplinary group, it is written in such a way that specific training in any one field is not a prerequisite to its use. Although it should also prove valuable for the layman who seeks authentic information on hyperactivity, it is *not* a guide to rearing the hyperactive child. In our opinion the best source of information on this topic is *Raising a hyperactive child*, by Mark A. Stewart and Sally S. Olds.

The purpose of this second edition is to provide a comprehensive picture of the current status of our understanding of hyperactivity within a behavioral context. Many topics that merited only brief mention in the first edition (e.g., the fetal alcohol syndrome) or were the subject of speculation (e.g., the psychological costs of being hyperactive) have now become part of the mainstream of hyperactivity with commensurate space in this text. Two new chapters have been added—one on assessment procedures, primarily the rapidly evolving group that are specific to hyperactivity, and the other on prediction. Until we can predict onset and outcome, efforts to cope with hyperactivity are little more than essential stopgaps. Closely allied to prediction is our careful consideration of etiological research as well as the delineation of established fact and unresolved problems in prevention. While one thrust of research attention has been directed to the problems of prediction and prevention, the major focus of empirical and clinical interest continues to be on the development and evaluation of procedures and combinations of procedures within the realms of pharmacotherapy, psychotherapy, and education. We have given critical attention to the many new developments within each of these areas. Throughout this text special emphasis has been placed on one facet of this complex spectrum of behavior, one which is only now beginning to receive some attention in contemporary treatments of hyperactivity: the viewpoint of the hyperactive child.

DOROTHEA M. ROSS
SHEILA A. ROSS

San Francisco, California
Palo Alto, California
March 1982

Acknowledgments

We wish to express appreciation to our many colleagues who generously made their prepublication materials available to us: Russell Barkley, James Bosco, Susan Campbell, Dennis Cantwell, Keith Conners, Charles Cunningham, Thomas Dalby, Lloyd Daniels, Philip Drash, Dennis Dubey, Kenneth Gadow, Barbara Henker, Marcel Kinsbourne, Nadine Lambert, Benjamin Lahey, Jan Loney, Eric Mash, Richard Milich, Stephen Porges, Ronald Prinz, Judith Rapoport, Stanley Robin, Donald Routh, Jonathan Sandoval, Esther Sleator, Robert Sprague, Mark Stewart, James Swanson, Gabrielle Weiss, Paul Wender, and Carol Whalen. We would also like to thank several investigators who took the time to talk to us and, in some cases, went back to their original data to answer our questions: Susan Campbell, Dennis Cantwell, Philip Drash, Marian Diamond, Henry Dunn, Abba Kastin, Y. D. Lapierre, Jon Levine, and Curt Sandman.

The material in this book was also greatly enhanced by the inclusion of case studies and verbatim comments of a number of hyperactive children. Warmest thanks are extended to the children, parents, pediatricians, and psychiatrists who permitted us to reproduce these otherwise unobtainable materials.

Special thanks are due to Herb Reich for his amiable tolerance of deadline delays; to our long-time research colleague, Peggy Satterlee, and to Eileen Cassidy for their help in locating books and articles relevant to hyperactivity; and to Win Vetter and Sally S. Cotter who typed the manuscript in its various forms with skill and enthusiasm.

It is also a pleasure to acknowledge the encouragement and support that Walter J. Maytham, III, has provided throughout both editions of this book. We greatly value this association.

D.M.R.
S.A.R.

Contents

CHAPTER 1

Hyperactivity—An Overview

Hyperactivity is one of the most common symptoms of disordered behavior in childhood.* In this text hyperactivity is defined as a high level of activity that is manifested in situations in which it is clearly inappropriate and cannot be readily inhibited upon command. Although hyperactivity can exist as a single functional disturbance, such as a manifestation of chronic anxiety, it more often occurs as a primary symptom in a variety of medical and psychological disorders. One of the latter group is a symptom complex with a diversity of diagnostic labels—hyperkinetic syndrome, minimal brain dysfunction, and attention deficit disorder with hyperkinesis—which we will refer to as *childhood hyperactivity* or simply *hyperactivity*. The fact that one of the symptoms of this disorder, the inability to restrain inappropriate activity, is also referred to as *hyperactivity*, has created a situation in which the same label is used to name the disorder and describe one of its behavioral symptoms. This terminological inadequacy has been a source of confusion and has probably contributed to the proliferation of attempts to describe the disorder more precisely.

Childhood hyperactivity is variously regarded as a medical problem that is a discrete clinical entity, a behavioral disorder of a heterogeneous nature, a variant of the category of behavior problems known as conduct disorders, and as a myth. It has been defined by Routh (1978, p. 3) as a child's consistent failure to comply in age-appropriate fashion with situational demands for restrained activity, sustained attention, and inhibition of impulsive response. Although the basic terminology of this behavior disorder is a matter of dissent, there is remarkable consensus among clinicians and researchers concerning primary and secondary symptomatology and exclusionary criteria (Cantwell, 1979; Douglas & Peters, 1979; Dubey, 1981; Minde, 1977; Rapoport & Zametkin, 1980; Satterfield, Cantwell, & Satterfield, 1979; Whalen & Henker, 1980a). The most frequently cited primary or core symptoms include chronic hyperactivity, short attention span, marked distractibility, emotional lability, and impulsivity, all of which are likely to be characterized by cross-situational

*We are well aware of the supposedly sexist language controversy that has made fashionable clumsy variations on the he/she theme. To avoid this variant of unnecessary clutter, we have throughout this book referred to the hyperactive child in general as "he" and the elementary school teacher as "she" on the grounds that most hyperactive children are boys and the majority of elementary school teachers are women.

1

and cross-temporal variability (Langhorne, Loney, Paternite, & Bechtoldt, 1976). Descriptions of the hyperactive child will vary as a function of the reporting source and context of the behavior, with not all children described as hyperactive exhibiting all of the symptoms (Loney, 1980a; Schleifer, Weiss, Cohen, Elman, Cvejic, & Kruger, 1975; Sleator & Ullman, 1981). Traditionally, a high level of inappropriate activity has been viewed as the common denominator of this behavior disorder, but now, primarily as a result of almost a decade of intensive research by two groups of long-time collaborators (Douglas and her research team at McGill University and Ackerman, Clements, Dykman, and Peters at the University of Arkansas), the emphasis has shifted from hyperactivity to a new central diagnostic concept: impaired attention (Douglas & Peters, 1979). Whereas in the *Diagnostic and statistical manual of mental disorders II* (1968) of the American Psychiatric Association, hyperactivity and impaired attention were viewed as almost inseparable facets of the descriptor Hyperkinetic Reaction of Childhood, in DSM III (1980) the descriptor Attention Deficit Disorder with and without Hyperactivity firmly established impaired attention as the central diagnostic concept that may or may not be accompanied by hyperactivity. Among the secondary symptoms are deficits in academic performance despite normal intelligence, low self-esteem, sleep-related problems, difficulties in social interaction particularly with peers, fluctuations in performance, and aggression. These less salient symptoms are frequently referred to as resultant symptoms because they are attributed to the hyperactive child's flawed interactions with his social environment, but there is no empirical basis for this causal relationship (Milich & Loney, 1979a). Categorizing aggression as a secondary symptom is debatable in the light of recent research (Loney, 1980b) suggesting that hyperactivity and aggression are essentially independent dimensions and that, for the hyperactive child, childhood aggression is an important determinant of outcome in adolescence. If preliminary findings on childhood aggression and adolescent outcome are replicated, DSM IV may include a classification with all possible combinations of Attention Deficit Disorder, Hyperactivity, and Aggression.

Included in the exclusionary criteria for hyperactivity are other conditions and environmental events that could cause children to exhibit short-term or chronic inappropriate activity, attentional difficulties, and other behavioral characteristics associated with hyperactivity. Conditions and events to be ruled out prior to diagnosing hyperactivity include mental retardation, psychoses, severe sensory defects, gross neurologic disease, autism, serious developmental delays, and severe psychological stressors. The exclusionary criteria do not imply that children in the foregoing diagnostic categories cannot also be hyperactive; there is unequivocal evidence, for example, that mental retardation and hyperactivity frequently coexist (Gadow, 1981). Children with the problems subsumed under exclusionary criteria may exhibit clusters of hyperactive behavior, but these kinds of hyperactive problem behavior are secondary to conditions that differ markedly from childhood hyperactivity in etiology, symptomatology, and outcome.

The literature abounds with descriptions of the vagaries of the hyperactive child. Loney (1980a, p. 265) has aptly described the prototypical hyperactive child as one who is

notably long on motility and short on restraint . . . a child who flits around and blurts out but who doesn't finish assignments or chores; a child with a short and highly flammable fuse; a child of the present, who neither benefits from the past nor plans for the future.

Levine and Oberklaid (1980, p. 411) have portrayed hyperactive children as

not energy efficient. Their activity is misdirected, purposeless, fidgety, and seemingly random. . . . They tend to be chronically impulsive . . . in their overall behavior, in their social interactions, and in their efforts at problem solving. They tend not to reflect, plan, organize, or monitor their own productions. Many such youngsters feel very much out of control. Their impulsivity is constantly getting them into trouble. Often they seem not to believe what they have done, feeling unaccountable for their unpremeditated acts because things seem to happen so fast.

Hyperactivity is the single most common chronic behavior disorder in the preadolescent group (Wender, 1975). Although the early school years are the period when most children are identified as hyperactive, there are definite precursors in infancy (Thomas & Chess, 1977), and the constellation of problem behaviors often persists with changing symptomatology into adolescence and young adulthood (Bellak, 1979; Weiss & Hechtman, 1979). Like most childhood behavior disorders, it is more common in boys than in girls, with sex ratios ranging from 5:1 to 9:1. Although educators (Yanow, 1973) often cite 15 to 20 percent as the prevalence rate for hyperactivity in the elementary school population, several recent prevalence studies of large representative populations of public school children have reported rates well below 10 percent depending upon the social defining systems used. The most comprehensive of these prevalence studies (Lambert, Sandoval, & Sassone, 1978) reported rates in the 1 to 6 percent range. Childhood hyperactivity is not unique to this culture or to one school system: it has been reported in other major Western countries as well as in some rapidly developing Third World countries. However, the sweeping conclusion by the Office of Child Development (1971, p. 2) that "hyperkinetic disorders are found in children of all socioeconomic groups and in countries throughout the world" receives little support from the literature: children in Tokyo, Salt Lake City, primitive Pacific cultures, and Chinese-American children in New York City represent some of the groups in which hyperactivity is reported to be virtually nonexistent.

The diversity of descriptors for this behavior disorder reflects the existing uncertainty about etiology. Hyperactivity has been tentatively linked to a variety of causal factors including medical, neurological, and psychological disorders, as well as cultural and environmental forces. In the early literature it was generally attributed to innate or acquired organic pathology. However, in the past decade the familial, but not the genetic, nature of hyperactivity has been definitively established; the etiological search has intensified and diversified with attention focusing on a variety of potential nonsocial and social causal factors including asymptomatic lead poisoning, deviations in level of arousal, food additives, maternal gestational alcohol intake, environmental constraints, child rearing methods, and academic problems. Concurrently, the focus of etiological research has shifted from single causative determinants to an interactionist position that accommodates the contributions of multiple etiological factors including the influence of the immediate social and nonsocial environment (Bell & Harper, 1977; Porges & Smith, 1980).

There is no critical diagnostic test for hyperactivity; there are few exclusionary criteria, and no unequivocal positive markers (Conners, 1975b). Table 1.1 contains the operational criteria for the Attention Deficit Disorder with Hyperactivity (DSM III, 1980). The history, observations of immediate behavior, and reports of adults in the child's environment form the basis for the diagnosis (Sandoval, Lambert, & Yandell, 1976). Psychological tests and neurological and anatomical abnormalities may be corroborative, but the absence of such supportive data in no way rules out the diagnosis of hyperactivity. The behavior of the hyperactive child differs from that of his nonhyperactive peers in intensity, persistence, and clustering of symptoms rather than in presence or absence of specific symptoms. In marked contrast to the general consensus concerning symptomatology is the notable disparity in diagnostic practices within this country as well as between the United States and Britain.

Of all the chronic childhood behavior disorders, hyperactivity responds most readily to relatively minimal intervention. In terms of short-term improvement the most effective single treatment is stimulant medication. The response is often so dramatic that for some time after the introduction of stimulant medications, drug response was erroneously considered to be a diagnostic test. The general consensus concerning frequency of positive drug response is that about 75 percent of the hyperactive children treated with stimulants manifest behavioral improvement; the remaining 25 percent either appear unchanged or become worse (Barkley, 1977a; Cantwell, 1980). The favorable effects of stimulants appear to be attributable to an improvement in the child's attentional skills. When drugs were first introduced on a wide scale they were hailed as a panacea, and their success, coupled with the incorrect belief that hyperactivity was a time-limited disorder, resulted in a general complacency among researchers and clinicians concerning optimal management with a consequent lassitude towards developing other treatment strategies. In the past decade it has become apparent that a number of unresolved issues exist that call for a more critical scrutiny of the drug treatment approach: No convincing demonstrations have been made of positive long-term effects of drug treatment; the effects of long-term drug usage on linear growth, cardiovascular functioning, and the psychological well-being of the

Table 1.1. Diagnostic Criteria for Attention Deficit Disorder with Hyperactivity

The following signs of developmentally inappropriate inattention, impulsivity, and hyperactivity should be reported by adults in the child's environment, particularly teachers and parents. The symptoms are variable: they may be absent in new or one-to-one situations, but may worsen when self-application to a task is required as in the school situation. The number of symptoms specified here is for children between the ages of eight and ten. In younger children more symptoms are usually present and in more severe forms, whereas in older children the severity and number both tend to diminish.

Inattention.. At least three of the following:

1. Often fails to finish things he or she starts.
2. Often doesn't seem to listen.
3. Easily distracted.
4. Has difficulty concentrating on schoolwork or other tasks requiring sustained attention.
5. Has difficulty sticking to a play activity.

Impulsivity. At least three of the following:

1. Often acts before thinking.
2. Shifts excessively from one activity to another.
3. Has difficulty organizing work (not due to cognitive impairment).
4. Needs a lot of supervision.
5. Frequently calls out in class.
6. Has difficulty awaiting turn in games or group situations.

Hyperactivity. At least three of the following:

1. Runs about or climbs on things excessively.
2. Has difficulty sitting still or fidgets excessively.
3. Has difficulty staying seated.
4. Moves about excessively during sleep.
5. Is always "on the go" or acts as if "driven by a motor."

Onset before the age of seven.

Duration of at least six months.

Not due to schizophrenia, affective disorder, or severe or profound mental retardation.

Adapted from the *Diagnostic and Statistical Manual of Mental Disorders*, 3rd Edition, American Psychiatric Association, 1980.

hyperactive child, as well as the potential for drug abuse, are matters of concern (Cantwell & Carlson, 1978; Roche, Lipman, Overall, & Hung, 1979; Werry, 1977). Other forms of treatment intervention include traditional psychotherapy, behavior therapy, biofeedback, environmental manipulation, and special classroom programs. Each of these modes of intervention has proven useful over the short term, but long-term evidence of their efficacy is still lacking. There is an increasing trend towards multimodal treatment in which drugs are seen as synergistic to other forms of intervention. At the present time, no prediction of outcome for a specific child can be made regardless of mode or duration of treatment (Cantwell, 1978a; Weiss & Hechtman, 1979).

Although no treatment has been shown to influence the long-range prognosis of hyperactivity, in some children this behavior disorder disappears spontaneously with increasing maturity; in others it persists into adolescence and early adulthood, often to the detriment of social and vocational functioning. There is reason to believe that hyperactivity may be a precursor of a number of psychiatric disorders in adult life, including alcoholism, sociopathy, and hysteria, although the recent identification of childhood aggression as a potential major predictor of outcome may show that the crucial factor in the childhood behavior-adult disorder link is childhood aggression rather than hyperactivity (Loney, 1980b; Stewart, 1980). Of increasing concern to researchers and clinicians are the prevalence and persistence of hyperactivity, as well as the pervasiveness of its effects upon the child, his family, and the community.

Unique Aspects of Hyperactivity

Hyperactivity is unique among the childhood behavior disorders in that the whole field is characterized to an unusual degree by uncertainty, contradictions, the unexpected, and the bizarre. By contrast, most other childhood behavior disorders have a stability, predictability, and overall low profile that does not elicit an excessive amount of uninformed attention from most sections of the public. The very existence of the disorder is surrounded by a diffused uncertainty. While scores of researchers and clinicians study and treat hyperactivity in the United States, others (Barkley, 1981; Lahey, Green, & Forehand, 1980; Quay, 1979; Shaffer & Greenhill, 1979) question whether hyperactivity exists as a clinical entity, and this concern is echoed by experts in Great Britain (Sandberg, Rutter, & Taylor, 1978) who contend that hyperactivity is a variant of the conduct disorders. Added to this uncertainty about existence is the troubling question of whether some of the socialization procedures of this culture, particularly those in the classroom, *cause* hyperactivity (Bax, 1972; Bettelheim, 1973; Cunningham & Barkley, 1978b; Henker & Whalen, 1980a).

Some children have the symptoms of hyperactivity, but these create no problems for either the children themselves or those around them, whereas for other hyperactive children the symptoms are a continuing burden that has a disruptive effect on all their major social environments (Lambert, Sandoval, & Sassone, 1978). There is no cure, but for some the symptoms disappear spontaneously in early adolescence; for others they persist in various forms into adolescence and young adulthood. The child's personality often changes suddenly and dramatically with little justification. He is given to wide mood swings, from contentment one minute to a violent tantrum the next. Often he behaves so well in one-to-one situations that physicians and others who see him on an individual basis find it hard to reconcile the compliant child with parental and teacher reports (Cantwell, 1979). On other occasions in the same situation the child may be impossible. He is often capricious, uneven, and unpredictable in general behavior and academic performance. He tends to respond atypically to both negative *and* positive reinforcement. Novelty may quiet him, but adapting to changes in familiar routines is difficult for him. He sometimes has as much difficulty sleeping at night as he does remaining alert in situations, such as the classroom, that demand a response. Although the impact of his behavior on those around him may be tremendous, with deleterious effects on family harmony, in fact hyperactivity is regarded as only a moderately serious behavior disorder in the spectrum of childhood psychopathology (Henker & Whalen, 1980a).

An astonishing number of decisions and directions concerning the treatment of hyperactivity has stemmed from precarious, undocumented, or even incorrect premises. *Stimulant medications* (the amphetamines) were approved for pediatric use in the absence of the careful and extensive testing that is supposed to precede the approval of drugs for unrestricted public usage. These drugs were approved when virtually nothing was known about their long-term effects (Gallagher, 1970). *Traditional psychotherapy* was firmly rejected as a part of the treatment armamentarium for hyperactivity, the major basis for this drastic stance being one methodologically inadequate study (Eisenberg, Gilbert, Cytryn, & Molling, 1961). The *minimal stimulation* classroom was set up on the basis of circular reasoning (Sarason, 1949) on the part of its proponents (Strauss & Lehtinen, 1947) and subjected to an inadequate experimental test (Cruickshank, Bentzen, Ratzeburg, & Tannhauser, 1961) that was accepted by many educators as unequivocal evidence of its efficacy, despite the fact that the experimenters reported negative results and acknowledged some major methodological and interpretive faults. Similarly, the *Feingold diet* (Feingold, 1975a) has been used widely with hyperactive children although there is not now, nor has there ever been, any conclusive evidence of its efficacy (Conners, 1980; National Advisory Committee on Hyperkinesis and Food Additives, 1980). This treatment regimen stemmed from Feingold's personal convictions concerning the hyperactivity-food additives link, and became popular as a result of unusual publicity, extravagant and unsubstantiated claims concerning its efficacy, and the evangelical fervor of the developer. *Biofeedback* has had widespread clinical use with hyperactive children in the absence of any firm empirical evidence of its efficacy. Experienced investigators (Miller, 1978b; Blanchard & Young, 1974) have emphasized that with one or two exceptions there is no compelling evidence that the reported efficacy of biofeedback is produced specifically by the biofeedback treatment.

Most pediatric problems, particularly those of a chronic nature such as allergy, juvenile diabetes, epilepsy, and childhood autism, do not attract active participation and interest on the part of adults other than the parents and those directly involved with the child. Indeed, the lack of interest is often a serious deterrent to progress in understanding the disorder or controlling it; and publicity and education campaigns often have little effect. In the case of childhood hyperactivity the reverse has been true, with an incredible amount of interest being shown in all aspects of this behavior disorder. Powerful, vocal national and state organizations, such as the Feingold Association and the

California Association for Neurologically Handicapped Children, have shown a vigorous and continuing interest in the problem of hyperactivity. By 1979, the National Feingold Association had 30,000 members, 120 local affiliates, and an impressive amount of media coverage, and had become the self-appointed advocate of the hyperactive child. At least one parent group has won a major lawsuit against a school district that pressured uninformed parents to have their children put on medication, and the case, *Benskin* v. *Taft City School District* (1975), received widespread national attention (e.g., Bell, 1977; Bruck, 1976) long before the courts had rendered a decision. In professional journals an unusual number of editorials and commentaries on hyperactivity, and sharp critical exchanges have appeared (e.g., Mayron, 1978, vs. O'Leary, Rosenbaum, & Hughes, 1978b; Whalen & Henker, 1977, vs. Conrad, 1975); and professional debates have been aired by intercontinental radio for the benefit of the laymen listeners (Feingold, 1976b). Several panels of respected scientists have been convened to consider the effects and efficacy of certain treatment procedures. With its multimillion dollar processed food market in jeopardy, the Nutrition Foundation assembled a National Advisory Committee on Hyperkinesis and Food Additives. The Food and Drug Administration organized an expert professional committee, the Inter-Agency Collaboration Group on Hyperkinesis, to review the evidence on the Feingold diet (Bierman & Furukawa, 1978). The American Academy of Pediatrics established a high-level review panel to consider the effects of stimulant medication on linear growth (Roche et al., 1979).

Hyperactivity has had tremendous and unremitting publicity and visibility in the mass media. The Omaha incident (Maynard, 1970), which in many ways is representative of the more bizarre aspects of the whole field, began with an erroneous account of the wholesale drugging of Omaha school children that set in motion a wave of public outrage undiminished by subsequent corrections in the initial report. Hyperactivity has consistently been treated as prime space news in major newspapers, such as the *Washington Post, Chicago Tribune, New York Times,* and *San Francisco Chronicle,* has had an unusual amount of TV coverage, and has been the subject of an unprecedented number of articles in major magazines such as *The Saturday Review, Time, Redbook,* and *Newsweek,* and books for the layman (e.g., Bittinger, 1977; Schrag & Divoky, 1975; Stewart & Olds, 1973; Taylor, 1980). At the government level, the topic attracted considerable interest in the early 1970s that has continued unabated. Testimony concerning hyperactivity and stimulant medication was made to several Congressional Committees (Gallagher, 1970; Points, 1970); a "blue ribbon" panel was convened by the Department of Health, Education, and Welfare to report on stimulant medication (Freedman, 1971); and Feingold's 1973 statement was read into the U. S. Congressional Record (Beall, 1973). Before the Feingold hypothesis could be formally tested, it was the subject of Senate hearings and a presidential decree directed the Food and Drug Administration to review all food additives in current use (Taylor, 1979).

Freeman (1976, p. 5) has described the field of hyperactivity as "character-ized by . . . a strangely seductive attractiveness." A factor contributing to the persistent and pervasive interest in hyperactivity may be that in terms of con-troversy potential this behavior disorder offers something for everyone: the general public, with their strongly held but often uninformed views on drug treatment, the role of the school, and the school as an etiological factor in hyperactivity; physicians, who contend that the school's role is not one of diagnosing and treating children; psychologists, who insist that the schools should have these functions; and those who view hyperactivity as a myth. Many of the problems of the hyperactive child are centered in the school, a setting that most people feel highly qualified to comment on. In addition, anxiety about drug addiction in general has heightened attention to the ad-ministration of any drugs to children, particularly those whose behavior is sometimes indistinguishable from their nonhyperactive peers.

The onslaught of publicity of the 1970s was accompanied by a sharp in-crease in investigative interest in hyperactivity. Although the result was a sub-stantial increment to our knowledge and understanding of this disorder, it is our opinion that the advances have not been commensurate with the amount of investigation. Two problems that have had a detrimental and pervasive ef-fect on progress in the field as a whole are the marked lack of consensus on basic terminology and the issue of syndrome status for hyperactivity. Because a grasp of these problems is basic to an understanding of the state of the field, each will be discussed in some detail.

TERMINOLOGICAL CONFUSION

There never has been a universally accepted descriptor for the behavior disor-der that we are calling hyperactivity, and some experienced clinicians (Wend-er, 1979) think that there will not be one in the near future. Instead, there has been a proliferation of terms (DeLong, 1972), some of which imply pathology and its hypothesized basis, while others avoid etiological implications by describing the kind of behavior exhibited. In terms of frequency of recent usage the major descriptors are *hyperactivity, minimal brain dysfunction, brain damage,* and *learning disability.* There is no consensus about either the definition of these terms or their diagnostic criteria; the confusion is further confounded by a tendency to use a variety of behavioral and academic prob-lem descriptors synonymously with hyperactivity (Rie, 1975). The behavior that we are calling hyperactivity may be referred to by others as brain dam-age, learning disability, developmental hyperactivity, conduct disorder, mini-mal brain dysfunction, overactivity, postencephalitis behavior disorder, or attention deficit disorder with hyperkinesis. Far from being a semantic game of strictly academic interest, the lack of a common terminology has a direct bearing on research and, as Rie (1980) has noted, is costly in several respects. It is difficult to compare the results obtained by different investigators because there is often no way of establishing comparability of samples across studies. Some investigators are scrupulous about providing detailed descriptions of their subject selection criteria, but many are not. Inadequate subject descriptions limit the generality of the results and make replication difficult if not impossible. In the clinical domain the lack of a common terminology lowers the probability that recommendations will be implemented, and impedes the communication among professionals treating a specific child and between professionals and parents. We know of one instance in which the parents were dismayed when a pediatric neurologist diagnosed their hyperactive child as having minimal brain dysfunction, because it suggested brain involvement. On seeking a second opinion, they were elated when the neurologist interpreted the earlier diagnostic data as evidence of a neurological handicap, which they perceived as unrelated to any problem with the brain. They were jubilant when school personnel reviewed the neurologists' reports and categorized the child as learning disabled, a school placement term.

In the contemporary literature on hyperactivity the terminological confusion is sometimes treated as a problem that has only recently evolved. This is a totally inaccurate view. The historical equivalents of the major categories, that is, hyperactivity, brain damage, minimal brain dysfunction, and learning disability, were described in 1902 by Still, and their use has been perpetuated and strengthened by subsequent events whose diversity is indicative of the variety of influences that has contributed to the problems of terminology. Their effect on the accumulation of knowledge about hyperactivity and treatment of it has been profound and for that reason it is worthwhile to trace these events briefly.

The foundation for the terminological confusion that has plagued the field was laid at the turn of the century when Still (1902) described a behavior pattern characteristic of children with "defects in moral control" that was remarkably similar to the symptom complex that we call hyperactivity. This pattern occurred more often in boys than girls, a disproportion that Still did not consider to be accidental. It was sometimes accompanied by peculiarities of physical conformation, often appeared to be a function of temperament, generally showed little relationship to the child's training and environment, was frequently apparent early in the school years, and often was associated with learning difficulties. Still linked the hyperactivity behavior pattern to a variety of etiological factors, including genetic transmission and child rearing procedures, and reported that it was remarkably resistant to punishment. Regardless of whether demonstrable brain damage was present, Still viewed the behavior pattern as a medical problem to be treated in a hospital and having a fair and often poor prognosis. The combination of a range in the degree of uncertainty concerning the etiology of the behavior and variations in the extent and timing of the onset of learning difficulties provided a logical basis for the separation of these behavior-disordered children into subgroups. Still distinguished between children with demonstrable gross lesions of the brain; those with a variety of acute diseases, conditions, and injuries that would be expected to result in brain damage although none could be demonstrated; and those with hyperactive behavior patterns that could not be attributed to any known cause. Thus in one fell swoop Still laid the groundwork for the three major diagnostic categories—brain damage, minimal brain dysfunction, and hyperactivity—and for the place of learning disabilities as a cross-category phenomenon. In the next 60 years a series of clinical observations, empirical investigations, the natural disasters of epidemics, and several wars served to delineate these categories more clearly.

Brain Damage

In terms of a medical disease model framework, Still (1902) had logically used the descriptor *brain damage syndrome* for children with demonstrable gross lesions of the brain. The link between the hyperactive behavior pattern and demonstrable brain damage was strengthened by the 1918 encephalitis epidemic, in which hyperactive behavior patterns, catastrophic changes in personality, and learning difficulties in school were among the predictable sequelae of the disease (Hohman, 1922; Strecker & Ebaugh, 1924). This link was confirmed in subsequent observations of children with encephalitis (Bender, 1942; Gibbs, Gibbs, Spies, & Carpenter, 1964; Sabatino & Cramblett, 1968). Further evidence of a causative link between brain damage and hyperactivity was provided by studies of epilepsy and other brain disorders (Clark, 1926; Lord, 1937; Preston, 1945). Children who had suffered demonstrable brain damage from head injuries or other causes, particularly anoxia during delivery, also exhibited a heterogeneous group of behavior problems, including hyperactivity. The causative link theory was also supported by reports from ablation studies in animals (Cromwell, Baumeister, & Hawkins, 1963; French & Harlow, 1955) and of military injuries in World War II, although some subsequent investigations have minimized the etiological role of head injuries in behavior disorders (Harrington & Letemendia, 1958).

In the early 1960s the concept of brain damage was extended and refined. Birch (1964) made a useful distinction between the fact of brain damage, that is, pathological changes in the nerve tissue of the brain with diverse functional consequences, and the concept of the brain damaged child, and emphasized that although some children with verified brain damage also exhibited behavior problems, there was no consistent correlation between the two. There was firm empirical evidence for the existence of many categories of brain damage in children, with children across categories having widely differing problems (Birch, 1964). The consensus was that the brain-damaged child's symptoms could be a direct result of tissue damage, or they could be attributable to his reactions to his environment. Despite this conceptual stance and its supporting empirical data, a substantial group of researchers and clinicians has firmly maintained that brain damage is a unitary phenomenon, a misconception that has proven detrimental to progress in understanding the role of brain damage in hyperactivity (Fish, 1971).

Minimal Brain Dysfunction

To support Still's reports (1902) of a hyperactive behavior pattern occurring when brain damage was expected but could not be demonstrated, Tredgold (1908) hypothesized that some forms of brain damage, such as birth injury or relatively mild anoxia, passed unnoticed at the time but became apparent in the form of behavior and learning difficulties when the child was faced with the demands of the early school years. The belief that brain damage could be inferred laid the foundation for the concept of minimal brain damage (Doll, Phelps, & Melcher, 1932; Ehrenfest, 1926; Smith, 1926). The idea that hyperactivity was caused by minimal brain damage gained the status of an entrenched belief as the result of the publications and minimal stimulation classroom programs of Strauss and his associates (Strauss & Kephart, 1955; Strauss & Lehtinen, 1947), despite the fact that their methods and views were based on circular reasoning (Sarason, 1949).

A substantial body of fetal and animal research strengthened the validity of the concept of minimal brain damage, with evidence from epidemiological studies demonstrating a strong association between maternal and fetal factors and behavioral problems (Lilienfeld, Pasamanick, & Rogers, 1955; Pasamanick, Rogers, & Lilienfeld, 1956), and data from animal studies supporting a relationship between behavior disorders and minimal degrees of brain damage (Cromwell, Baumeister, & Hawkins, 1963). Empirical evidence of a significant link between histories of anoxia and subsequent developmental deviations (Graham, Caldwell, Ernhart, Pennoyer, & Hartman, 1957), and the introduction of the concept of a continuum of degrees of damage (Knobloch & Pasamanick, 1966; Lilienfeld et al., 1955) also contributed to the status of this concept. The idea of minimal degrees of damage was bolstered by theoretical statements (Ingalls & Gordon, 1947) as well as by the erroneous assumption that the efficacy of stimulant medication in cases of minimal brain damage constituted evidence of the existence of minimal degrees of brain damage. Meanwhile the Oxford International Study Group of Child Neurology (Bax & MacKeith, 1963) contended that brain damage should not be inferred from behavior signs alone (Strother, 1973) and recommended that the descriptor *minimal brain damage* be replaced with *minimal brain dysfunction*, and also that attempts be made to classify into more homogeneous subgroups the heterogeneous group of children subsumed under the label minimal brain dysfunction. A national task force formulated an official definition of the disorder (Clements, 1966, pp. 9–10):

> The term "minimal brain dysfunction syndrome" refers . . . to children of near average, average, or above average general intelligence with certain learning or

behavioral disabilities ranging from mild to severe, which are associated with deviations of function of the central nervous system. These deviations may manifest themselves by various combinations of impairment in perception, conceptualization, language, memory, and control of attention, impulse, or motor function.... During the school years, a variety of learning disabilities is the most prominent manifestation.

This definition was welcomed by those who believed hyperactivity to be an unequivocal diagnostic sign of brain damage, but bitterly criticized by opponents of this view. The objections were to the definition of minimal brain dysfunction, particularly to its "umbrella term" quality and other shortcomings, rather than to the existence of the problem. The intensity of the criticism moved Clements and Peters (1973, p. 46) to protest that "the (1966) concept of minimal brain dysfunction ... was not intended as a final statement on the subject." Previously, Clements (1966) had emphasized the protean nature of minimal brain dysfunction and urged the specification of subcategories.

Hyperactivity

Three decades elapsed between Still's (1902) description of children with hyperactive behavior patterns unrelated to either demonstrable brain damage or a history suggestive of damage and the first comprehensive discussion in this country of hyperactive children. In 1935 Childers noted that only a small proportion of cases with the hyperactive behavior pattern seemed etiologically related to demonstrable or inferred brain damage or central nervous system disorder. His discussion of children with no evidence of brain damage is notable for the differentiation made between the hyperactive child and the brain-damaged child, the specificity of criteria used in selecting for study the truly hyperactive as opposed to highly active, normal children, the emphasis on the need to develop appropriate treatment procedures, and the similarity between the hyperactive child described in 1935 and his 1980 counterpart. The influential papers by Laufer and his associates (Laufer & Denhoff, 1957; Laufer, Denhoff, & Solomons, 1957), which introduced the descriptors *hyperkinetic behavior syndrome* and *hyperkinetic impulse disorder,* signaled the onset of the current period of final acceptance of the construct of hyperactivity. Their work served as the stimulus for a series of empirical investigations (Smith, 1962; Werry, Weiss, & Douglas, 1964), critical comments on organicity (Smith, 1962), and clinical descriptions (Bakwin & Bakwin, 1966; Werry, 1968) of cases of hyperactivity with no known organic base, with the result that this concept gained increased recognition in the scientific community. Further support came from reports of behavior problems with no known organic base in war veterans (Goldstein, 1942). In addition, the rapidly accumulating evidence of the efficacy of psychotropic drugs for behavior problems with nonmedical antecedents undermined the belief that a positive response constituted evidence of minimal degrees of brain damage. By the late 1960s, the concept of hyperactivity was firmly established in the literature.

Concern about the validity of all three descriptors—brain damage, minimal brain dysfunction, and hyperactivity—as diagnostic categories, as well as the considerable overlap among them, remained at an all but unobtrusive level in the literature until the Omaha incident (Maynard, 1970) catapulted the problems of definition and terminology into national prominence. Interest in the terminology problem was sustained throughout the 1970s by a diversity of events ranging from empirical investigations of terminological validity (e.g., Routh & Roberts, 1972) and school placement controversies (Gallagher, 1973; Ryor, 1978; Sapir, 1980), to federal, state, and local concern with the drug intervention issue, all of which focused attention on the descriptors used. A number of critical discussions of the terminology problem appeared (Clements, 1966; DeLong, 1972; Grinspoon & Singer, 1973; Minde, 1977; Satz & Fletcher, 1980), culminating in the publication of the American Psychiatric Association's new diagnostic categories in DSM II (1968) and again, with further revisions, in DSM III (1980). Terminology has continued to be problematic in this decade despite some monumental efforts to clarify the situation (e.g., Rie & Rie, 1980).

In this text, hyperactivity is conceptualized as a class of heterogeneous behavior disorders in which a high level of activity that is exhibited at inappropriate times and cannot be inhibited upon command is often the major presenting complaint. These behavior disorders, which range from mild to severe, are characterized by some or all of the following behavioral symptoms: hyperactivity, short attention span, distractibility, impulsivity, emotional lability, low frustration tolerance, aggressiveness, destructiveness, poor school performance, and poor peer relationships. Hyperactivity is not generally associated with demonstrable brain damage, cannot be attributed to chronic medical or neurological disease or to severe behavioral disturbances such as childhood psychoses, and may be etiologically linked to a variety of genetic, medical, social, and nonsocial environmental factors. The term *hyperactivity* is used to refer to any of the heterogeneous patterns of behavior that are manifested in individuals with this behavior disorder, and we emphasize here that diagnostic acumen and research have established that hyperactivity is a problem that can appear early in infancy (Routh, 1978) and persist through adulthood (Bellak, 1979; Wender, 1979).

We recognize that as we are using them, *hyperactive child* and *hyperactivity* are not ideal descriptors. However, we prefer the core-symptom approach that our definitions imply to that of the umbrella term. Consequently we will treat *brain damage* and *learning disability* as core-symptom terms. As used here, brain damage implies demonstrable damage to the brain tissue as a result of some specific prenatal or postnatal trauma but, as Birch (1964) emphasized, does not necessarily imply a resultant behavior problem or an intellectual deficit. Learning disability refers to learning difficulties that occur as a result of disturbances in cognition, perception, or motor functioning, and that result in performance discrepant from apparent ability despite adequate intelligence, sensory and motor capacity, and emotional adjustment in the child. A child with a learning disability is assumed to have normal capacity for learning, and normal outcome is anticipated. The considerable overlap between the category of learning disabilities and brain damage, minimal brain dysfunction, and hyperactivity has contributed to the terminological confusion that characterizes the field.

It is our opinion that use of the term *minimal brain dysfunction* should be discontinued because it contributes more than its share of confusion in this area. It is neither a specific disease nor a disorder with a specific symptomatology. Children with particular brain dysfunctions differ markedly from one another, and there are as many dysfunctions as there are functions of the human brain. Minimal brain dysfunction may coexist with hyperactivity or may occur independently of this or any other behavioral or physiological disorder (Rie & Rie, 1980). It is a presumptive diagnosis that should not be used synonymously with hyperactivity, but instead should be limited to children with considerable suggestive evidence of minimal neurological dysfunction, such as several of the following problems: well-documented prenatal or paranatal birth complications, head injuries, EEG abnormalities, abnormal neurological examination, perceptual and motor deficits. In this text we will use the term *minimal brain dysfunction* only when it is used in a particular study or article. For an excellent critique of the minimal brain dysfunction concept see Rie (1980).

THE SYNDROME ISSUE

The second problem that has impeded progress in the understanding of hyperactivity has been the assignment of syndrome status to this disorder. Any disorder described as a syndrome can be expected to have certain characteristics that form a framework delineating the direction and range of research and treatment for that disorder. In the event that the disorder is in fact *not* a syndrome, but is viewed as being one by researchers and clinicians in the field, the framework will continue to impose both directions and limits on their work. The result will be a narrowing of investigative interests, with the concomitant tendency of overlooking alternatives not encompassed by the framework, and the artificial forcing of disparate elements of the disorder into the homogeneous categories delineated by the framework of syndrome status. The effect will be a lack of continuing refinement in clinical treatment and a failure to advance on the research front at a rate commensurate with the ongoing expenditure of investigative time and energy. The criteria for syndrome status include the existence of a unitary cluster of symptoms, a common cause or having major etiological factors in common, a consistent response to treatment or a predictable course in the absence of treatment, and demonstrable differences between those with the disorder and other diagnostic groups or nonclinical groups. In respect to hyperactivity, assigning syndrome status implies that there is only one type of hyperactive child, and this child is characterized by a unitary cluster of symptoms sharing a common etiology, or at least having major etiological factors in common, and also by a consistent response to treatment with other hyperactive children. If left untreated this child will follow a predictable and uniform course and, whether treated or not, a group of these children would be demonstrably different in terms of behavior or other attributes from children with other psychiatric syndromes and from nonclinical comparision groups (Loney, 1980b).

Since Laufer and Denhoff (1957) first invoked the descriptor *hyperkinetic behavior syndrome,* the term *syndrome* has been an integral part of many of the labels designating this behavior disorder. In the 1960s, Task Force I advocated the descriptor *minimal brain dysfunction syndrome* (Clements, 1966), Stewart and his colleagues used the term *hyperactive child syndrome* (Stewart, Pitts, Craig, & Dieruf, 1966), and the World Health Organization included *hyperkinetic syndrome* in its classification scheme (Rutter, Lebovici, Eisenberg, Sneznevskij, Sadoun, Brooke, & Lin, 1969). The term has continued to be widely used (e.g., Goodwin, Schulsinger, Hermansen, Guze & Winokur, 1975; Klein & Gittelman-Klein, 1975; Margolin, 1978; O'Malley & Eisenberg, 1973; Routh, 1980; Stewart, 1980), and many clinicians and researchers have prescribed treatment regimens and conducted empirical investigations within the conceptual framework of syndrome status. Clinicians have tended, for example, to show minimal interest in the identification of causal factors, and to use the identical treatment intervention for all hyperactive children regardless of the behavioral symptoms that occasioned referral. In these terms a child who exhibits sustained overactivity for no apparent reason and one with the same pattern of behavior stemming from a heavy body-lead burden are both likely to be treated identically, although the former would probably benefit from stimulant medication combined with other forms of treatment, and the latter from chelation therapy. Within the research domain the effect for hyperactivity of a belief in syndrome status has been substantial. For the most part, the interpretation of research findings on pharmacologic, behavioral, and educational intervention has treated hyperactive children as a homogeneous group of subjects. Numerous empirical investigations, for example, have shown that only a percentage of hyperactive children in any one study benefit from a particular type of intervention. Yet there is rarely any suggestion that those who benefited might have differed from those who did not in underlying etiological factors. Exceptions here include the studies of Bugental, Whalen, and Henker (1977), Conners, (1970), David, Clark, and Voeller (1972), and Loney, Langhorne, and Paternite (1978).

The interest generated by the syndrome issue has led a small but determined group of investigators to search for empirical support for a hyperactive syndrome. Their conclusion, that there is no evidence that the existing body of knowledge about hyperactivity supports syndrome status, is based on studies relevant to each of the syndrome criteria listed above and discussed as follows:

A Unitary Cluster of Characteristics. Although the clustering of symptoms such as hyperactivity, distractibility, and impulsivity is frequently described by clinicians (Groover, 1972; Laufer & Denhoff, 1957) and is forced through subject selection in empirical investigations, the empirical attempts to demonstrate that these clusters are statistically interrelated have generally failed. One exception is a factor analytic study by Lahey, Stempniak, Robinson, and Tyroler (1978), which showed that the symptoms defining hyperactivity do cluster. Lahey et al. attributed other failures to demonstrate a unitary cluster of symptoms in hyperactivity to nonsubstantive reasons, for example, the size and breadth of the item pool, and the factor analytic procedures used. Using a variety of factor analytic methods, none of the following investigators was able to demonstrate interrelationships among the various components of the hyperactive child syndrome: Dreger (1964); Paine, Werry, and Quay (1968); Rodin, Lucas, and Simson (1963); Routh and Roberts (1972); Werry (1968). Instead of producing one or two major factors containing all or most of the various posited components of hyperactivity/minimal brain dysfunction, these studies yielded numerous relatively small factors that were independent of one another and that corresponded to the source of information. Werry (1968) concluded that the pattern of results in his study did not suggest a syndrome, that is, a single unitary dimension of minimal brain dysfunction, but rather a series of developmental dimensions, each of which might reflect different etiological factors and singly, or in combination, might be implicated in minimal brain dysfunction. Even when Langhorne, Loney, Paternite, and Bechtoldt (1976) confined their analysis to the primary behavior symptoms of hyperactivity, a procedure designed to maximize the possibility of a single syndrome cluster, the results were similar to those of Werry (1968): a relatively large number of rather small source-related factors were indentified that were not impressively related to each other. Although this analysis was criticized on several grounds by Zukow, Zukow, and Bentler (1978), a separate analysis of the Langhorne et al. data (DeFillipis, 1979) confirmed the accuracy of the original conclusions. Taken together, these factor analytic studies provide little support for a unitary cluster of symptoms in hyperactivity, and instead indicate a considerable variety of source-related factors, along with symptom complexes that may overlap minimally or not at all.

In commenting on the finding of source-related factors, Loney (1980b, p. 34) has also cautioned against a tendency to rely solely on factor analytic studies in the issue of syndrome status for hyperactivity:

> ... it is necessary to notice the strong influence of procedural and methodological features upon the number and nature of factors that are obtained. The previously cited studies ... each used data drawn from numerous sources (e.g., teachers, parents, neurologists, and psychometrists). Naturally, much of the vari-

ance in such a matrix of intercorrelations will be that associated with differences between the sources, and data obtained from within a single source will tend to yield elevated intercorrelations because they were obtained at the same time, using similar measurement techniques (Miller, 1976) . . . the source factors that have been derived from such across-source matrices are merely what we should have expected from the method used; they do not form a sound basis for inferring that the HK/MBD syndrome does not exist.

When one moves to single-source matrices, such as those obtained from ratings made by a group of teachers, the source-factor artifact is of course eliminated. However, procedural and methodological features continue to exercise a strong influence on the nature and number of factors that will be obtained (Achenbach & Edelbrock, 1978; Quay, 1979). For example, some methods of factor analysis tend to produce more factors from a given correlation matrix. Matrices with many items tend to produce more factors. Analyses that iterate communalities in order to produce their solutions will result in fewer factors. Decisions about subject variability, eigenvalue levels, item loading criteria, and item form and content will affect how many and what kind of factors are ultimately obtained. Therefore, although factor analysis is indispensable for data reduction (Langhorne, 1977; A. Wilson, 1976), decisions about . . . the existence of a syndrome should not rest solely on factor-analytic studies.*

A Common Cause. There is little evidence that the symptoms of hyperactivity have a common cause. The low degree of interrelatedness reported in the factor analytic studies suggests that different etiological factors are involved, or at best, that the clusters of symptoms reflect particular etiologies. The major symptoms have been linked to such diverse etiological factors as genetic transmission, brain damage, maternal alcohol intake, lead poisoning, metabolic dysfunction, exposure to radiation, allergy, child rearing practices, school stress, and environmental restraints. Furthermore, subgroups of hyperactive children have been identified through clinical acumen (Bender, 1942; Chess, 1979; Howell, Rever, Scholl, Trowbridge, & Rutledge, 1972; Marwit & Stenner, 1972; Ney, 1974) and empirical procedures (Conners, 1975b; David, Clark, & Voeller, 1972; Fleischmann, 1977; Lambert, 1981; Loney et al., 1978; Schleifer et al., 1975).

A Consistent Response to Treatment. There is no evidence of either a consistent response to treatment or a distinctive and uniform outcome to a lack of treatment. A substantial percentage of hyperactive children treated with stimulant medication or behavior modification procedures show varying degrees of improvement in short-term manageability, but consistent long-term improvement is not an established outcome for any of the procedures. Hyperactivity and the related symptoms disappear spontaneously in some children

*From Loney, J. Hyperkinesis comes of age: What do we know and where should we go? *American Journal of Orthopsychiatry*, 1980, *50*, 28–42. Reprinted, with permission, from the *American Journal of Orthopsychiatry*; copyright 1980 by the American Orthopsychiatric Association, Inc.

in early adolescence, but persist in others, and these varying outcomes appear to be unrelated to type or duration of treatment (Cantwell, 1979; Whalen & Henker, 1980b).

Demonstrable Differences between the Hyperactive and Other Groups. The requirement of differences between children diagnosed as hyperactive and those with other behavior disorders is the most researched criterion of syndrome status, with empirical interest focusing on the validity of the diagnostic distinction between childhood hyperactivity and conduct disorder. One group (e.g., Lahey, Green, & Forehand, 1980; Sandberg, Rutter, & Taylor, 1978; Shaffer & Greenhill, 1979) contends that childhood hyperactivity and conduct disorder are essentially similar with regard to behavioral characteristics, etiology, and prognosis. Representative of this view is Shaffer and Greenhill's argument (1979) that the frequency of both disorders is greater in males, and both disorders are associated with more psychiatric disturbances in parents, are more likely to lead to later social, academic, and psychiatric maladjustment, and have similar etiologies. In view of the paucity of established etiological knowledge, the latter point is dubious at best. The opposition (e.g., Barkley, 1981; Loney, Kramer, & Milich, 1981; Milich, Loney, & Landau, 1981; Offord, Sullivan, Allen, & Abrams, 1979) maintains that there are important behavioral and prognostic differences between the two disorders. In a convincing rebuttal of the research underlying the view of hyperactivity and conduct disorders as essentially similar, Barkley (1981) has focused on several methodological shortcomings, for example, the lack of rigor in the diagnostic parameters, inadequate factor analytic procedures, and total reliance on rating scale data. Barkley (1981) has also stressed the recently documented differences between the two disorders in demographic and familial antecedents and eventual outcome (Loney, 1980b). We concur with Barkley's conclusion that it would be premature to collapse these two diagnostic categories. The same pattern of dissent surrounds hyperactivity and learning disabilities, but here the supportive evidence is more conclusive, with both empirical investigations of a general nature (e.g., Cantwell & Satterfield, 1978; Trites, 1979) and factor analytic studies (Blouin, Bornstein, & Trites, 1978; Lahey et al., 1978) acknowledging that the two disorders do coexist but clearly supporting the validity of viewing hyperactivity and learning disabilities as relatively independent behavior dimensions.

One beneficial offshoot of this facet of the syndrome controversy has been an intensification of empirical and clinical interest in the identification and study of subgroups. Sandberg, Rutter, and Taylor (1978) and Schleifer et al. (1975), for example, have presented evidence suggesting that *cross-situational* hyperactives might be a distinctive diagnostic group from *situational* hyperactives, and follow-up studies of the Schleifer et al. subjects (Campbell, Endman, & Bernfeld, 1977; Campbell, Schleifer, Weiss, & Perlman, 1977) have supported this distinction. Conners and Blouin (1980) have distinguished between *externalizers*, who are impulsive, disorganized, and have a low frustration tolerance, and *internalizers,* who are immature and have notable attentional difficulties. Loney and her associates (Loney et al., 1978) and others (Prinz, Connor, & Wilson, 1980) have differentiated between *pure hyperactives, pure aggressives,* and *hyperactive aggressives.*

Taken together, the foregoing clusters of studies on the syndrome status issue suggest that there is great heterogeneity in the group of children who currently are labeled as hyperactive, and that they do *not* make up a single clinical entity, although as data accumulate from this high density research area there may prove to be several hyperactivity syndromes. It is our opinion that the progress to date on the issue of syndrome status generally does not justify the continuance of the foregoing directions of investigative effort (an exception being the research on subgroups). Researchers should consider the conceptual framework implicit in the critical review of the hyperactivity syndrome by Shaffer and Greenhill (1979) and more explicitly stated by Achenbach and Edelbrock (1978). They suggest that the utility of a syndrome or a diagnosis is not so much in its covariation of symptoms but rather in its ability to provide prognostic and prescriptive information that will differentiate children with the syndrome from those in other diagnostic categories.

Meanwhile, belief in *one* hyperactivity syndrome has been reaffirmed by some researchers and clinicians even in the face of relatively strong evidence to the contrary. In a recent conference on hyperactivity in adulthood (Bellak, 1979), no consensus was reached on the relative merits of descriptors such as adult brain dysfunction (Mann & Greenspan, 1976) and paroxysmal episodic dyscontrol (Gallant, 1979), but the chairman, Leopold Bellak (1979, p. 201) concluded, "My one suggestion is that we call it a syndrome, whatever else we call it." As long as this thinking persists, it will continue to impede progress in the field.

MAJOR ADVANCES

Despite the ubiquitous problems of terminological confusion and syndrome status, there is, for the most part, agreement that notable advances in our knowledge of hyperactivity have been made in the past decade (Barkley, 1978; Cantwell, 1979; Loney, 1980a, 1980b; Whalen & Henker, 1980b). Some investigators view the increased complexity of the current research topics as constituting the major advance. Douglas (1976, p. 307), for example, described the status of hyperactivity research as being past the preliminary period of empirical study "to a second, more difficult, stage of research in this disorder," and in a comprehensive review of the field, Loney (1980b, p. 40) concluded that "we have seen the end of some speculations about childhood hyperkinesis—and the sketchy beginnings of several lines of research that may lead to answers for our more complex and subtle questions." Among the dissenters is one of the most respected investigators in the field. In Freeman's (1976, p. 5) terms. "There is only one phrase for the state of the art and practice in the field of minimal brain dysfunction (MBD), hyperactivity (HA), and learning disability (LD) in children: a mess." We strongly disagree with this pessimistic view. There are far too many methodologically weak studies, but we think that they are offset to a considerable extent by the rapidly increasing number of methodologically sophisticated investigations. In the 1970s the field was characterized by increasing productivity in the broadest sense, and during this period there were three truly significant advances, whose effect on progress in the field has far surpassed that of any other developments in hyperactivity over the past decade.

One of these is a fundamental and long overdue change in the conceptualization of hyperactivity, from a disease model and medical problem that fostered the notion of *one* hyperactive child to a broader concept of hyperactivity as a behavior disorder. Hyperactivity is now seen as a diffuse and nonmedical phenomenon that is heterogeneous in its manifestations and thus requires a multifaceted approach to research and treatment. The acceptance in the full scientific sense of this broader concept is apparent in a group of diverse spheres of activity: The American Psychiatric Association (DSM III) has recommended two new diagnostic categories, Attention Deficit Disorder with Hyperactivity and Attention Deficit Disorder without Hyperactivity. Researchers (Bugental et al. 1977; Conners, 1975b; David, Clark, & Voeller, 1972; Fleischmann, 1977; Lambert et al. 1978; Loney et al. 1978; Porges & Smith, 1980; Schleifer et al., 1975; Sleator & Ullman, 1981) and clinicians (Bender, 1942; Chess, 1979; Howell et al., 1972; Marwit & Stenner, 1972; Miller, 1978a; Ney, 1974) have shown increased interest in the classification of hyperactive children into homogeneous subgroups. Perhaps most significant of all has been the trend towards the empirical identification in initial investigations of subgroups, which then are designated as primary groups in subsequent research on the same topic (David, Hoffman, Sverd, Clark, & Voeller, 1976; Harley, Ray, Tomasi, Eichman, Matthews, Chun, Cleeland, & Traisman, 1978). Acceptance of a broader concept of hyperactivity is also apparent in the shift from the standarized drug regimen, in which a trial of medication signified an automatic (and often unmonitored) age-weight dosage (Solomons, 1971, 1973) to the carefully calculated individually titrated dosage long advocated by pharmacological experts (e.g., Cantwell, 1978a; Sprague, 1978; Werry, 1977) but only recently accorded widespread acceptance. The procedure of studying the effect of nondrug interventions on individual children and developing highly specialized treatment programs for them (Diller & Gofman, 1981; Hirst, 1976; Pelham, 1977; Satterfield, Satterfield, & Cantwell, 1980; Thelen, Fry, Fehrenbach, & Frautschi, 1979; Varni & Henker, 1979; Walker, 1974) is a further offshoot of this broader concept. The extent to which hyperactivity has begun to be particularized is evident from recent documentation that it can vary from not being a problem for either the child or those in his ecosystem (Lambert et al., 1978; Shelley & Riester, 1972) to being a problem in some or all settings (Schleifer et al., 1975), and that the duration varies markedly from that of a relatively brief period for some to a lifelong affliction for others. Furthermore, there is new concern (Henker & Whalen, 1980a; Loney, 1980a) that the manifestations and effects of this disorder in girls appear to be quite different from those in boys (Battle & Lacey, 1972; Mainville & Friedman, 1976; Prinz & Loney, 1974; Waldrop, Bell, & Goering, 1976). The concern that hyperactive girls should become a focus of study (Henker & Whalen, 1980a; Loney, 1980a) is in marked contrast to the procedure of including small subsets of hyperactive girls with hyperactive boys in statistical analyses under the assumption of homogeneity.

Another major advance over the past decade has been a radical change in the perception of the role played by the hyperactive child in the problems created by his behavior disorder. In much of the first half of the century the hyperactive child was generally viewed as the hapless recipient of a disease or pathological process with diverse and disruptive behavioral consequences. In the turmoil associated with this disorder, the role of the child was essentially that of a passive victim (Bond & Appel, 1931; Ebaugh, 1923; Still, 1902). As the concept of minimal brain dysfunction gained acceptance in the 1940s, the perception of the hyperactive child changed subtly to that of a helpless victim in a fruitless struggle with powerful internal and undocumented forces. The child was often depicted as "driven" (Kahn & Cohen, 1934), and this view has persisted in many quarters (Strauss & Lehtinen, 1947; Wender, 1971) through the 1970s. In the last decade, particularly in the last half of it, theoretical (Bandura, 1974; Bell & Harper, 1977; Bronfenbrenner, 1979a; Chess, 1979; Klaus & Kennell, 1976; Pederson, 1976) and empirical developments (Barkley & Cunningham, 1979; Henker & Whalen, 1980a) have led to the perception of the hyperactive child as an active force in creating and maintaining the often chaotic social environments associated with this behavior disorder. A rapidly accumulating body of empirical data attests to the powerful and often adverse influence of the child on the early intrafamilial dyadic relationships (Campbell, 1979a; Drash, 1975; Mash & Johnston, 1981; Thomas & Chess, 1977), school-age peer group (Battle & Lacey, 1972; Campbell & Paulauskas, 1979; Whalen, Henker, Collins, McAuliffe, & Vaux, 1979), ecology of the classroom (Klein & Young, 1979; Schleifer et al., 1975; Whalen et al., 1978), and harmony of the household (Barkley, 1978; Diller & Gofman, 1981; Lyness, 1977). The effect of this change in the understanding of the role of the hyperactive child has been to focus increased investigative and clinical interest on the factual interactions of the hyperactive child and his family and peers (Bax, 1978; Minde, 1977).

The third of the major advances concerns the importance of childhood aggression to adolescent outcome for the hyperactive child. Although there has been continuing resistance in this past decade to the use of stimulant drugs, this opposition has been tempered by the belief that the untreated hyperactive child is at risk for antisocial aggression in adolescence, which proponents of drug intervention claimed could be averted by stimulant treatment. When the first of a cluster of follow-up studies (Weiss, Kruger, Danielson, & Elman, 1975) reported that stimulant treatment was *not* associated with improved outcome in adolescence and when, in fact, the treated and untreated children in most of the studies did not differ at all, these findings were totally unexpected, particularly in the light of the often dramatic improvements that occurred in childhood with stimulant treatment. The explanations for the follow-up phenomenon were as diverse as they were ingenious, but with one major exception were lacking in any true substance. Advocates of drug intervention remained unshaken in their conviction, arguing that the function of drug treatment was to modify the child's behavior and that what was needed was intervention, such as social skills training, that would elicit the reactions from the social environment necessary to maintain the newly acquired good behavior. Interactionists contended that the poor outcome in adolescence was attributable to a variety of social learning and experiential factors, such as parenting variables and live and media models, and cited a diverse group of theoretical and empirical support sources (Bandura, 1969; Olweus, 1973; Robins, 1966, 1978) for this viewpoint. Cunningham and Barkley (1978b), who attribute hyperactivity to achievement deficits, suggested that intervention directed at hyperactivity leaves the child's primary problem of achievement untreated, so that the continuing deficit in achievement makes the child vulnerable to social forces that are conducive to the development of antisocial aggression.

The exception to the above explanations is the empirically derived model for explaining adolescent outcome, that is, symptomatology and antisocial behavior, that has been developed by Loney and her associates (Loney, Kramer, & Milich, 1981; Loney, Milich, & Maurer, 1979; Milich, Loney, & Landau, 1981). This model is based on their own research (Loney et al., 1978; Langhorne & Loney, 1979; Paternite & Loney, 1980) and the follow-up data and work of other investigators (Blouin, Bornstein, & Trites, 1978; Minde, Weiss, & Mendelson, 1972; Robins, 1966, 1978; Weiss & Hechtman, 1979; Weiss, Hechtman, & Perlman, 1978; Werner & Smith, 1977). We consider this model to be an extraordinary contribution to the field and, although it will be described in detail in Chapter 5, a brief discussion of it as a major advance is relevant here. The basic rationale for the Loney model can be summarized as follows: Childhood aggression and hyperactivity are assumed to have markedly different antecedents and consequents; the former is associated with subsequent adolescent difficulty and delinquent behavior, whereas the latter is not associated with these problems. Childhood aggression is not responsive to stimulant medication, so no matter how effective stimulant medication is in modifying the constellation of primary problems of hyperactivity, it leaves the aggressive component of the child's behavior untouched and free to lead to such problems as antisocial aggression in adolescence. It follows that for drug treatment that has been associated with the successful reduction of hyperactivity in the middle childhood years to be linked with positive outcome at adolescence, an essential condition would be that the child not be aggressive; and where childhood hyperactivity is accompanied by aggression, drug treatment alone is unlikely to be associated with positive outcome. Within this framework the target of intervention for the aggressive hyperactive child should be the reduction of both kinds of behavior by means of stimulant medication for the hyperactivity and behavioral treatment for the aggression. Environmental factors associated with aggression, such as poor parenting and the correlates of low socioeconomic status, should also be targets of intervention, because research on adolescent aggression suggests that treatment focused on the child alone has little effect.

The potential impact of this tentative model is tremendous. If subsequent independent investigations do confirm it, the direction of research in the field will be significantly changed and many existing "facts," explanations, and procedures modified, including the following: the theory of primary and secondary symptoms in which childhood aggression is currently classified as a secondary symptom and the *result* of hyperactivity; the recently developed category of Attention Deficit Disorder with Hyperactivity in DSM III (1980); the achievement deficit etiological theory of Cunningham and Barkley (1978b); assessment routines at referral for hyperactivity that have barely touched on aggression; the proposed genetic link between childhood hyperactivity and adult psychiatric disorders; single-pronged treatment strategies that focus almost entirely on the primary symptoms; and the assumption of a stimulant medication-adolescent drug abuse link. In view of the fact that this model is by far the most exciting development of the past decade, Loney and her colleagues have shown commendable restraint in their discussion of it (Loney, 1980b; Milich & Loney, 1979a) and admirable concern for methodological rigor with their replication and further validation of the findings (Milich et al., 1981). Also, they have emphasized the need for independent empirical documentation of their findings. While this model focuses on the impressive predictive potential of childhood aggression for adolescent outcome, Loney and her colleagues (Loney et al., 1981; Milich & Loney, 1979a) are not suggesting that aggression is the only significant predictor of adolescent outcome for their population of hyperactive boys.

With this overview of the field as a background, we will now proceed with the purpose of this text, which is to provide a comprehensive review and evaluation of the current status of empirical knowledge of hyperactivity, synthesize research and clinical examples, discuss the implications of empirical knowledge for prevention and management techniques, and specify new directions for research and treatment.

CHAPTER 2

Clinical Description

The major developmental periods of infancy, preschool, middle childhood, adolescence, and adulthood provide a convenient, if compartmentalized, framework for a clinical description of hyperactivity. The behaviors subsumed under each of these periods represent a composite of the behaviors likely to occur in the hyperactive individual of that age. It would be most unusual for a specific hyperactive individual at any one stage to exhibit the entire constellation of behaviors described here for that stage, and highly unlikely that the behaviors exhibited would all be of equal intensity. It is the cumulative effect of a number of difficult behaviors of varying intensity that leads parents and pediatricians to suspect hyperactivity. The prototypical description that follows of hyperactivity at different developmental periods may be inconsistent with the reader's concept of hyperactivity. In evaluating such discrepancies it should be remembered that the cluster of behaviors characteristic of hyperactivity is not a stable response pattern that occurs regularly in diverse stimulus settings. Both the cross-situational and temporal variability of the hyperactive child's behavior are well documented (Campbell & Redfering, 1979; Loney, 1980b; Schleifer, Weiss, Cohen, Elman, Cvejic, & Kruger, 1975). Pediatricians, clinicians, and experimenters, who are relatively unfamiliar to the child and whose interactions are confined to one-to-one office or laboratory settings, are likely to see the behavior of the hyperactive child as far less extreme than do those who interact regularly with him in his natural habitats of home, school, and neighborhood. Familiarity of personnel, setting, and procedure often exert a disinhibitory effect on the child, whereas strangeness of personnel and situational or procedural novelty may have a marked inhibitory effect (Cantwell, 1979; Whalen, Henker, Collins, McAuliffe, & Vaux, 1979); and group interactions are more likely to elicit hyperactive behaviors than are one-to-one interactions. In short, the social-situational context is a major determinant of the hyperactive child's immediate behavior.

ACROSS AGE STAGES

Although there is some clinical (Barkley, 1978; Routh, 1978) and empirical evidence (Campbell, Schleifer, & Weiss, 1978) for continuity of hyperactive behaviors across age stages, at the individual level both the time of onset and the duration of symptoms can vary markedly. For some individuals the infancy period may be a serene and untroubled one, with the onset of hyperactivity coinciding with beginning to walk or entering preschool, and the duration of symptoms being relatively brief. For others, the onset of symptoms predictive of hyperactivity may occur in infancy and persist, with changing symptomatology, throughout childhood, adolescence, and young adulthood (Campbell, et al., 1978; Weiss & Hechtman, 1979; Wender, 1979).

Within any one response modality, the form of the behavior also changes from one developmental stage to the next, paralleling the changes in maturation and functioning. Level of activity may manifest itself in infancy as almost ceaseless thrashing about in the crib, in the preschool setting as dashing from one free-play activity to another, in the school years as the inability to remain seated throughout a seatwork period, in adolescence as unusual restlessness in situations in which same-age peers remain still, and in adulthood as endless pacing up and down in a situation in which most adults would remain seated. A similar sequence of changes occurs in the realm of social functioning (Barkley, 1978, p. 160):

> ... the overactive, temperamental infant becomes the hyperactive, noncompliant preschool child, and eventually the child who has trouble following rules and teacher commands in the classroom during school years. As the child enters adolescence and participation in a larger social sphere, problems with peer relationships become paramount, as does difficulty in obeying the rules of society. With entry into adulthood, these problems persist and may affect the adult's social adaptation and ability to obtain and hold employment.

The behavior seen as the most serious problem also changes from one age period to the next, with parents viewing sleep problems and crying as the salient problems in infancy, hyperactivity as the most conspicuous problem in middle childhood, and rebelliousness and antisocial behavior as the predominant problems in adolescence. A behavior that remains unchanged across age levels may be seen as serious at some levels and not at others. Teachers generally are not disturbed about a short attention span in a preschool child, but begin to show concern about such a problem in the primary grade child, and consider it a serious problem requiring remedial intervention in the elementary school child.

WITHIN AGE STAGES

Within each of the major developmental stages quantitative and qualitative characteristics differentiate the behavior of the hyperactive child from that of his same-age, same-sex normal peers. In infancy, for example, this child often cries more than the average infant, and his crying has a strange and inconsolable quality that clearly distinguishes it from the normal crying of infancy. In the school years the child engages in more inappropriate activity than the normally active child; sometimes this activity has a curiously precipitous quality that seems to make it almost impossible for the child to stop on command to do so, and often elicits sympathy from adults despite their aggravation (Nichamin, 1972; Pincus & Glaser, 1966).

The impact of these various patterns of hyperactive behavior on the child's social environment can be described within an interactional perspective (Chess, 1979). According to this model, the child's physiological and psychological characteristics interact with forces in his social environments to determine whether or not he is viewed as hyperactive. It has been well documented in prevalence (Lambert, Sandoval, & Sassone, 1978) and preschool studies (Schleifer et al., 1975) that a child with a particular combination of physical characteristics and psychological traits may be considered hyperactive under certain environmental conditions and not under others. It follows that having a cluster of hyperactive behaviors will not automatically cause problems for the child. In some children the hyperactivity pattern is clearly present in the preschool years, yet it is not a problem because environmental social pressures that could accelerate it to the problem level are absent, or the household is so chaotic that the behavior passes unnoticed, or the parents are so tolerant or inexperienced that the behavior is not viewed as unusual. Problems develop when there are repeated negative interactions between the child's hyperactive behavior and the demands and expectations of his social environment. The following case study describes a child in conflict with a new social environment and the reciprocal impact of this confrontation:

A four-year-old boy, the youngest child and only boy in a family of five children, exhibited an extremely high activity level almost from birth. Before he was a year old he could bounce up and down so vigorously in his crib that he had bounced out on several occasions and he wore out the crib that all of his sisters had used. He was termed "a mobile disaster area" and provided with an escort whenever his mother took him to the local supermarket, and was regarded by the neighbors as a well-meaning threat to any small child or animal. He was noncompliant, constantly in motion, unusually unruly and impulsive in free play situations, and was prone to such rapid changes of mood that he was described by the teachers at a nursery school that he attended for one week as "a time bomb that might explode at any minute and disrupt the entire preschool setting." These behaviors were not perceived as cause for concern by his parents, who expected boys to be difficult. His mother dismissed his misbehavior as "a bit rambunctious but just what a regular boy should be like," and his father was inordinately proud of him and predicted that he would be "a real pace-setter once he got it all worked out." Both parents were genuinely perplexed when they were asked to remove him after his first week at preschool, disconcerted when a second school refused to keep him, and astonished and dismayed when their pediatrician assured them that the actions of both schools were justified.

The above example illustrates the immediate effects within Chess's (1979) interactional model. A long-term and more serious effect of such behavior is that it has the potential to impede the hyperactive child's cognitive and social development. The rationale for this statement is as follows: The cluster of hyperactive behaviors would be categorized as strong response patterns along a strong-weak continuum. One of the salient features of such responses is that they prevent other intrinsically incompatible behavior from occurring. When the latter behavior is essential for an adequate social or cognitive behavior repertoire, the child needs all the opportunities for practicing them that he can get. Deprivation, particularly at critical periods, can have serious effects on the child's psychosocial development. The infant who is chronically restless, irritable, and crying cannot at the same time be engaged in positive interaction with his mother. The day-in and day-out handling of the difficult behavior, particularly on the part of the mother, is a crucial determinant of outcome. If she is skilled, patient, and tolerant, much of the difficult behavior will be defused, because up to a point, it takes two to make a potentially unpleasant interaction into an actuality. If the mother reacts with anger, irritation, and withdrawal, and begins to feel anxious and defeated, one possible result will be a diminishing of the overall quality of the mother–child relationship (Campbell, 1979a), with a consequent deleterious effect on the attachment process as well as a significant long-term effect on the cognitive and perceptual motor development of the child (Scholom & Schiff, 1980). Similarly, the school-age child whose restlessness and impulsivity prevent him from participating in peer-group games is deprived of a sequence of peer group experiences that would help him acquire critically important social interaction competencies. From an interactional perspective, it can be seen that to a considerable extent the child's hyperactive behavior can shape his environments, and in so doing can impede his cognitive and social development.

INFANCY

Patterns of behavior predictive of hyperactivity sometimes are present early in infancy (Fidone, 1975; Rapoport, Quinn, Burg, & Bartley, 1979; Routh, 1978; Salter, 1977). By *predictive* we mean that the probability is increased that infants who consistently exhibit certain difficult behavior patterns will be diagnosed as hyperactive in the preschool or school years (Thomas & Chess, 1977). We consider these infants to be at risk for later hyperactivity, and will use the descriptor *hyperactive infant* rather than the more precise but cumbersome *infant at risk for later hyperactivity*. However, from a clinical viewpoint, no definite diagnostic label should be attached at this point because the difficult behaviors are exhibited by all infants to some extent and may be transient ones that disappear with increasing age. However, lending a certain validity to the predictive value of persisting patterns of difficult behavior are the retrospective reports from parents (Barnard & Collar, 1973; Stewart, Pitts, Craig, & Dieruf, 1966) and experienced clinicians (Drash, Stolberg, & Bostow, 1977; Weiss & Hechtman, 1979) about the infant behavior of children who were subsequently diagnosed as hyperactive.

If we were limited to a single descriptor for the infancy period, *difficult* might be the best choice. All aspects of his response repertoire, including activity patterns, vocalizations, sleep patterns, and feeding behavior, are likely to be hard for the mother to contend with, thus imposing a severe strain on the dyadic relationship.

Activity. Often the infant is so active that even an experienced maternity nurse has difficulty holding him comfortably as he turns, twists, arches his back, wriggles, and thrashes about in her arms. If he is left unattended for a few seconds on a table he is likely to roll over and fall off. During routine care he often shows surprising strength in resisting activities that most infants appear to find pleasurable. Mothers describe him as kicking more forcefully both prenatally and postnatally and showing more strength of grip than the average infant. He usually shows normal progress in growth and general development, but exhibits advanced motor activity that tends to be characterized by a jerky quality rather than by a rhythimic flow (Nichamin, 1972; Stewart & Olds, 1973). He often climbs out of his crib in the first year of life and sometimes wears out the crib mattress with his constant rocking about. Once he leaves the crib of his own volition he begins to crawl almost immediately, and from then on his mother knows little peace.

Vocalizations. Throughout the first year of life the hyperactive infant often cries readily with either a distinctive high-pitched cry or an angry monotonic scream. In a study of the morphology of early vocalizations, Wolff (1969) noted that the cry is typically shrill and piercing, and of a fundamental frequency significantly higher (650–800 cycles per second) than that of the normal cry of a healthy infant (400–450 cycles per second). Distraught parents have described it as "a sound like a siren," "an animal in acute distress," and "the high thin note of static on a radio." Although the crying is often mistaken for colic, it differs in several important respects: the time of onset is earlier, it lacks the painful piercing quality of the colicky cry, and it is not paroxysmal (Nichamin, 1972). The excessive crying can have two results costly to the child's development. It may exceed the tolerance limits of the mother, causing her to feel inadequate as a mother followed by withdrawal from the infant in disappointment over him. This cycle of events seriously jeopardizes the early mother–child relationship. A second effect is that frequent distress and crying maintains a state of arousal in which the infant is bombarded by internal stimuli, with the result that he has less time than he should have to explore his external environment and so creates an experiential deficit having important implications for cognitive development (Schaffer, 1977).

Sleep. The infant's sleep patterns sometimes resemble those of the premature infant in respect to the ratio (1:3) of quiet sleep (no rapid eye movements [REM] or body movements and normal respiration and heart-rate) to active sleep (REM, many small limb and head movements, irregular respirations and heart rate). The lower than normal amount of quiet sleep exhibited by the hyperactive infant is of relevance because the area of the brain that controls quiet sleep is also involved in the maintenance of attending behavior (Barnard & Collar, 1973). The infant does not fall into a pattern of regular sleep times, nor does he fall asleep quickly. When his sleep periods do occur, they are of short duration (Campbell, 1976), and he awakens easily with a startled reaction often followed by screaming (Nichamin, 1972).

Feeding. The hyperactive infant is notable for the unusually long time that it takes him to eat, his tendency to eat very lightly, and a reluctance to try new food. He cries for food at irregular temporal intervals and does not become quiet even when he is lifted to the feeding position. His feeding behavior has been described by weary mothers as "obstinate, obstructive, and picky, with every meal being more like a battle than a social event." This pattern of feeding behavior is more important for the negative effect it has on the mother–child relationship than for any predisposition to later feeding problems (Campbell, 1976).

In addition to the generalized difficulty of the hyperactive infant's behavior, he is often characterized by a pervasive kind of irregularity that extends to his physical appearance as well as his personality. Physiologically. the infant may exhibit asymmetrical reflex responses (Denhoff, 1973), and his features, especially his eyes, are sometimes asymmetrical, a fact that in infancy often elicits negative comments from tactless adults and later, derogation from peers. No contribution is made to this problem by attaching labels such as Wender's (1971) FLK (Funny Looking Kid) to the hyperactive child. Physical examination may reveal the presence of one or more characteristics that appear to be irregularities, such as head circumference out of the normal range and widely spaced eyes; low-seated, malformed, or asymmetrical ears; and a wide gap between the first and second toes. These are minor physical anomalies, and their presence has been shown to be positively associated with hyperactivity in the early preschool years (Waldrop, Bell, McLaughlin, & Halverson, 1978). These minor physical anomalies are described in more detail in the section on the physical examination of the hyperactive child in Chapter 9. Psychologically, the infant may exhibit wide variations in mood states and affectional patterns. He may be yelling and almost apoplectic one minute then suddenly switch to a period of calm, possibly lasting for several days. This unpredictability makes it difficult for his mother to enjoy even his calm periods, because she knows they are fleeting and likely to be interrupted momentarily by explosive outbursts. Heightening the problem further is the fact that the infant's personality is often not an engaging one: he is described as intense, jittery, hypertonic, querulous, irritable, demanding, and unsatisfied.

One particularly telling characteristic is that he rarely smiles or looks directly at his mother. Absence of this social response is important because eye contact serves as a catalyst in the development of social expressiveness in the infant (Bloom, 1975; Schaffer, 1977). Ambrose (1969, p. 198) believes that, in addition, the absence of smiling has potentially serious implications for the mother-child relationship as well as for the infant's cognitive development:

> I should like to emphasize the importance of the infant's smiling as a communication signal that has a powerful effect on the mother. In my earlier studies of this response in the natural setting I was very struck by the enormous delight shown by the mother when her baby first smiles at her face. Furthermore, if her infant doesn't smile at her when she feels it should be starting to do so, usually during the second month, some mothers go to considerable lengths in trying to elicit the response such as by tickling the sides of the mouth. When the infant's smiling responsiveness has really developed, one can see that this behavior does increase the chances that the infant will get longer durations of playful interaction with the mother. I believe that this kind of interaction provides important sensory inputs and early cognitive structuring for the infant which are not provided adequately in the feeding situation alone.

A consistent theme implicit in the foregoing discussion is that of an increasingly unsatisfactory mother-child relationship accompanied by a lessening of maternal responsivity to the difficult infant that is not easily reversed. Campbell (1979a) reported that mothers who perceived their 3-month-old infants as extremely "difficult," according to Thomas and Chess's categories (1977), and were less responsive to them than control mothers, continued to be less responsive when the infants were eight months old, even though the formerly "difficult" infants were now virtually indistinguishable from the control infants. Continued maternal unresponsivity may have potentially serious consequences for the infant's subsequent social adjustment: Pastor (1981) has suggested that one precursor of diminished or inadequate sociability with peers in the early preschool years is a poor mother-infant relationship. These findings underscore the powerful effects that the daily behavior of the parents, particularly the mother, may have on long-term outcome for the difficult infant. The serious consequences for the infant of a deteriorating relationship can best be understood by examining the stages that characterize the interactions of normal infants and their mothers. In a longitudinal study on the emerging mother-child relationships in young mothers and their normal first-born infants, Sander (1969) identified and defined a sequence of five levels of adaptation, common to all the mother-infant pairs, that occurred according to a temporally orderly sequence and for predictable durations of time in the first 18 months of life. To obtain his data, Sander used recorded mother interviews conducted at regular intervals, standardized situational and free-play observations of the infants, and periodic developmental tests. The resulting levels conceptually are very close to the developmental tasks of Havighurst (1972) in that both investigators believe that one level or one task should be mastered if the next level or task is to be accomplished without unusual difficulty. In the Sander investigation it was found that a degree of harmony in the mother–child relationship at any level was dependent on the successful resolution of adaptation at the previous level. The relatively short duration of each level created problems for mothers and infants who had difficulty achieving synchrony at a particular level, because it meant that they would soon be faced with the demands of the next level without having accomplished the tasks of their current level. Sander's levels of adaptation that are shown in Table 2.1 specify the behavioral changes at each level that are prerequisite to the progressively more differentiated degrees of regulation, reciprocation, and initiation of behavior essential for harmony in the mother–child interaction. In the first level the task concerned the regulation of the infant's rhythms of feeding, sleeping, and elimination, so that a certain predictability in daily routines occurred, which in turn resulted in feelings of confidence and competence in the mother. Occurring in the second level was the spontaneous

Table 2.1. Sander's Five Levels of Adaptation

Issue	Title	Span of Months	Prominent Infant Behaviors which Became Coordinated with Maternal Activities
1	Initial regulation	Months 1–2–3	Basic infant activities concerned with biological processes related to feeding, sleeping, elimination, postural maintenance, etc. including stimulus needs for quieting and arousal.
2	Reciprocal exchange	Months 4–5–6	Smiling behavior which extends to full motor and vocal involvement in sequences of affectively spontaneous back and forth exchanges. Activities of spoon feeding, dressing, etc., become reciprocally coordinated.
3	Initiative	Months 7–8–9	Activities initiated by infant to secure a reciprocal social exchange with mother or to manipulate environment on his own selection.
4	Focalization	Months 10–11–12–13	Activities by which infant determines the availability of mother on his specific initiative. Tends to focalize need meeting demands on the mother.
5	Self-assertion	Months 14–20	Activities in which infant widens the determination of his own behavior often in the face of maternal opposition.

Reprinted, with permission, from Sander, L. W. The longitudinal course of early mother-child interaction: Cross-case comparison in a sample of mother-child pairs. In B. M. Foss (Ed.), *Determinants of infant behavior* IV. London: Methuen, 1969, pp. 189–227.

development of smiling play and reciprocal coordination of caretaking activities with an overlay of mutual affection and well-being. The third level was characterized by a marked increase in the infant's initiation of social exchange and bids for attention. In the fourth level an increase in independence occurred that was facilitated by the mother's knowing when to intervene. In the final level there was an increase in genuine independence as the infant began to achieve both psychological and physiological separation from his mother. It is reasonable to conclude that a hyperactive infant and his mother would have an exceedingly difficult time accomplishing the tasks described by Sander (1969).

Supporting this supposition are findings for the first three years of life from a longitudinal study (Battle & Lacey, 1972) of the maternal and child correlates of motor activity.* These data suggest a high degree of asynchrony and a lack of harmony in the early mother–child relationships. During this period the mothers of hyperactive boys were critical of them and showed a lack of affection, and these behaviors continued to be manifested in a variety of forms, including a low intensity of interaction, throughout the entire preschool and elementary school period. In turn, the hyperactive infant boys were characterized by noncompliance toward their mothers and adults in general, a lack of achievement striving, and a failure to exhibit the increase in independence specified by Sander's (1969) fourth and fifth levels of adaptation.

In the literature on early socialization, the tendency has been to interpret correlations between mother–child characteristics, such as the Battle and Lacey (1972) findings, in a unidirectional fashion from mother to child. A more accurate interpretation would be one in which the powerful influence of the infant is also acknowledged, that is, the interaction becomes one of bidirectionality of effect (Bell & Harper, 1977). In this reciprocal framework, infant temperament characteristics interact with parental personality and adjustment to partially determine the degree of harmony in the early mother–child relationship. For example, a chronically difficult infant, such as the hyperactive infant, usually will elicit negative affect from his mother, and an indifferent or rejecting mother may produce a fretful, restless, or unresponsive

---

*The Battle and Lacey (1972) data on the correlates of motor activity were collected during the period from 1939 to 1957 as part of the Fels Longitudinal Study. At the end of this period hyperactivity was just beginning to be recognized as a diagnostic category (Laufer & Denhoff, 1957; Laufer, Denhoff, & Solomons, 1957), so none of the 74 subjects in the study had been diagnosed as hyperactive. However, the definition used by Battle and Lacey was similar to that used by other investigators: Hyperactivity was the degree to which the subject's motor behavior was described cross-situationally (home, nursery school, and day camp) as impulsive, uninhibited, uncontrolled, and at the high end of the motor activity dimension. Children who were described as hyperactive were characterized by constant running, fidgetiness, restlessness, impulsive motor acts, and inappropriate touching. Although attention span, inappropriateness of behavior, and distractibility were not specifically mentioned, they were implicit in the behavioral descriptions. If these subjects were in a clinic situation today, it is our opinion that they would be diagnosed as hyperactive.

infant. Once such a pattern is established, whatever its origin, both members of the dyad usually will contribute to the problem through an interactive process that maintains and exacerbates it. In this way a cycle of mutually reinforcing negative interaction is set in motion, gaining momentum as the infant's feelings of disequilibrium are superimposed on the disappointment, indifference, or outright dislike of the mother. For management purposes what is needed is one set of specific procedures, defined operationally and adaptable to individual differences, for preventing this destructive cycle from getting started, and a second set for interrupting an already existing cycle.

PRESCHOOL

The pervasive irregularity of both function and mood that characterized the infancy period continues to predominate in the preschool period. The child is often very tense and then abruptly and with no intervention suddenly relaxes. He has violent fits of rage and temper tantrums that are well above average in frequency and intensity, and the frequency of these reactions is increased by a low tolerance for frustration. When frustrated he may cry or scream with rage for as long as an hour. Even in sleep these abrupt changes are apparent: he often awakens suddenly for no apparent reason, and is immediately wide awake, alert, and noisy.

Speech. Although the preschool hyperactive child's progress in physical growth and development is usually normal, he often exhibits delayed speech development (Safer & Allen, 1976; Wender & Wender, 1978). He may still be jabbering in his second year, saying only single words in his third year, and not using short sentences until his fourth year, so that even before the end of this period his speech development is far behind that of his same-age peers. This delay in overt speech has two consequences, both of which are likely to exacerbate the child's difficulties. One effect is a concomitant slowness in the acquisition of covert speech skills, which enable the child to observe events in his environment and verbally code them for later usage. Any child who lacks the verbal repertoire prerequisite to such mediational activity is at a marked disadvantage in the acquisition of a variety of skills and cognitions that facilitate daily functioning. A second effect of slower speech development is that the shift from tactual to visual dominance, which is dependent in part on naming, may be delayed. The child remains touch-dominated, and this serves as an increasing source of difficulty not only in peer relations (children typically dislike being held or grasped while being spoken to or played with) but also in the increased probability of breakage of objects through handling. The verbal difficulty may be due in part to the quality of the early mother–child relationship: Kagan (1971) has reported that mothers of normal children typically engage in less social talk with infant boys than with girls, a predisposing factor in the verbal superiority of girls in the preschool years, and clinicians have noted that weary and exasperated mothers of young hyperactive children infrequently engage in social talk, thus partly setting the stage for the child's verbal deficit.

Management Problem. The difficulties of infancy do little to prepare the parents for the serious management problems of the preschool period. The child is so much more mobile, is impulsive, noncompliant, fearless, quite unresponsive to discipline, discussion, or persuasion, and generally does not learn from experience. A combination of apparently boundless energy and poor judgment means that he must constantly be supervised. His distracted caretakers regard him as accident-prone, a subjective opinion with empirical support from a study by Stewart, Thach, and Freidin (1970) in which a significant proportion of preschool boys who were accidentally poisoned were diagnosed as hyperactive at a follow-up six years later. The association between instances of accidental poisoning and hyperactivity is a predictable one. Hyperactive children are impulsive, more prone to get into things, and often more persistent than normal children, so the probability is higher that they will come into contact with a greater percentage of dangerous household items, including poisonous substances.

The difficulty of effectively managing the preschool hyperactive child is evident in clinical and parental reports (Cantwell, 1979; Drash, 1975; Nichamin, 1972; Stewart & Olds, 1973). A mother of a 4-year-old boy reported that he would dash about the house wreaking havoc if she did not forcibly restrain him. He had to be physically restrained in stores and on the street because of his tendency to run out into the traffic if he saw a car that interested him. On one occasion he ran the elevator in their apartment building up and down for 20 minutes without stopping, and on another he climbed up a telephone pole and refused to come down. He could never be left alone in any room with a manipulable appliance. On several occasions he had overturned pots on the stove. Neither the threat of punishment nor the promise of reward had more than a momentary effect on him. He could not remain in preschool for more than 30 minutes a day without falling apart, stay seated throughout even a short meal, or watch a 15-minute television program. No babysitter ever came twice. His mother said sadly that they could never do anything as a family and was seriously concerned about the effect of this child on their marriage. The validity of such concern is evident from clinical reports (Barkley, 1978), and experienced clinicians agree that the hyperactive child is more likely to be the cause of marital disharmony and family psychopathology than the result of it (Firestone, Peters, Rivier, & Knights, 1978).

Peer Relations. In this period the hyperactive child moves into the neighborhood peer group and preschool. With this expansion of his social world the ramifications of his hyperactive behavior patterns assume considerable importance. For the first time he is in social situations in which his parents and siblings are not available to act as buffers, and the adults and children that are present have no emotional ties to him. Although his behavior in new situations at first may appear subdued, he soon comes to be viewed as a stressor, particularly in peer group play. In a study of 4-year-old hyperactive children, a majority of mothers reported that their children had problems playing with others, were aggressive with peers, and had difficulty in group situations, whereas fewer than one-fifth of the control mothers had similar complaints (Campbell & Paulauskas, 1979). In peer group play the hyperactive child is sometimes aggressive, dominating, and destructive, thus evoking negative reactions from his preschool teachers and peers (Battle & Lacey, 1972; Campbell & Paulauskas, 1979). He shows little concern for others' feelings and seems to be genuinely unaware when he has hurt another child. At the same time, he is very responsive to peer disapproval and sometimes responds very aggressively at being excluded. He has difficulty in establishing early peer relationships, so in order to gain some peer recognition he may resort to teasing, showing off, name calling, deliberate destruction of others' work, shouting, and blatant aggression (Battle & Lacey, 1972). The irregularity pervading his behavior as an infant continues into the preschool period, but is seen by peers as unpredictability, and this characteristic imposes a severe strain on peer relations. The child may be playing harmoniously one minute and having a violent tantrum seconds later. The abruptness and extent of these changes of mood and behavior are frightening to other young children. Often he is excluded after a few sessions from one preschool after another and this series of failures, plus his difficulties in peer relations, lay the groundwork for the development of a poor self-concept (Cantwell, 1979).

Despite the obvious importance of information about hyperactivity at this age level, there has been only one major study (Schleifer et al., 1975). The subjects were 28 3- and 4-year-old children of normal intelligence, all of whom were characterized by chronic, sustained overactivity, and 26 matched control children. The hyperactive group was dichotomized into *true* hyperactives ($n = 10$), whose mothers' complaints of hyperactivity were confirmed by teachers' and psychiatrists' ratings, and *situational* hyperactives ($n = 18$), who were reported to be hyperactive at home but were not considered to be hyperactive in the nursery school setting. Schleifer et al. considered the true, but not the situational, hyperactive children to be more typical of the group of hyperactive primary school children who are referred to clinics shortly after entering school. They speculated that this dichotomy represented severe and milder forms of the same basic condition, but another possibility is that the home environments of the situational hyperactives were characterized by poorness of fit, whereas the nursery school environment represented goodness of fit for these children (Chess, 1979). Each of the 54 children was placed in a group of six children (three hyperactive and three controls) and participated in two-hour nursery school sessions once a week for nine weeks. The data used to compare the hyperactive and control groups consisted of observations of the children in free play and structured play activities, individual psychological tests, psychiatric interviews with the mothers, and home assessments by the psychiatrists. In the free-play observations, no differences were found among the true hyperactives, situational hyperactives, or controls, a finding that is consistent with Pope (1970) and Routh and Schroeder (1976). Furthermore, the two psychologists who were doing blind ratings of the free play were unable to identify the hyperactive children in each group, which suggests that hyperactive and normal preschool children exhibit similar levels of activity and social behavior in a free play setting. However, in the structured table activity the hyperactives as a group were more aggressive and more likely to be out of their chairs and away from the table than were the controls, and the true hyperactives were less attentive but not more active than were the situational hyperactives. Schleifer et al. noted a parallel between this finding and one with older children (Douglas, Weiss, & Minde, 1969; Sroufe, Sonies, West, & Wright, 1973) showing that school-aged hyperactive children differed from controls in exhibiting more irrelevant behavior and poor conduct in the classroom, but did not differ on measures of overactivity per se.

Of three cognitive style dimensions that were assessed, the hyperactive group differed from the controls on reflection-impulsivity but not on field independence-dependence or motor impulsivity. True hyperactives were more field-dependent and less impulsive than situational hyperactives. It should be noted that the status of these cognitive style constructs is somewhat controversial, with Block and others (Block, Block, & Harrington, 1974, 1975; Weisz, O'Neill, & O'Neill, 1975) questioning their validity and applicability to different age groups of children, and Kagan and Messer (1975) and Douglas (1972, 1974) defending their use. Psychiatric interviews showed that the homes of all the hyperactive children were more tense, with the mothers talking and playing less with their children than did the control mothers. The mothers of true hyperactives exhibited more frustration and used more physical punishment than did mothers of the other two groups. Causal direction cannot be inferred here, however, because these maternal behaviors could result from the children's hyperactivity or be a contributing cause to it.

The hyperactive preschool child generally is not referred for treatment until the point of formal school entry, yet it is clear from the foregoing empirical and descriptive data that he is already exhibiting a set of behaviors that will impede the development of satisfactory peer relations and cause continuous problems in the school setting. Furthermore, outcome data on hyperactive preschool children indicate that in the early school years these children are still perceived by adults as having more behavior problems than nonhyperactive controls have (Cohen, Sullivan, Minde, Novak, & Helwig, 1981; Schleifer et al., 1975). Consequently, whether or not a diagnosis of hyperactivity is eventually made, it should be clear to the pediatrician that *immediate intervention* is indicated. We are assuming of course that the pediatrician has been taking the time to really listen to the mother. If he brushes aside the mother's attempts to explain the difficulties she is having with her child, it is to be hoped that she will seek help elsewhere. Certainly in recent years parents have become more aware of the symptomatology of hyperactivity as a result of more articles in the mass media, and have shown increasing interest in early intervention with hyperactivity (Campbell, 1976; Cantwell, 1974; Drash, Stolberg, & Bostow, 1977; Routh, 1978). The two or three years available to the pediatrician before the child goes to school should enable him to markedly improve the probability that the child will be capable of entering school and handling the demands of peer relations and academic tasks. From the hyperactive child's point of view, this period is the optimum time to halt the onset of the downward spiral that so often characterizes his school years.

MIDDLE CHILDHOOD

The pattern of physiological and psychological irregularity of the preschool years continues into middle childhood, becoming more clearly delineated and consequently more readily identifiable as a clinical entity than is the case at any other developmental period. In fact the prototypical hyperactive child in the clinical literature is a middle childhood child. For descriptive purposes we will discuss the hyperactive child within the context of his major social environments of home, school, and neighborhood peer group, but it will be clear that much of the behavior described in one setting is characteristic of the child in the other settings.

Home

Although to an outsider it would seem that the child would be less of a problem now than he was in the preschool years because he spends substantially less time at home, to his parents he is now a serious problem, in part because they have begun to worry about his future. Behavior that could be dismissed as immature in the preschool years can no longer be ignored. Comparisons with same-age peers emphasize that he is lagging behind in important respects. The child himself now begins to feel anxious about his peer status and school performance; often he is depressed (Brumback & Weinberg, 1977; Salter, 1977). Just as in the previous age periods, he has a Jekyll and Hyde quality marked by sudden extreme fluctuations of behavior, performance, and mood. He has some days when, as one mother put it, "he acts like an ordinary child and we all enjoy a brief period of normal living," but these periods of good behavior only make it more difficult for his family to be tolerant of his bad days. The inconsistency itself acts as a stressor because of the high degree of uncertainty about how the child will behave in a specific situation. The pattern of physiological irregularity also continues in middle childhood. He is often a reluctant, light eater and a light sleeper. He does not fall asleep easily and he awakens early. His sleep patterns are qualitatively different from those of nonhyperactive children (Luisada, 1969) in that he is likely to spend less of his total sleep time dreaming, have fewer dreams per sleep period, and more frequently disrupt his dream periods by awakening.

The child is now an abrasive force in the household, a source of anxiety, and often a hazard. He may be extremely active, and his activity has a precipitate quality and an underlying clumsiness. This combination, plus his own anxiety about his capabilities, is almost certain to cause problems. His activity level and short attention span combine to make it difficult for him to remain seated throughout a meal or short television program. At the same time, he is disruptive, excitable, easily upset, notably lacking in self-control, and impulsive without stopping to evaluate all aspects of a situation (Campbell, Schleifer, Weiss, & Perlman, 1977). An unfortunate and familiar sequence is the impulsive, spur of the moment, well-intentioned decision to give unsolicited and unmonitored assistance → mishap, accident, or damage → parental or sibling exasperation and anger → bewilderment, misery, and often deep resentment on the child's part at the total disregard of his good motive. The following account by a 9-year-old boy provides a graphic illustration of such a sequence:

> Well, see, Linda and my mom were rushing round getting ready for Linda's party and my mom was being frantic like she always gets before parties. . . . And I thought I'd really surprise them and get the balloons blowed up, see, with this electric blowing thing my dad has. . . . So the first two blowed up *just super* and I thought Jumping Jody but Mom will get a surprise! Then these colored paper things got caught in the blower and before I could turn it off the whole colored paper thing came down from the ceiling and the tablecloth got caught too and some plates and things got broken. . . . Linda cried a lot and said I spoil everything and why did she have to have a brother like me.

Although there is extensive research on the hyperactive child himself, there has been relatively little interest in the analysis of his interactions with parents or other individuals of importance to him (Cunningham & Barkley, 1979). This lack of interest represents a serious omission in view of the powerful shaping effect that daily interactions with his parents and teachers can have on his behavior. Recently, however, both theoretical as well as research interests have focused on reports (Battle & Lacey, 1972) that hyperactivity in boys was associated with maternal coolness, disapproval, and criticism, over several developmental periods, but particularly in the middle childhood years. The speculation by Bettelheim (1973) that the foregoing maternal response style is a primary etiological factor in the child's hyperactivity was firmly rejected by Bell and Harper (1977), who contended that this cluster of maternal behavior was a response to the hyperactive child's pattern of behavior rather than a principal cause of it. A small group of empirical studies by three different teams of researchers working in temporal sequence on this issue illustrates the value of building up a body of research findings that lead to new studies built on existing data, and permit between-study comparisons. This body of research is notable for the consistency of results, despite differences in several important independent variables including comparison subjects, experimental tasks, instructions to mothers, and extent of use of stimulant medication. In the pioneer studies on this topic, Campbell (1973, 1975) compared the behavior of unmedicated hyperactive and nonhyperactive children, each paired with their mother, in structured problem-solving situations. Each child was presented with a series of tasks varying in difficulty, and the mother was instructed to give as much or as little help as she wished. On easy tasks there were no differences between the hyperactive and nonhyperactive group mothers. However, on difficult tasks the hyperactive group mothers provided more help, encouragement, structure, and suggestions about impulse control. Campbell attributed this controlling, structuring maternal response to the hyperactive child's pattern of behavior, but lacked empirical support for such an antecedent-consequent relationship between the child's and his mother's response set because the behavior of mother and child was coded independently of each other, although simultaneously, so that the coding yielded parallel sets of data rather than antecedent-consequent behavioral sequences.

Cunningham and Barkley (1979) built on the Campbell series by adding a drug and a placebo condition and an unstructured free-play activity, and by using a response class matrix coding method (Mash, Terdal, & Anderson, 1973) to describe antecedent-consequent sequences in mother-child interactions. With this method there was unequivocal confirmation of the antecedent-consequent relationship that Campbell et al. had hypothesized, with the child's off-task behavior being the antecedent, and the mother's behavior the consequent. Maternal intervention was optional across conditions and activities. Maternal management with unmedicated children was similar to the controlling, intrusive maternal management strategy reported by Campbell (1973, 1975) and Battle and Lacey (1972) in both free-play and task situations, although more apparent with the tasks. With the medicated children, a marked increase occurred in compliance, independent play, and prosocial behavior, with a decrease in activity level and dependency bids. The concomitant maternal responses were a marked decrease in directiveness and increase in positive reactions.

To eliminate the possibility that mothers in the Cunningham and Barkley (1979) study may have biased the results by their reluctance to intrude in the child's activity (since maternal intervention was optional), Humphries, Kinsbourne, and Swanson (1978) assigned equal responsibility to the mother and child for completion of the task, again under both drug and placebo conditions. The impressive drug-related changes in the children in the previous study were supported. However, both Humphries et al. and Cunningham and Barkley agreed that in terms of theoretical and treatment implications, the most important finding was the mothers' sensitivity to their children's (medication-based) control: the mothers immediately relinquished the directive role, and their subsequent behavior was appropriate for their children's improved behavior. This drug-related shift in maternal response style supports Bell and

Harper's (1977) position on the bidirectional influence of effect in mother–child interaction, and the role of the child in determining the quality of his social environment. These findings are basically optimistic: they suggest that noticeable improvement in the hyperactive child's behavior can elicit reciprocal positive changes in maternal behavior. The significance of these drug-related shifts in maternal response style is enhanced by a parallel in medication-related changes in teacher behaviors. In a series of studies by Whalen and her colleagues (e.g., Whalen, Henker, & Dotemoto, 1981) to be discussed later in this text, teachers were less intense and controlling with behaviorally improved medicated hyperactive boys than with those on placebo. Whalen et al. concluded that the effect of stimulant medication (methylphenidate) was to normalize both hyperactive children's classroom behaviors and teacher-student interchanges.

The foregoing research on mother-child interactions has been extended by Mash and Johnston (1981) to include sibling interactions. In this important extension of intrafamilial social interactions of hyperactive children, the subjects were 22 hyperactive boys and 22 nonhyperactive boys, ranging in age from four to nine, and their mothers and siblings. In the hyperactive- and nonhyperactive-sibling interactions the pairs were comparable across the two groups with respect to ordinal position, number of children in the family, number of siblings who were older than the target children, and sex of siblings. Observations were made in a laboratory-playroom situation of the following interactions: mother-target child, mother-sibling, target child-sibling, and target child-sibling with the mother present. With the mother–child dyads the interactions were partly social play and partly measures of child compliance to maternal requests (command situations); the target child-sibling interactions were a combination of social play and cooperative tasks; and in the triadic interactions the mother was present in a supervisory capacity. The results showed that the sibling interactions of the hyperactive children were characterized by a higher rate of social conflict than were the nonhyperactive-sibling dyads. The hyperactive-sibling dyads exhibited high rates of negative behavior during play, with less conflict during the mother-supervised situations. In the mother–child interactions the hyperactive boys and their siblings initiated less interaction and showed more independent play than the nonhyperactive boys and their siblings. One of the most interesting findings was that the mothers of the hyperactive boys were less responsive, interactive, and rewarding, and more negative, than mothers of the nonhyperactive children, and these characteristics applied to their interactions with the siblings as well as to the hyperactive children. Although this reaction could be due to the siblings of hyperactive children being more difficult and generally less attractive than those of the nonhyperactive boys, it is more likely that this finding is an instance of the spread of negative affect phenomenon in the hyperactive child's social environment that has often been reported by clinicians (e.g., Barkley, 1978; Cantwell, 1979), and suggested (Campbell, Endman, & Bernfeld, 1977) and, more recently, documented by researchers (Whalen et al.,

1981). This study represents a major contribution to our knowledge of the hyperactive child's interactions with his family, particularly his siblings. The results underscore the role of the hyperactive child in determining the quality of his social environment and suggest that remediation directed towards improved sibling-interaction skills in the early school years might be an essential prerequisite for subsequent satisfactory peer relationships.

School

The active, inquisitive, impulsive behavior of the hyperactive child is sometimes regarded by parents as evidence of a vigorous personality, but these characteristics become a handicap when the child is expected to conform to classroom constraints and routines. Hyperactive boys are more active than their classmates even when compared to teacher-nominated high active boys (Klein & Young, 1979; Whalen, Henker, Collins, Finck, & Dotemoto, 1979). The accompanying disruptive behavior, even at the preschool level (Buchan, Swap, & Swap, 1979), has led Klein and Young (1979) to speculate that it may be the combination of high activity level and high disruptive behavior that distinguishes hyperactivity from high normal activity in a teacher's mind. An extreme of either behavior might be tolerable in the classroom, but not the combination of the two extremes. The following account by a grade three teacher illustrates the effect of the hyperactive child's disruptive behavior on even the simple classroom routines:

> Things go smoothly enough when they are milling around first thing in the morning and getting settled. Ricky [the hyperactive child] may jostle the others a bit but nothing serious. It's as though the others' tolerance is high at that point. Then one group has oral reading while Ricky's group does seatwork. It takes him at least five minutes to settle in. He'll sharpen his pencil, look around, whistle under his breath, grunt, and still he doesn't get the others going. Then he starts clowning, giggling, shuffling his feet and some of the others start looking at him and, of course, he likes attention in any form. When he gets bigger he'll probably do things that get him police attention if he keeps on his present track. Then he goes a little further and the silly element in the class join in. I reprimand them but of course that focuses attention on Ricky. If I ignore him the whole situation gets worse quickly. If I isolate him he's impossible. I feel as if there's no right way of handling it. Once I reprimand him the whole situation escalates, the tension in the room increases, and even the best ones in the seatwork group get restless and I have to stop the reading. When Ricky is absent it's a completely different classroom.

This behavior contagion pattern has both theoretical and empirical support. In social learning theory terms (Bandura, 1969), the child exhibits attention-directing misbehavior that elicits relatively weak negative reinforcement from the teacher, which serves to focus attention upon the misbehavior rather than terminating it. Exposure to the misbehavior has a disinhibitory effect on a subgroup of observers for whom the competing task (seatwork) has little appeal, and they exhibit the same or similar misbehavior. There is increasing empirical support for the disruptive effects of the unmedicated hyperactive child on the classroom (Campbell, Endman, & Bernfeld, 1977; Cohen et al., 1981; Klein & Young, 1979; Whalen et al., 1979; Whalen et al., 1981; Whalen, Henker, & Finck, 1981). For example, Campbell et al., (1977) found that the presence of one hyperactive child seemed to have a negative influence on the ecology of a classroom. In a study comparing hyperactive boys on placebo with their nonhyperactive peers (Whalen et al., 1979), the hyperactive boys' repertoire of potentially disrupting behavior included high rates of gross motor movement, regular and negative verbalizations, noise making, physical contact with classmates, overtures to other children, energetic responding, and unexpected acts. Although this list is rather formidable, it should not be concluded that the children's behavior consisted solely of an unbroken string of inadequacies. The annoyance value of the activity level is heightened by a lack of efficiency which teachers frequently describe as being nonproductive. One teacher reported that even when the child was conforming in a waiting situation, such as standing in line or sitting at his desk, he would engage in a series of nonproductive acts including foot tapping, hitting the side of his lunch pail, and zipping and unzipping his jacket. In the same situation, his peers used cognitive mediators rather than physical mediating behaviors (which underscore the hyperactive child's immaturity) to fill an interval of waiting (Gordon, 1979).

The hyperactive child is unable to sustain attention for any length of time so that considerable teacher effort is required to keep him on task. When he is off task he is disruptive, engaged in disorganized behavior, negative-attention-getting, and the like. Because he does not handle reinforcement as well as his normal peers (Douglas, 1975; Parry & Douglas, 1976), teacher intervention of his disruptive behaviors may serve to prolong rather than halt them. Related to the problem of a short attention span is the child's deficit in selective attention: he has difficulty focusing on what is important. He may have a rapt look of attention, but in fact be listening to hallway or heating system noises. A curious attribute contributing to the child's attention problem is an inability to accurately estimate time (Cappella, Gentile, & Juliano, 1977); consequently many teacher comments or warnings of a time-related nature have little meaning for him.

Impulsivity is another characteristic leading to problems for the child on the playground and in the classroom. In free play he seldom stops to consider beforehand whether something is a good idea. He pushes into games, plays out of turn, and interrupts play. As a result, he has many more negative social interactions than do even his high-active peers. In the primary grades he is not behaviorally isolated and ignored by his peers (Klein & Young, 1979), but in the upper elementary grades his peers often actively dislike him and exclude him from their activities in the school setting (Riddle & Rapoport,

1976). Impulsivity is particularly costly for the child's image in the classroom. He makes many errors in both oral and written work because he does not stop to think, and may even start a task before being given the instructions. His impulsivity is irritating to his teacher because he does not seem to care about his mistakes; his hand is often the first to be raised in answer to a question, and the answer is almost always incorrect. Teachers are seldom tolerant of this behavior; the peer group picks up the teacher's attitude and tends to make fun of the child when he impulsively blurts out a clearly incorrect answer. Sometimes the hyperactive child welcomes even this negative attention, because it is the only peer attention that he gets, and then makes a game of giving wrong answers. Once the teacher sees this behavior as intentional she comes to resent the interruptions and misbehavior, an attitude that is soon transmitted to the other children, with the result that school becomes an increasingly intolerable experience for him.

The unpredictability that characterizes the child's behavior and academic performance also works to his disadvantage. A teacher who sees a child act like a disorganized tornado one minute and then suddenly switch to being obedient and industrious has a hard time believing that the child's behavior is out of his control. His grades often fluctuate from high to low, so that the teacher usually concludes that having done it once he could do it again if he tried. He does not do as well in school as his intelligence score would predict: In the elementary grades he is often underachieving in the core subjects of reading, spelling, and arithmetic, and when compared to peers of equal intelligence, he is behind in more subjects and in more grade levels within subjects (Cantwell & Satterfield, 1978; Minde, Lewin, Weiss, Lavigueur, Douglas, & Sykes, 1971; Salter, 1977).

The cumulative effect of the elementary school experience on the hyperactive child is to further demolish his tattered self-esteem and to subject him to a barrage of deficit-amplifying feedback (Wender, 1971), the result being an uninterrupted downward spiral of worsening performance.

Peer Group

Learning how to form and maintain peer friendship is one of the most difficult and important tasks of childhood. During the middle childhood stage of psychosocial development, peer acceptance becomes increasingly important because the peer group gradually assumes a major socializing role. It provides a child with an opportunity for learning how to develop self-control, interact effectively with same-age children, acquire appropriate social behavior skills, and develop age- and sex-appropriate skills and interests, all within the context of a group sharing similar feelings, concerns, and problems (Hartup, 1976). In the middle childhood years, satisfactory peer relationships have long been considered the best single index of adjustment (Cowen, Pederson, Babijian, Izzo, & Trost, 1973; Robins, 1966).

There is general agreement that the hyperactive child rates poorly on this aspect of general adjustment. Parent ratings or reports (Battle & Lacey, 1972; Conners, 1970; Patterson, Jones, Whittier, & Wright, 1965; Schleifer et al., 1975; Stewart, Pitts, Craig, & Dieruf, 1966) and structured interviews (Campbell & Paulauskas, 1979) consistently show that parents perceive hyperactive children as having more difficulty than nonhyperactive controls in initiating and maintaining close peer relationships. Teacher ratings vary somewhat on this issue, with some (Riddle & Rapoport, 1976) seeing the child's peer acceptance as relatively less of a problem for him, and others (Campbell & Paulauskas, 1979) rating it as more inadequate than did the parents. These parent-teacher differences are consistent with source-related differences (Langhorne, Loney, Paternite, & Bechtoldt, 1976). They also underscore the importance of distinguishing between peer ratings by a fixed group of same-age peers in the structured setting of a classroom, where inadequacies stand out, and peer acceptance in the neighborhood peer group with its unsupervised play, its own behavior code, and a wider age range that gives the hyperactive child the option of playing with younger children. Self-report (Campbell, Endman, & Bernfeld, 1977) and sociometric data (Mainville & Friedman, 1976) also agree with the low rating for peer relationships of hyperactive children. In the Mainville and Friedman study, for example, the correlation between peer rejection (classroom sociometric data) and hyperactivity (teacher ratings on the Conners Abbreviated Teacher Questionnaire) was .74 for boys.

We attribute the poor peer adjustment of the hyperactive child to two related conditions, namely, social and emotional immaturity, and incompetency in the prerequisites for positive peer interactions. The child typically exhibits a conglomerate of immature behaviors that are perceived by children of both sexes as undesirable. He engages in a considerable amount of negative-attention-getting behavior, such as showing off and clowning, that may have a temporary appeal for the less-accepted segment of the peer group (Battle & Lacey, 1972). He has outbursts of temper, and sometimes genuine temper tantrums, if his demands are not met immediately. The explosive responses and the pervasive unpredictability of his behavior have little appeal for the middle childhood peers, who at this stage are notable for their need of stability and predictability. Similarly, his misguided attempts to dominate his peers are rarely tolerated by this age group, and when rebuffed, he may use more anti-social ways to gain attention, such as deliberately bothering other children, name-calling, and teasing. As would be expected, such behavior is aversive to peers: Pelham (1980) has reported that hyperactive boys were firmly rejected by nonhyperactive peers within two hours of becoming acquainted. One complicating aspect of this whole problem is that the hyperactive child, like much younger children, is unable to understand the experiences and particularly the affect of other people (Paulauskas & Campbell, 1979), so his perception of the effects of his behavior on others is close to zero. His attention-seeking behaviors are often interpreted by adults however, as hostile, aggressive, and deliberately intended to provoke counteraggression. With the model of children's friendship proposed by Selman and Selman (1979), an alternate interpretation is that much of this aggressive behavior is the child's ill-conceived strategy for interacting with others, a way of initiating social interaction that developmentally is far behind the interaction norms of his same-age, same-sex peers.

A second condition, that of incompetency in the prerequisites for positive peer interactions, underlies the hyperactive child's peer problems. He is unable to play games properly and often disrupts them. His inability to play well is due in part to problems of a general nature, such as his clumsiness and his attention deficit, which causes him to lose interest in a game long before his peers do. Extended games of Monopoly, for example, would be out of the question on both counts. His incompetency may also distort his intentions: Often when he is genuinely trying to be friendly and helpful, the result is disastrous and the peer group, who tend to judge the outcome rather than the motive, react punitively. This response to good intentions is highly confusing to the child and contributes to his feelings of anger and resentment at the injustice of others' treatment of him. A cluster of specific behavioral difficulties that could jeopardize the outcome of any cooperative peer group activity has been identified in a recent major study (Whalen et al., 1979) of the interactions of hyperactive boys with their nonhyperactive peers. These interactions were assessed within the context of an ingenious and highly appealing dyadic referential communication game called "Space Flight." The hyperactive boys experienced marked difficulty in forming and maintaining an appropriate task set, settling in and learning the routines during the early stages of the task, and responding appropriately to changes in task demands when inhibition of ongoing or habitual behavior was required. Patterson et al. (1965) have hypothesized that the acquisition of essential peer interaction skills is precluded by high activity level. According to their intriguing explanation, activity level has a curvilinear relationship to the acquisition of social skills: children who are hyperactive as well as those who are hypoactive will be less socially skilled due to the lack of opportunity for the extended social interactions that children of moderate activity level enjoy.

The peer interaction problems of the hyperactive child are more than just a deficit, in that they constitute a potentially damaging psychological force, and as such must be considered actively harmful. Few children or adults are unmoved by peer rejection. Most judge their own worth in terms of others' assessments of them. Peer rejection often results in a self-defeating cycle of diminished self-esteem → inappropriate efforts to gain a place in the peer group → more peer derogation and rejection → further curtailment of normal social interaction → reduction of opportunities for developing acceptable patterns of behavior. One possible outcome of this cycle of negative interactions is the development of a conglomerate of secondary symptoms, such as poor self-esteem, defiance, and sadness. These secondary symptoms have considerable prognostic importance because, once established, they are often more difficult to correct than are the primary symptoms (Cantwell, 1979). Perhaps the most serious consequence of all is the possibility that the hyperactive child may acquire anxious avoidant responses to social situations that will prove difficult to extinguish and will make it exceedingly difficult to gain acceptance in adolescence (Cantwell, 1979).

Despite the critical importance of adequate peer relationships to socialization in the middle childhood years, little direct interest has been shown in the peer relationships of the hyperactive child. However, two recent developments suggest a reversal of this trend. One is the appearance of a cluster of papers on the hyperactive child's peer interaction difficulties; some of these studies have already been discussed, but new additions to this cluster center on hyperactive-nonhyperactive dyadic interactions (Cunningham, Siegel, & Offord, 1980; King & Young, 1982; Mash & Johnston, 1981) and peer interaction skill training (Pelham, 1980). The other noteworthy development is a critical and comprehensive review by Milich and Landau (1981) of research on general peer socialization, within a developmental framework, that succeeds in putting the cluster of studies on hyperactive children into perspective. Methodological issues related to the assessment of peer relations are subjected to critical scrutiny, patterns and consistencies in the existing literature are noted, and the resultant potentially productive directions for research are delineated in generous detail along with specific research strategies for their implementation. The Milich and Landau (1981) review provides the conceptual as well as the methodological framework prerequisite to unraveling the intricacies of the hyperactive child's peer interaction problems, and as such, constitutes a major contribution to the goal of understanding the hyperactive child.

ADOLESCENCE

Prior to 1970 clinical reports of a subjective nature presented a positive prognosis for the hyperactive child in adolescence (Bradley, 1957; Eisenberg, 1966; Laufer & Denhoff, 1957; Lytton & Knobel, 1958). Distinguishing symptoms, such as inappropriate activity, tended to diminish sharply (Routh, 1978; Weiss & Hechtman, 1979) so that the child was no longer a member of a clearly defined and conspicuous group, and his residual behavioral and emotional problems were not unlike those of his age group who were experiencing difficulties in adolescent adjustment (Milich & Loney, 1979a). Clinicians cited maturational lag as the primary causative factor and reassured parents that all would be well in adolescence (Chess, 1960; Eisenberg, 1966; Laufer & Denhoff, 1957). Occasional reports appeared that contradicted this optimistic view by stating that hyperactive children often did not outgrow their problems in adolescence (Anderson & Plymate, 1962; Laufer, 1962) and in fact sometimes developed serious psychiatric difficulties (Hartocollis, 1968; Quitkin & Klein, 1969), but these warnings had little impact on the established prognostic view and, in the absence of supporting empirical data, remained at the level of disregarded minority opinion. The lack of research on outcome in adolescence was consistent with the prevailing view of hyperactivity as a time-limited disorder, and this view was further strengthened by the often dramatic effects of stimulant medication, causing many clinicians to conclude that the cure was at hand.

Since 1970, interest in outcome in adolescence has increased sharply as the result of growing concern about the prevalence of hyperactivity (Milich & Loney, 1979a; Whalen & Henker, 1980b), emerging theoretical and empirical evidence of an association between hyperactivity in childhood and specific psychiatric disorders in adulthood (Cantwell, 1972; Morrison & Stewart, 1971, 1973b), and an urgent need for an empirical basis for making informed decisions about intervention prior to and during adolescence. Most sobering of all, however, has been the conclusion that neither stimulant medication nor any other form of intervention used to date has had any discernible long-term effect on hyperactivity (Loney, Kramer, & Milich, 1981; Weiss, Kruger, Danielson, & Elman, 1975). The result has been a surge of interest in the form of prospective follow-up studies, which have shown a remarkable consistency in results despite wide variations in type of subject, composition of control groups, assessment procedures, and methodological rigor. The most important studies in this category are the series initiated by Weiss at McGill University (Hechtman, Weiss, Finkelstein, Wener, & Benn, 1976; Hechtman, Weiss, & Perlman, 1980; Hoy, Weiss, Minde, & Cohen, 1978; Weiss, Kruger, Danielson, & Elman, 1975; Weiss, Minde, Werry, Douglas, & Nemeth, 1971; Weiss, Hechtman, & Perlman, 1978; Weiss, Hechtman, Perlman, Hopkins, & Wener, 1979) and Loney at the University of Iowa (Kramer & Loney, 1978; Langhorne & Loney, 1979; Loney, Kramer, & Milich, 1981; Loney, Langhorne, & Paternite, 1978; Loney, Langhorne, Paternite, Whaley-Klahn, Blair-Broeker, & Hacker, 1976; Loney, Prinz, Mishalow, & Joad, 1978; Paternite & Loney, 1980; Paternite, Loney, & Langhorne, 1976). In both series the subjects were children who had originally been diagnosed in the university clinics of the investigators, with overlapping samples in the McGill studies and children from the same data pool in the Iowa studies. Both series are notable for their methodological rigor, data sources tapped, and significance of findings. The important difference between them lies in their primary focus of interest, with the McGill series centering upon the *natural history* of hyperactivity from early childhood through young adulthood, and the Iowa team concentrating on identifying potential *predictors of outcome* in adolescence. In pursuit of these topics both series have made substantive contributions to each other's area of interest. For example, an ongoing study by Loney and her team (personal communication, 1981), which is almost certain to contribute substantially to the knowledge about the natural history of hyperactivity already gained from the Weiss series, involves following 200 medicated and 100 nonmedicated hyperactive boys from referral (at six to 12 years) to young adulthood. Classmates and nonhyperactive full brothers will provide comparison data for addressing various questions about prognosis and treatment. The Iowa search for variables from the referral and early treatment periods predictive of outcome in adolescence will be described in detail in Chapter 5. Our discussion here concerns the natural history and clinical description of the hyperactive adolescent.

Other studies in the category of natural history include those of the teams of Dykman (Dykman, Peters, & Ackerman, 1973; Dykman & Ackerman, 1975; Ackerman, Dykman, & Peters, 1977), Huessy (Huessy, Metoyer, & Townsend, 1974), Sassone, Lambert, and Sandoval (1981), and Stewart (Mendelson, Johnson, & Stewart, 1971; Stewart, Mendelson, & Johnson, 1973), as well as those of individual investigators (Denhoff, 1973; Milman, 1979). With the exception of the Dykman series and the Sassone et al. study, these studies are characterized by major methodological shortcomings, such as a lack of concern for exclusionary criteria resulting in more loosely defined and heterogeneous groups, and failure to use control groups. The study by Sassone et al. was a model of methodological rigor. The procedure used for the selection of subjects was specifically designed to avoid selecting a sample based on etiological preconceptions (as would be the case if only hyperactives who were stimulant drug responders were selected), and to provide a generalizable procedure. The criteria for subject selection were identification of the child as hyperactive by three defining systems (home, school, and physician), measures of the child's home and school behavioral characteristics, and any hyperactive symptoms of long standing. The controls were randomly selected from representative school classrooms in the same area. With respect to the possibility of apparently spontaneous remission of hyperactivity in adolescence (Eisenberg, 1966), Sassome et al. reported that 20 percent of the 59 hyperactive boys in their study were no longer considered to be hyperactive or to have learning, behavioral, or emotional problems by the time they reached their teenage years; 37 percent were no longer hyperactive, but their parents did report learning, behavioral, or emotional difficulties; and 43 percent were still hyperactive and had persistent learning, behavioral, or emotional difficulties.

The composite picture of the hyperactive adolescent that emerges from the follow-up studies is not an encouraging one. Adolescence is not the symptom-free period it was believed to be by clinicians of the 1960s, and equating the reduction of activity level and other primary symptoms to a positive prognosis has proven to be a gross oversimplification of the problem. The primary symptoms do diminish in intensity but continue to be troublesome enough to differentiate between hyperactive and nonhyperactive adolescents (Ackerman et al., 1977; Loney, 1980a; Weiss et al., 1971). In addition, two other sets of problems confront many hyperactive adolescents: One is the cluster of hyperactivity-related secondary problems, such as poor self-esteem, aggressiveness, academic difficulties, and peer interaction difficulties that are generally attributed to the interaction in the childhood years between the primary symptoms of hyperactivity and the social environment, although as Milich and Loney (1979a) have noted, there is no empirical evidence for this concept of resultant symptomatology; the other set includes the developmental tasks that beset adolescents in our culture and that may or may not become problems, for example, concern about one's identity and future, physiological changes, peer acceptance, and heterosexual adjustment. We view adolescence as a period of storm, stress, turmoil, restlessness, and rebellion for only a minority of adolescents. Taken as a whole, adolescents manage these years well (Nicholi, 1978). These developmental tasks can accurately be labeled as problems only when an adolescent is ill-equipped to handle them, as is the case for the typical hyperactive adolescent whose social interaction, academic, and emotional deficits and antisocial tendencies are almost certain to impede effective coping with the developmental tasks of this age period.

Social Interaction Problems

The best single descriptor for the social adjustment of the hyperactive adolescent is _lonely_. He generally has few if any close same-age friends and spends much of his spare time either alone or with younger children (Battle & Lacey, 1972; Hoy et al., 1978; Minde, Weiss, & Mendelson, 1972; Weiss et al., 1971), whereas the most common activities of nonclinical adolescent boys are of a social nature, such as peer conversational and recreational interactions (Csikszentmihalyi, Larson, & Prescott, 1977). The only report negating this picture of psychological isolation comes from an uncontrolled interview study by Stewart et al. (1973), in which hyperactive adolescents' accounts of popularity with their peers were refuted by the respondents' mothers. Stewart et al. attributed the discrepancies to the enormous importance of peer acceptance in adolescence as well as to the possibility that the whole topic of peer acceptance was too sensitive for the respondents to face objectively.

Several alternative explanations have been offered for the peer interaction problems of the hyperactive adolescent, all centering on a deficit in social interaction skills. Battle and Lacey (1972) and Patterson et al. (1965) view his aberrant behavior as impediments to opportunities for acquiring competency in peer interaction, whereas Hoy et al. (1978, p. 323) believe that his well-documented attentional and stimulus-processing deficits are at the root of the problem:

> .... successful social interaction requires both the simultaneous monitoring of several informational sources (e.g., contextual, partner, and self-produced stimulus sources) and the in-depth processing of relevant stimuli, followed by the selection and emission of an appropriate social strategy.... Failure, for example, to monitor continually the effect of one's behavior on others or to process in depth existing social rules and implicit conventions, would produce immature and aberrant social behaviors. Such behaviors would be objectionable to peers (but perhaps less so to younger children) and would lead, for example, to more frequent police contacts and school detentions as well as possibly to a recognition of the unsuccessfulness of one's strategies (i.e., to low self-esteem).

It is our opinion that an important contributor to the peer interaction problem is the hyperactive adolescent's lack of competency in any of the major areas valued by the peer group, for example, academic skill, athletic prowess, or heterosexual social success. For most of these adolescents, the high school years can be conceptualized as an almost classic example of poorness of fit (Chess, 1979) between the adolescent with conspicuous deficits on the one hand, and relatively immutable school demands, family expectations, and requirements for peer acceptance on the other; and with no prospect of reconciliation or intervention that might at least partially narrow the gap. The core of the problem, as well as one approach to a solution, is contained in the competence-deviance hypothesis (Gold, 1968), which states that the more deviant an individual is in some areas, the more competent he must be in others if he is to gain the acceptance of the group. It follows that if the hyperactive adolescent could develop some skill or attribute valued by the peer group, the probability of a degree of acceptance by them would be increased. There is no empirical support for this hypothesis, but we have seen occasional instances in which a modicum of success was followed by increased acceptance.

It is obvious from the follow-up studies that the peer interaction and acceptance problem, *whose precursors were often identifiable at the preschool level*, persists, intensifies, and becomes increasingly complex and difficult to modify when it is carried over from one developmental stage to the next. It is for this reason that we stressed the preschool period as the optimum point for intervention by the pediatrician.

Academic Performance Problems

The academic difficulties experienced by most hyperactive children in the elementary grades result in serious scholastic problems for the hyperactive adolescent despite his adequate or more than adequate intellect. By the junior high school level hyperactive adolescents can be differentiated from their nonhyperactive peers on most aspects of academic performance including number of grades repeated and special class placement. Typically they score two or more years below grade level in the basic subjects (Loney et al., 1981; Minde et al., 1971) and in achievement test scores (Ackerman et al., 1977; Sassone et al., 1981). A particularly discouraging finding in the Weiss series was that the hyperactive group exhibited the same pattern of cognitive difficulties that they had at earlier periods (e.g., Cohen, Weiss, & Minde, 1972), which suggests a pervasive deficit that would put the child at a serious disadvantage on most academic tasks. These various findings underscore the conclusion of Weiss et al. (1971) that only 20 percent of their hyperactive adolescents had made a satisfactory academic adjustment, and add validity to self-reports of hyperactive adolescent boys indicating poor opinions of their academic performance and ability (Battle & Lacey, 1972; Mendelson et al., 1971). This pattern of school performance has led some educators to conclude, we think erroneously, that hyperactive adolescents are probably more disabled academically than any other way. It is our opinion that the social difficulties of the hyperactive adolescent far outweigh his academic problems in terms of present misery and future difficulties. They are potentially far more serious because social inadequacy extends into areas beyond school, whereas poor grades, with astute choice of work setting, can be left behind.

Emotional Adjustment

Adolescence is frequently a very unhappy period for the hyperactive child, perhaps the unhappiest period of his life. He is beset by major problems, and often feels that he has no one to turn to. Immediate prospects are grim, with no reason for optimism about the future. After his history of failure on most fronts, he is singularly lacking in ambition and confidence (Battle & Lacey, 1972; Weiss et al., 1971), and his isolation from the peer group deprives him of a source of support that by rights should be his in the adolescent years. It is not surprising that he is usually depicted in the literature as being sad and depressed, having poor self-esteem, and sometimes considering and occasionally committing suicide (Cantwell, 1979; Mendelson et al., 1971; Sassone et al., 1981; Stewart et al., 1973). Although there is no firm evidence of increased prevalence of severe psychiatric disorders among hyperactive adolescents (Milich & Loney, 1979a), there is a substantial empirical and clinical base for viewing them as highly vulnerable in this regard. The following verbatim response by a 15-year-old boy to the question, How are things in your life right now? exemplifies the feeling of aloneness and the total absence of social support systems that many hyperactive adolescents experience:

> *What* life? I don't have no life, no friends, not even a girl friend. Most kids at school don't hardly know my name . . . when they pick up teams I'm always last one to get picked and they say like, "uh–you." . . . My family wishes I'd get out, I heard my Dad talking to my Mom about jobs I could get and *every one of them* was way out of town, like far off some place. . . . I hate school but I can't leave yet, I'm not ready. . . . Sometimes I call in to this talk-show guy on the radio, you know? Like you can tell him your problems or anything. And he says to me, "Hey, Benny, hey, man, this bad spell is just a *stage*, man. This time next year it'll all be over." . . . Well, this isn't no *stage*, this is my whole life so far, but I *surely* do like it when he says that.

Antisocial Behavior Problems

The difficulties in conforming to the social demands of home and school in middle childhood continue to be a problem in adolescence and sometimes assume more serious forms. The findings in general are suggestive of more antisocial behavior in hyperactive adolescents than in their nonhyperactive peers, but given the methodological weaknesses in many of the studies, it is impossible to state unconditionally that such a difference does exist. One problem is the failure to use control groups, as is the case in the Mendelson et al. (1971) study; another is the lack of exclusionary criteria, which weakens the data of Mendelson et al. (1971) and Huessy et al., (1974) by increasing the possibility of erroneously including nonhyperactive subjects in the hyperactive group. Schuckit, Petrich, and Chiles (1978) have cautioned that difficult-to-handle children may be treated for hyperactivity in childhood, because there is a high degree of similarity in the early clinical pictures of hyperactive adolescents and those with antisocial personalities. When less than rigorous criteria are used in subject selection, adolescents with antisocial personalities who have been previously mislabeled as hyperactive could be included in follow-up studies of hyperactivity. The effect would be to attribute a spuriously high incidence of antisocial behavior and legal encounters to the hyperactive adolescent. A third problem is the failure to provide sufficient information about significant outcome-related variables, such as socioeconomic status and type of parenting (Milich & Loney, 1979a) and to adequately define key terms such as "trouble with the law" or "legal encounters."

Several methodologically sound follow-up studies attest to the fact that a substantial number of hyperactive adolescents engage in antisocial behaviors, such as arson, carrying illegal weapons, and threatening members of their families, that result in juvenile court referrals and other police contacts (Laufer, 1971; Milich & Loney, 1979a; Weiss et al., 1971). Ackerman et al. (1977) reported that over one-third of the hyperactive 14-year-olds in their follow-up study had had recent trouble with school authorities or had at one time been in serious trouble with the police, whereas only 3 to 4 percent of the normoactive and control groups had a record of socially deviant behavior. Similarly, in the study by Sassone et al. (1981), 20 percent of the 59 hyperactive boys had had trouble with law enforcement agencies as opposed to 4 percent of the control boys; 28 percent of the hyperactives had been suspended from school at least once, as compared to 14 percent of the controls; and 10 percent of the hyperactives, but none of the controls, had been committed to a juvenile facility or were on probation. In addition, two of the hyperactives had tried to commit suicide, one had attempted murder, five had repeatedly attempted burglary, and two were in psychiatric institutions. Other studies present a somewhat more optimistic picture. Comparisons by Blouin et al. (1978) and Hechtman, Weiss, Finklestein, Wener, and Benn (1976) of hyperactive and nonhyperactive adolescents similar in academic difficulties showed that the two groups did not differ in reported police contacts, although the latter study found that the offenses committed by the hyperactive group were against others, for example, theft and familial violence, whereas the nonhyperactive controls engaged in victimless crimes such as the use of illicit drugs. Loney et al. (1981) also concluded that hyperactive children are no more likely than their peers to become juvenile delinquents or to be involved with alcohol or illegal drugs.

Since these studies do not support the widely held belief (Milich & Loney, 1979a) that the hyperactive adolescent exhibits more antisocial behavior than his normal peers, it is possible that this belief has been fostered by the cumulative effects of a bad reputation stemming from years of misbehavior and other difficulties in the school setting. Or, as the Hechtman et al. study (1976) would suggest, it could be because the antisocial acts that the hyperactive adolescent does commit tend to be more conspicuous or attention directing than those of his nonhyperactive peers. Whatever the reason, it is during adolescence that antisocial behavior for the first time becomes a major problem leading to police contact and court referral in a significant number of the hyperactive group.

ADULTHOOD

General acknowledgment of the persistence of hyperactivity into adolescence has led logically to clinical and research interest in outcome in adulthood. Evidence for the existence of this disorder at the adult level comes from a diverse group of publications, including a report of the first major conference on hyperactivity in adulthood (Bellak, 1979), prospective follow-up studies (Beck, 1976; Hechtman et al., 1976; Hechtman, Weiss, & Perlman, 1980; Milman, 1979; Weiss et al., 1978; Weiss et al., 1979), retrospective follow-up studies (Borland & Heckman, 1976; Shelley & Reister, 1972), de novo diagnoses of hyperactivity in adulthood (Gross & Wilson, 1974; Wood, Reimherr, Wender, & Johnson, 1976), case histories of young adults who were diagnosed as hyperactive in childhood (Morrison & Minkoff, 1975; Packer, 1978), and skilled clinicians (Arnold, 1979; Borland, 1979; Hartocollis, 1979; Huessy, 1978; Mann & Greenspan, 1976; Morrison, 1979, 1980b; Wender, 1978). The behavioral picture of the hyperactive adult that emerges from these clinical and research data is remarkably similar to that of the hyperactive adolescent, although the symptoms may change in relative importance, form, mode of expression, and intensity. Restlessness, attentional difficulties, impulsivity, affect lability, temper outbursts, poor self-esteem, and a deficit in social interaction skills continue to be significant problems. The hyperactive adults in the foregoing reports fall primarily into a category that Cole (1980) has designated *simple adult minimal brain dysfunction.* Our description of hyperactivity in adulthood will be limited to this group. For an interesting discussion of hyperactivity in schizophrenia and other psychiatric states in adulthood, see Cole (1980).

For the most part, interest in the question of adult hyperactivity has been tempered by commendable restraint in the form of concern for empirical documentation. Note, for example, Wender's conclusion following careful evaluations of empirical findings, that tentative support for the validity of adult hyperactivity did exist, but that the hypothesis of adult hyperactivity should be viewed "not as one of ultimate or absolute truth but as a working model" (Wender, 1979, p. 12). His statement documenting the series of events leading to this conclusion (Wender, 1979, p. 9) is relevant here:

> ... it followed from clinical observation. In talking to the parents of MBD children, I routinely inquire which parent was temperamentally most like the proband when he or she had been a child. A frequent maternal response was, "What do you mean, 'was'? His mother says he was just like that as a boy and he still is that way. He still never finishes anything he starts, fidgets all the time, gets upset easily, does dumb things without thinking, and won't listen." ...
>
> Clinically, I had to take notice when several parents of MBD children told me they had taken diet pills, "speed," or their children's medicine and reported that it calmed them down even though they expected it to pep them up. That was an acute treatment response and could not be disregarded; however, a few parents told me they had taken diet pills or amphetamine (Dexedrine) for years—ostensibly for weight control—and had for only that period in their life been able to control distressing psychological symptoms.
>
> The final input came when I began to consult at the community mental health clinics, where I found that there were a fair number of outpatients who had no clear syndromal status but who presented with many signs and symptoms that would be considered diagnostic of hyperactivity if they were younger. Dr. Johnson, Dr. Reinherr, Dr. Wood, and I decided to take the syndrome by the horns, constructed some rating scales ... and conducted a double-blind crossover study of the effects of methylphenidate on this population. Many of them got better.*

Of particular interest here, because the diagnosis of childhood hyperactivity was not dependent on retrospective accounts, is Packer's case description (1978, p. 501) of a young hyperactive man:

> There were no known complications while his mother was pregnant with him, but labour was prolonged. Milestones were reached at an appropriate or an early age. During his school years he had experienced no problems with reading or mathematics, but there were possibly some coordination problems present since he felt himself to be awkward during childhood and adolescence. He stated that during these years he "drove everybody nuts," not being able to sit still when at home or school. Also described were incidents in which he would begin to "joke around" with friends, and these situations would escalate until he would become very active, and often ended in his having an angry outburst. It was this hyperactivity and labile affect that led to his parents consulting a child psychiatrist when he was twelve years old. A diagnosis of minimal brain dysfunction was made and stimulant therapy was prescribed; however, for unknown reasons the

*Reprinted, by permission, from Wender, P. H. The concept of adult minimal brain dysfunction. In L. Bellak (Ed.), *Psychiatric aspects of minimal brain dysfunction in adults.* New York: Grune & Stratton, 1979.

patient never returned for follow-up visits. Because it seemed that the patient's present complaints might be a persistence of symptoms of MBD, a trial treatment with methylphenidate was initiated, beginning with 10 mg per day and increasing in one week to 25 mg per day. On this latter dosage there occurred a marked diminution of his irritability, a decrease in his moodiness and restlessness, and an increase in his ability to study for longer periods of time. Over the succeeding four months the improvement was maintained on the same dosage of methylphenidate, which was being taken approximately every other day.*

Similar results from treatment of adults with stimulant medication were obtained by Wood, Reimherr, Wender, and Johnson (1976). They offered the interesting suggestion that the cluster of hyperactive behaviors observed in adults could be either symptoms *or* habits, that is, that adolescent hyperactivity persists into adulthood, or that it is outgrown in adulthood but behaviors such as restlessness and low self-esteem are learned responses that have become habitual. The adults treated with stimulant medication responded positively to it, thus providing support for the validity of adult hyperactivity.

Despite the fact that hyperactive adults typically undergo treatment of their own volition and generally experience marked symptomatic relief, they tend to be difficult patients and are often noncompliant or actively resistant to the treatment regimen. This unexpected reaction in the face of apparently successful treatment serves to underline the importance of an holistic approach to the patient's problems. The elimination of one set of symptoms often reveals another set whose presence now begins to be felt. Gallant (1979, p. 187) has complained that "some of my patients will only take it when they feel like it. When they feel like they want to explode and enjoy it, they'll stop their medication." Mann and Greenspan (1976) note that one effect of symptomatic relief, particularly of the increased ability to focus attention, is depression as the patient looks objectively at himself and becomes more aware of his feelings and his life situation. Many adults elect to omit or discontinue drug therapy in order to avoid these painful confrontations—an option that is not open to children in similar circumstances. In discussing this phenomenon, Preis and Huessy (1979, p. 170) noted that the usual drug abuser uses stimulants to try to "tune out," but with hyperactive adults stimulants cause them to "tune in":

> . . . a crucial dimension in hyperactivity . . . has to do with the individual's relationship to time . . . (hyperactive) adults live in the moment. It seems that with the medication working on "tuning in," it prevents the individuals from being able to live in the moment. We conclude that if one has not grown up with an internal tolerance for stress and frustration, when the medicine suddenly gives one this privilege, it is not particularly attractive.

*Packer, S. Treatment of minimal brain dysfunction in a young adult. *Canadian Psychiatric Association Journal*, 1978, *23*, 501–502. Reprinted by permission from the *Canadian Psychiatric Association Journal, Vol. 23: 501–2, 1978.*

An interesting point in the above reasoning is the implication that hyperactive adults tend to have a different relationship to time than do nonhyperactive adults. This problem may well have its roots at least as far back as middle childhood, where, as Cappella, Gentile, and Juliano (1977) have noted, a factor contributing to the child's attention problem is an inability to accurately estimate time so that he fails to grasp the significance of warnings of a time-related nature.

Although many hyperactive adults are resistant to treatment, others report great difficulty in finding practitioners who will consider hyperactivity seriously as a diagnosis. Such reluctance has been attributed to unwillingness to accept a new concept (Bellak, 1979) and to failure to notice the symptoms because they are scattered through the clinical picture and do not present as a cohesive problem, or, if noticed, are not interpreted as evidence of hyperactivity (Hartocollis, 1979). The following is an example of failure to diagnose hyperactivity in adulthood:

> A 20-year-old student who was enrolled in an art school reported that she believed that she had symptoms suggestive of hyperactivity but was unable to find a doctor who would take her seriously. She described herself in childhood as "always bouncing round, couldn't sit still for 15 minutes in school, often got into trouble because I never stopped to think, always lost the place in seatwork because I couldn't help looking round, and had terrible temper tantrums until age ten." She reported that these difficulties were accepted as temperament by her teachers in the convent she attended throughout her school career. These teachers made commendable efforts to accommodate her restlessness without stigmatizing her; for example, she was often sent on errands and could leave the room of her own volition if she felt unable to cope with sitting still. Other girls accepted her and, although her family were exasperated at times by her behavior, they viewed her as "God's wishes for them."
>
> As soon as she entered art school she was in trouble. Her restlessness and impulsivity were annoying, and she was ignored by some of her fellow students, ostracized by others, and finally advised by her teachers to leave. At this point, through reading, she was exposed for the first time to the concept of hyperactivity and, believing that stimulant medication might help her to cope with the school demands, she sought medical help. After seeing three doctors, all of whom discounted the possibility that she might be hyperactive, she contacted a psychologist who referred her to a psychiatrist. He diagnosed her almost immediately as hyperactive, prescribed stimulant medication, and enrolled her in a group of young adults who had experienced peer problems. Her problem behavior improved dramatically, and at the beginning of the next semester she reenrolled in the art program, and subsequently made excellent progress and exhibited good social adjustment.

Reports of outcome of hyperactivity in adulthood range from moderate optimism to deep pessimism. The prospective series by Weiss et al. (Hechtman et al., 1980; Weiss et al., 1978; Weiss et al., 1979) report a generally favorable outcome, with the qualifier that the young adults are still experiencing social and emotional difficulties but not to the extent that they did in adolescence. The hyperactive adults in Weiss et al. were rated by teachers as markedly inferior to the nonhyperactive controls, but differed only slightly from them in level of education attained, and not at all in employer ratings of job status, satisfaction, and performance (Weiss et al., 1978). Although the two groups did not differ in amount of antisocial behavior, nonmedical use of drugs, or serious psychiatric disturbances, restlessness and impulsivity continued to be a problem for the hyperactive group, with geographical moves, car accidents, and early deaths having a higher incidence. The fact that the behavioral problems characteristic of hyperactivity do not affect the major facets of the hyperactive adult's life to the extent that they did in adolescence may be partly due to a lessening of some of these symptoms with maturity (Wood et al., 1976), as well as to the fact that he rarely is at odds with his work setting to the extent that he was with his academic environment during adolescence. In noting this improvement, Weiss (1975, p. 224) commented:

> It is our impression . . . that the previously hyperactive young adults have adjusted surprisingly well once they have left those environmental circumstances with which they could not cope (for most this included secondary school, and for some it included rejecting homes). It seems that young adult life offers a wider range of life-styles, including varieties of continuing education . . . large choice of jobs, and so on.

Few of the hyperactive subjects were married, and Weiss has expressed her intention of following the two groups into an older age period in order to assess their ability as husbands and fathers (only a few are female), their final work adjustment, and the presence or absence of psychosis or criminal behavior. Weiss et al. concluded that in young adulthood the adjustment of the previously hyperactive child is considerably closer to the normal in early adulthood than it was in the elementary and secondary school years.

The ability of the hyperactive adult to find a job environment that is harmonious with his particular needs determines to a considerable extent his overall social adjustment. Consider, for example, the following case description of a young hyperactive man who had finished high school with the worst possible references from his teachers, but was able to make an astute judgment concerning the kind of job he could handle:

> One of the authors wished to obtain several dozen assorted tiles, a tedious and time-consuming order to fill because it involved opening a large number of crates. When she offered to pick up the order in ten days, the manager assured her that it could be filled immediately and invited her to come to the warehouse to watch a new employee, a recent high school graduate, who was "exploding with energy all the time." The manager then gave the order to a young man who literally trotted off, sped up and down ladders with great agility, and filled the order accurately in less than 15 minutes. The manager commented on his puzzle-

ment about the refusal of the local high school to give the employee a good reference and recommendation because, in the manager's opinion, he was an unusually hard worker, who was dependable and courteous and got on well with the warehouse crew. That he rarely sat down, jigged about while others stood still, and jogged in the noon hour "after being cooped up all morning" was interpreted by the manager as evidence of energy. In fact, the author subsequently found out by accident that this young man had been in classes for the hyperactive throughout most of his school years and that high school had been an exceedingly difficult experience for him, socially, academically, and emotionally.

Three years later he was in charge of the warehouse and was considered to be highly efficient; he was happily married, was attending night school courses, and gave every indication of being a well-adjusted adult.

Two studies of previously undiagnosed hyperactive adults provide further information in support of a favorable prognosis. Although the use of retrospective diagnosis has its limitations, the quality of early data available in these studies, coupled with the methodological rigor of the subsequent assessment, justifies their inclusion here. Borland and Heckman (1976) compared men who had been referred to a guidance clinic 20 to 25 years previously, and who appeared to conform to the diagnostic criteria of hyperactivity, with their nonhyperactive brothers. Most of the hyperactive men were married with children, and many had spent time in military service. Although their level of education did not differ from that of their brothers, they had entered the work force at a lower level and had lower socioeconomic status. All were steadily employed and self-supporting. They worked more hours per week, partly out of genuine interest and as an antidote to restlessness, and changed jobs more often. Nearly half had problems of a psychiatric nature, but Borland and Heckman did not consider either their social or psychiatric problems to be serious ones. They had experienced more difficulties than their brothers in military service, the work setting, their marital situations, and formal as well as informal social affiliations. Problems in these areas were generally associated with the persistence of major symptoms of hyperactivity. Those with fewer than three symptoms did not differ significantly from their brothers in either social or vocational adaptation.

The second of these studies (Shelley & Riester, 1972) represents the most optimistic report of hyperactivity in adulthood. The subjects were 16 cases (M = 14, F = 2) of previously undiagnosed minimal brain damage located as a result of psychiatric referral for difficulty in coping with the basic tasks of military training at an Air Force base. A careful evaluation included psychological testing with the Wechsler Adult Intelligence Scale (WAIS), Bender-Gestalt, and Rorschach; a psychiatric evaluation; a neurological evaluation including an EEG; and a Child Development Questionnaire completed by the subjects' parents. Some of their test results were consistent with a minimal brain damage diagnosis. Both the psychiatric examination and the parents' responses to the questionnaire were consistent with a retrospective diagnosis of hyperactivity in childhood. Most of the group had had problems in school, but all had been able to complete high school and some had finished college prior to enlisting. The results of the evaluation of these 16 young adults suggested that their hyperactivity was of a relatively mild type; that the problem was handled well in childhood by their families, who combined helpfulness with the children's motoric problems with firm demands for achievement; and that the subjects themselves were reasonably intelligent, motivated to do well, and astute at avoiding areas in which they performed badly. Apparently this combination of attitudes and behaviors carried them along until they entered the Air Force and were thrust into a situation that demanded precise and effective visual-motor skills, one of this group's weakest performance areas.

A more pessimistic outcome is supported by a diverse group of studies linking retrospectively reported hyperactivity to adult psychopathology in the form of alcoholism, antisocial behavior, and hysteria. Evidence that psychiatric disorders in adulthood may be preceded by childhood hyperactivity comes from clinicians' reports (Bellak, 1979; Greenspan, 1979; Hartocollis, 1979; Morrison, 1979; Morrison & Minkoff, 1975; Quitkin & Klein, 1969; Schuckit et al. 1978), as well as from two family studies (Cantwell, 1972; Morrison & Stewart, 1971) that report a higher frequency of psychiatric disorders, especially alcoholism, in first and second degree relatives of hyperactive children than in control adults, and more reported childhood hyperactivity in the former group. It is unfortunate that these studies have two avoidable methodological weaknesses, which have been noted by Stewart (1980). Neither study used blind interviews, and neither included a control group of children with psychiatric problems rather than pediatric ones. The data fail to establish unequivocally a link between adult psychiatric disorders and childhood hyperactivity. Psychiatric disorders are common in the parents of children attending psychiatric clinics, and alcoholism is one of the more common psychiatric disorders in men. It follows (Stewart, 1980) that the association could be between adult psychopathology and child psychiatric problems in general, rather than specifically with hyperactivity. However, support for a link between adult alcoholism and childhood hyperactivity does come from data (Goodwin, Schulsinger, Hermansen, Guze, & Winokur, 1975) that alcoholic adoptees were more often reported to have been hyperactive than nonalcoholic adoptees, and that alcoholics with severe symptoms and early onset were more likely to have had symptoms of childhood hyperactivity than alcoholics with milder symptoms and late onset (Tarter, McBride, Buonpane, & Schneider, 1977).

Further evidence that childhood hyperactivity may be a precursor of adult psychiatric disorder comes from a follow-up study (Huessy, Metoyer, & Townsend, 1974) on a group of 84 hyperactive children who had been placed on medication 8 to 10 years previously. Of the total group, 10 had required hospitalization in late adolescence or early adulthood for psychiatric treatment, and 18 had been institutionalized, a rate that was 20 times the expected rate. Other data supportive of this view include three case reports (Morrison

& Minkoff, 1975) that suggest that an explosive personality in adulthood may be one of the sequelae of hyperactivity in childhood. In pursuing this line of thought further, Morrison (1979) found that comparisons between adult psychiatric patients who had reportedly been hyperactive in childhood, with carefully matched patients having no history of hyperactivity, showed significantly more personality disorder problems, sociopathy, and alcoholism in the former group. He also reported (1980b) that hyperactive children are at greater risk than their nonhyperactive peers for psychiatric disorder, a not surprising finding in view of the stressful and difficult time that most hyperactive children have. Support for a strong association between childhood hyperactivity and significant antisocial behavior in adulthood is contained in a careful review (Cantwell, 1978b) of retrospective and follow-up studies of hyperactive children, studies of the childhood histories of adults with antisocial disorders, and treatment studies linking these two behavior disorders; but the mechanism mediating this association is as yet unidentified.

In an intriguing theoretical statement on disinhibitory psychopathology, Gorenstein and Newman (1980) have proposed that several traditionally separate psychological categories—psychopathy, alcoholism, hyperactivity, hysteria, impulsive personality, and antisocial behavior—are in fact separate manifestations of the same genetic diathesis. The task for researchers is to identify the common diathesis as well as the different experiential factors that produce these separate manifestations. Another possibility for the specific link between hyperactivity and antisocial behavior is suggested by the finding (Loney, 1980b; Loney, Langhorne, Paternite, Whaley-Klahn, Broeker, & Hacker, in press) that childhood aggression is a more powerful predictor of outcome in adolescence than are the primary symptoms of hyperactivity. The reasoning here is that childhood aggression may serve as a powerful mediator of antisocial behavior and other negative outcomes in adulthood. This possibility has suggested several interesting lines of investigation to Stewart (1980) about the role of the primary symptoms of hyperactivity in adult outcome. For example, if childhood aggression serves a major mediating role in adult psychopathology, does this association rest on aggression in combination with hyperactivity, that is, is hyperactivity an essential factor in the association? Also, what adult psychopathology, not associated with a major aggression component, is related to childhood hyperactivity?

Despite methodological shortcomings, the foregoing body of research, clinical reports, and theoretical statements does suggest that with the intervention tools available, substantial numbers of hyperactive children are likely to have serious psychiatric problems in adulthood. There are large pockets of ignorance in the existing body of work. It is not known, for example, if the presence of adult psychopathology in some and its absence in others represents different outcomes of the same disorder, or if adults with psychiatric problems had an etiologically different form of childhood hyperactivity (Cantwell, 1978b), or if the major determinants of adult psychopathology are the secondary symptoms that are apparently unrelated to etiology (Stewart,

1980). Nor is it known if serious psychiatric problems will afflict one-third of all adults diagnosed as hyperactive in childhood, as Huessy (1974) has speculated on the basis of extrapolations from existing epidemiological data (Robins, 1966). What is clear, however, is that in less than a decade the field of hyperactivity has widened to include infancy through adulthood. High priority must be assigned to a search for empirically derived predictors of outcome, the development of intervention strategies, and their dissemination to clinicians and other professionals who work with the hyperactive child.

CHAPTER 3

Etiology

The paucity of etiological knowledge at the beginning of the 1970s was underlined in two comprehensive and influential reviews of hyperactivity (Werry, 1968; Werry & Sprague, 1970) whose conclusion was that there was insufficient empirical support for *any* etiological hypotheses, whether genetic, organic, or psychogenic. In the space of one decade the field has changed significantly on the empirical as well as the theoretical level. The role of genetics has been subjected to intensive study by investigators from several disciplines, a new genetic hypothesis has been proposed (Gorenstein & Newman, 1980), and a cluster of excellent review articles has appeared (e.g., Cantwell, 1975b, c; De Fries & Plomin, 1978; Dubey, 1976; McMahon, 1980). Two organic agents, high blood-lead levels and maternal alcohol intake during pregnancy, have been shown to be etiologically implicated. Biochemical alterations have been subjected to intensive investigation, and the role of food additives has generated sufficient research and clinical interest to warrant a comprehensive text (Conners, 1980) on this topic. Similarly impressive changes have occurred on the theoretical front. The unifactorial medical disease model view of hyperactivity, in which discrete factors originate in the child or are generated from the environment, has shifted in the last five years to a multifactorial etiological view based on the concept of a child *x* situation interaction (e.g., Chess, 1979; Loney, 1980b; Weiss, 1980; Whalen & Henker, 1980b; Williamson, Anderson, & Lundy, 1980). Porges and Smith (1980, p. 76) have conceptualized this interaction process as one in which continua of organic and environmental factors cause, to varying degrees, the cluster of behaviors characteristic of hyperactivity. Taking a sociological approach to this multifactorial view, Block (1977) has proposed a cultural theory of hyperactivity. Although some of the etiological explanations in the contemporary literature are of a fragmentary nature due in part to their comparative recency, others have already generated sufficient research to suggest productive new directions in etiological thinking, and a small number have substantial empirical support. In view of the obvious progress and vigor characteristic of current theory and research, it is difficult to see any justification for Barkley's (1978, p. 158) conclusion that "we appear to be no closer now than we were ten years ago in our understanding of the etiology of hyperactivity."

Equally incomprehensible is the well-entrenched pragmatic clinical viewpoint downgrading the necessity for etiological models, the rationale being that given our present limited state of knowledge, the symptomatic treatment of the child is likely to be the same across models. Representative of this viewpoint are the comments by Kinsbourne and Swanson (1979, p. 1) that

> with the present state of knowledge, the question of etiology is only indirectly relevant to the management of hyperactive children. At this time, insofar as we can help these children, it is only through symptomatic treatment. . . . The time will come when matters of etiology become of practical importance, but etiological models do not as yet have implications for diagnosis and treatment.

And those of Loney (1980b, p. 32):

> . . . etiology remains problematical. Although sophisticated theories about brain metabolism and arousal have been proposed and tested, many have abandoned the search for organic determinants (Dubey, 1976). . . . There have been no convincing demonstrations of psychogenic causation. . . . Fortunately, knowledge of etiology is not often required for treatment. It is generally accepted that organic etiology does not preclude response to psychological treatment, nor do disorders of psychogenic etiology fail to respond to pharmacological treatment.

The opposing view reflects the scientific perspective that an understanding of etiology is of critical importance to prevention and optimal management. Its influence is evident in the complexity, breadth, and overall quality of the etiological research of the past decade and the enthusiasm, focus, and vigor of the investigators. As Conners (1979a, p. 21) states:

> From a scientific point of view, I think that we really do want to know something about the different ways these children become hyperactive. From the perspectives of ultimately developing preventions as well as developing more targeted treatments that are specific to each child, we need to understand etiology. The treatment for a child suffering from developmental delays could be rather different in some respects from those for a child who has static limitations of the nervous system that aren't going to change. We do not in fact have good differential methods for segregating children with respect to their specific long-term needs.

Porges and Smith (1980, pp. 76–77) also stress the specificity of treatment value of a solid etiological base:

> It is our belief that the interaction of these two continua (organic and environmental factors) cause, to varying degrees, the collection of behaviors associated with hyperactive children. Thus, if one could identify the individual organic and situational factors associated with the specific etiology of hyperactivity in a child, a more individualized treatment might be developed.

The clinical and research factions have created a curious dichotomy in the hyperactivity literature of the past decade, with both pursuing their relatively independent ways. As one would expect, the search for sources of symptoms has been responsible for much more of the progress made to date in the treatment of hyperactivity than has concern primarily for the treatment of immediate symptoms. Even in our present limited state of knowledge, the progress made through the scientific pursuit of an etiological base has led to refinements in treatment unlikely to have occurred otherwise. A child with no identifiable cause for his hyperactivity constitutes a different clinical problem from one with a heavy body-lead burden (David, 1974); a trial of medication may be justifiable in both cases, but chelation therapy is mandatory for the latter child. If a hyperactive child on stimulant medication is experiencing a growth delay, it is essential for the clinician to know if the delay is likely to be attributable solely to the drug regimen or if it preceded the use of stimulants, as would be the case of the child whose hyperactivity is a manifestation of the fetal alcohol syndrome (Smith, 1979a). For the clinician, the crucial difference here is that growth retardation associated with stimulant medication is likely to correct itself with a growth rebound (Safer, Allen, & Barr, 1975), whereas the growth disorder in the fetal alcohol syndrome is irreversible (Gordon & Lieber, 1979). We have no quarrel with the clinical group's choice of specialty, that is, the treatment of the child's immediate symptoms. What we do strongly object to is the tendency of respected investigators to brush aside as relatively unimportant the necessity for the continued pursuit of etiological bases.

GENETIC FACTORS

Although there has been substantial investigative interest in behavioral genetics for the last 30 years (DeFries & Plomin, 1978; Lindzey, Loehlin, Manosevits, & Thiessen, 1971), it is only in the past decade that attention has turned to the possibility of genetic heritability in hyperactivity. The question remains undecided. To date, only tentative empirical support exists for a genetic component in hyperactivity because the crucial genetic studies have not yet been done. The only way to prove a genetic component is to specify the precise genetic mechanism, and to do this would require segregation or linkage analyses, both of which are difficult to conduct (Cantwell, 1975c). The research that has been done falls within the context of family, twin, and adoption methodologies. Its contribution has been lessened by inadequacies in experimental design, but it has had a certain impact in that the results overall are consistent in supporting the genetic component position. In his review of research on possible biologic determinants of hyperactivity, Stewart (1980, p. 160) commented that the research to date

> has made the idea of heredity taking a part in the origins of hyperactivity respectable and the connection with adult psychiatric disorders an interesting lead.

Family Studies

The finding that a disorder runs in families is usually the first major body of evidence suggesting that genetic factors may be operative, and this evidence can be considered grounds for *proposing* a genetic mechanism (Cantwell, 1975b; Omenn, 1973). Although familial resemblance is not proof of genetic influence, it must be demonstrated for a genetic component to be considered. In the early stages of genetic research in hyperactivity, the general approach in establishing familial resemblance was to determine whether first degree relatives of the proband (the hyperactive child) were more likely to have been or be at higher risk of becoming hyperactive than were control groups of comparable individuals from the general population. If adhered to, this general approach would have been quite productive. However, its implied criteria were often ignored, thus limiting the conclusions that could be drawn from the data. In a systematic evaluation of the biological parents of hyperactive children and nonhyperactive controls, Morrison and Stewart (1971) reported a significantly higher prevalence of retrospectively reported hyperactivity in the parents (particularly the fathers) and second-degree relatives of the hyperactive children that was the case for the controls. Contrary to acceptable standards of experimental design, the interviewers knew whether the parents being interviewed were those of a hyperactive or a control child, and consequently, the possibility existed that the retrospective diagnosis of childhood hyperactivity was influenced by experimenter bias. Cantwell (1972) reported similar findings, but these too were marred by a failure to establish blind interviewing conditions, as well as a failure to adhere to acceptable procedures for control group selection. In this study, the pediatrician who located the control group had been asked to recommend families in which there were no known cases of hyperactivity, thus increasing the probability of group differences. These weaknesses in design, which the investigators themselves have recognized (e.g., Cantwell, 1975b; Stewart, 1980), are violations of long-established standards for sound experimental design in behavioral research and are not a function of either the recency of genetic research or the problems specific to it. By contrast, certain validity problems are intrinsic to the family study approach. These problems range from those that are common to all family studies, for example, the need to accurately quantify the population of interest within each family (Thompson, Kidd, & Weissman, 1980), to those that are specific to family studies of hyperactivity, for example, the fact that the recency of this diagnostic category makes it unlikely that adequate records would be available to confirm retrospective parental diagnoses of hyperactivity in childhood. In addition, these diagnoses are confounded by the fact that the typical symptomatology of hyperactivity in childhood is differently expressed in adulthood with a far more variable behavior pattern (Bellak, 1979; Weiss & Hechtman, 1979). As Dubey (1976) has noted, fathers of male probands may identify with their sons and associate their old behavior patterns with those of their hyperactive children; or some fathers may be more likely to think of themselves as having been problem children if they are currently exhibiting undesirable behavior patterns such as alcoholism or antisocial behavior. The problems with retrospective parental diagnosis could be avoided and unequivocal evidence of familial resemblance obtained by conducting a prospective follow-up study of the offspring of probands who had been diagnosed as hyperactive in childhood. To date, such a study has not been done.

Some of the pitfalls of parental reports of childhood hyperactivity have been bypassed by studying the siblings of hyperactive children, a group offering major matching and other advantages as compared to parental diagnosis (Offord & Jones, 1976). However, these data too are weakened by the same disregard for principles of experimental design noted above. Welner and her associates (Welner, Welner, Stewart, Palkes, & Wish, 1977) used the proband-sibling design to determine if the full siblings of hyperactive elementary school boys were at a higher risk of being hyperactive than were the siblings of a matched control group of nonhyperactive boys. One-quarter of the brothers of the probands were themselves hyperactive, a total that was three times greater than was the case for the control group brothers, but some of these evaluations were made on a nonblind basis.

Some investigators have looked for links between childhood hyperactivity and personality disorders with a known genetic base in adults. Evidence has been reported for a hyperactivity-alcoholism link in a group of studies of adopted (Cadoret & Gath, 1982) and nonadopted individuals (Goodwin, Schulsinger, Hermansen, Guze, & Winokur, 1975; Tarter, McBride, Buonpane, & Schneider, 1977). In the latter two studies, however, the data were based on retrospective diagnosis of childhood hyperactivity. The studies of Cantwell (1972) and Morrison and Stewart (1971) mentioned earlier also reported a high prevalence rate of alcoholism in the biologic parents and adult relatives of the hyperactive children (as well as a high rate of antisocial disorders and hysteria), as compared to the family members of the nonhyperactive controls. In both studies the comparisons with the control group data were invalidated because, as Dubey (1976) and Stewart (1980) have noted, the use of nonclinical controls leaves open the possibility that the disorders that occurred more often in the relatives of hyperactive children would also be more common in the relatives of any children who were patients in a child psychiatry clinic. To eliminate this possibility, Morrison (1980a) compared the family histories of 140 hyperactive children and adolescents with those of 91 nonhyperactive psychiatrically ill children matched on age and sex with the hyperactive group. He found that parents of the hyperactive group were more likely to have antisocial personality and hysteria, whereas endogenous psychoses occurred more often in the control group parents, but the diagnosis of alcoholism did not differentiate the two groups. Further evidence against the specificity of the relationships between hyperactivity in children and psychiatric disorders in their adult relatives comes from studies by Stewart and his associates (Stewart, deBlois, & Cummings, 1980; Stewart, deBlois, & Singer, 1979) comparing the prevalence of psychiatric disorder in the parents of hyperactive boys with prevalence in parents of boys with conduct disorders who were attending a psychiatric clinic. Here again, the results suggested that the differences reported earlier (Cantwell, 1972; Morrison & Stewart, 1971) were probably not related directly to hyperactivity in children, but instead were characteristics of families coming to a child psychiatry clinic.

In the Stewart et al. (1980) study, an additional refinement involved the assignment of the hyperactive boys to two subgroups of hyperactive only, and hyperactive plus aggressive, noncompliant, and antisocial. This breakdown proved to be an important one. The hyperactive plus aggression combination tended to be associated with psychiatric disorders, particularly that of the antisocial personality, whereas no such association existed for the hyperactive only group. These findings were consistent with an earlier pilot study (Stewart & Leone, 1978), but more important here than the reported trend in the data is the contribution to the only recently initiated methodological procedure of using subgroups of hyperactive children. The importance of separating out children who are hyperactive only from those who are both hyperactive and unsocialized aggressives is consistent with the viewpoint of El-Guebaly and Offord (1977) as well as with recent research by Loney and her associates (Loney, Kramer, & Milich, 1981; Milich & Loney, 1979a) linking unfavorable outcome in adolescence to childhood aggression rather than to hyperactivity. The Loney et al. research represents a milestone in current research. In any future research designed to establish a childhood hyperactivity-adult psychiatric disorder link, a mandatory criterion for inclusion in one experimental group should be childhood aggression, and in another, nonaggressive hyperactivity.

Twin Studies

The comparison of identical with fraternal twins, when at least one member of each pair exhibits the characteristic under investigation, is a method that has had widespread use in determining the role of genetic factors in a specific condition (Cantwell, 1975c). In this method the basic assumption is that differences between monozygotic (MZ) twins are a result of environmental factors, whereas those in dizygotic (DZ) twins reflect both genetic and environmental factors. Therefore, the greater the resemblance of MZ twins, and the smaller the resemblance of DZ twins for that characteristic, the stronger the assumption of a genetic contribution. In hyperactivity, if genetic factors are important in transmission, one would expect to find that when one MZ twin is hyperactive the probability would be high that the co-twin would also be hyperactive, that is, a concordant relationship would exist. However, the rate of concordance in DZ twins would be significantly lower, resembling that for same-sex singleton siblings. If environmental factors are important, the rate of concordance in MZ twins should not differ significantly from that in DZ twins.

A valid criticism of the use of this method in studying hyperactivity is that MZ twins are more at risk than DZ twins for some of the prenatal and perinatal problems that appear to be etiologically related to hyperactivity, and these environmental factors could spuriously increase the concordance rate for hyperactivity in MZ twins (World Health Organization, 1966). A second criticism, which has not been supported by research, is that MZ and DZ same-sex twins may differ in the homogeneity of their social and nonsocial environments, which could reduce interpair differences in MZ twins and thus provide spurious support for a genetic hypothesis. In respect to similarity of prenatal environments, Munsinger (1977) has identified an "identical twin transfusion syndrome," which makes identical twins *less* similar than fraternal twins; in the case of postnatal twin environments, the landmark National Merit study (Loehlin & Nichols, 1976) suggested that a reasonable degree of differential treatment does not result in personality differences. However, the whole issue in respect to hyperactivity remains an academic one at this point, because only one twin study has been reported with children diagnosed as hyperactive (Lopez, 1965) and its findings were invalidated by methodological weakness. There have been several studies of activity in normal twins (Scarr, 1966; Vandenberg, 1962; Willerman, 1973) that suggest a substantial genetic component to activity level, but not necessarily to hyperactivity. It is essential in this respect that researchers distinguish between the most active in a subject population and the truly hyperactive. There is a regrettable tendency to treat a high level of activity as synonymous with hyperactivity (e.g., Willerman, 1973) and as we have already pointed out, hyperactivity is qualitatively different from a high level of activity.

Adoption Studies

By studying genetically unrelated individuals living together (environmental influences) and genetically related individuals living apart (genetic influences), adoption studies separate out genetic and environmental factors common to members of biological families. DeFries and Plomin (1978) regard the adoption study method as the most powerful tool for studying complex human behavioral disorders. If an adoption study is to provide a stringent test of a disorder such as hyperactivity, two criteria must be met. The first of these, that the children in the study should have been separated from their biological parents at birth or in early infancy and have had no further contact, poses little problem. However, the second one, that there must be certainty about the accuracy of the retrospective parental report of hyperactivity in childhood, is difficult to meet because of the self-report aspects discussed earlier. Despite this problem, and the proliferation of avoidable methodological errors, adoption studies have yielded results consistent with a theory of genetic influence upon hyperactivity.

One adoption study design that has been used involves comparing pheno-typic similarity for biologically related families who have genes and familial environment in common, with phenotypic similarity for adoptive families who share only familial environment. Morrison and Stewart (1973b) interviewed the legal adoptive but not the biological parents of 35 hyperactive children who had had no contact since birth with their biological parents, and who had been permanently placed in infancy. The results of the interviews were then compared with previously reported groups of biological parents of *other* hy-peractive children and control parents (Morrison & Stewart, 1971), a proce-dure used by Cantwell (1975b) in a similar study. This procedure of substituting the biological parents of one group of hyperactive children for the biological parents of a second group of hyperactive children, so that the bio-logic and adoptive parents being compared do *not* in fact share the same off-spring, has as its only advantage economy of experimenter time and money. Furthermore, as McMahon (1980) has pointed out, the procedures used in these two studies to diagnose children for inclusion in the original hyperactivi-ty groups were inadequately described; the diverse sources from which sub-jects were drawn raises doubts about the comparability of the adoptive and nonadoptive groups; and inadequate procedures were used to diagnose par-ents and second-degree relatives. Keeping in mind the considerable limita-tions of the two studies, one of their findings provides some support for the role of genetic transmission in the development of hyperactivity. The biologi-cal first- and second-degree relatives reported a significantly higher prevalence of childhood hyperactivity than did the adoptive relatives or controls (who did not differ on this measure), which is consistent with a genetic transmission hypothesis. A second finding, that the adoptive parents did not have the high prevalence rate for alcoholism, sociopathy, and hysteria that had occurred in the biologic parents, makes no contribution to the genetic issue because the careful screening that prospective adoptive parents undergo probably elimi-nates the majority of those with existing psychiatric disorders or propensities for them.

Another type of adoption study involves comparisons between twins, sib-lings, or half siblings who have been reared apart. Using this approach, Safer (1973) reviewed the medical histories and social service charts of the full sib-lings ($n=19$) and half siblings ($n=22$) of 17 index children with minimal brain dysfunction, all of whom had been assigned to foster homes at an early age. The major difference in group description was that the full siblings had the same fathers as did the index minimal brain dysfunction children, but the half siblings did not. The results appeared to support the genetic transmission hypothesis, with 10 of the 19 full siblings classified as having minimal brain dysfunction as compared with two of the 22 half siblings. However, once again these results must be treated with caution. The sample was small; the families were characterized by seizure disorders, congenital anomalies, and low intelligence levels, and therefore the children were not representative of the hyperactive child population; information was lacking about the quality of the home environments of the two groups and about the psychiatric state of the stepfathers; the relationships between the children called for verification by means of paternity tests, because in families as deviant as these full sibling status requires further substantiation. One research topic that merits investigation is the significance, if any, of the finding (Swanson, personal communication, 1981; Trites, personal communication, 1981) that there appears to be a disproportionate number of adoptees in the hyperactive population.

Although the foregoing data concerning genetic transmission are far from conclusive, they are compelling enough to justify the consideration of a genetic influence operating in combination with environmental factors. The question of how such a genetic influence might be mediated has led to two markedly different approaches to the problem of identifying a genetic mechanism of transmission. In the first of these Morrison and Stewart (1973a) point out that the well-established excess of affected males argues against a single autosomal dominant gene pattern, because for this pattern there should be no sex differences in prevalence, no generations should be skipped, and one parent should have been hyperactive; and there is considerable clinical evidence that these events do not occur with any consistency. If a reduced penetrance explanation is invoked, generations could be skipped with a single autosomal dominant gene pattern. With a single autosomal recessive gene both parents would be carriers but neither should have been affected, and approximately one-quarter of the siblings of the hyperactive child should be hyperactive. The number of affected parents in the Morrison and Stewart (1971) and Cantwell (1972) studies, coupled with the lack of evidence of the prevalence rate in siblings, excluded this mechanism of transmission. The well-documented evidence of apparent transmission of hyperactivity from father to son (Cantwell, 1972; Omenn, 1973) is inconsistent with a sex-linked mode of transmission. In the only chromosome study of hyperactive children in the literature, Warren, Karduck, Bussaratid, Stewart, and Sly (1971) reported no evidence of any chromosome aberrations. Chromosomal studies should be conducted with families with multiple cases of hyperactivity because of the increased probability of evidence of metabolic, biochemical, or chromosomal abnormalities specific to hyperactivity occurring in these families. [If the preliminary findings (Lubs & Smith, 1981) of an inherited genetic defect in dyslexia are confirmed, there may be increased interest in the search for hyperactivity-related chromosomal abnormalities.] Morrison and Stewart (1973a) concluded that the high ratio of males to females afflicted with this syndrome suggests some sort of polyfactorial transmission in which a sizable number of different hereditary and environmental influences interact to produce the behavior, with the hereditary component being polygenic, that is, reflecting the activity of many genes rather than that of a single major gene. Wender (1971) considered the fact that minimal brain dysfunction did not "breed true" to be support for a theory of polygenetic transmission.

Polyfactorial transmission implies a genetic predisposition to hyperactivity that puts the individual at risk so that the extent to which he is affected by hyperactivity, if he is affected at all, is determined by various environmental influences that operate on the substrate of the genetic predisposition. A polyfactorial hypothesis would be consistent with the sex differences in hyperactivity as well as with its variability. To test the hypothesis of polygenetic transmission, Morrison and Stewart (1973a) reexamined the data of a previous study (Morrison & Stewart, 1971) that had demonstrated an association between hyperactivity and the adult psychiatric disorders of alcoholism, hysteria, and sociopathy. Two aspects of the polygenetic hypothesis were tested, the first being that the greater the number of individuals in a family who are hyperactive, the higher the risk component for related conditions in that family. Thus if hyperactivity is linked with alcoholism, families with several cases of hyperactivity in the immediate or extended families of the hyperactive child would be expected to have a higher incidence of alcoholics than families with no secondary cases of hyperactivity. This hypothesis was supported: the incidence of alcoholism in first- and second-degree relatives was nearly twice as high in families with secondary cases of hyperactivity as in families with no secondary cases. According to the polygenetic theory, if a proband has a first-degree relative who is hyperactive, that family probably has a higher dose of the genes responsible, and hence would be more likely to have more remote relatives affected than would a family in which only the proband is hyperactive. This hypothesis was also confirmed. Of the 15 families with an affected first-degree relative, seven had an extended relative with hyperactivity and eight had none. Of the 44 families with no affected first-degree relatives, eight had an extended relative with hyperactivity and 36 had none. Although these data do not rule out other modes of genetic or social transmission, they are consistent with a polygenetic transmission model.

In a second study Morrison and Stewart (1974) used Slater's method (1966) to distinguish between polygenetic transmission and dominant gene transmission with reduced penetrance. With this method family histories are analyzed to determine whether secondary cases occur almost exclusively on one side of the family, as would be expected with a single dominant gene, or whether a significant number of affected persons have both paternal and maternal ascendant relatives so affected, which would support polygenetic transmission. When the family histories of 12 hyperactive children were examined, relatives affected with hyperactivity or adult psychiatric disorders were found on both sides of the families, a finding congruent with a polygenetic mode of transmission.

Although these results are consistent with a genetic mechanism of transmission, particularly a polygenetic model (Cantwell, 1975c), they have not proven it. The crucial genetic study of hyperactivity (or any trait, condition, or disorder) must specify the precise genetic mechanism involved. The only procedures that can precisely define a genetic mechanism are segregation studies, which could only be done with humans under very unusual circumstances, and linkage studies, which would require the identification of the genetic marker associated with hyperactivity (Cantwell, 1975c).

The second approach to the problem of identifying a genetic mechanism of transmission takes an entirely different direction. Gorenstein and Newman (1980) have proposed that hyperactivity is part of a broader constellation of disinhibitory syndromes that traditionally have been regarded as separate. They view these syndromes, which include psychiatric disorders such as alcoholism, psychopathy, hysteria, antisocial behavior, and impulsive personality, as single manifestations of the same genetic diathesis modified by differential early life experiences. Taking psychopathy as the prototypical syndrome of disinhibition by reason of it being the most extreme form, Gorenstein and Newman (1980) provide convincing empirical and clinical support for this cluster of disinhibitory syndromes being behaviorally and genetically related. Psychopaths and hyperactives, for example, have several behavioral characteristics in common: they both engage in an unusual amount of stimulation-seeking, are characterized by deficits in the mediation of time intervals, are unusually impulsive, are unresponsive to punishment, and show a total disregard (psychopath) or notable unawareness (hyperactive) of any suffering or hardship on their own part or that of others as a result of their actions. Evidence of a psychopathy-hyperactivity genetic relationship comes from clinical reports that psychopaths are often hyperactive as children, a finding that led Tarter (1979, p. 59) to suggest that "hyperactivity may be the behavioral substrate for what later emerges in a significant proportion of persons as sociopathy or alcoholism." Investigations of psychiatric disorder among relatives of hyperactive children have also provided evidence supporting this relationship.

The idea that hyperactivity is one of a number of disinhibitory syndromes arising from a common diasthesis, rather than the final common pathway for a variety of conditions, is lent credence by Gorenstein and Newman's (1980) proposal that the syndrome produced by lesion of the septum in animals can serve as a functional research model of human disinhibitory psychopathology. Such a model has the potential to cast new light on the psychological antecedents of disinhibition. These researchers do not imply that human disinhibition can be traced to septal dysfunction. Rather, they are proposing that behavioral analysis of the septal syndrome in animals may elucidate basic psychological components of human disinhibition. The research task is clear, but in terms of our present understanding of such phenomena, monumental. The diasthesis common to this cluster of syndromes must be identified along with the differential environmental social and nonsocial forces that produce the separate manifestations. Gorenstein and Newman (1980, p. 307) propose that such a diasthesis is likely to be

a disposition to a particular behavioral style, which may or may not be rooted in a neurophysiological irregularity, and which entails more or less serious consequences for psychological adjustment depending on environmental circumstances.

ORGANIC FACTORS

The possibility that hyperactivity may have an organic base has been proposed by many investigators (e.g., Still, 1902; Strauss & Lehtinen, 1947; Wender, 1971). For organic factors to play an etiological role in hyperactivity, one or other of the following lines of investigation would have to prove supportive: Either there should be evidence of genetic transmission occurring, as Wender (1971) has suggested, on the basis of altered structure or as biochemically mediated—and, as we have noted in the previous section, these are possibilities for which there is as yet no evidence—or certain types of biochemical and neurological abnormalities should occur. The issue is of more than academic interest, because the demonstration of organicity in hyperactivity would have a number of implications for the hyperactive child (Dubey, 1976). Organicity suggests a medical disorder and so logically would require medical intervention, probably in the form of stimulant medication. If medication is prescribed and proves to be effective, there could be a diminished emphasis on other kinds of intervention, particularly of essential social, educational, and other therapeutic help. Neither the child nor his parents would be "to blame" for the disorder, but on the other hand organicity implies a permanent problem, a view that could have negative long-term effects on the child and undermine efforts to effect changes. In this section we will examine the evidence from the second line of investigation, involving biochemical and neurological abnormalities, as possibly supportive of an organic basis for hyperactivity.

Biochemical Factors

There is evidence for abnormalities of the monoamine (serotonin, dopamine, norepinephrine) systems in clinical disorders (Shaywitz, Cohen, & Shaywitz, 1978). Wender (1971) has speculated that a biochemical imbalance involving one or more of these central nervous system neurotransmitters may be etiologically related to hyperactivity. The basis for this proposal is that the amphetamines influence both the behavioral symptoms of hyperactivity and the levels of brain monoamines. More specifically, activity level is assumed to be a function of the comparative levels of the inhibitory and excitatory systems, and both systems are assumed to be monoaminergic, so that both respond to amphetamine. In children, the activity level commonly viewed as normal represents a balance between the two systems: if the excitatory system is at a higher level of activity, the child is more active; if the inhibitory system is higher, the child is more controlled. A low monoamine level decreases activity in the inhibitory system and thus results in a high level of activity. Because the amphetamines and the clinically related agent, methylphenidate, are chemically similar to the monoamines, they can substitute for them as modifiers of the low monoamine level, with a consequent calming effect on the hyperactive child. In a discussion of Wender's (1971) theory, Sroufe (1975) has noted that it rests on two dubious assumptions, that of a high arousal level and of defective reward mechanisms. A third assumption, concerning the paradoxical drug effect in the hyperactive child, was seriously questioned by Sroufe (1975) and has since been disproven (Rapoport, Buchsbaum, Zahn, Weingartner, Ludlow, & Mikkelsen, 1978).

Dubey (1976) has noted in his excellent critical evaluation of organic factors in hyperactivity that the influence of the amphetamines on both hyperactivity and monoamine levels does not necessarily prove that the two are functionally related. Since they could be independent, it follows that an important step would be a comparison of the monoamine levels of hyperactive and nonhyperactive children.

Serotonin. Ninety percent of body serotonin is found in the gastrointestinal tract, with lesser amounts ranging from 8 to 10 percent in the blood platelets, and a minimal amount of perhaps 1 to 2 percent in the cerebrospinal fluid (Shaywitz et al., 1978). Urinary concentrations of the metabolites of serotonin were found not to differ in hyperactive and nonhyperactive children (Wender, Epstein, Kopin, & Gordon, 1971). However, as Wender et al. noted, differences in the relatively minute central serotonin levels might have been obscured by this method because urinalysis reflects total body production of monoamines. As an alternative to urinalysis, Coleman and her associates (Bhagavan, Coleman & Coursin, 1975; Coleman, 1971) have measured blood platelet serotonin levels in hyperactive children. Although the 25 hyperactive children in the latter study had consistently lower levels than a cohort of 150 age-matched nonhyperactive controls, under stressful situations the levels of many of the hyperactive children were similar to those of the nonhyperactive group. Furthermore, in two of the children the serotonin levels were shown to be clearly related to environmental manipulation. Bhagavan et al. (1975) reported a decreased blood platelet serotonin in hyperactive children as compared to the controls. However, Rapoport and her associates (Rapoport, Quinn, Bradbard, Riddle, & Brooks, 1974; Rapoport, Quinn, Scribanu, & Murphy, 1974) have reported strongly conflicting results: the platelet serotonin levels in hyperactive boys did not differ from those of their nonhyperactive peers, and platelet serotonin concentration was not related to severity of hyperactivity. Administration of methylphenidate improved the behavior of the hyperactive boys, but contrary to Wender's (1971) model, did not reduce the serotonin levels, the assumption here being that the platelet is a functional model for the serotonergic CNS neuron, as Pletscher (1968) has claimed. A more direct approach, the determination of serotonin metabolites in the cerebrospinal fluid, failed to demonstrate differences in serotonin levels of hyperactive and nonhyperactive children (Shaywitz, Cohen, & Bowers, 1977; Shetty & Chase, 1976). As a group, these studies provide little support for an association between serotonin metabolism and hyperactivity. Furthermore, the fact that it has never been proven that an abnormality in peripheral serotonin is evidence of an abnormality in central serotonin metabolism (Shaywitz et al., 1978) suggests that most of these studies rest shakily on an uncertain basic premise.

Catecholamines—Dopamine and Norepinephrine. The evidence for a hyperactivity-catecholamine link is based primarily on the finding that the stimulant medications improve behavior in hyperactive children. Pharmaco-logical data have suggested that the action of the stimulant medications in the CNS is mediated by brain catecholaminergic mechanisms (Heikkila, Orlansky, Mytilineous, & Cohen, 1975). Although these data suggest abnormalities of brain catecholamines in hyperactivity, such a relationship has not been demonstrated. Wender et al. (1971) found no difference between hyperactive and nonhyperactive children in urinary concentrations of homovanillic acid, the major metabolite of dopamine. Similarly, in an investigation of dopamine-B-hydroxylase (DBH), the last enzyme involved in the synthesis of norepinephrine, Rapoport, Quinn, and Lamprecht (1974) reported that DBH levels did not correlate with hyperactivity.

The optimum procedure for demonstrating that hyperactivity is a disorder of CNS monoaminergic function would be the impossible task of examining concentrations of monoamines in the human brain. An alternative that has been used is the examination of neurotransmitter substances in the cerebrospinal fluid. There is considerable evidence that the concentrations of the major metabolites of dopamine and serotonin can be reliably determined on small samples of spinal fluid (Shaywitz et al., 1978). A study by Shetty and Chase (1976) yielded inconclusive results (Shaywitz et al., 1978). A second study, however (Shaywitz et al., 1977), using the more sensitive technique of probenecid loading, suggested that central dopaminergic systems may play a role in hyperactivity. Neither study provided any support for a disorder of central serotonin. Further, the support for the role of dopaminergic mechanisms in hyperactivity should be viewed with caution in the light of the small number of subjects involved. Altogether, this cluster of empirical findings provides no firm evidence for a biochemical abnormality in hyperactivity. Hyperactive children are not characterized by abnormal levels of peripheral monoamines, and as Dubey (1976) has noted, brain monoamine levels in children are unexplored and likely to remain so.

Evidence consistent with the dopamine hypothesis is contained in a thoughtful review by Mattes (1980) of data linking hyperactivity to frontal lobe dysfunction. Mattes (1980, p. 364) notes that dopamine pathways have recently been found in the frontal lobes so central dopaminergic systems could be etiologically implicated in hyperactivity. Several investigators (Newlin & Tramontana, 1980; Rosenthal & Allen, 1978) have discussed a possible relationship between hyperactivity and frontal lobe dysfunction. However, the most persuasive evidence for the implication of dopaminergic mechanisms in childhood hyperactivity comes from experimental animal models of hyperactivity (Shaywitz, Yager, & Klopper, 1976; Sorenson, Vayer, & Goldberg,

1977) in which the dopaminergic pathways of developing rat pups have been pharmacologically destroyed with a resultant profound and permanent reduction of brain dopamine, while leaving norepinephrine concentrations unaltered. The behavioral profile of the rat pups showed several similarities to the behavior characteristic of the hyperactive child. The rat pups exhibited high activity levels that abated with maturity, reduction of activity level with stimulant medication treatment, some difficulty in adjusting to a novel environment, and cognitive difficulty in mazes (Shaywitz et al., 1976, 1978). Shaywitz et al.'s research appears to represent an important step towards the establishment of a biochemical basis for hyperactivity.

Neurological Damage

Hyperactivity has often been attributed to some form of neurological damage such as brain damage. It has been assumed that if brain damage did exist, it could be demonstrated with either electroencephalogram (EEG) tracings or the presence of an unusual number of soft neurologic signs. The evidence concerning brain damage, EEG abnormalities, and soft signs will be briefly considered here.

Brain Damage. The earliest descriptions of hyperactivity (Still, 1902; Strecker & Ebaugh, 1924) usually attributed the condition to brain damage that had occurred as a result of traumatic events, such as severe illness, injury, and prenatal and perinatal problems. Although hyperactivity does occur in children with severe and demonstrable brain damage, there is little empirical evidence to support the view of brain damage as a major etiological factor in hyperactivity (Routh, 1978). Stewart and Olds (1973) estimate that less than 10 percent of the referrals for hyperactivity have histories suggesting brain injury, and point out that the frequency of birth process complications is no greater among the hyperactive than the general population; even when such complications do occur they are not necessarily significant. Evidence from the Kauai pregnancy study (Werner, Bierman, French, Simonian, Connor, Smith, & Campbell, 1968) and other major studies (Lilienfield, Pasamanick, & Rogers, 1955) showed little relationship between severe perinatal stress and later performance. Werry and Sprague (1970) state that when the criteria for subject selection are either demonstrable brain damage or brain damage inferred from noxious events, such as severe perinatal anoxia, that carry a high probability of causing significant damage, the research produces little evidence that brain damage causes hyperactivity. There is a higher incidence of minor abnormalities in the hyperactive group than is usually the case for the nonhyperactive control children. The bulk of the evidence suggests that although hyperactivity can result from brain damage, it is not the typical behavior manifestation of brain damage (Birch, 1964; Routh, 1978; Satterfield, 1973; Stewart, 1980).

EEG Abnormalities. If brain damage is present in a hyperactive child, one indication of it might be EEG abnormalities. However, the research during the 1970s on EEG patterns in the hyperactive child provided little support for a clear association between hyperactivity and EEG abnormality. Although a relatively high percentage of EEG abnormality has been reported in hyperactive children, these studies have often lacked comparative control data from nonclinical children, and in addition have included children who ordinarily would be excluded from a study of hyperactivity, that is, those with known neurological disease and severe intellectual handicaps (Dubey, 1976). When comparisons were made with appropriate controls, the results were equivocal, with some investigators (Satterfield, Cantwell, Lesser, & Podosin, 1972; Werry, Minde, Guzman, Weiss, Dogan, & Hoy, 1972) finding no differences between hyperactives and controls and others (Werry, Weiss, & Douglas, 1964) reporting differences in type of abnormality but not in incidence of it. There is no evidence of EEG abnormalities specific to hyperactivity: the EEG records of hyperactive children are indistinguishable from those of other diagnostic groups (e.g., Werry et al., 1972; Wikler, Dixon, & Parker, 1970); and hyperactive children with EEG abnormalities do not differ from those with normal tracings (Satterfield, Cantwell, & Satterfield, 1974). The most stable and best documented EEG difference between hyperactive children and nonhyperactive nonclinical controls is an excess of slow-wave activity (Werry et al., 1972; Wikler et al., 1970), whose interpretation is a matter of dispute.

One problem with EEG indexes has been that when abnormalities have been found in specific children, their significance has been unclear. In two recent studies, Ahn and his associates (Ahn, Prichep, John, Baird, Trepitin, & Kaye, 1980; John, Ahn, Prichep, Trepitin, Brown, & Kaye, 1980) have taken a major step towards eliminating this problem. They have derived developmental equations for the frequency composition of the resting EEG that describe the development of the electrical activity of the normal human brain as a function of age and independently of cultural, ethnic, socioeconomic status, and sex factors. The equations based on large groups of healthy children (aged 6 to 16) in the United States and Sweden are almost identical. The frequency composition of the EEG reflects the age and the functional status of the brain. With maturation, the dominant frequency becomes more rapid, whereas brain damage, dysfunction, or deterioration causes a slowing of frequency in the brain regions involved (John et al., 1980). The developmental equations derived by these investigators predict the values of 32 EEG parameters and have been validated with EEG records from normal children and those with known neurological disease. When the equations were tested with three large groups, normal children, those with disabilities, and those who were considered at risk for brain dysfunction, there was a low incidence of false positives in the normal group and significant deviations from the predicted norms in the other two groups. This line of investigation represents an important step in establishing the diagnostic and evaluative functions of EEG records for hyperactive children.

Soft Signs. Neurological signs are considered soft (as opposed to hard) when either their actual presence is uncertain or the relationship between their presence and specific central nervous system damage is unclear. The signs occurring most frequently are motor impersistence, incoordination, impaired alternating movements of the forearms, ataxia, inability to hop, Babinskis, synkinetic movements, involuntary movements, graphesthesia, and speech impairment. Soft signs have been considered to be either a reflection of minimal brain damage or of immature development of nervous system structures. Their presence is age-dependent, and they are present in approximately 50 percent of hyperactive children (Casey, 1977; Kenny, Clemmens, Hudson, Lentz, Cicci, & Nair, 1971).

The significance of soft signs is highly controversial (Ingram, 1973; Wender, 1971). Some investigators (Gross & Wilson, 1974; Lerer & Lerer, 1976; Millichap, 1975; Safer & Allen, 1976) view them as being of some diagnostic value, particularly if five or more are observed (Renshaw, 1974), whereas others (Casey, 1977; Varga, 1979) regard them as minor neurological abnormalities of little clinical significance and point to the problems of examiner subjectivity, the lack of age-specific standards, and the frequent presence of the same signs in nonhyperactive children. In an excellent short editorial on the significance of soft signs, Touwen and Sporrel (1979, p. 528) state in part:

> ... soft signs may mean anything or nothing, and in clinical diagnosis they are rightly discarded as trivial, i.e., they are considered to offer no real contribution to the solution of the diagnostic problem ... terms like soft ... should be discarded ... a neurological sign which can be properly assessed must be called a sign, whatever its significance may be.... The attempt to explain disorders of complex behavior only on the basis of neurological minor signs testifies to an objectionable kind of reductionism.

AROUSAL LEVEL

Arousal level is viewed here as a quantitative dimension that reflects an organism's immediate capability for processing external stimuli, characterized by degrees of complexity, intensity, and novelty; and internal stimuli whose source is in muscular and cognitive activity (Rosenthal & Allen, 1978). According to Berlyne (1960, p. 194), arousal level has motivating properties and operates according to a homeostatic model in that there is an optimal level of arousal that the organism strives to maintain:

> Arousal potential which deviates in either an upward or downward direction from this optimum will be drive-inducing or aversive. The organism will thus strive to keep arousal potential near its optimum.

Within this conceptual framework, overarousal results in a state of psychological discomfort, analogous to overexcitement, that causes the organism to

withdraw in an effort to lower the state of overstimulation; underarousal results in a state resembling boredom that leads to an active search on the part
of the organism for sources of stimulation. Ferguson and Pappas (1979) have
noted two substantive sources of support for the etiological role of abnormality in the arousal level of the hyperactive child: first, a degree of abnormality
in arousal is consistent with some of the salient characteristics of this child,
particularly his attentional deficit and deviant activity, and second, the efficacy of stimulant medications is associated with their effects on the neurotransmitters, which in turn appear to be closely related to central nervous system
(CNS) arousal level. Several psychophysiological models have attributed
hyperactivity to an abnormality in the arousal level of the CNS, but the direction of this abnormality is a matter of dispute. The models viewing it as one
of overarousal (e.g., Freibergs & Douglas, 1969; Kahn & Cohen, 1934; Laufer,
Denhoff, & Solomons, 1957; Strauss & Lehtinen, 1947) interpret hyperactivity
as a behavioral manifestation of an overaroused or highly aroused CNS,
whereas the underarousal models (e.g., Bradley, 1937; Satterfield et al., 1974;
Werry & Sprague, 1970; Zentall, 1975) conceptualize hyperactivity as a compensatory response by a suboptimally aroused individual that is designed to
increase arousal level through increased proprioceptive sensory input (Porges,
1976).

Overarousal Models

One of the earliest statements on overarousal came from Laufer et al. (1957),
whose model was based on the finding that hyperactive children had lower
photo-Metrazol thresholds than controls, which Gastaut (1950) has attributed
to dysfunction of the diencephalon. According to the Laufer et al. model, the
diencephalon acts as a switch or filter that determines how sensory inputs are
projected to various cortical areas. The low photo-Metrazol threshold of the
hyperactive child, presumably an indication of dysfunction, could result in
difficulty in selectively filtering information, with a resultant oversensitivity to
peripheral stimulation. Dysfunction of the diencephalic structures permits the
following sequence to occur: it alters resistance at the synapses, impulses are
then allowed to spread out beyond the usual pathway, the consequence being
cortical overarousal (or, as Knobel, Wolman, and Mason [1959] termed this
process, "critical overfunctioning"), which, in turn, results in hyperactivity
(Ferguson & Pappas, 1979). Central to this model is the idea that hyperactive
children have difficulty in selectively filtering incoming information and are
particularly sensitive to peripheral stimulation, a characteristic that was basic
to the Strauss and Lehtinen (1947) minimal stimulation classroom. The effect
of amphetamine on the hyperactive child with a low photo-Metrazol threshold
is to raise the threshold to the level of the nonhyperactive child. The Laufer et
al. model accounts for the tendency of hyperactivity to decrease with age as

Hyperact or control-
anti-social person stimulation study

being due to the fact that as the cortex develops with increasing age, expanding cortical control enables more inhibition and discrimination.

Underarousal Models

A representative model here is the one proposed by Satterfield and his associates (Satterfield et al., 1974; Satterfield & Dawson, 1971), which is based on data that suggest the presence of lower than normal arousal indices and insufficient CNS inhibition in hyperactive children. In this model both arousal and inhibitory functions are conceptualized as originating in the reticular activating system (RAS). The high activity level is seen as secondary to a lower than normal excitation level in the reticular formation, and represents an attempt on the part of the hyperactive child to optimize arousal level through increasing the proprioceptive and exteroceptive sensory input (Satterfield & Dawson, 1971). The reduction of activity that is associated with drug intervention is not paradoxical in this model, but is seen as the effect to be expected from optimizing the arousal level: hyperactive children are presumed to have low levels of electrical discharge at the reticular formation, and the effect of stimulants is to reduce hyperactivity by increasing arousal. According to Satterfield and Dawson (1971), stimulant medication modifies hyperactivity by facilitating norepinephrinergic transmission. Although there is no firm evidence as to which catecholamine mediates these stimulant effects, there are some data (Heikkila et al., 1975) that suggest that the positive effects of the stimulants may be due to the facilitation of dopamine transmission. Thus the Satterfield and Dawson (1971) model could provide a parsimonious explanation for hyperactivity as well as for the hyperactive child's response to drugs.

The justification for tracing any arousal-related dysfunction to specific brain structures has been questioned by Ferguson and Pappas (1979), who contend that hypotheses about the location of brain dysfunction are premature in the light of available empirical knowledge, and by Rosenthal and Allen (1978), who believe that underarousal cannot be adequately accounted for as simple underactivity of the RAS. Both pairs of investigators agree that there is a sufficient psychophysiological data base for considering the issue of overarousal versus underarousal of the CNS in hyperactivity. Rosenthal and Allen (1978) recommend that investigators focus on the fact that many other brain structures exert an influence on arousal primarily by modulating RAS activity, and point to a dysfunction of forebrain inhibition as a promising alternative to a simple RAS-arousal theory of hyperactivity. The emphasis on psychophysiological data stems from dissatisfaction with behavioral data: many of the behavioral investigations (e.g., Forehand & Baumeister, 1970; Reardon & Bell, 1970) have used severely retarded subjects who would not ordinarily be included in hyperactivity research; in addition, the behavioral data in themselves offer no reliable information concerning the central arousal state of the hyperactive child because the behavior of the child can be interpreted, according to Ferguson and Pappas (1979), as resulting from either over- or underarousal. Two exceptions are the methodologically sound behavioral studies of Horner (1977) and Ives (1977), neither of which supports an arousal-hyperactivity link.

Although the various models have a certain face validity, investigations of peripheral and central indices of arousal in hyperactive children have failed to yield conclusive evidence concerning the etiological role of over- and underarousal in hyperactivity. There is no firm evidence from electrodermal measures, for example, that hyperactive children suffer from a deficit in arousal level. Although some investigators have reported lower basal skin conductance levels (Kløve & Hole, 1979; Satterfield & Dawson, 1971), the majority have found no differences between hyperactive children and nonhyperactive control children (e.g., Firestone & Douglas, 1975; Ferguson, Simpson, & Trites, 1976; Montagu, 1975). The results continue to be inconclusive when the subjects are actively engaged in laboratory tasks (Ferguson & Pappas, 1979). Results from studies on the effects of stimulant drugs on arousal level have also been inconclusive (e.g., Satterfield & Dawson, 1971; Zahn, Abate, Little, & Wender, 1975). However, on a frequency basis the weight of the evidence for electrodermal measures, as well as for cardiovascular measures (e.g., Porges, Walter, Korb, & Sprague, 1975; Zahn et al., 1975), leans towards underarousal that can be normalized in hyperactive children with stimulant medication.

In respect to the central indices of arousal, studies of EEG records of hyperactive children showing a positive response to stimulant medication (Knights & Hinton, 1969; Satterfield, Cantwell, Lesser, & Podosin, 1972) generally provide no support for the view that behavioral improvement from drug intervention reflects an increase in central inhibition. The data on EEG response to photic stimulation are equivocal (Ferguson & Pappas, 1979; Laufer et al., 1957; Shetty, 1971). In addition, the evoked potential literature is inconsistent on the arousal issue, with some research (Buchsbaum & Wender, 1973; Prichep, Sutton, & Hakerm, 1976) supporting the low arousal hypothesis and other studies failing to do so. The issue is further complicated by reports of interactions between age and evoked potential differences (Satterfield & Braley, 1977).

The studies of peripheral and central indices of arousal, taken together, are inconclusive on the arousal issue. Those differences that do occur appear to favor the underarousal hypothesis, the sole exception in the psychophysiological research being the Laufer et al. (1957) study that clearly supported the overarousal position. When the issue is approached from the point of view of predictions that could logically be generated from the underarousal hypothesis, the results are unacceptable. In both the Satterfield and Dawson (1979) and Zentall (1975) models, for example, the primary dysfunction in hyperactive children is underarousal of the RAS. This explanation would lead one to predict lower cortical and autonomic indices of both tonic and phasal arousal. However, hyperactive children do not exhibit consistent differences in tonic skin conductance levels and heart rates which suggests, contrary to the underarousal hypothesis, that their levels of autonomic arousal are not below normal. A second line of reasoning critical to the low RAS theory is that stimulant medications are beneficial because they increase arousal. The data do show that stimulants increase tonic autonomic levels (Cohen, Douglas, & Morgenstern, 1971; Zahn et al., 1975), as well as the magnitude of cardiac deceleration responses (Porges et al., 1975; Zahn et al., 1975), but they also appear to decrease skin conductance responses (Cohen et al., 1971; Montagu, 1975; Zahn et al., 1975), a result that is clearly inconsistent with the model of Satterfield and Dawson (1971). One possible explanation for the differing results may be that Satterfield and Dawson used Cambridge electrode jelly as the contact medium, and this hypertonic jelly is specifically formulated to increase skin conductance (Montagu, 1975). If the efficacy of stimulants is due to their ability to compensate for a phasic arousal deficit, then their effect should be an increase in skin conductance responses. Although the low arousal hypothesis in its present form is consistent with some of the empirical data, the failure to find tonic autonomic deficits, coupled with the amphetamine-induced reduction of skin conductance responses, presents a strong argument against an underarousal view of hyperactivity (Rosenthal & Allen, 1978).

INCREASED BODY-LEAD BURDEN

Lead is a trace element that has no known essential role in the human body. This useful but toxic metal occurs naturally and so widely in the ecosystem that exposure to it is almost inevitable even for fetuses (Lin-Fu, 1972; 1979). Its toxic significance for adults has been recognized for centuries: Pliny warned of the dangers of using lead pots in wine making (Gilfillan, 1965), and in the latter half of the eighteenth century Baker traced the cause of colic among cider drinkers in Devonshire to lead poisoning that developed as a result of the cider being transported in leaden pipes (Needleman, 1973). With the Industrial Revolution the dispersion of lead in the environment increased markedly, and this upward trend sharpened further after World War II (Lin-Fu, 1979). Although lead poisoning has long been recognized as an industrial disease, an increased body-lead burden, whether symptomatic or asymptomatic, is now an acknowledged residential as well as occupational hazard justifying public health concern.

Lead poisoning in children was not described until 1926, when Aub, Fairhall, Minot, and Resnikoff published a monograph on the diagnosis and treatment of this syndrome. Lead in the environment (in industrial discharge, gasoline, and food) is a far more serious and widespread pediatric problem than has previously been acknowledged (Chaiklin, 1979). The prevalence of cases of undue lead absorption in the United States is greater than that of most other pediatric health problems (Lin-Fu, 1979). Most cases of lead poisoning or elevated lead levels are associated with the eating of lead-pigment paints in deteriorating urban housing areas by preschool children characterized by pica, the tendency to ingest nonedible materials. Although lead-based paints have not been used since World War II, there are many deteriorating inner-city urban housing areas where peeling paint still contains lead pigment. A chip of paint the size of a penny can contain between 50 and 100 mg. of lead, and the repeated ingestion of a few chips a day over a 3-month period can lead to clinical symptoms and eventually to the absorption of a potentially lethal body burden of lead (Chisolm, 1976).

Another major source of lead is high octane gasoline. In the United States almost all of the 240,000 tons of lead emitted into the atmosphere each year results from the combustion of gasoline containing lead. Inner-city and suburban children may inhale lead from this source or may ingest it by eating roadway dust or snow on busy city streets (Air Quality Criteria for Lead, 1977; Minerals Yearbook, 1976). But there are other factors operating here, because children in the heavily trafficked, old homes area of Honolulu have unusually low blood lead levels, whereas those in another heavily trafficked American urban area with an acknowledged "lead belt," Newark, New Jersey, have unusually high blood lead levels (Joselow, 1974). Treatment is with a compound known as a chelating agent, which removes lead atoms from the body tissues for excretion through the kidneys and liver. Even high lead levels can be rapidly reduced to levels approaching normal with chelating agents (Chisolm, 1976).

The diagnosis of lead poisoning can be a difficult one to make because the onset of the disease is insidious in that the symptoms (e.g., fatigue, pallor, irritability, headache, anorexia, and nausea) are not distinctive, and they occur in many childhood diseases (Needleman, 1973). Consequently, a child with lead poisoning might easily be incorrectly diagnosed and treated unless the pediatrician is alert to the possibility of lead poisoning. The body-lead burden can be determined by the analysis of blood, teeth, and head hair. The blood test is simple and quick, and requires only a fingertip blood sample. The analysis is done by a nurse or paramedic using an inexpensive portable instrument developed by Bell Telephone Laboratories. However, the use of blood-lead concentration as an index of previous exposure has one serious disadvantage: it is a marker of recent exposure, and it may return to a normal level following even excessive exposure, so that as an index of past absorption or of toxicity per se it is unreliable (Chisolm, 1976). If blood-lead level is relied on to classify subjects after exposure has ceased, false negatives could be reported in clinical practice, and errors in assignment to experimental and control conditions could occur (Lin-Fu, 1979). Blood-lead levels that exceed the upper limits of normal, designated in the early 1970s as 40 μg (micrograms) per 100 ml (deciliter) of blood and later revised to 30 μg/100 ml blood (Center for Disease Control, 1978), are considered cause for concern; levels of 60 μg/100 ml or higher are viewed as diagnostic evidence of lead poisoning. However, this threshold view of toxicity is questionable, because the designation of 60 μg/100 ml blood as toxic is quite arbitrary, having been based historically on the correlation between this blood-lead level and obvious symptoms of lead poisoning (David, Clark, & Hoffman, 1979). Chaiklin (1979) has stated incorrectly that the tolerance of children for lead is probably zero, when in fact there is unequivocal evidence of great individual differences. Some children appear to be unaffected by massive blood-lead levels in the 90–100 $\mu g/100$ ml range, whereas others may suffer severe effects from relatively small blood-lead level elevations. For this reason David et al. (1979) recommend the adoption of a continuous rather than a threshold view of lead toxicity.

Dentine lead concentration is considered a more reliable lead marker because lead exists in dentine in a closed storage system. A number of studies have validated the classification of earlier lead exposure according to dentine lead levels (Needleman, Gunnoe, Leviton, Reed, Peresie, Maher, & Barrett, 1979). The dentine test requires a recently shed tooth, and is more expensive and complicated than the blood test. Hair analysis is a relatively unobtrusive procedure generally performed by neutron or photon activation analysis, atomic absorption spectometry, or particle-induced X-ray emission analysis. There are several problems with hair analysis: measurements made in different laboratories often show large variations in absolute values; the accessibility of hair to the external environment allows trace elements in addition to lead to be deposited on the surface of the hair but there is dispute concerning the optimum method for removal of these external contaminants. The concentration of trace elements generally increases with increasing distance from the scalp, so there may be a 30-fold difference in concentration of some elements on opposite ends of a single hair (Maugh, 1978).

Children with confirmed lead poisoning often sustain severe neurological and psychological sequelae, one of the latter being a behavioral pattern of hyperactivity, short attention span, and impulsivity (Byers & Lord, 1943; Rummo, Routh, Rummo, & Brown, 1979). Children with elevated body-lead burdens below the level needed to produce overt symptoms of toxicity also exhibit hyperactive patterns of behavior, a finding that has unequivocal support in the series of studies by David and his associates (David, 1974; David, Clark, & Hoffman, 1979; David, Clark, & Voeller, 1972; David, Hoffman, & Koltun, 1978; David, Hoffman, Sverd, & Clark, 1977; David, Hoffman, Sverd, Clark, & Voeller, 1976). In 1972 David and his colleagues (David et al., 1972) provided the first well-documented evidence that lead absorption at even relatively low levels might be implicated in the etiology of hyperactivity. In this study children were designated as hyperactive on the basis of one or more of the following: a doctor's diagnosis, a teacher's rating scale, and a parent questionnaire. The hyperactive children were then assigned to the following groups: *pure hyperactive*, with no evidence of any event known to be associated with the hyperactivity; *highly probable cause of hyperactivity*, such as prenatal or perinatal complications; *possible cause*, in which there was a history of an event that could have resulted in hyperactivity; and a *history of lead poisoning* that had been treated. In addition to these hyperactive subgroups, there was a control group of nonhyperactive children. Overall, the hyperactive children had significantly higher values than the controls on blood and urine measures of body lead taken after challenge by a single oral dose of the chelating agent penicillamine and on ratings on a lead exposure questionnaire, thus supporting the hypothesis of a relationship between hyperactivity and a concomitant condition of increased body lead stores. Since these findings suggested that many of the hyperactive children had probably had increased, but not toxic, lead stores for some time, and that one consequence of such a long-term minimal poisonous assault might be hyperactivity, David and his colleagues examined the subgroup results for support for the assumption that lead poisoning might cause hyperactivity and found two comparisons supporting this possibility. First, the *highly probable cause group* did not differ in lead values from the controls, a finding that would be expected since there was a likely cause of the hyperactivity in this group and it was not lead poisoning. Second, the *pure hyperactives* (no known cause but no reason why it could not be lead-associated) showed significantly raised lead levels as compared to the controls. A sobering finding about the eight children in the *lead poisoning group*, all but one of whom had had chelation therapy five years previously, was that they all had elevated blood and urine levels, indicating that the chelation therapy and follow-up procedures had been inadequate, or that the children had subsequently been reexposed to lead, or as David et al. (1972) have suggested, that hyperactivity may not be an after-effect of lead poisoning, but might instead be a condition dependent upon continuing nontoxic elevations of body lead.

The possibility that chronically elevated body-lead burdens below the level considered to be toxic (25 to 40 μg/100 ml blood) might be directly etiological in some cases of hyperactivity received further support from a study (David et al., 1976) of behavioral response to chelation. Of the 13 hyperactive school children with elevated blood and urine lead levels treated with chelating agents, six had histories of etiologically relevant perinatal or developmental complications and showed relatively little improvement, whereas the remaining seven, with unremarkable histories that allowed a lead etiology explanation, showed marked improvement. David et al. concluded that lead could be etiologically related to some cases of hyperactivity and urged that lead level measurements be included in the medical workup of hyperactivity.

Although the above data constitute support for an elevated body lead-hyperactivity causal association, the data are equivocal as to the direction of causality. Is lead the causative agent of the hyperactivity? Or does being hyperactive lead to the acquisition of an elevated body-lead burden (David et al., 1972; Lansdown, Shepherd, Clayton, Delves, Graham, & Turner, 1974)? If being hyperactive predisposes a child to accumulate undue body lead, then all hyperactive children, regardless of etiology, should manifest increased body-lead burdens. The data in the original study (David et al., 1972) and a subsequent one (David et al., 1977) provide no support for this hypothesis. Children with probable causes for their hyperactivity had significantly lower body-lead burdens than did children with no known cause. However, an intriguing finding in the latter study was that these two groups did not differ on amount of exposure to situations in which body-lead burdens could have been acquired. Assuming that the lead-exposure questionnaire had validity as an index of lead exposure, this similarity suggests that the group differences in lead levels may be a function of differences in ability to excrete lead that has been ingested, or of some inadvertent differential intervention such as mothers in the low-lead group feeding their children foods with naturally occurring chelating agents.

In a study using dentine lead content as a marker of previous exposure, rather than the less stable blood-lead analysis, Needleman et al. (1979) found that amounts of lead well below those previously considered hazardous could adversely affect the school behavior and intelligence of young children. The frequency of nonadaptive classroom behavior such as hyperactivity, impulsivity, daydreaming, distractibility, and poor attention span was not limited to children in the high lead level group, but instead increased in a dose-related fashion to dentine lead content. In addition to exhibiting these kinds of behavior, those children with high dentine lead content performed significantly less well on the Wechsler Intelligence Scale for Children (Revised) (WISC-R), and high lead was also associated with lower paternal education. An earlier study (MacIsaac, 1976) showed similar results with black school children living in the lead belt of Newark, New Jersey, who were tested with the Wechsler Preschool and Primary Scale of Intelligence (WPPSI). In a follow-up of these children, Duva (1977) found poorer performance on the WISC-R and an association between increased body lead and lower parental educational level. Rummo and his colleagues (Rummo et al., 1979) reported that preschool and primary grade children with increased body-lead burdens were more hyperactive, more retarded intellectually, and also had a higher incidence of neurological deficits than a matched control group. The results of this cluster of studies suggest that many young urban school children who exhibit adverse behavior and impaired intellectual functioning may be suffering from the effects of asymptomatic lead poisoning.

A causal relationship between high levels of activity and lead has been reported in animal studies by Silbergeld and Goldberg (1973, 1974). In the first of these, one group of mice was given one of three concentrations of lead in their drinking water from birth, and a second group was given sodium acetate. Activity level was measured for four consecutive days when the mice were between 40 and 60 days old. Mice who had ingested lead were more than three times as active as the controls, and similar findings with rats were obtained by Sauerhoff and Michaelson (1973). Silbergeld and Goldberg consider this finding to be conclusive evidence of a causal relationship between chronic ingestion of lead and a high level of activity in mice. The fact that the lead-induced high level of activity was not dose-related, at least in the range of doses used, coupled with the fact that there were no deaths in the experimental group, suggests that increases in motor activity may be a symptom that occurs early in the period of exposure when the body level is increased but not toxic. Also, increases in the amount of lead given to the mice produced other sequelae of lead intoxication, such as peripheral ataxia and splayed gait. In a second study, Silbergeld and Goldberg (1974) replicated the causal relationship between lead ingestion and hyperactivity in mice and then administered to both the lead-treated and control group mice three stimulant drugs (dextroamphetamine, levoamphetamine, and methyphenidate) that are used in the treatment of hyperactivity, and also chloral hydrate and phenobarbital, which is contraindicated in hyperactive children because it exacerbates their hyperactivity. Lead-treated mice responded with decreased hyperactivity to the three stimulant medications and with increased levels of activity to the phenobarbital. Controls showed an increase in activity with the amphetamines and a decrease with phenobarbital. Chloral hydrate effected an equal decrease in activity level in the experimental and control groups. Related work by Sobotka and Cook (1974), in which rats were subjected to early lead exposure, has demonstrated a reduction of motor activity and an alleviation of a performance deficit on a two-way shuttle task with amphetamine treatment. These investigators concurred with Silbergeld and Goldberg (1974) that perinatal lead exposure might be etiologically related to some forms of minimal brain dysfunction. The parallels between this animal model of hyperactivity and the clinical description of hyperactivity suggest that lead may be an etiological agent in the hyperactivity of children in urban areas. The fact that Silbergeld and Goldberg (1973, 1974) have produced and replicated a lead-induced animal model of hyperactivity, and demonstrated a striking parallel between the efficacy of stimulant medication at the infrahuman level and at the human level, represents a potentially major contribution to knowledge about the etiology and treatment of hyperactivity. An extension of their animal model would be of value in determining if the toxic effects, particularly the hyperactivity, are reversible with chelation therapy, and if this reversal, once accomplished, is maintained as long as there is no further exposure to toxic levels of lead.

The mechanism that might mediate an association between increased lead absorption and hyperactivity has not yet been identified. It is likely that neuropsychological impairment is involved because, as Silbergeld and Adler (1978) have pointed out, even a low concentration of lead can penetrate the neuron and have adverse effects on neuronal ion metabolism. The pathways that mediate inhibition in the brain are also highly sensitive to lead and use gamma-aminobutyric acid (GABA) as a transmitter. There is evidence that the disinhibitory effects of lead may be mediated by increased levels of delta-amino-levulinic acid (ALA), which itself can inhibit GABA-ergic function (Lin-Fu, 1979). At this point, however, the possibility of neuropsychological impairment in children with increased lead absorption and no clinical symptoms is difficult to detect because sensitive biochemical indicators of the effects of lead on the nervous system have not yet been identified.

The relationship between many neuropsychiatric disorders and metabolic abnormalities of the biogenic amines has led to investigations of a possible disorder in the monoamine (serotonin) system. Conclusive evidence for such a disorder is lacking. Some fragmentary support for a relationship between disorders in serotonin metabolism and hyperactivity has been reported (e.g., Coleman, 1971; Bhagavan et al., 1975) but the majority of investigations (e.g., Rapoport, Quinn, Scribano, & Murphy, 1974; Shaywitz et al., 1977; Shetty & Chase, 1976) provide no support for such an association.

Silbergeld and Chisolm (1976) have reported data on both animals and children that support an association between increased lead absorption and the enhancement of catecholamine (dopamine and nonepinephrine) function. Long-term postnatal exposure of mice to lead resulted in a marked increase of urinary output and brain levels of two catecholamine metabolites—vanillymandelic acid (VMA) and homovanillic acid (HVA). These results, which are consistent with other reports of enhanced catecholamine function in experimental lead poisoning in animals (Golter & Michaelson, 1975; Silbergeld & Goldberg, 1974), are interpreted by Silbergeld and Chisolm (1976) as evidence of alterations in both peripheral and central catecholamine metabolism. Preliminary clinical data from children are consistent with the foregoing findings of increased urinary output of HVA and VMA. Asymptomatic and mildly symptomatic children with increased lead absorption excreted five times as much HVA and VMA in their urine (collected quantitatively under controlled dietary conditions) than did controls without undue lead exposure. In the latter group the values of these metabolites were in agreement with published data for healthy nonclinical children; in the increased lead absorption group the degree of metabolite elevation was comparable with that reported for children with tumors of the sympathetic nervous system. These data suggest that the altered catecholamine metabolism demonstrated in mice with experimental subclinical lead poisoning also occurs in children with increased lead absorption. The value of these preliminary data lies in their identification of neurochemical indicators of the effect of lead on the sympathetic nervous system. Further research is needed to determine the nature of the change in catecholamine metabolism, its significance to catecholamine function, and a dose-effect relationship for this change (Silbergeld & Chisolm, 1976).

In a critical review of the research on increased lead levels Rutter (1980) concluded that the quality of the research was singularly lacking and that the findings did not point specifically to a hyperactivity-increased body lead link but rather to a possible association between more general behavior problems and raised lead levels. We disagree with this conclusion. The research in this relatively new area of investigation has been beset with methodological difficulties and questions of prime importance, for example, the mechanism mediating a hyperactivity-increased lead level link remains to be identified. Despite these problems, it is our opinion that there has been sufficient research of a methodologically sound nature in the past decade to support the assumption that undue lead absorption is *implicated* in childhood hyperactivity. Further, we contend that the existing body of clinical reports and empirical data demands intensive activity on the research front, particularly in the arena of pediatric care. Although the identification of the mechanism linking undue lead absorption to hyperactivity is of theoretical as well as practical importance, the crucial task is prevention. Lead poisoning and undue lead absorption in children are preventable. As Needleman (1973) has pointed out, the economic costs of prevention are formidable. A program of lead-poisoning prevention would require cooperative and persistent action at federal, state, and local levels. The notable absence of such a program reflects the national philosophy of emphasis and dependence on treatment rather than prevention. The issue also comes down to one of priorities, of balancing the economic and social costs of having an increasing number of temporarily and permanently impaired children living in various degrees of avoidable misery, against the cost of implementing a nationwide prevention program for which all the essential information is available now.

RADIATION STRESS

Ott (1968, 1976) has hypothesized that hyperactivity may be a radiation stress condition that results from exposure to conventional fluorescent lighting and certain conditions of television viewing. According to this radiation stress hypothesis, the conventional fluorescent lighting typically used in schools and offices is harmful because it gives off soft X-rays through the cathode ray guns at the ends of all fluorescent tubes, and it is inadequate because it lacks certain of the long ultraviolet wavelengths of the natural light spectrum that are essential to humans. Ott believes that the conventional fluorescent lighting and unshielded TV cathode tubes may result in sufficient radiation exposure to directly cause hyperactivity, or may serve as environmental stressors that alter the body so that hyperactivity results (Ott, 1968). His premise that these sources of radiation might directly or indirectly cause hyperactivity is based on research with animals. Frey (1965) found that animals experienced behavioral changes and transient effects in the central nervous system following repeated exposure to radio and television frequencies; Hartley (1974) reported that rats who were placed in front of a color television set with standard (unshielded) cathode tubes became hyperactive within three to 10 days, remained hyperactive until the thirtieth day of radiation exposure, and then became lethargic and died, whereas rats who were exposed to the same conditions with lead-shielded cathode tubes showed no change in either behavior or physical well-being. These findings were replicated in two subsequent studies in the same laboratory. Further support for an association between radiation and hyperactivity comes from a case study (Hartley, 1974) in which an exceedingly hyperactive girl was found to be exposed for long periods to the radiation leak from a television set that was placed against a living room wall so that the set was separated from the head of her bed by the wall between the adjacent rooms. When lead shields were put on the television tubes, the girl's behavior began to calm down and eventually returned to normal.

These and similar findings led to an investigation of the effects of shielded versus standard unshielded fluorescent lights on established cases of hyperactivity in children. In a 90-day experiment with primary school children, Mayron, Ott, Nations, and Mayron (1974) compared the effects of conventional and improved fluorescent lighting in four windowless first-grade classrooms. Two were illuminated with standard cool white fluorescent lights and two with fluorescent lighting having three special features: long ultraviolet wavelengths present in sunlight, lead foil shields over their cathode ends to keep X-rays from escaping, and a wire grid screen over their entirety to ground radio frequencies. In all four classes there were some hyperactive children who were scheduled for transfer to special classes because they were unable to function in the regular class setting. Time-lapse pictures and teacher reports showed that the disruptive behavior, irritability, and poor attention spans of the hyperactive children working in full spectrum, shielded fluorescent lighting diminished so sharply that special class placement was not required. No change occurred in the behavior of the hyperactive children in the two classes with conventional fluorescent lighting. Mayron et al. concluded that the improvements in the hyperactive children could be attributed to the full spectrum lighting rather than to other environmental or social factors, such as differences in teacher efficiency.

Several serious methodological weaknesses make it difficult to accept this conclusion. The criteria for labeling a child as hyperactive were not provided, and hyperactivity in the classroom is a quantitative change-in-activity variable with no consideration being given to the appropriateness of the activity. The observational methodology was not specified with respect to film rater blindness, reliability of ratings, and other details. There were no controls to ensure equivalence of illumination level and brightness across conditions, both of which could affect attention (O'Leary, Rosenbaum, & Hughes, 1978a), and the use of procedures to minimize teacher differences over the 90-day period was not specified.

O'Leary et al., (1978a) investigated the effect of full-spectrum lighting in a study that differed from that of Mayron et al. (1974) in several critical respects: type of subject, length of intervention, observational procedures, lighting system, and use of controls for illumination levels and teacher differences. The subjects were seven first-grade children with conduct disorders or hyperactivity who were attending full-day sessions in a laboratory school classroom. During an 8-week period the classroom lighting conditions alternated every week as follows: in odd-numbered weeks illumination was provided with a standard cool white fluorescent system; in even-numbered weeks a broad-spectrum daylight-simulating illumination was used that was functionally equivalent to the full spectrum lighting used by Mayron et al. (1974). To ensure equivalent illumination at each desk and across conditions, additional lighting was included. Lighting conditions had no effect on hyperactive behavior as measured by ratings of activity level and independent observations of task orientation. There was increasing evidence across time of an association between full spectrum lighting and sensory visual fatigue.

In a commentary on these findings, Mayron (1978) stated that the differences in subject population, length of study, type of lighting, and experimental design made comparisons between the two studies pointless, but added that a replication of his group's study would be welcomed. In a sharp rejoinder to the Mayron commentary, O'Leary et al. (1978b) pointed out that they did not feel that the replication of a methodologically flawed study was advisable. Further, they described their study as a *systematic* replication, that is, intended to extend the generality of the lighting effect with population and procedural variations, as distinguished from a *direct* replication which can establish the generality of a phenomenon with a particular population (Sidman, 1960). It is our opinion that the Mayron et al. (1974) study has weaknesses that invalidate the conclusions, and that the O'Leary et al. (1978a) study has not clarified the issues of concern here. At this point, a systematic replication is premature since documented information about effect of lighting on hyperactivity is virtually nonexistent. One reason for the relatively slow progress in understanding the etiology of hyperactivity is that interesting possibilities are investigated but no attempt is made to first document the preliminary findings. Instead of doing this, other investigators go off in new directions and then interpret negative findings as grounds for refuting the original findings. What is needed in the case here is a direct replication of the Mayron et al. procedure but with the methodological weaknesses remedied within the framework of the initial experiment. The 90-day period under unchanging conditions, for example, would be an essential factor since the cumulative effects of long-term exposure may be critical. In any event, rigorous investigation of the radiation stress hypothesis (Ott, 1968) is needed not only to determine whether radiation stress is etiologically related to hyperactivity but also to investigate the amount of radiation exposure that occurs for any child who works under fluorescent lights at school followed by long hours at home of television viewing close to the set.

FOOD ADDITIVES

In a 1973 report (Feingold, German, Brahm, & Simmers, 1973) to the American Medical Association, Feingold proposed that naturally occurring salicylates in fruits, vegetables, and other foods, artificial food colorings, and preservatives could in genetically predisposed children produce a toxic reaction of cerebral irritability with the behavioral symptoms of childhood hyperactivity. In subsequent revisions of this hypothesis (Feingold, 1975b, 1976a), the relative importance of naturally occurring salicylates lessened, and the role of two antioxidant preservatives BHA (butylated hydroxyanisole) and BHT (butylated hydroxytoluene) was emphasized (Feingold & Feingold, 1979). The hypothesized food additive-hyperactivity link represents a *toxic* rather than an *allergic* effect; evidence for the latter effect for a small proportion of hyperactive children remains equivocal (Conners, 1980; Taylor, 1979; Trites, Tryphonas, & Ferguson, 1980). Taylor (1979, p. 357) has also stressed the distinction between these two effects:

> . . . the intolerance of food additives . . . is not an allergy, but a toxic effect. The difference is worth emphasizing. A toxin causes damage to the body directly. An allergy, by contrast, is an alteration of the body's response to a substance. It is produced by the immunological defense mechanisms. It is not shown in the first encounter with the allergen, but only in later contacts. In Feingold's hypothesis, the toxic effect is supposed to be apparent only in predisposed individuals and so the notion of an idiosyncratic response is still present.

The mechanism underlying this toxic effect has been the subject of considerable speculation (Feingold, 1975a, 1975b, 1976a). There is some evidence that children who appear to be affected by food additives may differ biochemically from those who are unaffected (Brenner, 1979). Further evidence for a biochemical factor in the food additive-hyperactivity link comes from reports (Augustine & Levitan, 1980; Lafferman & Silbergeld, 1979; Logan & Swanson, 1979) that low concentrations of a food dye, called Red No. 3 or erythrosin B, which is widely used in candy, powdered desserts, and beverages, partially prevents brain cells from taking in dopamine, a substance that is known to have profound effects on motor activity. Lafferman and Silbergeld (1979) concluded that the food dye's blocking of dopamine is consistent with the idea that this dye can induce hyperactivity in some children.

The primary focus of clinical and research interest, however, has not been on the mechanism of toxic effect but rather on the effects of the Feingold diet on behavior. Feingold has repeatedly made dramatic, highly specific, and empirically unsubstantiated claims concerning the efficacy of the diet: the extent of reported improvement varies in different statements but a representative figure is the report (Feingold, 1975a) that 30 to 50 percent of the hyperactive children in his practice displayed complete remission of symptoms as a result of following the diet. The degree and rapidity of response to it appeared to be a function of age: the younger the child, the more rapid and complete the improvement. On the basis of his own nonempirical data and that of other investigators, Feingold (1973, 1975a, 1975b) also stated that the diet-induced reduction in hyperactive symptoms was followed by markedly improved academic achievement and motor coordination, particularly in writing, drawing, speech, and gross motor activities, and by a lessening notably in younger children of perceptual-cognitive disturbances.

The immediate effect of Feingold's statements was a surge of newspaper and television publicity followed directly by public acceptance of them as established fact (Bierman & Furukawa, 1978). They were also read into the U.S. Congressional Record (Beall, 1973). The food industry, however, perceived the claims as a threat to its multimillion dollar processed food market and quickly assembled a committee to review the evidence; the Food and Drug Administration organized a second committee for the same purpose. Both groups cautiously concluded that there was no empirical evidence for the hyperactivity-food additive link or the behavioral improvement ascribed to the diet, and recommended further empirical investigations of the diet (Bierman & Furukawa, 1978). The resulting clash of vested interests created extensive research interest in the Feingold diet on the part of the scientific community (Taylor, 1979). The attempts at evaluating the diet's efficacy fall into three groups: uncontrolled studies and clinical reports, diet crossover studies, and specific challenge experiments.

Uncontrolled Studies

For the most part the studies in this group (e.g., Cook & Woodhill, 1976; Crook, 1980; O'Shea, 1979; Salzman, 1976) reflect a consistent phenomenon in Feingold diet research, namely, striking improvement when the Feingold diet is initiated nonblind (Conners, 1980), coupled with serious methodological shortcomings. For example, Salzman (1976), in a methodologically weak study of 15 hyperactive children placed on the Feingold diet, reported significant behavioral improvement. Although his selection procedure was excellent, information concerning the diagnosis of hyperactivity, identification of allergies, and diet compliance was insufficient; and the preliminary instructions to parents (Salzman, 1976, p. 249) were virtually certain to cause expectancy effects:

> ... if the diet was going to have an effect, they would see the results within four weeks, and if the child violated the diet his behavior would return to the pre-diet condition within two to four hours and remain that way for up to 96 hours.

The flagrant methodological defects in the Salzman (1976) study and in one by Cook and Woodhill (1976) led Werry (1976, p. 282) to comment that "their conclusions ... are susceptible to alternative explanations of spontaneous remission, placebo effect, measurement drift or even straight-out random error." One very interesting uncontrolled study was a case report (Stine, 1976) of two hyperactive preschool boys who, as a last resort, were treated with the Feingold diet. Both boys showed a slow, gradual amelioration of the target symptoms, rather than the sudden dramatic effect that Feingold (1975a) has described.

Diet Crossover Studies

In this design two groups of hyperactive children are randomly assigned by group to two different experimental diet conditions, one of which is the Feingold diet. The groups remain on each diet for a specific period of time, usually several weeks, without knowing which diet they are on; both diets appear to be the Feingold, but only one contains salicylates, artificial food colors and flavors, and antioxidants. While they are on each diet, measures are obtained of the subjects' behavior: if hyperactivity diminishes when a group is on the Feingold diet, then this constitutes support for this diet. Inherent in this design are a number of methodological difficulties: there is the problem of ensuring that neither parents nor children break the blind, of evaluating carryover effects, and of controlling for placebo factors and social environmental effects. This design was used by a team from Wisconsin (Harley, Ray, Tomasi, Eichman, Matthews, Chun, Cleeland, & Traisman, 1978) in a study, with 36 school-age and 10 preschool boys. Extraordinary care was taken to ensure compliance and to maintain blindness, and multiple outcome measures were obtained in classroom and laboratory settings. There was no evidence of an advantage for the Feingold diet for the 36 school-age boys. The frequency of reported positive diet effects was highest in the parent ratings, but declined sharply in the teacher ratings. There was no evidence of a favorable diet response in the objective tests and observational data. Also, favorable parent reports occurred only in the placebo-challenge sequence, not in the challenge-placebo sequence. The results for the group of 10 preschool children showed some support for the efficacy of the Feingold diet regimen on one of the dependent variables, mothers' reports, but not on the other dependent variable, neuropsychological tests. In addition to the failure to obtain strong support, the small sample size and other methodological problems caused the Wisconsin group to view the results with extreme caution and withhold a conclusive judgment pending the outcome of a specific challenge experiment, a more rigorous procedure for investigating the possibility of improvement in subgroups.

Two other crossover studies should be briefly noted. In the first one a Pittsburgh team of investigators (Conners, Goyette, Southwick, Lees, & Andrulonis, 1976) reported improvement in five children in the control diet-Feingold sequence and then *only* on teacher ratings. Although Conners et al. (1976) viewed these findings as providing some support for the Feingold diet, Sprague (1976) questioned this interpretation on the grounds of methodological shortcomings in diet comparability and blindness of parents and teachers and, most serious of all, inadequacies in the statistical analyses. For these reasons the findings should not be interpreted as support for the Feingold diet. The second study was a careful 10-week, double-blind multiple crossover study conducted by Mattes and Gittelman-Klein (1978) with a 10-year-old hyperactive child who had a history of marked positive responsiveness to the Feingold diet and of dramatic deterioration with diet violation. The child's behavior was rated by his mother, teacher, and himself on the Conners Abbreviated Teacher Rating Scale and each participant also tried to guess each week if the color-containing cookies were active or placebo. The mother guessed correctly beyond chance throughout the study. Preliminary trials were used to establish the dose-response relationship, and an intensive multiple crossover procedure permitted statistical analysis. The results failed to support a causative link between food colorings and hyperactivity symptomatology, an outcome all the more surprising because the design of the study favored the possibility of demonstrating a diet effect.

Specific Challenge Studies

In the basic methodology for a specific challenge study a group of children is selected who have been rated as responding with reduced hyperactivity to the Feingold diet. They are then divided into an experimental and a control group, both of which are fed the Feingold diet. The experimental group is also fed a challenge food that appears to meet the Feingold diet guidelines, but in reality contains prohibited ingredients such as food colorings; the control group is fed a matching food with none of the prohibited ingredients. The behavior of the groups is observed, tested, and compared. Often there is a second testing period, during which the treatment conditions for the two groups are reversed so that every child in the study is challenged. There are two modifications of this basic challenge methodology: In the first of these a single group of children is given the challenge and placebo food in a random sequence throughout a single testing period; and in the second, a diet crossover study and a specific challenge experiment can be carried out sequentially as a two-stage research project. The subgroup of children in the crossover study who show a reduction in hyperactivity on the Feingold diet then become the entire sample for the specific challenge experiment.

Two specific challenge experiments were carried out by the Pittsburgh group (Goyette, Conners, Petti, & Curtis, 1978). In the first of these, 15 school-aged hyperactive children who had previously shown a reduction in hyperactivity on the Feingold diet and who continued to demonstrate less hyperactivity in the Feingold condition, showed no significant challenge effect either on a visual motor tracking test or according to teachers' and parents' observations when Nutrition Foundation challenge cookies containing 27 mg of food colors (the amount estimated to equal the American child's daily consumption of artificial food colors) were included in their diets. Because three of the younger children in the study did appear to be responsive to food colors, a second smaller specific challenge study was conducted with eight young hyperactive children, all of whom had improved on the Feingold, according to parental report. With only the parents as observers, this study supported the Feingold theory, leading Goyette et al. (1978) to conclude that artificial food dyes may be particularly disruptive to younger children.

In the second phase (Harley, Matthews, & Eichman, 1978) of the earlier Wisconsin study (Harley et al., 1978) the nine hyperactive boys who had shown the most favorable response to diet manipulation in the earlier study were repeatedly challenged with specified amounts of placebo and food items containing artificial color, while being maintained on a strict Feingold diet over an 11-week period. Classroom behavior observations, teacher and parent ratings, and neuropsychological test scores obtained during the baseline, challenge, and placebo conditions, showed no adverse effects of challenge materials. Teachers as well as parents frequently rated the children as *more* hyperactive during the periods in which color-free food was ingested. In considering the conflicting conclusions from the Wisconsin and Pittsburgh studies, it should be noted that the Wisconsin study offered closer diet supervision, was more effective in disguising the diet, used more dependent measures, and had a larger sample. These methodological strengths would suggest that the Wisconsin results have the greater validity.

Several other challenge experiments merit consideration. A carefully conducted study by Mattes and Gittelman-Klein (1981) with reported Feingold diet responders yielded no evidence for the food coloring-hyperactivity link in evaluations made by parents, teachers, psychiatrists, and psychologists. The investigators used procedures designed to maximize the probability of demonstrating behavioral effects: attempts were made to exclude placebo responders, for example, and a high per diem dosage of coloring (78 mg) was used.

Weiss and his associates (Weiss, Williams, Margen, Abrams, Caan, Citron, Cox, McKibben, Oga, & Schultz, 1980) conducted an 11-week test of the Feingold diet with 22 children ranging in age from two to seven years, none of whom had been diagnosed as hyperactive. The study was conducted as a double-blind trial with each child serving as his own control and parents' observations providing the criteria of response. At a specified time on each of the 77 days, each child drank a bottle of the challenge material or substitute, both of which were disguised as a soft drink. The challenge drink had 35.6 mg of artificial colors, a slightly higher content than that used in previous studies. The finding that one child responded mildly and one dramatically to the challenge led Weiss et al. (1980, p. 1488) to conclude that "modest doses of synthetic colors can provoke disturbed behavior in children." The Weiss et al. study has elicited an incisive critical analysis from Wender (1980) centering on the diagnostic procedures used, the possibility that the parents could distinguish between the active and placebo challenge, the dependence on parental opinion, and the somewhat sweeping conclusions. A sharp rebuttal by Weiss (1980) implied that Wender's position was based, among other things, on "misleading allegations," "invalid insinuations," "an uncritical appraisal of the literature," and "insensitivity to the toxicological issues." We agree with Wender's major points. Further, we do not dispute the importance of research on the issue of behavioral toxicity from food additives; we merely wish to emphasize that an issue of such "societal importance" merits a methodologically rigorous test, beginning on a small scholarly scale with carefully conducted single-subject studies, rather than with a cluster of "22 separate experiments" (Weiss, 1980, p. 1488).

Meanwhile, Swanson and Kinsbourne (1980b) conducted a 6-day challenge study in which the subjects were 20 children who had been classified as hyperactive on the Conners Rating Scale and whose hyperactivity was known to be modifiable by stimulant drugs, and 20 children for whom the diagnosis of hyperactivity had been rejected on the basis of a Conners score of under 15, and who were known to react adversely to stimulant drugs. Following three days free of food dyes and other additives, counterbalanced heavy loads of food dyes (100 or 150 mg) or placebo were administered on the fourth and fifth days. The performance of the nonhyperactive group on paired-associate learning tests the day they received the dye blend was reported as not affected by the food dye challenge relative to their performance after placebo. By contrast, the performance of the hyperactive children was reported as impaired: their scores began to show the effects of the high dose of food dyes in 30 minutes, reached a maximum in 90 minutes, and lasted at least 3½ hours. Swanson and Kinsbourne interpreted their data as suggesting that a large dose of food dye decreases attention span in hyperactive children as reflected in increased errors on a paired-associate learning task.

The methodology in the Swanson and Kinsbourne (1980b) study has been sharply criticized by Wender (1980), Ferguson, Rapoport, and Weingartner (1981), and others (e.g., Mattes & Gittelman-Klein, 1981), with major criticisms centering on the use of drug response as a confirmatory criterion for a diagnosis of hyperactivity, the criteria for medication response, the failure to show that the hyperactive children in the challenge test had previously responded favorably to the Feingold diet under controlled conditions, and the fact that the performance of the nonhyperactive controls appeared in the final test session to be as affected by the food dye challenge as that of the hyperactive children. Swanson and Kinsbourne (1980c) countered with a defense of their procedure and an additional data analysis showing that even when all 70 children were treated as one group, there was statistical support for the conclusion that a large dose of a blend of food dyes impaired performance on a learning test; but the fact remains that their study has serious flaws. Yet the methodological shortcomings in the Swanson and Kinsbourne study should not be allowed to denigrate the potential importance of the fundamental question addressed, which is whether food dyes can induce disordered behavior *at all*. With increasing numbers of nonnutritional substances being used in foods, the neurobehavioral effects of chemicals is rapidly becoming an investigative area of some importance.

Taken together, the specific challenge data suggest that a small number of hyperactive children, but many fewer than the 30 to 50 percent figure claimed by Feingold, reportedly benefit by showing a reduction in hyperactivity while on the Feingold diet. This small group *appears* to include many young children. If true, this effect would be highly advantageous because hyperactive preschool children do not respond well to stimulant medications, and most authorities (Cantwell, 1979; Werry, 1977) advise against prescribing them. In addition, the diet would present fewer management difficulties, since preschool children are under more stringent parental control and surveillance.

A larger group of hyperactive children reportedly benefit from the Feingold diet but do not react to the challenge, that is, the artificial food colors given these children do not make them more hyperactive, and therefore the elimination of these colors is not responsible for the reported improvement. The question then is, What is it about the Feingold diet that causes the improvement? Feingold attributes all observed behavioral changes to the food substances eliminated from the diet, a simplistic approach that ignores the impact that the diet has on other aspects of the child's life. One possibility concerns the effect the parents' expectations for the diet therapy might have on their perception of their child's hyperactivity. As Harley, Matthews, and Eichman (1978, p. 982) have pointed out, it is likely that

> the numerous Feingold associations that have been established across the country may also contribute to a positive expectancy effect and to a collective parental identity and conviction of making common cause against exploitation by a malevolent food industry complex.

The publicity issued by the Feingold Association strengthens these expectancies. After Goyette et al. (1978) concluded that artificial food dyes may be particularly disrupting for younger children and called for more research on why preschoolers react differently, the Feingold Association issued an enthusiastic press release announcing that these findings meant that a simple nutritious diet will turn a "problem-plagued existence" into a normal life for most hyperactive children (Divoky, 1978). Other possibilities include the placebo effect, the change for the better in nutritional status since this diet is probably better than what the family has been eating, aspects of family dynamics such as the impact on the child of all the attention and interest, the fact that the hypothesis itself is a parsimonious one and that the prescribed diet is characterized by relatively low cost and safety (as opposed to the danger of drugs). It provides parents with an alternative to medication and, because it is identified with outside causative agents, it helps to minimize their feelings of self-blame. Our culture, with its emphasis on diet, health food fads, and the like, is predisposed to accept this form of treatment.

Another question that should be raised concerns whether or not this major dietary change is justified in the light of the few children who appear to improve. On the negative side is the possibility that other kinds of helpful treatment for the child's hyperactivity may be ignored. Also the diet teaches the child that his behavior is controlled by what he eats and so focuses undue attention on food and eating, with the possibility that food could become a symbol of punishment to him. In a review of the relationship between diet and hyperactivity, Stare, Whelan, and Sheridan (1980) concluded that the danger of teaching the child that his behavior is controlled by what he eats far outweighs the possible benefits from the diet.

In 1980, two important evaluative statements on the Feingold diet were made. The National Advisory Committee on Hyperkinesis and Food Additives (1980) stated their conclusions in the following terms:

> It is our opinion that studies already completed provide sufficient evidence to refute the claim that artificial food colorings, artificial flavorings and salicylates produce hyperactivity and/or learning disability.

> We see no indication, based on the evidence, for the continuation of high
> priority, specially funded programs for further investigation in this area.

In a succinct, objective, and clearly written discussion of the Feingold controversy, Conners (1980, p. 109) concluded:

> On the basis of all the evidence available at this time, in answer to the ques-
> tion, "Is there anything to Dr. Feingold's hypothesis?" one might answer, "Yes,
> something—but not much and not consistently."

In general, Conners' findings agree with those of the National Advisory Committee. The difference between these two expert opinions lies in Conners' reluctance to close the door on further research. Instead he points to various
major and lesser research topics, for example, the need to establish empirically the level of food dye dosages that accurately reflects daily consumption of
such dyes and to study their effects on brain chemistry, and to look into the
suggestion that diet-related improvement occurs more frequently in children
without serious home problems, and recommends further limited empirical
investigations. We concur with Conners. It is important not to allow the
"gross overstatements by Dr. Feingold" (Conners, 1980, p. 109) and the excessive number of methodologically weak studies to blind investigators to
other possibilities: that for a subgroup of hyperactive children the Feingold
diet represents optimal management; that the effects of food dyes on brain
chemistry may have profound implications for the field of child psychopathology; that seemingly innocuous food substances such as milk (Trites et al.,
1980) or sugar (Prinz, Roberts, & Hantman, 1980) may be implicated; and
that megavitamin therapy and other orthomolecular approaches may benefit
some hyperactive children (Arnold, Christopher, Huestis, & Smeltzer, 1978b;
Trites, 1981). As such, these research topics merit careful investigation. The
Conners text will be of great value to researchers, clinicians, and interested
laymen. To date, it represents one of the most important contributions to the
Feingold controversy.

FETAL ALCOHOL SYNDROME

There is widespread evidence that prenatal exposure to certain drugs and environmental agents can cause abnormal embryonic development that results
in teratogenesis, that is, physical malformations. In the past decade there has
been increasing evidence that teratogens may induce behavioral abnormalities
in offspring as well as physical malformations (Vorhees, Brunner, & Butcher,
1979). Although alcohol has been a suspected teratogen for centuries, it is
only with the recent work of a French research team (Lemoine, Harrousseau,
& Borteyru, 1968) and the independent observations of an American investigator and his group (Jones, Smith, Ulleland, & Streissguth, 1973) that the

existence of a variable pattern of fetal malformation etiologically related to maternal alcohol intake during pregnancy has been established and described in the medical literature, with subsequent additional documentation in numerous reports from other parts of the world (e.g., Barry & O'Naullain, 1975; Ferrier, Nicod, & Ferrier, 1973). This pattern of malformation, termed the *fetal alcohol syndrome* by Jones et al. (1973), ranges from full to partial expression. In its most severe form, having a frequency between one and two live births per 1000 (Clarren & Smith, 1978b), an irreversible prenatal and postnatal growth deficiency for linear growth and weight occurs along with a characteristic cluster of facial abnormalities, neurologic dysfunction with mild to moderate mental retardation, and variable major and minor malformations of the extremities, heart, and genitalia (Streissguth, Herman, & Smith, 1978; Toutant & Lippman, 1980). Partial or atypical expression of the syndrome has a frequency of three to five live births per 1000 (Clarren & Smith, 1978b), with these children being smaller than usual, having borderline or low normal intelligence, and exhibiting aberrant motor function and behavior such as unusual irritability and restlessness in infancy and hyperactivity in childhood (Smith, 1979a; Streissguth et al. 1978). In addition, there is emerging evidence of a relationship between maternal gestational alcohol abuse and cancer in these children (Hornstein, Crowe, & Gruppo, 1977; Kinney, Faix, & Brazy, 1980; Seeler, Israel, & Royal, 1979).

The variability with which the fetal alcohol syndrome may be expressed has caused Smith (1979a, p. 121) to caution that

> strictly speaking, the term *fetal alcohol syndrome* may be somewhat misleading. It tends to limit one's thinking to one end of the spectrum, to the more severely affected patients in whom the basic diagnostic triad of growth deficiency, mental retardation, and facial abnormalities is fully expressed: yet, equally important to the diagnostician are the patients with only partial or atypical expression of the syndrome.

Clinicians should note, for example, that the hyperactive child with facial characteristics that are unusual enough to elicit unkind descriptors such as Wender's (1971) *funny-looking kid* may be a fetal alcohol syndrome child. With Smith's remarks in mind, perhaps the pertinent clinical question is not, "Does this child have the fetal alcohol syndrome?" but "Is this child's problem secondary to alcohol exposure in utero?"

The pathogenesis of this syndrome has not yet been precisely specified, but it appears to be related to maternal alcohol intake in the first trimester of pregnancy. Although it occurs most often in children of chronically heavy drinkers (Jones, Smith, Streissguth, & Myrianthopoulos, 1974), recent clinical reports suggest that even occasional binge drinking and to a lesser extent moderate but regular drinking during the first trimester can also have adverse effects on fetal development (Smith, 1979a; Toutant & Lippman, 1980). Of those women who drink heavily throughout pregnancy, it is estimated that one-third of their children will suffer some kind of damage, much of which will be irreversible (Jones et al., 1974). Smith (1979a) presents preliminary evidence of a dose-response curve for maternal alcohol intake relative to fetal well-being, which suggests that the risk of fetal alcohol syndrome characteristics increases proportionately with average daily alcohol consumption. One heartening finding from the available animal and human data is that there appears to be no carryover effect when heavy alcohol intake is stopped prior to conception (Smith, 1979a).

As one would expect considering the relatively short period in which the fetal alcohol syndrome has achieved the status of a well-documented clinical entity, a number of important questions remain unanswered. The amount of alcohol that is toxic (Clarren & Smith, 1978b; Dalby, 1978) and the effect of the timing of its intake on fetal development (Himwich, Hall, & MacArthur, 1977) are not yet known, nor has the mechanism by which alcohol produces the pattern of defects been identified. One possibility is that some characteristics result from acquired chromosomal damage (Gordon & Lieber, 1979). The possibility of using pharmacological prenatal intervention to minimize or off-set the effects of intrauterine exposure to alcohol is still to be investigated (Gordon & Lieber, 1979). It is not known whether the teratogen is ethanol or its breakdown product acetaldehyde (Mendelson, 1978; Smith, 1979a) or if the lead content of untaxed alcoholic beverages plays a contributory role (Sneed, 1978). There is uncertainty about the role of maternal nutritional factors (Toutant & Lippman, 1980) and whether the adverse effects of alcohol are increased by its interaction with other drugs such as caffeine and nicotine (Clarren & Smith, 1978b). Mendelson (1978) has suggested that the fetal alcohol syndrome may in fact be a polydrug abuse fetal syndrome or a polydrug abuse-nutritional deficit-stress-induced fetal syndrome. It would be particularly productive to do a comprehensive study of children who showed no fetal effects as a result of their mother's alcoholism compared with those who did show such effects.

The fetal alcohol syndrome has been described by Clarren and Smith (1978b, p. 1066) as "the most frequent known teratogenic cause of mental deficiency in the Western world," and by Gordon and Lieber (1979, p. 15) as "rapidly becoming the most common, yet preventable, congenital abnormality." The magnitude of the problem is evident from the fact that the experts regard the full manifestations of the syndrome as more serious than those of thalidomide. The recent sharp increase in chronic alcoholism in adolescent girls and young women (Langone & Langone, 1980; Norwood, 1980) should spur the development by behavioral teratologists (Buckalew, Ross, & Lewis, 1979) of educational programs aimed at the high school and young adult populations and emphasizing the established consequences of alcohol intake during pregnancy. In the interim, every young woman contemplating pregnancy should read _Mothering your unborn baby_ by Smith (1979b). In addition, pediatricians dealing with adolescents, family practice physicians, and obstetricians should make opportunities to convey the seriousness of such consequences. We advocate the severe, authoritarian, fear-arousing approach that is appropriate for the high probability of the serious lifetime consequences to the unborn child. We have pointed out that many gaps exist in our knowledge of the fetal alcohol syndrome. However, from a preventive point of view no further information is needed beyond the plain fact that alcohol intake during pregnancy should be avoided. It is our opinion that most obstetricians fail abysmally to convey to their patients and to the patients' families the serious probable consequences of alcohol ingestion during pregnancy. It is time for the medical practitioner to reassume the role of an authority, and the education of the patient in respect to her responsibilities during the prenatal period would be a productive place to start.

DELAYED OR IRREGULAR MATURATION

Some investigators have invoked a maturational lag explanation for hyperactivity, that is, a delay model that emphasizes the rate of acquisition of age-related skills and competencies. Such a model implies that the child's overall performance, or certain aspects of it, are abnormal only with regard to his chronological age and that there is always the possibility that he may catch up at some later date (Abrams, 1968; Bax & McKeith, 1963; Kinsbourne, 1973; Laufer, Denhoff, & Solomons, 1957; O'Malley & Eisenberg, 1973; Werry, 1968). In this framework the hyperactive child differs from the nonhyperactive child in the age at which he acquires certain capabilities rather than in the mode of their acquisition (Kinsbourne, 1973). The well-documented attentional problems, for example, are viewed as a delay in the development of attentional competence rather than as a defect; the hyperactive child is seen as being like a younger child—immature in respect to attentional skills—but not abnormal. The delay model has considerable face validity, in that many of the behavioral characteristics of the hyperactive child are consistent with immaturity rather than abnormality. The hyperactive child has been described (O'Malley & Eisenberg, 1973) as "normal but displaced chronologically to the right by four to six years," and data from neurological, physiological, and psychological research support this description.

Using a conventional neurological examination of hand, foot, and eye preference tests, as well as a timed coordination battery, Denckla and Rudel (1978) compared hyperactive boys of elementary school age with nonclinical controls. Discriminant function scores for speed and rhythm differentiated between the two groups, with the hyperactive boys performing at a more immature level. In addition, these boys showed significantly more overflow movements at all ages. Overflow, which refers to the inability to make discrete isolated movements, such as flexing a single finger, is of particular relevance to the question of developmental delay because it is characteristic of the lack of motor inhibition control of young children. Denckla and Rudel (1978) concluded that the descriptor *developmental delay* aptly described the immature coordination of the hyperactive group. Support for the concept of a neurophysiological maturational lag comes from the electroencephalograph (EEG) studies by Buchsbaum and Wender (1973) and other investigators (Satterfield, Lesser, Saul, & Cantwell, 1973; Shetty, 1971) who have demonstrated in hyperactive children the excessive EEG slow wave activity patterns characteristic of chronologically younger normal children. It is interesting to note that these EEG patterns are also consistent with a low central nervous system arousal model of hyperactivity (Satterfield & Braley, 1977). Additional evidence of a neurophysiological maturational lag comes from a study by Surwillo (1977) which showed that the mean age of hyperactive elementary school children predicted on the basis of the second, third, and fourth central moments of their EEG histograms was nine months lower than the group's actual mean age. Oettinger and his associates (Oettinger, 1975; Oettinger, Majovski, Limbeck, & Gauch, 1974) measured bone age of a substantial number of elementary school children diagnosed as minimal brain dysfunction and reported that they were significantly retarded on this dimension. The value of these findings is weakened, however, by a failure to use evaluators of bone age who were naive as to the subjects' status on this variable and to include nonclinical controls (Safer & Allen, 1975a). The latter failure is of particular importance because the Greulich and Pyle (1959) standards that are frequently used in bone age assessment apparently underestimate bone age to a significant degree. In a recent study (Schlager, Newman, Dunn, Crichton, & Schulzer, 1979) the average bone age of nonclinical control children was three months below their mean chronological age, and that of hyperactive children was eight months below it.

Clinical and research reports on psychological aspects of the hyperactive child also support the delayed maturation model. The child's tendency to seek out younger playmates, live in the present, and function best in one-to-one and novel situations, as well as his inability to change set and adjust to situational demands as ably as his same-age peers, are characteristics that have been noted in the literature (Cantwell, 1979; Henker & Whalen, 1980a; Loney, 1980a; Stewart & Olds, 1973). Peters, Romine, and Dykman (1975) reported that although younger children with minimal brain dysfunction showed significantly more lags or deficits at the highest levels of central nervous system functioning (language, fine motor coordination, cross-modality integrations) than did control children, many of these signs diminished or disappeared with age, so that older children with minimal brain dysfunction were more like the control children. Weithorn (1970) found greater similarity of performance on measures of impulsivity between older hyperactive and younger nonhyperactive boys than between same-age hyperactive and nonhyperactive boys. These differences were more clearly defined in comparisons between first- and fourth-grade groups than they were between fourth- and sixth-grade groups. Butter and Lapierre (1974) compared elementary school hyperactive boys with nonhyperactive matched controls on the Illinois Test of Psycholinguistic Abilities and found that the hyperactive group were from 18 to 24 months less mature than the controls. The playroom activity levels of hyperactive children have been reported by Routh and Schroeder (1976) as quantitatively equal to those of younger nonclinical children.

The maturational lag explanation has been criticized by Kinsbourne and Swanson (1979, p. 3) on the following grounds:

> One reservation is that the developmental lag model does not necessarily differ from the brain damage model. Brain damage can cause developmental delay. . . . Second, and more importantly, it is not clear that the behavior of hyperactive children is immature . . . the behavior patterns of some hyperactive children are clearly abnormal very early. . . . Evidence is accumulating that in some cases the symptoms of hyperactivity do not disappear at puberty. . . .

We question the validity of these reservations on several counts. Contending that the developmental lag and brain damage models do not differ because the outcome, delay, is the same in each is illogical and contrary to the fact that many medical problems and behavior disorders represent the final common state for a diverse group of etiological factors. Paralysis, for example, may result from physical injury, poisoning, pathogenic organisms, or psychological trauma. Using the fact that the behavior of some hyperactive children is abnormal to refute the developmental lag explanation shows a disregard for the heterogeneity of hyperactivity. The behavior of some hyperactive children may be abnormal and that of others immature; the age of onset of the abnormal behavior in no way discounts the possibility that similar behaviors, even those present at birth, may stem from other causes such as immaturity. A neonatal pattern of excessive restlessness could stem from pre- or perinatal brain damage or from neurological immaturity; or the behavior could be a normal variant of temperament—the difficult child that Thomas and Chess (1977) have described. In addition, the fact that the symptoms sometimes do not disappear in puberty does not invalidate the concept of maturational lag. As Routh (1978) has noted, a neurodevelopmental lag should not be taken to imply that the child *always* outgrows the problem. Within the interactionist framework adopted in this text a maturational lag could be exacerbated and maintained by social and nonsocial environmental factors (Porges & Smith, 1980). Or, as Routh (1978, p. 11) has speculated, the myelinization of the reticular formation may be a slower than normal process in the hyperactive child and one that fails to be completed in adulthood, with the result that symptoms might persist into adulthood.

Although there is clinical and research evidence for a maturational lag of a physiological and psychological nature in some children, the precise criteria for its diagnosis in a specific child have not yet been identified. For example, in how many areas should a hyperactive child be immature, and what other characteristics should be present for such a diagnosis to be made with a reasonable degree of certainty? Clarification is obviously needed if the maturational lag explanation is to be of clinical value. The problem here is analogous to that which exists in the case of minor physical anomalies: there are no norms to differentiate between an anomaly count that is within normal limits and one that is clearly of significance in hyperactivity.

A CULTURAL ETIOLOGICAL HYPOTHESIS

In the preceding etiological statements hyperactivity has been viewed as a problem either originating within the child or resulting from an interaction between the child and his immediate environment. Block (1977) has proposed that hyperactivity may also be a cultural phenomenon. In his cultural etiological view, "societal and cultural forces may be related to the problem of hyperactivity in both a primary (causal) and secondary (amplifying) manner" (p. 238). The causal relationship proposed by Block is dependent on the acceptance of two "facts": that the incidence of hyperactivity is increasing, and that the cultural tempo of our society has accelerated markedly in the past 50 years, the result being an increase in excitation that has interacted with the predisposition to hyperactivity in a causal fashion. Although Block's proposal is consistent with Leighton's (1959) more general statement that as societies become more urbanized and industrialized more people are at risk for behavior disorder, its premises do not stand up to scrutiny. The assumption that a significant increase in incidence of hyperactivity has occurred over the past 50 years is difficult to either substantiate or refute. Although hyperactivity was recognized at the turn of the century (Still, 1902) it has been a part of our culture for less than 25 years (Loney, 1980b) so there are no authoritative records or acceptable methods of estimating the annual incidence over the past 50 years (Spring & Sandoval, 1976). However, claims of a steady rise since 1965 (Feingold, 1975c) do not withstand objective investigation (Spring & Sandoval, 1976). Empirical findings from two reliable sources refute the belief that a sharp rise in the incidence of hyperactivity has occurred. The data from the methodologically excellent study of prevalence by Lambert, Sandoval, and Sassone (1978) provide no supportive evidence for a recent short-term increase in hyperactivity. Approaching this issue from a different viewpoint, standardization data for the Coding subtest of the Wechsler Intelligence Scale for Children (WISC) provide a second argument against the rise in incidence claim. Spring and Sandoval (1976) have noted that hyperactive children frequently show impairment in performance on the Coding subtest. This subtest is identical in both the 1949 and 1974 versions of the WISC (Spring, Yellin, & Greenberg, 1976). If hyperactivity had increased dramatically in the past 15 years, one would expect to see a drop in the mean raw scores for this subtest in the 1974 WISC standardization tables. In fact the 1974 means are significantly higher than the 1949 means, even after the latter were corrected for the inclusion of institutionalized mental retardates in the 1949 sample. Although the increased incidence belief has the support of several investigators who have stated that hyperactivity *appears* to be on the increase, it is our opinion that the increased incidence belief can be attributed to the heightened visibility of hyperactivity in the past decade being interpreted as increased incidence. The Omaha incident (Maynard, 1970), for example, resulted in a tremendous amount of media coverage, and this interest has been maintained by the continuing issues of drug treatment of hyperactive children and special class placement (Bruck, 1976) and by organizations such as the Feingold Association. The continuing publicity coupled with increasing research interest led Douglas (1976, p. 307) to comment that "During the past few years the hyperactive syndrome in children has emerged from relative obscurity to become one of the most diagnosed and researched of the disorders of children."

A second difficulty with Block's (1977) proposal concerns his conclusion that a causal relationship between increased cultural tempo and hyperactivity is a possibility. If such were the case, we would expect the prevalence rates in urbanized and rapidly developing countries to be higher than those in less developed countries, where the cultural tempo is likely to be slower. In fact prevalence rates do not relate systematically to urbanization and pace of daily life. A wide range of prevalence rates has been reported in urban and suburban centers of the United States (Bosco & Robin, 1980; Cantwell, 1975a; Huessy & Gendron, 1970; Lambert et al., 1978; Yanow, 1973), as well as in both relatively underdeveloped and industrialized countries in other parts of the world, including Canada (Minde & Cohen, 1978; Trites, 1979b), South America (Knobel, 1975), West Germany (Sprague, Cohen, & Eichlseder, 1977), as well as in Uganda (Minde & Cohen, 1978), the island of Kaui (Werner & Smith, 1977), and parts of the South Pacific (Werry, Sprague, & Cohen, 1975). In contrast, hyperactivity is reported to be virtually nonexistent in the People's Republic of China (Robinson, 1977, 1978), urban Japan (Cole, 1979), Salt Lake City (Richardson, 1978), and among Mexican groups in the Southwestern United States (Anderson, 1977).

Our position on this issue is that hyperactivity is to some extent culture bound, in that there are cultural factors related to the accelerated tempo of Western industrialized countries that may also be etiologically implicated in hyperactivity. We are not disputing the possible negative contribution of such factors as lead in gasoline, food additives, television, maternal gestational alcohol use, lighting, and inner city crowding; but we do not attribute causal importance to increased cultural tempo. Instead we offer the following hypothesis for the role of cultural factors in hyperactivity. In contemporary society cultures and subcultures differ in respect to the consistency of basic tenets across institutions (e.g., home, school, church, mass media, and major organizations), with some cultures having marked consistency across institutions and others being notable for their inconsistency. Cultures characterized by high consistency tend also to be high on group cohesiveness, emphasize group achievement (while still being responsive to individual efforts), require conformity that does not depend primarily on ability, and offer acceptance to individuals because of their membership in the cultural group rather than on the basis of their performance or other attributes. In the process, individual differences to some extent are minimized. Children and adolescents in these cultures tend to receive highly similar messages from socialization agents across institutions and usually these messages are further reinforced by a cohesive within-culture peer group. Cross-age interaction is the norm, that is, friendships and social activities cross age lines. (This pattern of friendship is not typical of modern Western countries, in which an age-segregated educational system prevails and age mates are viewed as appropriate friends by adults and the children themselves.) Examples of cultures having marked consistency across institutions are the People's Republic of China and, on a small scale, Salt Lake City; examples of subcultures are the lowest ranks of most armies and some residential schools with strong religious affiliations.

In contrast to these consistent cultures and subcultures are those marked by inconsistency across major institutions. These cultures tend to maximize individual differences, emphasize individual achievement, and segregate individuals from the earliest years on the basis of achievement, socioeconomic status, religion, and other attributes. Within these cultures many strong subgroups exist that differ greatly in beliefs, attitudes, and goals, and these subgroups reject some members of the cultural group and accept others. Children often receive quite contradictory messages from socialization agents in the home, school, church, and mass media, and personal attributes rather than cultural membership determine their acceptance and rejection by the various peer groups. Many major cities, particularly in the Western world, would fall into the category of inconsistent cultures; in the Far East, Tokyo is a notable exception (Cole, 1979). Note that the kinds of consistency and inconsistency being discussed here do not relate systematically to urbanization, sophistication of technology, or cultural tempo.

In our hypothesis consistent cultures represent rarefaction ecologies (Whalen, Henker, Collins, Finck, & Dotemoto, 1979) or goodness of fit situations (Chess, 1979) for the hyperactive child by providing a structure and clarity that minimize differences between the hyperactive child and his peers and in some cases result in his being virtually indistinguishable from his same-age peers. The cross-age interaction in these cultures is particularly beneficial for the child with hyperactive tendencies, because it permits him to play successfully with younger children without stigma or concern on the part of adults. Furthermore, as Whiting (1978) has pointed out, children in these cultures are less dependent on their parents, less individualistic and competitive, more concerned with the group's welfare, and more likely to accept and protect the child who is different, all of which would work to the benefit of the hyperactive child so that the effect of the rarefaction ecology would be to reduce the number of existing cases of hyperactivity. According to this framework, inconsistent cultures become provocation ecologies (Whalen et al., 1979) or poorness of fit situations (Chess, 1979) that serve to maximize hyperactive–nonhyperactive differences and increase the number of known cases. In our cultural hypothesis, therefore, the primary or causal link between cultural factors and hyperactivity is between inconsistency of the ecosystem and a predisposition to hyperactivity in the child. Of secondary, or as Block (1977, p. 238) says, "amplifying" importance, is the increased cultural tempo that often coexists with rapid urbanization and increased technological sophistication. The effect of an accelerated pace of life may be to exacerbate *existing* hyperactivity more than would a slower cultural tempo, but not to *cause* hyperactivity.

CHILD REARING

A functionally significant cluster of infant behavior has been identified by Thomas, Chess, and Birch, (1968) and categorized by them as *difficult*. Included in this cluster is a high activity level, biological and behavioral irregularity, nonadaptability, high intensity, and many negative mood responses. Longitudinal data from these investigators have shown that a substantial number of infants with difficult temperaments become hyperactive (Thomas & Chess, 1977), and these findings are supported by numerous other clinical reports. Lacking such consensus, however, are the theoretical explanations for the process by which a difficult infant often becomes a hyperactive child. Two explanations have been proposed, the first of which, the unidirectional view of the socialization process, has dominated research and theory on child rearing for most of this century. In this conceptual framework the direction of effect is from the socialization agent to the malleable and unformed child, with the child's behavioral characteristics largely attributable to the socializing influence of his parents, and later his teachers. The essence of this unidirectional view can be found in the radical behaviorism of Watson (1928), who strongly believed that the infant could be shaped into any pattern his caretakers desired, regardless of his own characteristics (other than physical health and reasonable intellectual functioning). A current formulation representative of the unidirectional view is the diasthesis-stress model proposed by Bettelheim (1973). According to this formulation, when children who are constitutionally predisposed to hyperactivity are stressed with environmental pressures that exceed their tolerance, they react with hyperactivity. Many difficult but potentially normal infants become increasingly restless and more difficult because their mothers are impatient or resentful of the trouble the infant causes them; presumably a mother with an unusual capacity for calming, or considerable tolerance for restlessness, would not react to the infant in a way that exacerbates his difficult temperament. Often the unhappy dyadic relationship deteriorates into a continuing battle, with the infant fighting back through restlessness and resistance as he finds himself unable to cope with his mother's demands for quiet compliant behavior (Minde, 1977). As he moves chaotically through the preschool and school years, his performance elicits increasing maternal anxiety and disapproval, and the demands at school for conformity and compliance, particularly inhibition of motor movement, are often far beyond the child's capacity, so that he is labeled as a failure by his teacher and peers. The result is an accelerating deterioration in both his behavior and his already battered self-concept.

An empirical example of this diasthesis-stress sequence appears in the Battle and Lacey (1972) report of the correlates of hyperactivity in boys. The mothers of hyperactive male infants were critical of their difficult babies during infancy and showed a lack of affection for them, continued to be disapproving and tended to use severe penalties for disobedience during the primary school years, and assessed their sons' intelligence as lower than did mothers of boys with a moderate level of activity. From an early age hyperactive boys were characterized by noncompliance with adults and a lack of achievement striving; by adolescence the boys had poor opinions of their intellectual ability. Although these correlates of hyperactivity are consistent with a diasthesis-stress sequence, the format of correlational studies does not permit the separating out of each participant's contribution.

According to Bettelheim, the inability to learn that so often characterizes the hyperactive child is partly a function of his low self-esteem and restlessness, but is primarily the child's way of defending himself against an environment that has been peopled since his infancy by rejecting agents of socialization. The increasing demands for achievement lead to an inability to perform at the level expected on the basis of the child's intelligence, or to an inability to perform at all. Bettelheim portrays the child as driven into a state of hyperactivity, and advocates more warmth, acceptance, and flexibility on the part of women in the child's environment. The implication here, that the same child would probably be able to maintain an acceptable pattern of behavior if the environmental stressors were modified, receives support from the following clinical description of two children, both of whom had difficult temperaments but whose parents differed greatly in child management practices (Chess et al., 1963, p. 145):

> The first pair of children, a girl and a boy, both showed the characteristics of irregularity, non-adaptability, negative mood and intense reactivity in the infancy period. Both were what are often called "difficult infants" to manage, with irregular sleep patterns, constipation and painful evacuations at times, slow acceptance of new foods, prolonged adjustment periods to new routines, and frequent and loud periods of crying. Adaptation to nursery school in the 4th year was also a problem for both children.
>
> In terms of parental attitudes and practices, however, the children differed greatly. The girl's father was unusually angry with her, in speaking of her gave the impression of dislike of the youngster, was punitive, and spent little or no recreational time with her. The mother was more concerned for the child, more understanding, and more permissive, but quite inconsistent. There were only two areas in which there was firm but quiet parental consistency, namely safety rules and choice of clothing.

The boy's parents, on the other hand, were unusually tolerant and consistent. The child's lengthy adjustment periods were taken in stride and his strident altercations with his younger sibling were dealt with good-humoredly. They waited out his negative moods without getting angry. They tended to be very permissive but set safety limits and consistently pointed out the needs of his peers at play.

By the age of five and one-half years, these two children, whose initial characteristics had been so similar showed qualitative behavioral differences. The boy's initial difficulties in nursery school had disappeared, he was a constructive member of his class, had a group of friends with whom he exchanged visits and functioned smoothly in the major routine areas of daily living. The girl, by contrast, had over the previous few years developed a number of symptoms of increasing severity. These included explosive angers, negativism, fear of the dark, encopresis, thumb-sucking, insatiable demands for toys and sweets, poor peer relationships, and protective lying. It is of interest that there was a lack of any symptomatology or negativism in the two areas where parental practice had been firmly and quietly consistent, i.e., safety rules and choice of clothing.*

According to the diasthesis-stress model, modification of environmental stressors should result in a concomitant improvement in the behavior of the hyperactive child. Support for this sequence is contained in parental and clinical reports of children being labeled as hyperactive by their teachers at some grade levels and not others (Bax, 1972; Grinspoon & Singer, 1973), a phenomenon aptly described by Lambert et al. (1978) as "moving in and out of the group considered to be hyperactive." Empirical support for the effects of modifying environmental stressors on a short-term basis is reported by Gelfand (1973) in a study comparing the task performance of children with minimal brain dysfunction under two conditions. In one condition the child was required to perform the experimental task in the presence of his mother; in the other he performed the task in the presence of an experimenter whom he knew well, and who created an interpersonal climate that was as different as possible from that of the child with his mother. The maternal climates were more nonresponsive and generally more negative then those of the experimenter. The hypothesis that the children would perform better with the experimenter was confirmed. They showed greater absorption in the task and more exuberance with the experimenter, whereas their behavior with their mothers was more distractible, angry, and anxious. These results are consistent with Bettelheim's view that the child's behavior and performance are not isolated variables; instead they covary with the general behavior and affect of socialization agents within specific interpersonal situations.

The second theoretical explanation for the difficult infant-hyperactive child sequence is a social interaction model that emphasizes a shared responsibility

*Reprinted by permission, from Chess, S., Thomas, A., Rutter, M., and Birch, H. G. Interaction of temperament and environment in the production of behavioral disturbances in children. *American Journal of Psychiatry*, 1963, *120*, 142–148. Copyright 1963, the American Psychiatric Association.

described as bidirectionality of effect. Advocates of the bidirectional position believe that a mother's behavior with her child is the complex endpoint of a variety of determinants, two of the most important being her attitudes, motives, and philosophy of child rearing on the one hand, and the child's temperament and behavioral competence on the other. Although the mother's behavior to the infant is guided by her beliefs and attitudes, it is also controlled to a substantial degree by the infant's behavior, just as the infant's behavior can be determined to a great extent by the mother's behavior. The mother may by her negative and rejecting attitude *cause* her infant to behave in a difficult manner, or she may become impatient, critical, and rejecting as a *result* of her infant's behavior, in which case her behavior and response patterns then serve to heighten and maintain the infant's negative behavior (Henderson, Dahlin, Partridge, & Engelsing, 1973). Evidence clearly supporting bidirectionality has been reported by many experienced clinicians and researchers (e.g., Barkley & Cunningham, 1979; Chess, 1979; Humphries, Kinsbourne, & Swanson, 1978; Prechtl, 1963). However, the major contribution comes from Bell (Bell, 1968; 1971; Bell & Harper, 1977), who described the mother–child system (Bell, 1977; p. 15) as

> a reciprocal relation involving two or more individuals who differ greatly in maturity although not in competence, in terms of ability to affect each other. . . . There is a certain balance of controls, in that the greater intentional behavior of the parent is offset by two features of the offspring's behavior: (1) the active short-range initiation of interactions, and (2) the organization of the behavior so that it is compelling and selectively reinforcing.

A classic example of the impact of a difficult infant upon his social environment and particularly his mother, has been described by Brazelton (1961). The mother, a young professional woman, and her husband were delighted with her pregnancy and both eagerly awaited the birth of their first child. The child, a boy, proved to be a bitter disappointment to both parents. From the day of his birth the infant was capable of only two extreme states. In one he appeared to be in a state of deep sleep during which his muscle tone was poor, he was difficult to rouse, and was unresponsive to external stimuli. In the second state he screamed continuously, was hyperactive, and overreacted to touch and other stimulation. Only forcible restraint and swaddling could calm him, whereupon he would lapse back to the first state of inaccessible deep sleep. From the start the mother felt depressed, rejected, despairing, and overwhelmed by the task of caring for an infant who could not be comforted when he was upset or contacted when he was in his withdrawal state. The mother finally sought psychotherapy, which enabled her to see her son's problems as his own rather than the result of mishandling on her part, and she went on to have a second child who was an easy infant with whom she had a rewarding mother–child relationship.

The basic disagreement between the unidirectional view, as represented by the diasthesis-stress model, and the bidirectional view concerns the source of eliciting stimuli for the mother's immediate behavior to her infant. There is no argument about the existence of the temperament pattern described by Bettelheim and supported by others. In our view, the weakness in the diasthesis-stress model is not that it is an incorrect description but that it is an incomplete one. It has persisted as the dominant explanation of the socialization process partly because of its initial entrenchment in socialization theory and practice, but also because the practical application of findings from clinical and research reports on behavioral problems to the pediatric setting lags far behind their publication. Despite the existence of a considerable body of work supporting bidirectionality, many pediatricians continue to treat dyadic problems from a unidirectional viewpoint. The issue is of far more than academic interest, because clearly the acceptance of one viewpoint rather than the other as a philosophical base determines the specific content of the intervention program planned for a particular child.

ACADEMIC FAILURE

Cunningham and Barkley (1978b) have proposed that persistent academic difficulties and failure are sufficient to generate hyperactive behavior in children. Within this framework academic problems assume primary status and hyperactivity is relegated to the status of a secondary or resultant symptom. According to this model the hyperactive behavior pattern once generated may be strengthened as a function of a heterogeneous group of inadvertent social reinforcers in the classroom, such as peer attention, and may persist because it effectively reduces the frustration and anxiety associated with academic difficulties. Aggression and impulsivity, which may coexist with hyperactivity, are regarded as responses to the frustration of classroom failure. The optimal treatment for this failure-related hyperactivity is intervention aimed at supplanting academic failure with classroom success experiences. Within this framework drug treatment and environmental manipulation, such as stimulus reduction, are viewed as adjunctive intervention designed to modify troubling secondary or related symptoms.

The academic failure model has difficulty in encompassing certain findings. Although drug or behavioral intervention that successfully modifies hyperactive behavior rarely results in improvement in academic performance (Barkley & Cunningham, 1978; Rie, Rie, Stewart, & Ambuel, 1976; Weiss & Hechtman, 1979), Sprague and Sleator (1977) contend that it is the drug dosage that is incorrect, and that the correct dosage can effect an improvement in academic performance in the absence of any manipulation of the child's success-failure experiences. The Barkley and Cunningham model accords secondary symptom status to aggression and other disruptive classroom behaviors but the work of Loney and her associates (e.g., Loney, 1980b; Loney, Kramer,

& Milich, 1979) suggests that aggression is independent of hyperactivity and therefore merits primary symptom status. However, Loney et al. have also shown that on an empirical basis hyperactive children can be categorized into subgroups of hyperactive only, and hyperactive with aggression. So it could be argued that the Cunningham and Barkley model applies to the former but not the latter group of hyperactive children. A more difficult problem for the model concerns an explanation for the uneven school performance characteristic of the hyperactive child. The model cannot accommodate the fact that the hyperactive child performs well in school on some days and poorly on others even when task content remains constant.

Despite these problems, there is a diverse group of empirical findings reported on by Cunningham and Barkley (1978b) as supportive of the academic failure model. Classroom studies in which the level of academic success experience is manipulated have shown that the cluster of off-task, disruptive behavior characteristic of the hyperactive child were inversely related to the level of task success (Ayllon & Roberts, 1974; Ayllon, Layman, & Kandel, 1975). Research in laboratory settings has shown that task failure or a sudden reduction in anticipated reward or reinforcing feedback (which is often perceived by the hyperactive child as an indication of failure) may severely disrupt his behavior; and it is an established fact that hyperactive and nonhyperactive children differ in their responses to certain reinforcers (Douglas, 1980).

In addition to these findings, Cunningham and Barkley could also have drawn on the following points as being explained by or consistent with their academic failure hypothesis:

1.   Battle and Lacey's (1972) finding that the mothers of hyperactive boys were critical and disapproving of them in infancy and the preschool years, and the boys were low on achievement striving in both periods.

2.   The fact that preschool hyperactive children were notably different (more restless, difficult, and off-task) from their nonhyperactive peers in a preschool situation when they were required to engage in academic-type pursuits, such as sitting at the table and listening, but were indistinguishable from their peers in free play (Schleifer et al., 1975).

3.   The finding that the onset of hyperactivity often coincides with the point of school entry and, as Weiss and Hechtman state (1979, p. 1353): "Whether or not the environment is for some children the primary etiology is not known, but in many hyperactive children the environment is a highly significant antecedent variable even when not the primary cause."

4.   The finding that hyperactive children move in and out of the hyperactive group in school from one year to the next (Lambert et al., 1978), which could be due to fluctuations in the ratio of success to failure, with some teachers offering a goodness of fit environment (Chess, 1979) and others providing a provocation environment (Whalen & Henker, 1980).

5.   The fact that hyperactive children often function quite adequately in terms of classroom behavior when their academic tasks are not challenging,

but tend to "fall apart" when given difficult assignments (Whalen, Collins, Henker, Alkus, Adams, & Stapp, 1978).

6. The reports that hyperactive children do best on self-paced tasks (when they can proceed at a rate commensurate with their own abilities), and that their behavior often deteriorates on other-paced tasks when they are required to modulate their academic-type performance in accord with external cues (Henker & Whalen, 1980a).

7. The fact that the hyperactive child tries to dominate situations and is at his best when he is in charge and presumably is able to keep frustration due to failure at a minimum (Battle & Lacey, 1972; Whalen, Henker, Collins, McAuliffe, & Vaux, 1979).

8. The reports that hyperactive children have a difficult time in school but particularly so in adolescence (Milich & Loney, 1979a; Weiss & Hechtman, 1979) when school work becomes more demanding and achievement becomes an important goal, and that the situation improves in adulthood (Weiss, Hechtman, & Perlman, 1978) when they can select for themselves a job in which they can succeed; as Weiss and Hechtman (1979, p. 1353) have pointed out "the degree to which hyperactives are viewed as deviant depends on the demands of the environment in which they function."

The academic failure model appears to be applicable to a subgroup of hyperactive children, one of whom is described in the following case study:

Several years ago, one of the authors observed a girl in kindergarten who after three months had become so restless and difficult to contain in the school setting that her teacher had labeled her as hyperactive. In fact, this particular kindergarten was highly academically oriented and the child, whose IQ on the Stanford Binet was 84, was seldom able to perform most of the tasks that were presented to her. However, she was also very achievement-oriented, and in order to avoid failure she learned to move from one activity to another to avoid aversive consequences. Her teacher frequently worked quite intensively with her in an effort to improve her performance, but these interactions produced a generalized anxiety reaction that increased when she persisted with a task because she had apparently recognized that the longer she stayed at a task, the higher the probability of failure. Terminating the task and moving to another for a period that was too short to result in failure reduced the anxiety and thus reinforced the high rate of motility. In this child hyperactivity was not a disturbance in motility; instead it could more accurately be regarded as perpetual avoidance behavior. It was recommended that she be moved to a less achievement-oriented kindergarten and that she be given special tutoring on readiness tasks, with the provision that the tutoring situation offer a very high proportion of success experiences, particularly in the early stages. Because her solution for avoiding failure at a task was at a higher level of problem solving that one would expect of a child with an IQ of 84, it was also recommended that she be tested again after a period of time in the new setting. With these changes, hyperactivity disappeared in a few weeks, and a subsequent follow-up revealed that she was quite successful in the first grade, and her Stanford-Binet IQ now measured 98.

ENVIRONMENTAL CONSTRAINTS

The effect of high density urban living on human behavior is one of modern society's critical problems (Freedman, 1975). An aspect of this problem that has been the focus of a group of empirical investigations is human crowding, described in terms of situations in which density or other related conditions restrict or interfere with the activities of individuals within the setting (Schmidt & Keating, 1979). The high density slum area of New York City is an example of a restrictive setting, with its overcrowded schools, lack of green space, almost total lack of recreational outlets, and high crime and accident rate. In settings such as this, parents are justifiably fearful for the safety of their children. The combination of this fear, the nonavailability of recreational services, and the "specialized withdrawal" (Baldassare, 1979) characteristic of high density neighborhood residents causes them to keep the children indoors as much as possible, thereby imposing a major restriction of physical activity. The possibility that this combination of environmental conditions, parental demands, and other stresses can result in the onset of situationally induced hyperactivity has been suggested by McNamara (1972) and Thomas, Chess, Sillen, and Mendez (1974). McNamara described the factors that he viewed as causative in the onset of hyperactivity in lower-class Puerto Rican children in the high density slums in New York City. According to McNamara, a typical day in the life of one of these children consisted of going to school, trying to learn in an overcrowded classroom from a teacher who often was not bilingual, returning home, doing homework, and watching television. Many of the children responded to this general curtailment of their physical activity with a pattern of behavior, particularly in school, that was characterized by hyperactivity, attention problems, lethargy, and indifference, and that resulted in a referral for neurological evaluation and subsequent drug intervention. McNamara's conclusion, however, was that the only remedy needed for this apartment-bound hyperactivity was the obvious one of adequate and safe outlets for the normal physical activity of childhood. Unfortunately, there is no empirical evidence of the efficacy of such a solution.

In the second paper, Thomas et al. (1974) reported a cross-cultural comparison, also in New York City, of the behavior patterns of Puerto Rican working-class children and non-Puerto Rican middle-class children. The economic, social, and cultural backgrounds of the two groups presented a sharp contrast, but there were also some striking similarities, with both groups being characterized by a relatively high degree of family stability, living in two-parent homes in which geographic and economic stability prevailed, and not differing in the incidence of prenatal and perinatal complications. Like their middle-class counterparts, the Puerto Rican parents were clearly concerned about the well-being of their children, but they were more demanding about compliance to rules, less child-problem oriented, and less prone to pressure their children for early achievement and independence, particularly in the preschool years. Of relevance here is the finding that in the Puerto Rican sample there was a signficantly higher incidence of parental complaints about excessive and un-controllable motor activity than in the middle-class group: 53 percent of the Puerto Ricans under nine years presented problems in activity level as compared to only one child in the other group who was brain damaged. Thomas and his colleagues attributed the hyperactivity to the fact that these East Harlem parents coped with the dangers of the street by keeping their children in and expecting them to restrain their physical activity. This restrictive method of coping and its resultant hyperactivity effects are precisely those described by McNamara (1972) in his Puerto Rican group. The problem was exacerbated by the fact that children who temperamentally had high activity levels were even more likely to be restricted to the home because their parents were already aware that they were more accident-prone (Stewart, Thach, & Freidin, 1970) and therefore in greater potential danger on the streets than their less active siblings. The children typically reacted to parental demands for restraint with disobedience that in turn elicited physical punishment and further disobedience, thus setting up a cycle that led to these children also being described as disciplinary problems. Thomas and his colleagues pointed out that the number of complaints about hyperactivity would almost certainly have been sharply diminished if these children had been in an environment with more space for physical activities and fewer hazards. Note that the cause of the restrictiveness was a lack of safe physical space for physical activity, rather than social crowding, but the effects were somewhat similar. As evidence for the effect of lack of physical space, Thomas et al. noted that one Puerto Rican boy who had been described as "uncontrollably active" at school and "a whirling dervish" at home improved markedly when the family moved to a house with a small yard. Their conclusion (Thomas et al., 1974, p. 63) was that

It is likely that this high motility did not represent pathological hyperactivity as such, but rather, the normal temperamental characteristics of high activity level which became exacerbated and the basis for a behavior problem development because of environmental constraints.

CHAPTER 4

Assessment

Two major groups of tests and measurement procedures are used in the clinical evaluation and empirical study of the hyperactive child. Of interest here is the group of measures specifically related to hyperactivity, for example, measures of activity level and attention, and temperament rating scales. The other group includes assessment procedures, such as intelligence and achievement tests and peer nomination inventories, that are widely used in pediatric, psychiatric, and educational settings. These will be discussed in Chapters 9 and 10. The two groups differ markedly in generality and, more important, in the extent to which the developers have conformed to the basic tenets of test construction. Unlike the more general measures, the hyperactivity-related measures usually do not meet the basic criteria of reliability, validity, and practicality. In a critical review of the assessment of hyperactivity, Werry (1978a) commented that research workers have tended to focus on the problem of reliability, very often at the expense of validity and particularly by ignoring practicality. For the reader unfamiliar with the basic principles of measurement, Werry's review provides an excellent summary statement on this topic. Despite their serious shortcomings, selected hyperactivity-related measures will be described here because they are frequently used in empirical investigations as well as in the clinical assessment of the child at risk for hyperactivity. Emphasis will be given to assessment procedures in the following categories: measures of the primary symptoms of hyperactivity, global rating scales, classroom observation schedules, and temperament rating scales. As Whalen (1982, in press) has noted, each of these assessment modalities has its own advantages and disadvantages:

> Rating scales are global measures that are as easily influenced by the cognitive and motivational characteristics of the respondent as by the behaviors of the child. Subjectivity and bias are less likely to plague direct behavior observations, but frequency counts of target behaviors may be too specific, time-limited, or reactive to provide a representative picture of the child's problematic patterns. Laboratory measures tend to be more objective than ratings, more sensitive than behavior observations, and perhaps the most comparable from study to study. However, they are often obtained under novel, artificial, and even anxiety-inducing conditions rather than in the child's natural environments. Thus their ecological validity—their relevance to everyday functioning—must be documented.

Given the tradeoffs involved in the selection of any single assessment approach, many investigators are now conducting multimodal evaluations that encompass diverse assessment sources and techniques.

MEASURES OF THE PRIMARY SYMPTOMS OF HYPERACTIVITY

A variety of tests and other devices is available for the assessment of the primary symptoms of hyperactivity. Included here will be those procedures that provide objective measures of discrete behaviors, that is, one kind of behavior to one test. With the exception of the primary symptom, activity level, investigators have been more interested in developing global measures such as rating scales for hyperactivity and classroom observation schedules for multiple hyperactivity-related behaviors.

Activity Level

In the clinical as well as the research literature of the 1960s and early 1970s, the hyperactive child has generally been depicted as consistently far more active than his nonhyperactive peers. This quantitative viewpoint has now been firmly refuted by empirical investigations (e.g., Douglas, 1972; Werry, 1978b) and has been replaced by the qualitative view that the salient characteristic of the activity level of the hyperactive child is inappropriateness rather than excessiveness and consistent overactivity. In terms of activity level, it is now established that the unmedicated hyperactive child is generally indistinguishable from his nonhyperactive peers in free-play unstructured situations (Barkley & Ullman, 1975; Routh & Schroeder, 1976); however, in settings requiring a degree of inhibition easily conformed to by nonhyperactive children, the behavior of the hyperactive child is more likely to be conspicuous, disruptive, and detrimental to group productivity, but even here his behavior cannot accurately be described as either excessive or consistent. Despite the empirical findings to the contrary, many clinicians and researchers (e.g., Salkind & Poggio, 1977; Van Osdol & Carlson, 1972) have continued to define hyperactivity quantitatively and to lament the lack of empirical interest in basic investigative topics, such as the establishment of activity norms, the implication being that the value of such norms for comparative purposes would markedly enhance our knowledge of hyperactivity. The fact is that activity norms have not been of interest because the complex effect of qualitative aspects of activity level has been recognized as a variable that allows many interpretations of a single activity level score. Which interpretation is made rarely depends on quantity of motor output per se, but rather on such variables as situational context, goal directedness, or cultural norms. Compare, for example, a child rocking contentedly in a rocker, with the mindless, perseverative rocking of an autistic child.

Instrumental Measures of Activity Level

Direct measures of activity in children have been obtained with actometers (Bell, 1968; Schulman & Reisman, 1959), electromagnetic movement meters (Kretsinger, 1959), by fitting a room with photoelectric cells (Ellis & Pryer, 1959), and by inserting a radio transmitter in a child's helmet (Herron & Ramsden, 1967). Particularly interesting is the biomotometer developed by Schulman, Stevens, and Kupst (1977) to provide the wearer with continuous feedback for self-control of activity level. The instrument consists of an electronic package that is worn at the waist and measures activity level by angular displacement of mercury switches. Because it is small and light and does not restrict the wearer's movements in any way, it is ideal for research with children. The biomotometer has proven to be a reliable measure of activity level in the classroom, and measures made with it correlate well in a variety of settings with the actometer, an activity measurement device with demonstrated validity (Stevens, Kupst, Suran, & Schulman, 1978). Werry (1968) has contended that technological requirements make it difficult to obtain data without distorting the child's normal behavior, but subsequent inventions, such as the biomotometer, and research have invalidated this opinion. Wade and Ellis (1971), for example, reported a study of the free-range activity of kindergarten children in which each child wore a telemeter and a pair of electrodes attached to his sternum, and played vigorously without being inhibited or distressed by these attachments. We have often seen children enthusiastically wearing the Holter apparatus for long-term measures of heart performance and radio monitors for recording verbalizations, and making no complaints that the apparatus inhibited their normal activities. Children will be willing and even eager to wear such attachments if the initial presentation of the task is done with ingenuity and sensitivity.

Observational Measures of Activity Level

Observational procedures allow the recording of ongoing behavior in the child's natural environment or in the experimental settings with minimal inference or data reduction. The advantage of these procedures lies in their objectivity, relative freedom from observer bias, and direct relevance to the child's problems (Werry, 1978a). They also have marked disadvantages, namely, the difficulty of ensuring unobtrusive observations, the costs as compared to procedures such as rating scales, and the problems of establishing and maintaining reliability and of procuring adequate samples of behavior from a representative set of environments. The latter problem is particularly troublesome because activity level varies as a function of the setting and time interval in which it is measured. The following observational procedures have been used successfully with hyperactive children both as diagnostic and effect measures, and all have proven to be drug sensitive. The ongoing record is the procedure in which all the instances of one or more kinds of behavior are noted for a specified period of time, an example being the parent diary method used by Rapoport and her associates (Rapoport, Abramson, Alexander, & Lott, 1971; Rapoport, Quinn, Bradbard, Riddle, & Brooks, 1974). In time sampling, one or more kinds of behavior are noted in consecutive intervals, usually of five or 10 seconds duration, in the classroom setting (Wolraich, Drummond, Salomon, O'Brien, & Sivage, 1978); in the nursery school (Schleifer, Weiss, Cohen, Elman, & Cvejic, 1975), where the observers record the frequency of actions such as out-of-seat behavior; or in a playroom that has been divided into equal areas to permit counting the number of times a child moves across an imaginary grid (Routh, Schroeder, & O'Tuama, 1974).

Attention

Although there is general agreement that the hyperactive child is characterized by a basic attentional deficit, there are relatively few discrete measures of attention for use in diagnosis and research on hyperactivity. The measures that are available are in the form of laboratory tasks that emphasize to varying degrees components of attention such as alertness, focusing, stimulus selection, and physiological and psychological readiness to respond, that is, vigilance (Rosenthal & Allen, 1978).

Choice Reaction Time Task. On this measure the hyperactive child is required to direct his attention for a few seconds to a screen on which two or more stimuli appear. The child's task is to push the press-button with the picture or geometric shape corresponding to the particular stimulus appearing on the screen, and the score is his reaction time. Prior to the onset of the stimulus the child is oriented to the screen and is warned that the stimulus is about to appear. The stimulus is not shown until the experimenter can see that the child's attention is directed toward the screen, so the task is self-paced. When these preliminary efforts are made to ensure the child's attention, he performs as well as nonhyperactive control children (Douglas, 1972; Sykes, Douglas, & Morgenstern, 1973).

Serial Reaction Task. This is a self-paced measure that requires sustained attention over a prolonged period of time. The child sits facing a screen with five lights, each of which has a push button. As the lights go on one at a time, the child's task is to turn off the light by tapping the button corresponding to the light. As soon as one light has been turned off in this way, another light automatically comes on, so that the child determines the rate of onset of the stimuli to which he is to respond. The score is the number of correct and incorrect responses. In the study by Sykes et al. (1973) there were no hyperactive–nonhyperactive differences in number of correct responses, but the hyperactive group made more incorrect responses, which might be an indication of impulsive responding (Douglas, 1972).

Continuous Performance Test. This measure, developed by Rosvold and his associates (Rosvold, Mirsky, Sarason, Bransome, & Beck, 1956) to assess brain damage, is the most sensitive measure of the impaired attention of the hyperactive child. In this experimenter-paced task the child is required to perform for 15 minutes to stimuli that appear automatically at fixed intervals. The test has two forms, visual and auditory, and the stimuli are letters that either appear one at a time on a screen or are spoken by a voice on tape. The stimulus duration is 0.2 seconds and the interstimulus interval is 1.5 seconds. The child's task is to respond only to the significant stimulus, the letter *X* when it is immediately preceded by the letter *A*. Sykes et al. (1973) reported hyperactive–nonhyperactive differences, with the hyperactive children making fewer correct and more incorrect responses. The latter appeared to reflect impulsive responding (Douglas, 1972).

For all three of the foregoing tasks there are practice trials prior to the test trials, and test–retest reliability is satisfactory. On the first two tasks there is a practice effect, but this is not the case for the Continuous Performance Test.

Vigilance Tasks. Anderson, Halcomb, and Doyle (1973) have developed a 30-minute vigilance task for the assessment of attentional deficits. This task involves having the child sit in front of a console that has a pair of lights that flash one of three combinations (red–red, green–green, or red–green) every two seconds for a duration of 0.2 seconds. The child is required to press a button only when the red–green combination appears. Correct and incorrect responses are scored; the console is under computer control so that response latency can also be measured. Stimulus complexity can be increased by introducing visual and auditory distractors. On the basic task hyperactive children make fewer correct and more incorrect responses than nonhyperactive controls. A vigilance task with several important advantages over such traditional vigilance measures as the Continuous Performance Test is Holland's (1958) Operant Vigilance Task (Goldberg & Konstantareas, 1981). The child is seated in front of a "television set" with two keys. Pressing the left key produces a clown's face on the screen (observing response). The child is told that the clown's nose is "missing" because "it likes to run away a lot." Whenever the clown's nose appears (lights up red) the child is asked to notify the clown as quickly as possible by pressing the right key (signal detection response). Holland's task is far more appealing than most vigilance tasks; in addition, its self-pacing aspect is analogous to many situational tasks in the child's daily life, and it permits a distinction between two components of vigilance—the decision to attend to the task and the decision to report detection of the salient feature. On this task hyperactive children differed from normal controls in several respects: They exhibited slower observing response rates, detected fewer signals, and made more false alarm responses. Hyperactive children demonstrated faster orienting responses under low-density schedule conditions, but their signal detection rates did not relate systematically to the density factor.

Yellin (1980) has proposed a standard visual stimulus test for the measurement of attention deficit. The visual stimulus consists of a white circle against a rectangular black background. The white circle has one black dot located a small distance in from its edge. The basic stimulus configuration is such that the black dot can be presented in various positions, for example, the black dot positioned high up in the circle can serve as a signal requiring an active response, and the same circle with the dot positioned down can then indicate that no response should be made. Studies of the efficacy of this standard visual stimulus test are currently underway.

Another type of discrete measure of attention, the observational measure, has been used occasionally within the context of school-type tasks and frequently in free-play settings. Kendall and Brophy (1981), for example, assessed attention in a one-to-one psychological testing session by rating the following kinds of behavior: off-task verbal and physical behavior, off-task attention responses, out-of-seat behavior, and verbal interruptions. Observational measures of attention used in free-play settings have not been included in this discussion because we disagree with the assumption that nomadic activity is indicative of attention span. Ellis, Witt, Reynolds, and Sprague (1974), for example, defined attention in terms of length of time on specific play equipment in an informal play setting that contained many options. The subjects were children aged 8 to 10 and they were free to play on any equipment that they wished. Many interpretations could be offered for the "short attention span" in this situation: some children systematically look at all alternatives, some select a favorite activity and stay with it, some imitate other children by going where they go.

Distractibility

The firmly entrenched belief that distractibility is one of the primary symptoms of hyperactivity has been the basis for the development of educational programs characterized by a reduction or elimination of distracting stimuli (Strauss and Lehtinen, 1947). Subsequent research on this educational approach (Cruickshank, Bentzen, Ratzeberg, & Tannehauser, 1961; Haring & Phillips, 1962; Rost & Charles, 1967; Shores & Haubrich, 1969) failed to support the efficacy of reduction of distractibility for the hyperactive child. Other investigations also failed to support the distractibility factor (Campbell, Douglas, & Morgenstern, 1971; Cohen, Weiss, & Minde, 1972), leading Douglas and her associates to question the assumption that hyperactive children are distractible. Douglas (1972, 1974) has noted on several occasions failure to demonstrate distractibility empirically under conditions that should have elicited this behavior.

Two of the tests used to measure distractibility are the Color Distraction Test (Santostefano & Paley, 1964) and the Stroop Color Distraction Test (Stroop, 1935). Both tests assess the extent to which a child's ability to quickly

name familiar items on a page is disrupted by the presence of other distracting pictures or contradictory cues. The child, for example, might be required
to read a color name in the presence of a distracting factor, the color of the
ink. These distractors have no greater effects on unmedicated hyperactive children than on the controls. However, there is one difference between the two
groups: the hyperactive children make more complete errors of commission,
that is, they blurt out wrong responses and do not correct themselves. Under
medication, the hyperactive–nonhyperactive differences in ability to inhibit
and correct inaccurate verbalizations disappear (Douglas, 1972).

The attention tasks described in the previous section can be readily converted to assess distractibility. For example, Hoy, Weiss, Minde, and Cohen
(1978) gave their hyperactive adolescent boys an 18-minute continuous performance task involving a taped recording of a list of common words. The
task was to tap with a pencil every time a word containing the letter s was
heard. Meaningful distraction accompanied the list of words for a randomly
distributed six minutes, and nonmeaningful distraction, also randomly distributed, accompanied the list for another six minutes. There were no hyperactive–nonhyperactive differences as a function of the distraction conditions:
when the distractors were introduced, both groups increased their rate of responding to non-s words. Similarly, Sykes (Douglas, 1972) piped intermittent
white noise into the experimental setting, while hyperactive children worked
on the Continuous Performance task, and introduced conflicting color cues on
the Choice Reaction Time task. In neither instance were the hyperactive subjects differentially affected.

A cognitive style, field independence-dependence, has also been studied in
the research on distractibility. It can be assessed with the Children's Embedded Figures Test (Witkin, 1959), which requires the subject to act on a problem such as locating a figure in a confused and distracting visual context.
Field independent subjects are better able to perform this task than are field
dependent subjects, and there is some evidence that hyperactive children are
more field dependent than nonhyperactive control children. On this test, performance by hyperactive subjects is not influenced by medication (Douglas,
1974). Sandoval (1977) does not consider the Embedded Figures Test to be as
unequivocal a measure of distractibility as the color distraction tests of
Santostefano and Paley (1964) and Stroop (1935).

Impulsivity–Reflectivity

Impulsivity–reflectivity refers to the extent to which an individual reflects on
the solution to a problem prior to action, when several possible alternatives
are present and there is uncertainty about which is the most appropriate
(Messer, 1976). Children who respond quickly generally make more errors in
comparison with those who reflect on the alternatives. The test that has been
most often used to measure impulsivity–reflectivity is the Matching Familiar

Figures Test (MFFT) (Kagan, Rosman, Day, Albert, & Phillips, 1964), which Keogh and Barkett (1980, p. 274) regard as "the operational definition of impulsivity–reflectivity." Using different forms for different ages, this matching-to-sample test involves the presentation of a standard figure along with four, six, or eight other highly similar figures that differ in only a few details from the standard figure. The subject is required to identify the figure that exactly matches the standard one, a task involving careful scanning of the alternates. Two dimensions of the construct are assessed: response latency, which is response time, and perceptual accuracy, which is number of errors. A child's score on each of these dimensions is interpreted relative to the median. He is termed *impulsive* if he is below the median on response time and above it on errors, and *reflective* if he is above the median on response time and below it on errors. The loss of statistical power inherent in this dichotimization of subject data has been noted by Ault, Mitchell, and Hartmann (1976). A solution for handling this loss, by using separate distributions for both latency and errors and using all subjects, has been suggested by Salkind and Wright (1977).

Test–retest reliability that ranges from .34 on error reliabilities to as high as .96 on response time reliabilities is not considered by critics to be satisfactory (Egeland & Weinberg, 1976). In nonclinical children under six years of age errors are moderately stable but response time is not, whereas in children over six the reverse holds true, with response time but not errors being stable over time (Berry & Cook, 1980). An extensive literature attests to the construct validity of the MFFT (Sandoval, 1977).

The MFFT has been widely used with hyperactive children and has consistently proven to be useful. In a review of the impulsivity–reflectivity construct, Messer (1976) concluded that there was no doubt about the empirical relationship of MFFT scores to hyperactivity. It has been verified (Campbell, Douglas, & Morgenstern, 1971) that hyperactive children represent the extreme example of Kagan's impulsivity (1966). There is extensive evidence that the test differentiates hyperactive children of various ages from control children (e.g., Cohen et al., 1972; Schleifer et al., 1975). The impulsivity score is influenced by stimulant intervention (Campbell et al., 1971; Cohen et al., 1972; Schleifer et al., 1975), and unmedicated hyperactive children "make their choices more quickly than nonhyperactive controls and give less consideration, in a less organized fashion, to the other alternatives" (Douglas & Peters, 1979, p. 296).

Although there has been general agreement concerning the utility of the MFFT for studying hyperactive children, there has been considerable controversy over the meaning of children's scores on it (Bentler & McClain, 1976; Block, Block, & Harrington, 1974; Messer, 1976). In addition, some serious criticisms have been raised concerning the psychometric properties of the test, including the failure to control for a general intelligence factor (Block et al., 1974), as well as the previously mentioned reliability and dichotomization of subject data problems.

A new and longer version of the MFFT has been developed by Cairns and Cammock (1978) and labeled the MFF 20. It is composed of 20 items selected from three earlier versions of the MFFT on the basis of their discriminant power. In a comparison of the reliability and validity of the two tests with learning disabled children, the MFF 20 was more consistent on both error and latency scores and was also more sensitive as a predictor of academic achievement and attention in a naturalistic setting, that is, it has better internal reliability and better validity.

RATING SCALES OF HYPERACTIVITY

Rating scales are inexpensive, simple to use, and particularly appropriate for parents, teachers, and others having long-term contact with the child. Ratings obtained from these sources are based on behavior exhibited by the child in his various natural environments over a substantial period of time. Data from rating scales may provide a basis for deciding whether a problem does exist, determining what aspects of the problem should have priority as targets for change, and evaluating the effectiveness of the management and change program. For the reader who is interested in the methodology of evaluating treatments for hyperactivity, a recent chapter by Loney (1981) should be mandatory reading. Loney's excellent treatise on this topic is further distinguished by a degree of telling levity that is unfortunately rare in the hyperactivity literature:

> Evaluating treatments for childhood hyperactivity turns out to be even worse than one fears. It's a lot like agreeing to put on a hair shirt—and then finding out that the arms tie in the back . . . (Loney, 1981, p. 77)

Criticisms of rating scales of hyperactivity have centered on some vital points such as instability over time. With the Conners Scale, for example, Werry and Sprague (1974) reported a general reduction in scores from the first to the second rating, by the same rater, but not from the second to the third rating. They attributed this significant drop to a practice effect, but recent research by Milich, Roberts, Loney, and Caputo (1980) suggests that statistical regression may be a more accurate explanation for the decreases that occur. A second problem, one of validity, is the poor correlation between rated and objectively observed behavior (Blunden, Spring, & Greenberg, 1974; Werry, 1978a). Rating scales have also been criticized for poor interrater reliability, although as Whalen and Henker (1976) have noted, the differences are not surprising when temporal and situational variables are taken into consideration. Finally, ratings are made on the basis of subjective judgments rather than on firm empirical findings (Sandoval, 1977) and there are opportunities for rater bias, halo effects, and other errors. The use to be made of the ratings determines how serious these subjective flaws are, for example, if it is the rater's view of the child that one wants, then the subjective aspects of it are of value; if an accurate rating is the goal, then these aspects become a negative factor. A recent study by Madle, Neisworth, and Kurtz (1980) underscores the importance of observer training for rating accuracy in general and particularly with respect to reducing the effects of diagnostic labels.

Despite the acknowledged difficulties, ratings of hyperactivity are widely used in both clinical assessment and empirical investigations, with teacher rating scales outnumbering those for use by parents and, of these, the Conners Teacher Rating Scale being by far the most widely used. In this section we will describe the teacher rating scales, scales that both teachers and parents can use, and parent rating scales.

Teacher Rating Scales

Conners Teacher Rating Scale

This 39-item behavior symptom checklist (Conners, 1969, 1973) is the most widely used and researched of the teacher rating scales and is regarded as a good assessment tool (see Table 4.1). The 39 items may be summed to yield a global score; scored on a topic basis, such as classroom behavior, group participation, and attitude to authority; or scored on a factor basis, for example, Conduct Problem–Aggressivity, Inattentiveness, Anxiety–Tension, Hyperactivity, and Sociability. Each item is rated on a 4-point scale with the following categories: Not at all (score=0), Just a little (score=1), Pretty much (score=2), and Very much (score=3). The test–retest factor reliabilities range from .70 to .90 (Conners, 1973). The scale has consistently proven to be drug sensitive (Werry & Sprague, 1970, 1974) and to correlate with classroom behavior; in addition, all the factors except Anxiety–Tension have differentiated between hyperactive and normal children (Sandoval, 1977). The six items that comprise the 1969 Hyperactivity factor (constantly fidgeting; hums and makes other odd noises; restless or overactive; excitable, impulsive; disturbs other children; teases other children or interferes with their activities) have frequently been used in assessment and research on hyperactive children in the classroom setting (e.g., Copeland & Weissbrod, 1978; Gittelman-Klein & Klein; 1975 Kendall & Brophy, 1981). The efficacy of the scale for assessing and diagnosing hyperactive children in this setting has been confirmed by many investigators (Douglas, Parry, Marton, & Garson, 1976; Kupietz, Bialer, & Winsberg, 1972; Sprague, Christensen, & Werry, 1974; Sprague & Sleator, 1973; Trites, Blouin, Ferguson, & Lynch, 1981). Norms have been developed for a variety of populations including New York (Kupietz et al., 1972), the Midwest (Sprague, Cohen, & Werry, 1974), New Zealand (Werry, Sprague, & Cohen, 1975), Australia (Glow, 1981), and Canada (Trites, 1979a).

A revision of the Conners Teacher Rating Scale has been made by Goyette, Conners, and Ulrich (1978). The scale has been shortened to 28 items and in

Table 4.1. Conners Teacher Rating Scale

IV. Listed below are descriptive terms of behavior. Place a check mark in the column which best describes this child. ANSWER ALL ITEMS.

Observation	Degree of Activity			
	Not at all	Just a little	Pretty much	Very much
CLASSROOM BEHAVIOR				
1. Constantly fidgeting				
2. Hums and makes other odd noises				
3. Demands must be met immediately—easily frustrated				
4. Coordination poor				
5. Restless or overactive				
6. Excitable, impulsive				
7. Inattentive, easily distracted				
8. Fails to finish things he starts—short attention span				
9. Overly sensitive				
10. Overly serious or sad				
11. Daydreams				
12. Sullen or sulky				
13. Cries often and easily				
14. Disturbs other children				
15. Quarrelsome				
16. Mood changes quickly and drastically				
17. Acts "smart"				
18. Destructive				
19. Steals				
20. Lies				
21. Temper outbursts, explosive and unpredictable behavior				
GROUP PARTICIPATION				
22. Isolates himself from other children				
23. Appears to be unaccepted by group				
24. Appears to be easily led				
25. No sense of fair play				
26. Appears to lack leadership				
27. Does not get along with opposite sex				
28. Does not get along with same sex				
29. Teases other children or interferes with their activities				
ATTITUDE TOWARD AUTHORITY				
30. Submissive				
31. Defiant				
32. Impudent				
33. Shy				
34. Fearful				
35. Excessive demands for teacher's attention				
36. Stubborn				
37. Overly anxious to please				
38. Uncooperative				
39. Attendance problem				

Reproduced, by permission, from C. Keith Conners.

some cases the wording of the items has been slightly modified to simplify administration and interpretation. Items not loading in previous factor analytic studies have been omitted, and some similar or redundant items have been combined into single items. Goyette et al. (1978, p. 222) have stated that in important respects the original and revised scales are the same. Factor analyses of the revised scale compared favorably with previous analysis of the original one, and interrater parent–teacher reliability was acceptable, with the comparison producing relatively high correlations on the hyperactivity items. It appears that investigators who wish to use this shortened version may do so without significant loss of information.

Conners Abbreviated Teacher Rating Scale

This scale (Conners, 1973a) consists of 10 overlapping parent and teacher items from the 39-item Conners Teacher Rating Scale shown in Table 4.1. The 10 items were selected from those most often checked by teachers, and they have proven to be reliable in identifying hyperactive children and assessing drug-induced effects (Conners, 1972; Sprague & Sleator, 1973). The items are rated on the same 4-point scale used in the full scales. On the basis of a normative study (Sprague et al., 1974) the cutting score for classifying a child as hyperactive is a mean item rating of 1.5 or a total score of 15 for the 10 items. Satisfactory correlations have been reported between this checklist and both the Hyperactivity factor and the mean of all factors of the Conners Teacher Rating Scale (Werry et al., 1975), and also between this checklist and the Conners Teacher Rating Scale (Sprague et al., 1974). When frequent follow-up assessments of the hyperactive child by parents as well as teachers are required, the brevity of the 10-item scale is viewed as a definite advantage over the longer scales.

Sprague, Ullman, and Sleator (1981) have expressed concern about the items on both the Conners Teacher Rating Scale and the Conners Abbreviated Teacher Rating Scale following an empirical investigation and a comparison of the items in the scales assessing attention with the DSM III criteria for attention deficit. Sprague et al. obtained teacher ratings on both the 39- and 10-item scales on 183 clinic referrals for hyperactivity and on 725 normal second- and third-grade children. Although the cut-off score of 15 did indeed identify the hyperactive children, the attention item scores of the hyperactive children fell into a normal distribution over the entire range and showed considerable overlap with those of the normal children. This finding raises doubts about the discriminatory capacity of the scales, but a more fundamental problem concerns item content. Sprague et al. (1981) note that "only three of the eight items in the Conners Inattentive-Passive Factor group seem to be describing characteristics usually thought of as inattention." The eight items involved here are: Distractibility or attention span a problem; Daydreams; Appears to be easily led by other children; Appears to lack leadership; Fails to finish things that he starts; Childish and immature; Easily frustrated in efforts; and Difficulty in learning. In support of this observation Sprague et al. (1981) cite the "striking" differences between these items and the characteristics listed in DSM III. Further they note that the Conners Abbreviated Teacher Rating Scale contains only one item corresponding with one of the attention criteria in DSM III—"Fails to finish things he starts, short attention span."

Further criticism can be made of both the items and the response choices. In the items the behavior is labeled but operational definitions are rarely provided, so the respondent must generalize rather than rate specific behaviors in specific contexts; for example, on the revision of the Parents Questionnaire Item 29—Cruel, and Item 14—Destructive, both require generalization. There is overlap, for example, Item 38—Disturbs other children, Item 36—Doesn't get along well with sisters or brothers, and Item 20—Quarrelsome. The wording is ambiguous and confusing particularly when a negatively worded item is considered in relation to the scale point Not at all, for example, Item 34—Doesn't like or doesn't follow rules or restrictions. Both descriptive and interpretive items are included, for example, Item 35—Fights constantly and Item 45—Feels cheated in family circle. More than one kind of behavior is included in one item, for example, Item 19—Denies mistakes or blames others and Item 4—Excitable, impulsive. The shortcomings of the response choice will be discussed later in this section.

Several other investigators (Loney & Milich, 1981; Sprague & Sleator, 1973) have developed revisions of the Conners Teacher Rating Scale by selecting items to meet their research needs, adding or eliminating items, or changing their wording. After Loney and her colleagues (Langhorne & Loney, 179; Loney, Langhorne, & Paternite, 1978) had arrived at three diagnostic subgroups of hyperactive children—exclusive hyperactive (high scores on hyperactivity and low scores on aggression), exclusive aggressives (high scores on aggression and low scores on hyperactivity), and aggressive hyperactives (high scores on both aggression and hyperactivity)—they sought an assessment procedure for separating clinic referrals into these diagnostic subgroups. To test the possibility that the Conners Teacher Rating Scale would fill this need, Loney and Milich (1981) had trained judges independently rate the psychiatric charts of 50 boys from six to 12 years of age who were clinic referrals. Hyperactivity and aggression factor scores were derived from each boy's chart ratings and then were correlated with scores on the Conners Teacher Rating Scale. The existing Conners factors of Hyperactivity, Conduct Problem, and Inattentive-Passive all correlated with *both* of Loney et al.'s criterion factors of Hyperactivity and Aggression, and so failed to discriminate children on the basis of these criterion factors. The Conners Hyperactivity Factor, for example, correlated .54 with the Hyperactivity Factor Score from the chart ratings, and .44 with the Aggression Factor Score, with both correlations being significant. Loney and Milich (1981) then developed a 10-item measure of the hyperactivity and aggression dimensions correlating each item on the Conners Teacher Rating Scale with both chart rating factors and retaining for the hyperactivity and aggression subscales only those items that correlated significantly with either the Hyperactivity factor *or* the Aggression factor, but not with both. These 10 items formed the Iowa Conners Teacher's Rating Scale shown in Table 4.2. A report of the assessment of the reliability and validity of this scale is contained in Loney and Milich (1981).

Other Teacher Rating Scales

The Illinois Classroom Assessment Profile (ICAP) is a 27-item teacher rating scale developed by Porges, Ullman, Drasgow, Sleator, and Sprague (1980) to describe the behavioral components that have been consistently observed in children diagnosed as hyperactive. The ICAP contains five empirically established subscales assessing the following dimensions (Porges, Drasgow, Ullman, Sleator, & Sprague, 1981):

1. Concentration—easily absorbed in academic tasks to great difficulty in focusing attention.
2. Interaction—cooperative, gets along well with others to aggressive, disruptive, and difficult to live with.
3. Patience—thoughtful, reflective to heedless and impulsive.
4. Anxiety—relaxed and likes being evaluated to tense and fears evaluation.
5. Coordination—excellent manual dexterity to clumsy.

Table 4.2. Iowa Conners Teacher's Rating Scale[a]

Check the column which best describes this child.

	Not at all	Just a little	Pretty much	Very much
1. Fidgeting				
2. Hums and makes other odd noises				
3. Excitable, impulsive				
4. Inattentive, easily distracted				
5. Fails to finish things he starts (short attention span)				
6. Quarrelsome				
7. Acts "smart"				
8. Temper outbursts (explosive and unpredictable behavior)				
9. Defiant				
10. Uncooperative				

[a] Items 1 through 5 are summed to provide a score on the Inattention-Overactivity (IO) subscale; items 6 through 10 are summed to provide a score on the Aggression (A) subscale. For both subscales, items checked *not at all* are scored 0, those checked *just a little* are scored 1, those checked *pretty much* are scored 2, and those checked *very much* are scored 3.

Reprinted, by permission, from Loney, J., and Milich, R. Hyperactivity, inattention, and aggression in clinical practice. In M. Wolraich and D.K. Routh (Eds.), *Advances in Behavioral Pediatrics*, (Vol. 2). Greenwich, CT: JAI Press, 1981.

Of particular interest was the finding in the early stages of development of this scale (Porges et al., 1981) that the factor analytic procedures did *not* identify an activity factor. The items associated with activity or descriptive of it were factor complex, which led the scale developers to conclude that teachers do not identify a unique trait of activity level but evaluate activity levels as correlates of other dimensions of behavior.

An important feature of the ICAP is that the child's behavior is rated on a continuum with anchors consisting of concrete behaviors that are typical of children at the associated point in the scale. Item 16—Does the child seek or demand excessive teacher attention?, for example, has the following anchor points:

0	Seeks attention appropriately, only when necessary.
50	Usually seeks attention appropriately; may make excessive demands if confused, will calm down when asked.
75	Demands attention when frustrated, becomes insistent if required to wait.
100	Constantly seeks attention by asking silly questions, badgering teacher or talking out.

The anchors are guides to the range of the behavior in question, and the rater may use any integer from 0 to 100, that is, he is not limited to response options as with the nonbehavioral anchors of the Conners Scales with the 0—not at all, 1—just a little, 2—quite a bit, and 3—very much format. Porges et al. (1982) report that the effect of their format is to minimize between-teacher idiosyncratic differences: the impact of such differences is approximately 50 percent greater on the Conners Teacher Rating Scale (1969) than it is on the ICAP. The ICAP can also be used as a clinical screening device for children at risk or for deviant children; scale scores that would place a child in either of these categories are provided.

The ICAP was standardized on 707 children from 32 second and third grade classrooms. Internal consistency measures yielded satisfactory reliability on all five subscales. Fidelity coefficients showed that all the subscales related strongly to the factors that they were intended to measure, the lowest fidelity coefficient being .92. The ICAP appears to have excellent psychometric properties and considerable potential as a research and clinical instrument. Independent assessments of its value remain to be conducted. In the meantime the sophisticated procedures used in developing this instrument constitute a model of fine psychometric technique of great value for other scale developers.

Three other teacher rating scales will be briefly described. The Bell, Waldrop, and Weller Rating System (Bell, Waldrop, & Weller, 1972) has often been used despite many faults. Two more recent and less well-known scales that are far superior to the Bell, Waldrop, and Weller are the Behavior and

Temperament Survey (Sandoval, Lambert, & Sassone, 1980) and the School Behavior Survey, (Lambert, 1977).

The *Bell, Waldrop, and Weller Rating System* (see Table 4.3) consists of six hyperactivity rating scales and three withdrawal rating scales. Each is an 11-point scale with descriptive statements provided for from three to five of the 11 scale points. The scales all involve direct behavior observation, so that the rater does not have to go beyond this level, a plus feature; however, the descriptive statements for points within a scale are ambiguous. For example, the Frenetic Play scale includes frequency, intensity, and location unsystematically placed along the scale. As the scale points are described, the selection of a point along the scale is arbitrary. The sixth point on the Induction of Intervention scale is defined as "three to four interventions per day required" and the first point as "never plays in such a way that requires intervention." If one or two interventions a day are required the rater has four scale points (2, 3, 4, 5) to choose from and still remain within the defined points. Having 11 points in each scale would appear to contribute to rater error. Behaviors within a scale do not all relate to the topic of the category so that two different continua are treated as one. For example, in the Nomadic Play scale, three scale points (11, 6, 3) concern amount of shifting from one activity to the next, but the first scale point (1) is a withdrawal-from-activity behavior, "Very hesitant to engage in play. Stands and watches or leans on mother or teacher." There is overlap between scales. Although the distinction between Frenetic Play and Nomadic Play is clear in the Bell et al. (1972) article (*frenetic* has an intense and disorganized quality, whereas *nomadic* concerns rapid movement from activity to activity), this distinction is unclear in the descriptions given the rater: the descriptions for the eleventh point on both scales are difficult to differentiate. The scales vary greatly in breadth. Frenetic Play is a characteristic applying to a wide range of activities, while Spilling and Throwing is a very specific kind of behavior. It is difficult to see how satisfactory full-scale reliability could be obtained by two raters independently rating one child on the entire scale, with the limited number of *defined* scale points and without excessive training for the observers. Full-scale interobserver reliability for behavior ratings should be in the high .90s, and this level is not difficult to achieve with operationally defined response categories and descriptive items. Some validity support is provided by the finding that most (no data given) but not all of the children identified by the staff as having definite adjustment programs had scores above the cutting point, signifying the presence of adjustment problems.

The *Behavior and Temperament Survey* (Sandoval et al., 1980) is a 32-item checklist of behavioral attributes that are characteristic of hyperactive children, for example, motor restlessness, inattentiveness, impulsivity, aggressiveness, and emotional lability. The scale was designed for research use in the early 1970s and is similar in format to the Conners Teacher Rating Scale. The respondent checks a 4-point scale with categories from "not at all characteristic" to "very much characteristic." Test–retest reliability and internal consis

Table 4.3 Definitions of Rating Scales Used in Preschool Hyperactivity and Withdrawal Factor Scales

Scale Points	Definitions Hyperactivity

Frenetic Play

11. Much more than others, shows impulsive, fast moving, ineffective, incomplete play.
9. During play and transitions shows behavior with only two or three of the components listed in 11, or play showing all components but with less intensity.
6. Only during transitions or in vehicle shows frenetic behavior.
4. During transistions shows mild frenetic behavior.
1. Never shows any frenetic behavior.

Scale	11	10	9	8	7	6	5	4	3	2	1
Percentage distribution[a]	0	.2	.2	1	1	2	2	4	8	16	64

Induction of Intervention

11. Very frequently plays in such a way as to make it highly likely teacher in area would feel compelled to intervene either to prevent injury to the child or others, or to prevent damage to physical objects.
6. Three to four interventions per day required.
1. Never plays in such a way that requires intervention.

Scale	11	10	9	8	7	6	5	4	3	2	1
Percentage distribution	0	0	.1	1	1	2	2	4	8	16	66

Inability to Delay

11. When waiting turn for food, toy or any other object which is of interest, or when waiting to take part in some activity, seems unusually unable to wait for gratification.
9. Same as 11, except behavior is shown only during certain situations, such as transitions, or in the car.
6. In only a few instances seemed unable to wait for gratification.
1. Under above circumstances seems definitely able to contain self and wait for gratification.

Scale	11	10	9	8	7	6	5	4	3	2	1
Percentage distribution	0	.2	1	1	2	7	10	13	17	20	30

Emotional Aggression

11. Frequently throws toys, tears things down, breaks toys, pushes objects over, attacks, pushes or hits, takes things from others even though not needed to achieve an objective and even though may or may not be upset.
6. Usually interested in other activities but will occasionally throw toys, tear things down, break toys, etc., as a reaction to frustration, when just wandering, or during transitions.
1. Never takes from others.

Scale	11	10	9	8	7	6	5	4	3	2	1
Percentage distribution	0	0	.1	.1	.1	2	1	2	6	10	80

Nomadic Play

11. Shifts rapidly from one setting or toy to another, typically trying out an item for only an instant and then moving on, showing no sustained play or engagement of interest unless assisted.
6. Shifts between toys or settings but finds two or three activities during the session which engage interest for approximately five minutes.
3. Goes straight to a single setting or toy on arrival and remains engaged for most of session.
1. Very hesistant to engage in any play. Stands and watches or leans on mother or teacher.

Scale	11	10	9	8	7	6	5	4	3	2	1
Percentage distribution	.1	.2	2	6	13	28	22	18	10	2	.2

Spilling, Throwing

11. Spills water, containers, salt or other substances and/or throws food or other objects much more often than others (playful throwing of a ball should not be considered under this heading).
9. In certain situations, such as in the car or in transitions, shows frequent spilling and throwing.
6. Usually interested in other activities, but will occasionally spill and/or throw either as a reaction to frustration or when just wandering.
1. Never spills water or throws objects.

Scale	11	10	9	8	7	6	5	4	3	2	1
Percentage distribution	0	1	2	3	6	14	18	21	18	12	5

Withdrawal

Vacant Staring

11. Is immobile and staring without apparent focus much more than others.
9. Spends a large amount of time staring in a single direction, at a single object, setting or area, or occasionally shows staring without focus. (This can accompany relatively disorganized or aimless play.)
3. Seldom shows fixed or vacant staring and then as a reaction to some specific strange or fearful incident.
1. Never shows fixed or vacant staring.

Scale	11	10	9	8	7	6	5	4	3	2	1
Percentage distribution	0	.1	1	1	2	6	10	14	20	24	24

Closeness to Adult Base

11. Spends an unusually large amount of time clinging tightly to mother or teacher, hiding eyes, not exploring the situation either visually or otherwise.
9. Almost continuously follows or remains close to mother or teacher.
6. Alternates staying close to mother or teacher with occasional efforts to play separately.
4. Plays separately, except during transitions.
2. Only comes to mother or teacher and stays close when there is something strange or novel in situation.
1. Never spends time in activities listed.

Scale	11	10	9	8	7	6	5	4	3	2	1
Percentage distribution	0	0	1	1	2	3	6	15	19	28	28

Chronic Fearfulness

11. Characteristically appears to be guarded, wary, defensive, apprehensive, frightened, or panicky.
6. Neither characteristically bold or guarded; shows some of each.
1. Seems to be bold rather than fearful; seldom, if ever, shows fearfulness, even in situations which might ordinarily be expected to produce this effect.

Scale	11	10	9	8	7	6	5	4	3	2	1
Percentage distribution	0	.2	1	1	2	8	12	18	23	20	14

ᵃSmoothed percentages for scale points 11 through 1, based on combined data for 43 males and 31 females (test samples).

Reprinted from Bell, R. Q., Waldrop, M. F., and Weller, G. M. A rating system for the assessment of hyperactive and withdrawn children in preschool samples. *American Journal of Orthopsychiatry*, 1972, *42*, 23–34. Copyright 1972 by the American Orthopsychiatric Association, Inc. Reproduced by permission.

tency measures are .89 and .96, respectively. Concurrent validity estimates showed a correlation of .89 with the Conners Abbreviated Symptoms Questionnaire, and .82 with the School Behavior Survey.

The *School Behavior Survey,* an unpublished rating scale developed by the Lambert team (1977), differs markedly from the foregoing teacher rating scales, with half of its 32 items being positive behavior and the rest negative behavior. Four attributes are measured: motor restlessness, impulsivity, attention–distractibility, and social aggressiveness, with eight items per attribute. The items are specific descriptors of children in school settings, for example, #3: At recess prefers games such as tag or spontaneous activities involving running; #4: Stays calmly seated during school assemblies or other programs; #12: In class discussions, blurts out answers without raising hand or following other procedures; #22: Cannot do seatwork when an unfamiliar child or adult is in the classroom. The 4-point scale descriptors are concerned with the frequency of specific behavior: (the child exhibits a particular response) every day or nearly always, once or twice a week, rarely, never. The test–retest reliability and internal consistency measures are both .95. Concurrent validity estimates were .76 with the Conners Abbreviated Symptoms Questionnaire and .82 with the Behavior and Temperament Survey.

Sandoval (1981, in press) compared teacher ratings on the Conners Abbreviated Symptoms Questionnaire, the Behavior Temperament Survey, and the School Behavior Survey. The latter scale resulted in more discriminating teacher ratings, because teachers were more willing to use the extreme rating categories on this scale (the greater the dispersion of ratings, the more discriminatory the measure). Categories indicating moderate and extreme deviance were more often used if items worded negatively were interspersed with the positively worded ones and if the items had more concrete descriptors. The categories indicating deviance were selected more often for negatively worded items than for positively worded items. Analysis of the data indicated that there would be more children identified as potentially hyperactive with the Behavior and Temperament Survey and there would be fewer false positive hyperactives identified with this scale than with the School Behavior Survey.

Although teacher ratings are considered to be of prime value in the diagnosis of hyperactivity as well as reliable and valid indicators of treatment effects (e.g., Rapoport et al., 1974; Sleator, von Neumann, & Sprague, 1974; Whalen & Henker, 1980b), Sandoval (1981, in press) has expressed concern about certain weaknesses in the rating scale format that tend to magnify further those attributes of teacher rating procedures that are known to reduce the precision of ratings. Most teacher rating scales contain leading questions worded in the negative and are thus subject to rater bias and response sets such as reverse halo effects or reverse generosity errors (Selltiz, Wrightsman, & Cook, 1976); many items consist of traits or symptoms lacking concrete descriptive anchors so that there are no firm standards for comparisons.

Parent and Teacher Rating Scales

The most important rating scale in this category is the Conners Abbreviated Teacher Rating Scale (see Table 4.4) that has already been discussed. Several other less well-developed scales include the Davids Rating Scale for Hyperkinesis (Davids, 1971) and the Hyperactivity Rating Scale (Blunden, Spring, & Greenberg, 1974).

Davids (1971) Rating Scale for Hyperkinesis

This scale assesses seven characteristics of hyperactivity on a six-point Likert scale ranging from "much less," "less," "slightly less than most children," to "slightly more," "much more than most children." The six traits are hyperactivity, short attention span, variability, impulsiveness, inability to delay gratification, irritability, and explosiveness. The possible score ranges from 6 to 36; scores of 24 or more suggest hyperkinesis, scores of 19 to 23 are in the suspicious range, and those of 18 or less indicate no significant hyperkinesis. The scale is similar in content and form to the Conners Abbreviated Teacher Questionnaire but has fewer items. No reliability data have been reported by the developer of the scale. The validity data are sparse. Schnackenberg (1973) found the scale to be drug-sensitive (caffeine), and Denhoff, Davids, and Hawkins (1971) reported that it differentiated between active drug and placebo. The most extensive research on this rating scale comes from Zentall and Barack (1979) in a study of the concurrent validity and inter- and intratest reliability for the Davids Rating Scale and the Conners Abbreviated Teacher Rating Scale. In this study 16 teachers from two special and two regular schools rated 211 normal children and 49 special class children in grades one to four on both scales. The Conners scale was more conservative in its criterion for labeling children as hyperactive. High correlations were found suggesting excellent predictability between scales and considerable stability across raters and over time. Interrater reliability for the Davids scale on seven children rated by two teachers five months apart was .94, which is impressive in view of the small number of subjects. Intrarater reliability was .89 for the Conners scale over a 2-week period, and .71 for the Davids scale over a 5-month period.

Davids (1971) presents the scale as a less than fully developed tool, lacking reliability, validity, and normative data, and hopes that these data will be forthcoming from scale users, a cavalier attitude at best. Specific weaknesses of the scale include categories that overlap, require the respondent to extrapolate well beyond direct observation because the behaviors are described in general contexts rather than in specific situations, and lack clear operational definitions. The response choices are ambiguous. The standard is "behavior displayed by other 'normal' children." The respondents' definitions of 'normal" and their experience with children would lead to fluctuating standards across raters. No attempt is made to define the scale points and an important

Table 4.4. Conners' Abbreviated Teacher Rating Scale

CONNERS' ABBREVIATED TEACHER RATING SCALE

Child's Name _____

TEACHER'S OBSERVATIONS

Information obtained _____ By _____

Month   Day   Year

Observation	Degree of Activity			
	Not at all 0	Just a little 1	Pretty much 2	Very much 3
1. Restless or overactive				
2. Excitable, impulsive				
3. Disturbs other children				
4. Fails to finish things he starts, short attention span				
5. Constantly fidgeting				
6. Inattentive, easily distracted				
7. Demands must be met immediately – easily frustrated				
8. Cries often and easily				
9. Mood changes quickly and drastically				
10. Temper outbursts, explosive and unpredictable behavior				

OTHER OBSERVATIONS OF TEACHER (Use reverse side if more space is required.)

_____

_____

_____

_____

_____

Reproduced, by permission, from C. Keith Conners.

scale point, "same as," is omitted so that the respondent is forced to use either "slightly less" or "slightly more," when in fact he may regard the child as "the same as other children."

Hyperactivity Rating Scale

Spring and his associates (Blunden et al., 1974; Spring, Blunden, Greenberg, & Yellin, 1977; Spring, Greenberg, & Yellin, 1977) have developed the Hyperactivity Rating Scale for use by parents and teachers. This rating scale contains 11 categories, such as restlessness, impulsivity, and distractibility, with three items per category. The items in the category Rapid Tempo, for example, are talks rapidly, does things quickly, and walks fast. Items are in random sequence and category names do not appear on the rating form. Each item is rated on a 5-point scale: never observed, infrequently observed, sometimes observed, frequently observed, and always observed. Category scores are computed by adding ratings for the three items within each category. Validity and normative data have been reported by Spring et al. (1977), and Sandoval (1977), in his review of measures of hyperactivity, describes the scale as having good reliability and validity data for hyperactive children.

New Scales Being Developed

Zukow, Zukow, and Bentler (1978) have developed parent and teacher rating scales for identifying hyperactivity in preschool and elementary school children and assessing intervention procedures. The 26 items used in developing the parent rating scale formed three clusters: classical hyperactive behaviors, motor coordination, and sustained attention. Each item requires a Yes or No response. The teacher rating scale was developed with 15 items described as covering a broad range of school activities: tapping, motor skills, attention, and impulsive–explosive behavior. Teacher ratings on each item were made on a 5-point scale. Limited teacher time was the reason given for restricting the scale to 15 items. Multivariate analysis of parent ratings of clinical and control subjects yielded three factors: Excitability, Motor Coordination, and Directed Attention; the teacher ratings yielded two factors: Attention–Excitability and Motor Coordination. Analysis of variance of each factor score showed significant differences between clinical and control subjects, and cut-off scores correctly identified a large percentage of clinical and control subjects.

The scales at this point have several faults, quite apart from various methodological weaknesses in their development. The Yes-No answer format for parents and the reduced length of the teacher scale both serve as unnecessary limitations on the amount of information potentially available from these sources. Some of the items on the parent scale describe behaviors that are not typically associated with hyperactivity ("Panics easily") and that have limited applicability ("Trouble with bicycle" overlooks the fact that not all children have bicycles, particularly at the preschool level). Some items describe more than one behavior or attribute ("Is child lazy—not trying to do well in school?" "Not learning in school although seems 'bright.'"). On the teacher scale the item "There are no activities that the child can focus his attention on" is a poor item because the item is not apparently restricted to school activities, and there are always some activities that the child can focus on. As Douglas (1980) and others (Klein & Young, 1979) have noted, the hyperactive child can focus on activities in the classroom, it is just that they are not teacher-designated activities. Altogether, considerable work would be needed if these scales are to have any possibility of contributing to the cluster of established scales already available. Unless a new scale makes some unusual contribution it would appear that research efforts would more profitably be directed to the development of normative data for subgroups of hyperactive children on existing rating scales (Sandoval, 1977).

Parent Rating Scales

Werry—Weiss—Peters Activity Scale

This parent rating scale (see Table 4.5) developed by Werry and his associates (Werry, 1968) was originally intended for use by a professional in interviewing parents. Used in this way the scale yielded an interrater reliability of .90 (Werry, Weiss, Douglas, & Martin, 1966). However, it is almost always used now for parent ratings. The scale consists of seven categories, five for specific contexts of activity (mealtime, watching television, doing homework, playing, sleeping) engaged in by the child, and two for more general areas of activity (behavior at school, away from home). The behaviors within a category are all directly observable so that the rater is rating specific behaviors in specific contexts. The scale has been shown to be drug sensitive (e.g., Conners & Rothschild, 1968; Knights & Hinton, 1969; Werry et al., 1966) and has been endorsed by experienced clinicians. However, in a review of this scale the senior developer (Werry, 1978a, p. 60) was unexpectedly negative:

> . . . recent studies have revealed some significant shortcomings. It does not correlate well with objective measures of activity (Barkley & Ullman, 1975; Gittelman-Klein & Klein, 1975; Routh & Schroeder, 1976; Routh et al., 1974; Shaffer et al., 1974) or with teachers' estimates of hyperactivity (Gittelman-Klein & Klein, 1975; Gittelman-Klein et al., 1976) and correlates with estimates of conduct disturbance rather than activity (Shaffer et al., 1974). . . . A factor analytic study (Routh et al., 1974) revealed that instead of a single homogeneous dimension of activity, the scale consists of 7 discrete factors, some specific to the kind of behavior (e.g., verbal) and some to the situation (TV behavior).

In summary then, the Werry–Weiss–Peters Scale is drug-sensitive, but appears to be less a measure of activity than of various kinds of motor behavior

Table 4.5. Werry–Weiss–Peters Activity Scale

	No	Yes–A little bit	Yes–Very much
During meals			
Up and down at table	—	—	—
Interrupts without regard	—	—	—
Wriggling	—	—	—
Fiddles with things	—	—	—
Talks excessively	—	—	—
Television			
Gets up and down during program	—	—	—
Wriggles	—	—	—
Manipulates objects or body	—	—	—
Talks incessantly	—	—	—
Interrupts	—	—	—
Doing home-work			
Gets up and down	—	—	—
Wriggles	—	—	—
Manipulates objects or body	—	—	—
Talks incessantly	—	—	—
Requires adult supervision or attendance	—	—	—
Play			
Inability for quiet play	—	—	—
Constantly changing activity	—	—	—
Seeks parental attention	—	—	—
Talks excessively	—	—	—
Disrupts other's play	—	—	—
Sleep			
Difficulty settling down for sleep	—	—	—
Inadequate amount of sleep	—	—	—
Restless during sleep	—	—	—
Behavior away from home (except school)			
Restlessness during travel	—	—	—
Restlessness during shopping (includes touching everything)	—	—	—
Restlessness during church/movies	—	—	—
Restlessness during visiting friends, relatives, etc.	—	—	—
School behavior			
Up and down	—	—	—
Fidgets, wriggles, touches	—	—	—
Interrupts teacher or other children excessively	—	—	—
Constantly seeks teacher's attention	—	—	—
Total Score	_____	_____	_____

Reprinted, by permission, from Werry, J. S. Developmental hyperactivity. *Pediatric Clinics of North America*, 1968, *15*, 581–599.

with an emphasis on those which are socially unacceptable. It is thus as much a "problem child" defining measure or measure of *hyperactivity* as we have defined it here as an estimate of activity level.

The above statement is surprising in view of certain considerations. The fact that Werry–Weiss–Peters ratings generally do not correlate well with objective measures of activity is to be expected on two counts. First, it is unreasonable to require that a global rating correlate with narrow or situation-specific objective measures. The Scale is a rating based on extensive observations of the child in multiple situations by a parent who knows him well. It is a global rating in the broadest sense as compared to the objective measures of activity, such as the open field measure of grid crossings by nonhyperactive children (Routh et al., 1974), which represent a very narrow sample of behavior usually obtained in a novel situation that in itself may result in atypically "good" behavior. The typical objective measure can lead to behavior data that are not representative of the child's general behavior. However, a study by Stevens et al. (1978) has shown that when objective data are representative of the child's everyday activities, then the Scale does correlate with them. Stevens et al. used actometers to measure the activity of hyperactive boys and boys with other problems, in four different settings (classroom, gymnasium, woodshop, and group therapy), and then correlated these four scores plus an overall score (a combined measure derived from actometer scores in the four settings) with mothers' ratings on a modified version of the Scale; the mothers' ratings correlated significantly with actometer data from gymnasium ($r = .67$), woodshop ($r = .77$), and with overall activity ($r = .65$). A second reason for the failure of Werry–Weiss–Peters ratings to correlate with objective measures of activity is that parental judgments of hyperactivity appear to be closely tied to the hyperactive child's level of noncompliance and the parent's need to supervise and direct the child (Barkley, 1981). Barkley and Cunningham (1979) correlated rating scores from the Werry–Weiss–Peters and the Hyperactivity Index of the Conners Parent Questionnaire with objective measures of mother–hyperactive child interactions. The results showed that measures of child noncompliance and maternal commands correlated highly with the rating scale scores, with correlations ranging from .40 to .70 depending on whether the observational data were based on free play or supervised task periods.

The failure of the Scale to correlate with teachers' estimates is reasonable because almost all items on it are unrelated to the school setting (behavior during meals, television, doing homework, play, sleep, behavior away from home but not including school). Although some of the play items could be rated by the teacher, there are only four specific school items on the whole scale. Teachers generally lack the knowledge necessary to rate a child on this scale, which was designed as a parents' scale. One final point concerns the correlation with estimates of conduct disturbance rather than activity (Shaffer, McNamara, & Pincus, 1974). When Werry et al. constructed the scale, hyperactivity was viewed as a quantitative problem of excessive activity. Currently it is viewed as inappropriate behavior. If hyperactive children were excessively active, then scores on the scale probably would correlate with activity. But this is not the case: the behavior of the hyperactive child is much closer to a conduct disturbance than it is to a consistently high level of activity. Because the scale measures a variety of inappropriate activities, it would have been most unlikely that Routh et al. (1974) would have identified a single activity factor. The Werry–Weiss–Peters Scale is really a measure of inappropriate activity rather than of total activity and as such is useful in the assessment of hyperactvity.

Conners Parents Questionnaire

Conners (1970) has also developed a 93-item parent symptom checklist that assesses a diverse group of problems including fears, worries, bowel problems, sex problems, and perfectionism. Factor analysis identified six factors—Antisocial, Enuresis-Encopresis, Psychosomatic, and Anxious-Immature. The items were rated on the same 4-point scale as that in the Conners Teacher Rating Scale. Children previously diagnosed as hyperactive were correctly identified as hyperactive in 74 percent of the cases ($n = 133$) rated by parents (Conners, 1970). No reliability data have been reported for this questionnaire, there is no firm evidence of its validity, and normative data are scarce (Glow, 1981). It has recently been revised by Goyette, Conners, and Ulrich (1978). The scale has been shortened to 48 items and the wording in some items has been improved. Interrater correlations (mother–father) were satisfactory. Normative data were presented for 570 children.

On rating scales a failure to define the response categories operationally results in respondents attaching different numerical values to the response choices. For example, Simpson (1944) reported great differences among raters in applying the category "frequently": 25 percent used this term to describe events occurring at least 80 percent of the time, whereas another 25 percent used it for events occurring less than 40 percent of the time. The same problem arises in the Conners scales with the categories Not at all, Just a little, Pretty much, and Very much, and in a number of other scales. The Infant Temperament Questionnaire (Carey & McDevitt, 1978), for example, has the following categories: almost never, rarely, variable usually does not, variable usually does, frequently, and almost always; and the Behavior and Temperament Survey (Sandoval, Lambert, & Sassone, 1980) categories are: Not at all characteristic, A little characteristic, Quite a bit characteristic, and Very much characteristic. In the case of the Conners, if one parent regards 10 instances of bullying (Item 39) over the previous month as sufficient for a rating of Very much (Scale Point 3) and another parent categorizes the same number of bullying incidents as Just a little (Scale Point 1), the diagnostic value of the information supplied by the rating scale is limited, as is the value of the scale for research in which the dependent variable is between-child comparisons based on parental ratings. To obtain some information on the numerical values that parents assign to the four categories, we conducted individual interviews with white, middle-class mothers of elementary school children. All of the mothers had attended college for two or more years. Following a brief explanatory statement and opportunity for questions, each mother was given a total of three items, one at a time. She was handed a card with a single item and the four categories on it and was asked how often in the past month her child would have had to exhibit the behavior described in the item for her to use each of the categories. For each of the three items the mother gave four numerical values that would result in her rating her child in the different categories. The three items given to each mother from the Conners Parent Questionnaire were Item 32—Wants help doing things he should do alone, Item 39—Bullying, and Item 57—Throws and breaks things. As can be seen from Table 4.6, the results from this rather homogeneous group of respondents showed a wide range of numerical values for each category except Not at all (Scale Point 0), to which the majority responded with a zero. We recognize that these mothers were stating how they thought a child would have to behave to be rated in each of the four categories and, as such, are clearly somewhat different from mothers who are completing the rating scale because their children do have problems serious enough to warrant a consultation. Nonetheless, the results suggest that the Conners scales and, indeed, most scales with this type of undefined descriptive category might be of more value to the professional if the respondent was simply asked, "Approximately how many times in the past week has your child exhibited this behavior?" This type of question could also be combined with categories, as Lambert and Hartsough (1979) did in their Pupil Behavior Rating Scale. For the question, How often does this child act this way? they provided the following categories: Never, Rarely, Once or twice a week, Every day (or nearly always).

Table 4.6. Numerical Values Assigned by Mothers (n = 40) to Categories on Conners' Parents Questionnaire

Item			Not at all	Just a little	Pretty much	Very much
32.	Wants help doing things he should do alone	Mean	1.58	14.73	33.30	51.60
		Range	0–15	2–120	3–200	7–300
39.	Bullying	Mean	0.75	7.60	15.45	29.17
		Range	0–10	1–80	2–100	5–200
57.	Throws and breaks things	Mean	0.50	3.65	6.70	12.02
		Range	0–10	1–30	4–60	5–90

Peer Ratings

Peer evaluations of hyperactive children have rarely been used despite the fact that they are a potentially valuable source of information and have some characteristics not present in other sources (Milich & Landau, 1981). They are obtained in the school, which is the major social setting encountered by the child outside of the home, and are based on observations by a large number of same-age children who view the child dispassionately from a variety of perspectives within a common observation base. Peer ratings are less subject to rater leniency effects than are adult ratings and are surprisingly free of a tendency to respond with prosocial evaluations (Campbell & Paulauskas, 1979; Glow & Glow, 1980; Pekarik, Prinz, Liebert, Weintraub, & Neale, 1976). Also, the use of peer raters can help to separate out context effects on ratings from rater effects or effects due to the relationship between the rater and the child being rated. At the same time, peer ratings are not without shortcomings. In a critical review of three peer assessment methods (peer nominations, ratings, and rankings), Kane and Lawler (1978) describe peer ratings as the most useful of the three methods for feedback purposes but also the one producing the least valid and reliable evaluation.

Glow and Glow (1980) have developed a 50-item scale, the Peer Rating Scale, based on the 35-item, "psychometrically robust" Pupil Evaluation Scale (Pekarik et al., 1976). Items added were in the areas of activity, restlessness, impulsivity, and inattention. All the items on the new scale are worded as questions, with answer categories restricted to Yes-No. In developing the scale Glow and Glow administered it to unselected seventh-grade students who first rated classroom peers and then rated themselves. Cluster analysis of these data resulted in six scales—Shy-sensitive, Inconsiderate, Hyperactive, Effective, Popular, and Bully—each of which showed high internal consistency. The Hyperactivity Scale items corresponded to the clinical concept of hyperactivity, for example, #2. Who fidgets with things? #6. Who is rude to the teacher? #8. Who can't sit still? #16. Who bothers people when they are trying to work? #25. Who always messes around and gets into trouble? #28. Who doesn't pay attention to the teacher? The finding that the items relevant to the clinical concept of hyperactivity emerged as a coherent set was interpreted by Glow and Glow (1980) as a refutation of the notion that hyperactivity is merely a perjorative term used by adults about children's behavior, since unselected school children had no difficulty recognizing a cluster of behaviors relevant to hyperactivity in themselves as well as in their peers.

Self-Ratings

There is a paucity of information in the hyperactivity literature on what the hyperactive child thinks about the whole problem, and attempts to obtain the child's view of his own behavior are almost nonexistent. Serious doubts about the clinical utility of input from the hyperactive child have been expressed even by experienced clinicians (Stewart, Mendelson, & Johnson, 1973), and in the motivational deficit model of hyperactivity proposed by Glow and Glow (1979) predictions were made that hyperactive children would be less accurate than nonhyperactive children in describing their own behavior. However, in the study described in the previous section (Glow & Glow, 1980) the derived Hyperactivity Scale showed substantial convergent and discriminant validity when peer and self-ratings of unselected school children were compared. The distinct overlap between peer and self-perceptions of hyperactive behavior supports the idea that self-assessment by hyperactive children may be a useful clinical tool. The assumption here of course is that the results obtained with unselected school children could be replicated with hyperactive children.

Among the few who are interested in the hyperactive child's perception of his problem is Loney (1980a), who has strongly advocated the use of information obtained directly from the child for both clinical and research purposes. The Teacher Approval–Disapproval Scale (TADS) (Loney, 1974a) is a behaviorally focused school attitude questionnaire that assesses the child's attitudes towards, and estimates of, the amount of teacher approval and disapproval that he receives for academic and social behaviors and that the class as a whole receives for these behaviors. The 22 items on the TADS (see Table 4.7) include 11 items that apply to the individual and assess his perceptions of the teacher's behavior towards himself and how happy or unhappy he is in the classroom. Each of these items has a counterpart that requires the child to make the same judgments concerning the class as a whole. The items are brief and clearly worded, with each rated as "none of the time," "some of the time," "most of the time," or "all of the time," and scored 0, 1, 2, and 3, respectively. Preliminary test–retest reliability data were satisfactory (Whaley-Klahn, Loney, Weissenburger, & Prinz, 1976).

To evaluate the perceptions of hyperactive boys, the TADS was administered to three groups: boys considered by their teacher to be hyperactive and referrable (hyperactive), those considered high active but not referrable (high active), and those within the normal range of activity (normoactive). As would be expected, the three groups differed markedly on the individual scale items, with the hyperactive group reporting less teacher approval for academic, motivational, and social behavior than did the normoactive group, and significantly more general disapproval. However, the three groups differed on only two of the 11 counterpart class items, which suggests that hyperactive boys are capable of a realistic assessment of their own status and that of the class as a whole, and provides further support for the utility of self-report from the hyperactive child.

Table 4.7. **Items of the Teacher Approval–Disapproval Scale (TADS)**

Student behavior	*Items* Teacher response	*The class as a whole*	*The individual student*
Academic	Approval	The teacher likes the school work the class does.	The teacher likes the school work I do.
Motivational	Approval	. . . the way the class works.	. . . the way I work.
Social	Approval	. . . the way the class acts.	. . . the way I act.
General	Approval	My teacher praises students.	My teacher praises me.
Academic	Disapproval	The teacher doesn't like the school work the class does.	The teacher doesn't like the school work I do.
Motivational	Disapproval	. . . the way the class works.	. . . the way I work.
Social	Disapproval	. . . the way the class acts.	. . . the way I act.
General	Disapproval	My teacher punishes students.	My teacher punishes me.
Student Attitude			
Enjoyment		Students enjoy being in this class.	I enjoy being in this class.
Happiness		The students in my classroom are happy.	In my classroom I am happy.
Unhappiness		. . . are unhappy	. . . I am unhappy.

Reprinted, by permission, from Whaley-Klahn, M., Loney, J., Weissenburger, F., and Prinz, R. Responses of boys and girls to a behaviorally focused school attitude questionnaire. *Journal of School Psychology*, 1976, *14*(4), 283–290. Copyright 1976 Human Sciences Press, New York.

CLASSROOM OBSERVATION SCHEDULES

Direct observation in the school environment can provide important data concerning the hyperactive child's behavior and the classroom environment, particularly the teacher's behavior. Observations can be made quite unobtrusively even in the classroom setting; it is best if the teacher is given only a general description of the purpose of the observation, without singling out any particular child or specific behavior, because it is virtually impossible for a teacher to remain unaffected by prior knowledge of the purpose of the observation. Whatever the focus of interest, the behavior categories are precisely defined and a selected time period for the observation is broken down into subunits, usually ranging from five or more seconds to a minute. To obtain as representative a sample of the child's behavior as possible, observations are made at different times during the day and over a period of several days. When the categories are well defined it is possible to obtain high interrater agreement. Although one full-time observer is required, an astute observer can provide additional information concerning general aspects of the classroom scene, and this information can be of substantial help in planning a management strategy.

Observation schedules offer several important advantages: the behavior to be observed can be defined with clear operational criteria with a consequent decrease in criterion error variance; interrater agreement can be established easily; specific kinds of behavior can be assessed without bias due to halo effects, or rater set (Madle et al., 1980); blind assessments of therapeutic teacher interventions can be made; and the approach is simple and requires a minimum of equipment (Werry, 1978a). The disadvantages are that multiple categories can be very demanding for the rater; observation schedule procedures are more expensive than rating scales; and vigilance is required in maintaining satisfactory standards. For example, the observations will be invalid if adequate samples of the behavior are not obtained, the observer is unskilled in remaining unobtrusive, and observer drift is permitted to occur (Johnson & Bolstad, 1973), that is, the tendency of one observer over a long period of time to shift from initial reliability to increasing inaccuracies. For a detailed discussion of the advantages and disadvantages of observation schedules for behavior assessment see Jones, Reid, and Patterson (1975).

Classroom observation schedules that can be used with hyperactive children have been reported by Abikoff, Gittelman-Klein, and Klein (1977), Blunden et al. (1974), O'Leary, Romanczyk, Kass, Dietz, and Santagrossi (1971), Vincent, Williams, and Elrod (1977), and Whalen, Collins, Henker, Alkus, Adams, and Stapp, (1978). A brief description of two of these schedules will be presented here to illustrate the differences in observation procedures and categories. Note, though, that these descriptions are not sufficient for using the schedules—their use requires a complete coding manual that is available from the schedule authors.

Classroom Observation System

The categories used in this coding system (Whalen et al., 1978) were derived from two major sources: the work of other investigators in hyperactivity and research findings regarding medication-responsive behavior that is characteristic of hyperactive children. The coding system included categories for discrete behavioral acts requiring present-absent judgments (e.g., vocalization), as well as categories for qualitative aspects of those acts (e.g., energy level) requiring inferential judgments on the part of the observers. For the latter categories specific criteria were developed to minimize inference level. The idea of developing a coding system that would separate global behavior into stylistic and topographical components stemmed from Whalen et al.'s conviction that the well-documented discrepancy between behavior observations and rating scale data on hyperactive children could be due in part to the differences between hyperactive children and their nonhyperactive peers being a matter of style rather than content.

With this coding system Whalen et al. used 30-second observation intervals each consisting of 5 seconds assigned to locate the child to be rated, 10 seconds of actual observation, and 15 seconds during which each category that occurred during the 10-second observation period was recorded. The team of observers were paced by a tape recorder and headphones. Interrater reliabilities were lower than the conventional minimum, but as Whalen et al. have noted, the reliability indexes in this study were for groups rather than pairs of raters, the estimates of reliability during the study were limited in number, and there was a heavy observation and coding burden for each 30-second interval. Also, the coding system included qualitative judgments which added substantially to the value of the observational data by highlighting differences that would otherwise have been obscured. The behavior categories shown in Table 4.8 are currently being reduced in number, the goal being to increase reliability without sacrificing validity. Whalen and her colleagues have also developed coding systems to assess the qualitative aspects of communications of hyperactive children and their peers (Whalen, Henker, Collins, Finck, & Dotemoto, 1979).

Revised Stony Brook Observation Code

This classroom observation code was a modification of the Stony Brook Code developed by Tonick, Friehling, and Warhit (1973). The latter code, which was intended for use with problem children, possessed several excellent features such as demonstrated resistance to rater bias, many categories relevant to hyperactivity, detailed scoring criteria, and a satisfactory interrater reliability (Abikoff, Gittelman-Klein, & Klein, 1977).

With the Revised Code the behavior categories are sampled every 15 seconds and are either timed or nontimed. Timed categories are scored only if the child engages in the behavior for more than 15 consecutive seconds, a restriction that is likely to reduce and distort the amount of data collected. In the category Extended Verbalization, for example, a child could engage in sporadic conversation throughout an entire 20- or 30-minute classroom period without ever being scored in this category. Nontimed behavior is scored as soon as it occurs in any 15-second interval, with only the first occurrence in that interval being noted. Interrater reliability reported for interval scores ranged from .34 to .93 with a mean ϕ of .76 for all 14 categories. Session reliability was determined by calculating the product-moment correlation between the total number of behavior occurrences reported by the experienced observer and a second observer over an entire observation period. Of the 45 correlations obtained, 35 exceeded .85. Abikoff et al. reported that their behavior categories were stable over time, based on the finding that only *one* of 28 correlated t tests between early and late observations was significant. Of the 14 classroom observation categories, 12 discriminated significantly between hyperactive and normal children. This finding is weakened somewhat

Table 4.8.   Brief Definitions of Behavior Categories of Whalen et al.

1. *Task attention:* On task is coded when the child is completing class assignments or following the teacher's directions.
2. *Out of chair:* Child is not supporting his weight with a chair.
3. *Translocation:* Child moves from one place to another a minimum of 2 steps or about 3 ft, for example, walking, scooting while seated in a chair.
4. *Movement:* Child moves his trunk or entire body while in a relatively stationary position, for example, wiggling, stretching.
5. *Fidget:* Child's hands, head or feet are in motion for at least 2 sec, for example, tapping fingers, poking holes in notebook, drawing on self.
6. *Regular verbalization:* Spoken words that are neutral in affective content.
7. *Positive verbalization:* Spoken words that are friendly, pleasant, approving, complimentary.
8. *Negative verbalization:* Spoken words that are threatening, derogatory, offensive, aggressive.
9. *Vocalization:* Nonverbal noise with mouth, for example, humming, throat clearing, tongue clucking.
10. *Noise:* Audible sound other than verbalization or vocalization, including tapping pencil, slapping face, banging chair.
11. *Physical contact:* (positive or regular): Nonaversive contact with another person, for example, shaking hands, hugging.
12. *Negative contact:* Aversive or unpleasant physical contact, for example, tugging, tripping, slapping. Includes clear entries into another's personal space, for example, grabbing a pen out of a shirt pocket or throwing objects within 6 in of another.
13. *Grimace:* Facial contortion or distortion, if child seems unaware of the behavior. Grimace is not scored when the facial expression appears to be a nonverbal message, for example, nose wrinkling in response to a teacher's demand.
14. *Bystand:* Nonparticipant observation or onlooking.
15. Social initiation: Clear attempts to begin a social interchange, for example, starting a conversation.
16. *Ignore:* Refusal to acknowledge a clear social bid.
17. *High energy:* Acts that are vigorous, effortful, intense, vehement, rapid, or loud.
18. *Disruption:* Action has observable consequences that interrupt other people's behavior.
19. *Stand-out or inappropriate:* Nonnormative behaviors that tend to violate the observer's expectations of appropriate behaviors in specific social settings.
20. *Sudden:* An abrupt change in the direction, quality, or type of activity that cannot be predicted from the ongoing stream of behavior.
21. *Accidental:* Coded in conjunction with noise or physical contact when behavior is clearly unintentional.

Reprinted, by permission, from Henker, B., and Whalen, C. K. The changing faces of hyperactivity: Retrospect and prospect. In C. K. Whalen and B. Henker (Eds.), *Hyperactive children.* New York: Academic Press, 1980.

by teacher reports that the children's classroom behavior was relatively atypical in 44 percent of the hyperactives but only 14 percent of the controls. Support for the discriminant validity of this instrument is further rendered questionable by two findings: overlap in the distribution of scores for individual behavior categories across hyperactive and control children, and a substantial number of false positive and false negative classification errors. In a subsequent study by the same team, some of the categories proved to be responsive to stimulant drug and behavior intervention (Gittelman-Klein, Abikoff, Pollack, Klein, Katz, & Mattes, 1980). Table 4.9 contains a brief description of the observation categories.

For any researcher who is contemplating the development of a classroom observation system there is a report by Vincent, Williams, Harris, and Duval (1981) describing the development of a classroom observation procedure—the Hyperactive Behavior Observation System (HABOS). This comprehensive coding system consists of 34 categories of social and motor behaviors, some of which capture the flavor of the classroom social context, for example, teacher and peer interactions with the target child, and teacher instructional style. The HABOS differs from the two systems (Abikoff et al., 1977; Whalen et al., 1978) described here in two respects: it was designed for laboratory use with videotaped samples collected in the classroom rather than for direct classroom observation, and it is divided into four subsets of categories (social context, social target, motor hand, and motor body head) to allow coding of one category on one pass through of the videotape.

Using data coded over three consecutive days on 11 hyperactive children and 11 matched nonclinical controls in open classrooms, the developers used

Table 4.9.   Brief Description of Behavior Categories of Abikoff et al.

1. Interference (nontimed) is a general measure of disruptiveness. Included are calling out, interruption of others during work periods, and clowning.
2. Solicitation (nontimed) reflects how often the child seeks out the teacher's attention (e.g., calling out to the teacher, going up to the teacher's desk.
3. Off task (timed) is a general measure of inattentiveness. It indicates attention to stimuli other than the assigned work *after* initiation of appropriate task-relevant behavior.
4. Minor motor movement (nontimed) is a general measure of in-chair restlessness. Only buttock movements and body and chair movements are included.
5. Gross motor movement—standing (untimed) refers to standing up without permission.
6. Gross motor movement—vigorous (nontimed) is scored when the child engages in vigorous motor activity (e.g., running, jumping).
7. Noncompliance (timed) indicates how often the child fails to comply with teacher commands.
8. Out of chair (timed) reflects how often the child *remains* out of his or her seat without permission.
9. Physical aggression (nontimed) indicates destructive physical behavior (e.g., hitting, pushing, throwing objects, etc.) and destruction of materials.
10. Threat or verbal aggression to children (nontimed) indicates abusive or threatening verbalizations and physical gestures directed toward other children.
11. Threat or verbal aggression to teacher (nontimed) indicates abusive or threatening verbalizations and physical gestures directed toward the teacher.
12. Extended verbalization (timed) is scored when the child engages in conversation.
13. Daydreaming (timed) is scored when the child is not attending to a specific stimulus while a task has been assigned.
14. Absence of above behaviors is scored when none of the above behaviors occur.

From Abikoff, H., Gittelman-Klein, R., and Klein, D. F. Validation of a classroom observation code for hyperactive children. *Journal of Consulting and Clinical Psychology,* 1977, *45* (5), 772–783. Page 775.

multiple strategies, all of which are reported in detail, to evaluate the reliability and validity of the HABOS. Overall, the results of this careful evaluation were disappointing. Only 14 of the HABOS categories proved to be highly reliable and to occur frequently enough to allow interpretation. Factor analysis yielded no empirical basis for groupings of the 14 categories. The two groups of children differed significantly on only four kinds of behavior. Support for convergence and discriminant validity between the HABOS category and the Conners Teacher Rating Scale (1969) Hyperactivity Factor scores was minimal. The most important findings related to the analysis of teacher cue usage. The developers stated (Vincent et al., 1981, p. 238):

> ... although teachers can rely on behavioral information to make valid judgements, the behaviors on which they rely most heavily are not necessarily the most valid ones. Rather, they seem to depend on highly visible motor behaviors or contextual social behaviors. They are quite knowledgeable about what behavior cues are valid indicators of hyperactivity, yet these are seldom the ones which actually emerge in the model of their policy. This discrepancy could be one reason why behavioral observation and teacher ratings are only moderately related.

Vincent et al. (1981) concluded that direct observations in their present form are not well suited to widespread clinical use but are still the method of choice for research purposes. We disagree with this conclusion. It is our opinion that the procedures used by Vincent et al. are too complex, too costly in terms of data collection, encoding and analysis, and too intrusive in terms of potential for effect on behavior. By contrast, both the Abikoff et al. and Whalen et al. observation procedures are within the bounds of practicality for classroom usage; Whalen et al. (1978) are subjecting their Classroom Observation System to further empirical tests following current modifications of it as a result of concern about the rater load. Although observers must be trained in using these two observational schedules, the costs for most school systems would be within bounds if a small team of observers conducted all classroom observations for an entire school district.

MEASUREMENT OF TEMPERAMENT

The pioneer research on the measurement of temperament is the New York Longitudinal Study (NYLS) of Thomas, Chess, and their associates (Thomas & Chess, 1977; Thomas, Chess, & Birch, 1968; Thomas, Chess, Birch, Hertzig, & Korn, 1963). Thomas et al. defined temperament operationally in terms of nine variables: activity level, rhythmicity, approach-withdrawal, adaptability, intensity, threshold, mood, distractibility, and attention-persistence, which were derived from parental interview data. Their prospective study is notable for the large sample (141 infants from 85 families), low attrition rate, young age of the children at the beginning of the study, evidence of satisfactory test-retest reliability and concurrent validity of the parental interview data, frequency of data collection, and length of follow-up period. The study was also characterized by a number of limitations: The sample consisted primarily of highly educated, middle-class, Jewish families from the New York City area, which limits the generality of the findings; in the case of sibling subjects, temperament could be interdependent; the age periods used in the pooling of data varied across subjects, and the temperament patterns were only partially substantiated through factor analysis (Rowe & Plomin, 1977). The interview procedure itself has some practical limitations in that it may require as long as several hours by a specially trained interviewer, and an additional 30 minutes for scoring by a trained scorer. However, the information generated from the interview has considerable relevance to developing management procedures for the at risk infant.

Infants

The past decade has seen the development of a spate of temperament measures for infants based on the nine variables of Thomas et al. Carey (1970) developed the *Infant Temperament Questionnaire* for 4- to 8-month old infants as a screening device for pediatricians to use in identifying reaction patterns in situations such as eating and sleeping. The 95 items describe infants' typical reactions and are randomized as to content area and temperament category. Each item has six options concerning the frequency with which the statement is true for a specific infant: Almost never (1), Rarely (2), Variable, usually does not (3), Variable, usually does (4), Frequently (5), Almost always (6). Sample items include the following:

4.   The infant sits while watching TV or other nearby activity.
10.   The infant takes feedings quietly with mild expression of likes and dislikes.
36.   For the first few minutes in a new place or situation (new store or home) the infant is fretful.

A supplementary page on the back of the questionnaire asks the mother to describe in her own words the infant's temperament, how it may have been a problem for her, and whether she regards the infant as about average, more difficult, or easier than average. She is also asked to give an overall estimate of the infant's behavior (high, variable, or low) in each of the nine categories of temperament identified by Thomas et al. The questionnaire takes 25 to 30 minutes to complete and 15 minutes to score.

Test-retest reliability averages around .75 to .85 over 2- to 3-week intervals. External validity data are not available, and would be difficult to obtain in the absence of standardized observational techniques for these phenomena.

The major criticism that can be made concerning the psychometric properties of the questionnaire concerns the unrepresentative standardization sample, which consisted of infants from highly educated, white, middle-class families in three private pediatric practices. The justification offered for the source of subjects for the standardization procedure was "our wish to collect a sample more quickly" (Carey & McDevitt, 1978, p. 736). Although not usually stated so frankly, this implicit criterion of fast data collection unfortunately characterizes many of the research papers in the current literature on hyperactivity.

A Parent Questionnaire for the measurement of Thomas et al.'s nine temperament variables in 6-month-old infants has been developed and standardized in Sweden by Persson-Blennow and McNeil (1979). The questionnaire consists of 44 items with five or more representing each treatment variable. The multiple-choice questions concern the infant's actual behavior in everyday activities and specified situations. The following item represents the temperament variable, rhythmicity: When does the baby wake up in the morning? (a) The time usually varies by more than an hour. (b) Quite often at the same time, but sometimes more than half an hour earlier or later (than usual). (c) At the same time (within half an hour of the usual time). The questionnaire takes approximately 15 minutes to complete and five minutes to score. Geographically stratified random sampling was used to obtain the standardization sample of 160 infants; there was a good balance between male and female infants, and satisfactory representation of different social levels.

For children of one to three years of age Fullard, McDevitt, and Carey (1978) have developed the Toddler Temperament Scale. This scale uses parental responses to 97 behavior descriptors, similar in format and topic to those used in the Infant Temperament Questionnaire (Carey & McDevitt, 1978), to assess the Thomas et al. temperament variables. Test-retest reliability and internal consistency are satisfactory but, again, the standardization sample was obtained from two private pediatric practices in which the majority of children were from white, middle-class families.

Preschool and School Children

McDevitt and Carey (1978) have extended their two previous questionnaires upwards in the Behavioral Style Questionnaire, for children aged three to seven. Structured interviews assessing the nine temperament dimensions of Thomas et al. (1968, 1970) have been developed by Garside, Birch, Scott, Chambers, Kolvin, Tweddle, and Barber (1975) and Graham, Rutter, and George (1973). The latter study provided some evidence for the validity of the theoretical framework of Thomas et al. Interviews were divided into three segments: in the first segment the mother was asked to describe the child's behavior over a wide range of everyday situations, in the next she was asked for details of the child's regularity of function over the previous two weeks, and in the third she was asked about the child's behavior in various nonroutine

situations such as change of demands, meeting new people, and fastidious-
ness. All interviews were tape-recorded and interrater reliability of the interviews was uniformly high. Tape recording as an interview method is time
consuming and also requires experienced interviewers; as a result, this interview method is used far less frequently than are the various parent rating
questionnaires.

Rowe and Plomin (1977) have developed the Colorado Childhood Temperament Inventory, a parent rating instrument for infants and children from one
to six years of age. This scale evolved from two sets of items: one set with 54
items was designed to assess the nine temperament traits identified in the
New York Longitudinal Study (Thomas et al., 1968; Thomas et al., 1963), the
other set consisted of all 20 items from a previously developed measure of
temperament called the EASI Temperament Survey (Buss & Plomin, 1975)
that was designed to assess emotionality, activity, sociability, and impulsivity.
The 74-item questionnaire was answered by 91 mothers of twins, who were
contacted by mail and asked to complete a questionnaire for each twin. Test-
retest reliability was obtained by having randomly selected mothers rate one
twin (also randomly selected) again one week later. Comparisons of the factor
structures of the two instruments making up the questionnaire supported two
of the nine NYLS dimensions (attention span–persistence and distractibility).
All four of the EASI dimensions were replicated. The NYLS and the EASI
systems were merged to form the Colorado Childhood Temperament Inventory, a 30-item measure of temperament with six scales: sociability, emotionality, activity, attention span–persistence, reaction to food, and soothability.
Items were rated from 1–not at all like the child, to 5–a lot like the child.
Reliability estimates showed high internal consistency for all scales and moderately high test-retest reliabilities for all scales except soothability. The question of the validity of this measure of temperament is as yet unanswered.

Thomas, Chess, and Korn (Thomas & Chess, 1977) have begun work on
parent and teacher questionnaires for the assessment of temperament in children aged three to seven. The goal has been to develop assessment instruments that are reliable, valid, and economical to administer and score. The
psychometric properties of these instruments have not yet been established,
but Thomas and Chess and other investigators are using the questionnaires so
these data should be forthcoming. The development process and problems of
developing temperament measures for older children are described in detail in
Thomas and Chess (1977). Their approach is notable for exemplary concern
for appropriate topic selection, unambiguous wording, item-category consistency, and emphasis on child behaviors rather than on child attitudes. The
parent questionnaire assesses all nine dimensions of temperament but the
teacher questionnaire omits the rhythmicity dimension because rating it requires a knowledge of the child's functioning over a 24-hour period. One criticism concerns ambiguity in the 7-point scale categories, Point 3–once in a
while, and Point 4–sometimes; and Point 6–very often, and Point 7–almost
always. In addition, the length of one questionnaire (132 items) possibly

should be pared down in view of the time that it would take a conscientious respondent to complete the form. Sample items from the two questionnaires are contained in Table 4.10.

Table 4.10.   Sample Items from Thomas and Chess (1977) Questionnaires

1 Hardly ever	2 Infre- quently	3 Once in a while	4 Sometimes	5 Often	6 Very often		7 Almost always	

Parent Items:

My child splashes hard in the bath and plays actively.

1 2 3 4 5 6 7

When with other children, my child seems to be having a good time.

1 2 3 4 5 6 7

Teacher Items:

Child seems to have difficulty sitting still, may wriggle a lot or get out of seat.

1 2 3 4 5 6 7

When with other children, this child seems to be having a good time.

1 2 3 4 5 6 7

From Thomas, A., and Chess, S. *Temperament and development.* New York: Brunner/Mazel, 1977, p. 223 and 239.

CHAPTER 5

The Search for Predictors

The value of prediction has long been recognized in medicine, and more recently in the behavioral sciences. The ability to predict the onset, response to treatment, and outcome of medical and behavioral disorders serves two major purposes: The knowledge prerequisite to prediction increases our understanding of the disorder under investigation, thus providing a tool for researchers to use in further extensions, and the probability of controlling a disorder is markedly enhanced by accurate prediction. This knowledge makes possible interventive action in limiting the severity of the disorder at critical points in its sequence of development, or at least facilitates preparation for its onset. Parents of Down's Syndrome or Tay-Sachs disease children can be counseled, for example.

Prediction is possible when two factors can be identified as coexisting. When correlational knowledge of a particular variable allows predictions to be made about a second variable, the prediction is described as *pragmatic,* examples being the association between increased maternal age and the occurrence of Down's Syndrome, or infants' cry behavior as predictive of at-risk status: Zeskind, Lester, and Eitzman (1977) reported that the initial cry sound, overall cry length, and pitch distinguished high-risk newborns from other infants. When a cause and effect relationship exists, a change can be effected in one variable by altering the second. A *causal* relationship exists, for example, between a specific combination of obesity and menstrual dysfunction, and sterility. Causal prediction is of particular value where preventive or ameliorative action is the goal.

Two different procedures are used in the prediction of disorders. The *statistical association* approach predicts how many individuals will contract a specific disease. Epidemiologists, for example, can predict with a high degree of certainty that peptic ulcers will attack 4000 new victims a day in the United States, but they cannot say which individuals will be so afflicted (Winter, 1980). However, with reliable information about the rate and duration of smoking in subgroups of a population, they can predict that the risk of peptic ulcer is increased in certain groups of heavy smokers having a long history of smoking. In the *personal prediction* approach to the peptic ulcer problem, the clinician gathers all possible information about a specific individual and then uses the data in a global manner to make a personal judgment about the probability of this individual developing an ulcer. The critical element in personal predictions is, as one would expect, accuracy, and the two types of prediction error that are devastating to the utility of an early warning prediction system are false positives and false negatives. A person who is incorrectly identified as one who either is at risk for a certain disorder, or will be afflicted, is a false positive. Although this type of error may seem rather innocuous, its ramifications can be quite serious because of the possibility of self-fulfilling prophecy. In fact, in making any personal prediction, the effect of the prediction must be weighed relative to the known benefits. Also it is naive in the extreme to think that correcting an error that has been made in predicting a disorder will erase the possibility of the disorder's occurrence from the individual's belief system. False negatives occur when individuals who are at risk or are already afflicted with the disorders are missed by the tests and other measures intended to identify them. Errors of the false negative type are obviously serious because the individual is deprived of possible preventive action and is also less likely to be alert to early symptoms.

What criteria should a disorder meet to merit attention to identifying predictors? The incidence of the disorder should be sufficiently high to warrant an intensive and probably expensive search for precursors that can serve as predictors. There should be some basis for thinking that prediction of onset, or prediction that results in early detection, offers the possibility of preventive or ameliorative efforts that will be effective. Even when such possibilities are nil, prediction may be of limited value in that it allows the clinician to attempt to prepare the individual for the final outcome. There should be specific medical symptoms or behavioral manifestations that characterize the disorder so that it is reasonable to seek possible antecedents for them. In lead poisoning, for example, the onset is insidious with vague symptoms such as pallor, nausea, and vomiting; because all of these symptoms could be associated with numerous disorders, searching for their antecedents in lead poisoning is pointless. However, it can still be predicted that in heavy lead belts a certain number of children are likely to develop lead poisoning, but refinements in prediction are elusive in this instance. In addition, the disorder should be more than a minor, annoying, transient one that disappears spontaneously with increasing age. It should be sufficiently serious in terms of immediate manifestations and long-term somewhat pessimistic outlook to warrant the allocation of scarce resources in the form of scientific attention, effort, and money.

Although childhood hyperactivity is one of the behavior disorders that meets these criteria, the search for hyperactivity-related predictors is relatively recent and has as yet met with only a modicum of success. It is unlikely that it will ever be possible to identify specific infants who will be hyperactive, but the current level of clinical acumen, relevant assessment procedures, and empirical information should make possible the identification of infants who appear to be at risk for hyperactivity. In addition to this cluster of information and procedures relevant to the prediction of infants at risk for hyperactivity, something is known about the prediction of response to drug intervention; and from a small but impressive body of research it is now possible to see how a diverse group of ecological, familial, and behavioral parameters may fit into the prediction of outcome equation. It should be emphasized that the interaction model that we advocate for understanding hyperactivity is rarely compatible with the existence of a single biological or behavioral predictor of onset or outcome, because in most cases these stages represent the endpoint of a person x environmental challenge interaction. In the case of prediction of onset, for example, the optimum expectation would be to establish that a certain biological or psychological characteristic in an infant or young preschool child means that the child has increased vulnerability. If the child is then subjected to the relevant environmental stressor, he is more likely to become hyperactive or have behavior difficulties than the child without that characteristic. The interaction model can accommodate the fact that a supportive environment in infancy and early childhood can often ameliorate or even suppress the consequences that should logically proceed from the at-risk status. Conversely, a highly disordered or nonsupportive environment can convert even a normal infant, not to speak of the at-risk infant, into what Sameroff and Chandler (1975) have termed a "caretaking casualty." The interaction model is compatible with predictions concerning the differential effects of supportive and nonsupportive environments, and the literature abounds with examples of these effects. A case study (Chess, Thomas, Rutter, & Birch, 1963, p. 145) of a boy and girl who were very similar in infancy, with both having difficult temperaments, and who subsequently differed markedly in behavior and adaptation as a result of differential parental practices in child management, is reprinted in Chapter 3.

It is only in the last five years that the search for predictors of hyperactivity has achieved even a modicum of status as a topic of investigation. Until the mid-1970s most investigators thought the stimulant medications were a panacea for almost all hyperactive children and believed that hyperactivity disappeared spontaneously in adolescence. The change in attitude on the part of the medical and clinical community has come about gradually in the light of recent data on prevalence, duration, and cost of hyperactivity, coupled with the factual results of considerable research effort, namely, that existing treatments provide only short-term manageability, there is as yet no long-term cure, and when hyperactivity persists into adolescence and adulthood it is often associated with psychiatric disorders. Although this change in attitude has so far resulted in only scattered and sparse research, prediction is of paramount importance and so merits consideration in this text as a topic in its own right. In this chapter we will describe the status of clinical and research findings in the three areas on which clinical and empirical investigation has focused, that is, infancy, response to drugs, and outcome in adolescence; highlight some of the methodological difficulties that have arisen in the search for predictors; and suggest possible directions for future investigations.

PREDICTING FROM INFANCY AND EARLY CHILDHOOD TO LATER FUNCTIONING

How well behavior in infancy predicts later behavior is a crucial question with major implications for any program whose basis is the assumption that early identification may prevent later problems. Prediction on the basis of assessment in infancy has been attempted in several physiological and behavioral areas, but in the main it is only the extreme aberrations that lend themselves to prediction with any significant degree of certainty. Pediatric neurological examinations of infants, for example, have generally failed to predict later pathology except in cases of gross neurologic disorder (Thomas, 1970). Even in the case of attributes such as linear growth the correlation between height at birth and yearly increments in height is close to zero except for gross abnormalities of tallness and shortness. Similarly, the prime value of tests of infant mental development appears to lie in their ability to identify severe intellectual retardation. Among children in the normal range of intelligence the correlations between infant and early childhood test scores are too small to permit useful predictions (Rutter, 1970). One explanation for the fact that prediction of outcome within the normal range of function has been largely impossible for most physiological and psychological functions is that significant correlations between early and later measures are thought to occur only to the extent of the overlap between what is already present of the function in infancy and of the function at maturity. When the function being tested in infancy differs from that at maturity, prediction is virtually impossible, but when the function is alike at different points in time, prediction can be made with accuracy. Barring accidents or illness, adult hearing states, for example, can be predicted with a fairly high degree of certainty on the basis of infant tests because the relevant aural structures attain mature status shortly before birth. Despite the uncertainties in specifying the relation between early and later functioning, prediction from infancy to later childhood has been pursued in several behavioral areas (e.g., Rosenblith, 1974; Serunian & Broman, 1975). Those relevant in the prediction of childhood hyperactivity are infant temperament and minor physical anomalies.

Infant Temperament as a Predictor of Hyperactivity

Thomas, Chess, and their associates (Thomas & Chess, 1977; Thomas, Chess, & Birch, 1968; Thomas, Chess, Birch, & Hertzig, 1960) have established an empirical framework for classifying temperament, which McDevitt and Carey (1978, p. 245) have defined as "the behavioral style of the child in interaction with the environment." Thomas, Chess, et al. have derived nine temperament characteristics from parental interview data: activity, adaptability, approach, distractibility, intensity, mood, persistence, regularity, and threshold. From these characteristics three functionally significant patterns of stylistic differences in behavior that appear early in life have been identified and labeled as *easy, slow to warm up, and difficult,* and other investigators have presented evidence for the validity of these temperament characteristics (Lambert & Windmiller, 1977; Persson-Blennow & McNeil, 1979) and typologies (Maurer, Cadoret, & Cain, 1980). The difficult temperament, which was identified in about 10 percent of the infants in the New York Longitudinal Study (Thomas & Chess, 1977), is of relevance to the prediction of hyperactivity because the description of the behavior patterns of the difficult child is remarkably similar to parents' and clinicians' reports and observations of the early behavior of children subsequently diagnosed as hyperactive. The cluster of traits characteristic of the difficult temperament consists of irregularity in biological functioning, predominantly negative withdrawal responses to new stimuli, nonadaptability to changes in routine, frequent negative moods, and predominantly intense reactions. The difficult infant temperament pattern was predictive of a disproportionately high incidence of behavior disorder later in childhood, with 70 percent of the difficult infant group developing a significant childhood behavior problem. Thomas and Chess concluded that the difficult temperament was sufficiently predictive of behavior problems in the childhood years to be designated as high risk, defined as an increased probability that this constellation of traits will result in children who will present with a variety of behavior disorders such as hyperactivity, learning difficulties, and antisocial aggression. Of particular interest was the finding that the group of children in the New York Longitudinal Study who developed behavior disturbances when they grew older had received higher than average scores on activity level in their first year of life.

Although these data suggest that a difficult infancy is likely to be associated with childhood problems such as hyperactivity, little interest has been shown in the empirical investigation of this sequence. However, the studies that have been done do support the Thomas and Chess (1977) findings. Carey (1970) developed a parental questionnaire using the categories of Thomas et al. (1968), and although its purpose was not to identify hyperactivity in infants, his later reports (Carey, 1972) demonstrated a relationship between the difficult temperament and clinical conditions such as colic, night waking, and accident proneness, all of which are characteristic of the hyperactive child. In a study of the relationship between infant temperament status and 2-year-old behavior, McInerny and Chamberlin (1978) reported that infants identified by their mothers as "difficult" at six months had higher total symptom scores, were more aggressive and noncompliant, and were generally more difficult to rear at age two than were "easy" infants. At the preschool level a study by Terestman (1980) has provided strong support for the predictive value of two characteristics of the difficult temperament, namely, negative mood and high intensity. Ratings of these characteristics in 58 preschool children were derived from interviews with the children's nursery school teachers and from direct observations. The children were followed up five years later, with results suggesting that the two characteristics are powerful predictors of developing behavior disorders. Placement in the lowest mood quartile, which was categorized as *unpleasant, negative*, was associated with behavior disorder for every 4-year-old child, either concurrently or before the age of nine; and for six out of seven children under the age of four. *High intensity*, which is defined as the energy level of a response, irrespective of its quality or duration, was almost as discriminating: all of the children in the highest quartile subsequently developed significant behavior problems. Combined placement in the two categories produced the dramatic finding that placement in the lowest quartile of mood and highest quartile of intensity predicted later behavior disorder in 10 out of 10 cases.

In an exploratory factor analytic study of temperament traits in a population of elementary school children classified as either hyperactive, poorly adjusted, low-achieving, or as having no identifiable problems (controls), Lambert and Windmiller (1977) identified six of the nine temperament traits proposed by Thomas et al. (1968). Using scores derived from this factor analysis, Lambert and Windmiller showed that hyperactive children had more extreme temperament patterns than children in the other three groups. In a subsequent study of the extent to which temperament traits differentiate hyperactive children of elementary school age from their nonclinical peers Lambert (1982) used retrospective parental reports to a carefully designed interview to establish that children identified as hyperactive by all major defining systems (parent, teacher, and physician) were reported to have all the temperament extremes identified by Thomas et al. (1968). The interview form that was designed by Lambert and Hartsough (1979) covered a range of topics including family characteristics, developmental history of the child, provisions for learning, and goals and expectancies for the child's future. For this study the questions on temperament in infancy and early childhood were selected out for analysis. One group of hyperactive children were classified as primary hyperactives, which meant that all three defining systems thought that they were hyperactive and there was no competing medical diagnosis, such as lead poisoning or some condition that the physician regarded as reason for hyperactivity. Of relevance here was the finding that these primary hyperactives were significantly different from randomly selected controls on four out of the five measures describing temperament during infancy and the first year of life (retrospective reports by the parents, usually the mothers).

Using retrospective parental ratings of temperament and cluster analysis, Maurer et al (1980) categorized adolescent adoptees into Thomas, Chess, et al.'s three temperament groups of difficult, easy, and slow to warm up. Membership in the difficult group in infancy and early childhood was predictive of later childhood behavior problems, including conduct disorder, emotional disturbances, and hyperactivity. The prevalence of hyperactivity was 21.7 percent in the difficult group, 7.7 percent in the slow to warm up group, and 3.2 percent in the easy group.

Thomas and Chess (1977) have repeatedly emphasized that the difficult temperament does not in and of itself lead to behavior problems. Instead it is the interaction between this behavior style and the child's environment that can eventuate in behavior disorder. They have analyzed parental response to difficult infants and young children in terms of three types of response: feeling threatened and having feelings of inadequacy as parents, blaming the children for the problems they present, and unconsciously (or not so unconsciously) rejecting the child. In their view any of these parental responses to the difficult child could initiate a negative parent–child interaction that could make the child vulnerable to other psychological and physical problems. The potential risks of the difficult temperament can thus be minimized if the parents take the child in their stride and react firmly, positively, and consistently to the problem behavior.

Empirical evidence for the Thomas and Chess position on outcome comes from research by Cameron (1977, 1978) on the relationships between parental characteristics and changes in children's temperament over time. Cameron used two sets of data from the New York Longitudinal Study: (a) familial–parental factors identified through cluster analysis of parental interviews at the time of the child's third birthday and covering parenting issues such as degree of warmth, protectiveness, and permissiveness towards the child; and (b) change scores derived from parental interview data for each area of temperament across the first five years of life. Starting with the difficult temperament–childhood behavior disorder link described by Thomas and Chess (1977), Cameron investigated parental behavior as a determinant of the strength of the link. He hypothesized significant correlations between familial–parental factors and early shifts in the temperament variables previously reported (Thomas & Chess, 1977) to be linked to increased risk for childhood behavior disorders. The hypothesis was confirmed, with three parental dimensions—parental conflict in child rearing, maternal rejection, and inconsistent parental discipline—being highly correlated with negative changes in temperament across the first five years. The finding that infant temperament data alone predicted mild behavior problems, but temperament patterns combined with parenting styles were needed for predicting more severe problems, was consistent with Werner's (1980) conclusions on the importance of environmental factors as determinants of hyperactivity, and also supports the position of Thomas and Chess and other experienced investigators (Bell & Harper, 1977) that parental behavior plus children's temperament forms the matrix from which children's behavior problems emerge (Cameron, 1977). Clearly the social environment makes a significant contribution to the early temperament–childhood behavior disorder link.

The question of what constitutes an optimum social environment for the difficult infant is an intriguing one that may not permit an absolute answer. A recent empirical investigation by Scholom, Zucker, and Stollak (1979) of the combination of infant and parent temperament factors that best account for child adjustment in the preschool years has underlined the complexity of the effects of social interaction upon outcome. In their study there were striking sex differences in the relationships between early childhood adjustment and the temperaments of family members. Positive adjustment was significantly related to similarity of temperament among infant, father, and mother in girls; and to dissimilarity between infant and father temperament in boys.

In summary, the implications of the difficult temperament for the prediction of hyperactivity are as follows: Being difficult has predictive value in that if the infant is difficult there is an increased probability of subsequent problems unless intervention occurs. The difficult infant is at risk, but it is not known for what; there is evidence that some difficult children become hyperactive. When the difficult temperament is combined with negative parenting, the probability is increased that more severe problems will result. Risk may be increased if there is a mismatch between infant and parent temperament.

Minor Physical Anomalies

Minor physical anomalies are defined as organs or structures that are abnormal with respect to form, structure, or position. They are developmental deviations such as a furrowed tongue, a high steepled palate, widely spaced eyes, malformed or asymmetrical ears, and palmar creases. These deviations are believed to result from some form of genetic transmission or insult in the first weeks of pregnancy that mimics genetic transmission (Rapoport, Quinn, Burg, & Bartley, 1979). Individual anomalies are commonly believed to occur in the general population on the average of two to four per person and are not considered to be reason for medical concern although, as Gallant (Bellak, 1979) has pointed out, knowledge about the incidence of minor physical anomalies typically elicits considerable concern because Down's syndrome and other major congenital defects are characterized by multiple anomalies. A list of the 17 anomalies of relevance here is contained in Table 9.1 in Chapter 9.

Research interest in the predictive potential of the anomalies for hyperactivity stems from several sources. The diagnostic value of minor physical anomalies in Down's syndrome is undisputed, and it is possible that they might have diagnostic value in other disorders. Minor physical anomalies are known to be associated with a variety of problems including school failure (Rosenberg & Weller, 1973), learning disabilities and autism (Steg & Rapoport, 1975), and schizophrenia. High anomaly scores occur more often in children who are not hyperactive but who exhibit hyperactive-type behaviors such as distractibility (O'Donnell, O'Neill, & Staley, 1979) and high activity level at the nursery school (Waldrop, Pedersen, & Bell, 1968) and elementary school levels (Waldrop & Goering, 1971) than in nonclinical children who do not exhibit these extremes of behavior. Hyperactive children typically have more minor physical anomalies than do their nonclinical peers (Firestone, Lewy, & Douglas, 1976; Firestone, Peters, Rivier, & Knights, 1978; Lerer, 1977), and high anomaly hyperactive children are more likely than low anomaly hyperactive children to have had early onset of hyperactivity, that is, before age three (Rapoport et al., 1979). Research interest has been further stimulated by the characteristics of the anomaly measurement procedure itself: it can be administered at birth, is simple to conduct, has high reliability when only presence or absence of a specific anomaly is the issue, and has high test–retest stability over a 5-year period (Waldrop & Halverson, 1979). The importance of this assortment of research findings and measurement characteristics lies in the possibility that the minor physical anomalies may provide a biological means for identifying, perhaps even as newborns, a high-risk group whose study could reveal new information about the developmental precursors of childhood hyperactivity.

Evidence for Multiple Physical Anomalies as Predictors. The most important findings to date come from the NIMH Bethesda Longitudinal Study (Waldrop, Bell, McLaughlin, & Halverson, 1978), in which the number of minor physical anomalies was assessed in 30 male newborn infants and followed up three years later with 23 of the original group. The anomaly score was found to be stable ($r = .86$) between the two periods. Observations and ratings made in two free play settings at age three yielded two factors, Short Attention Span and Peer Aggression–Impulsivity, both of which were significantly related to the minor physical anomaly scores. In order to obtain a single hyperactivity score, each child's scores on these two factors were summed. The resulting composite score correlated .67 with the newborn anomaly score. In other words, close to half the variance of a carefully obtained nursery school measure of hyperactivity was accounted for by its relation to the newborn anomaly score. Scatterplots of standardized factor scores against standardized newborn anomaly scores showed that there were very few false positives and none was extreme; there were some false negatives for both the Attention Span and Aggression–Impulsivity scores. Taken together, these findings mean that it was not unusual for boys who were seen as hyperactive to have low newborn anomaly scores, but it was very unusual for boys with high newborn anomaly scores not to be seen as hyperactive at age three. Waldrop et al. (1978) concluded that it may be possible to use a neonatal anomaly assessment to identify a subgroup of boys who are likely to be hyperactive in the preschool years.

Evidence against Multiple Physical Anomalies as Predictors. In a nonblind comparison of the anomaly scores of hyperactive boys, their siblings, and their parents with those of same-age retarded boys and their families, and of normal control children and their families, Firestone et al. (1978) reported that the hyperactive and mentally retarded children and families had similar anomaly scores that were significantly higher than those of the control children and their families, with the control children and families not differing from each other. Firestone et al. interpret the finding that the frequency of anomalies was similar in hyperactive and mentally retarded boys and their families as evidence that although atypical children may have more anomalies than normals, there is a lack of specificity as far as the topography of the disorder is concerned. Of particular interest was the finding that the hyperactive boys and their families had similar anomaly scores, but there were apparently no other hyperactive children in these families. In this connection Rapoport and Quinn (1975) have suggested that it may only be children with minor physical anomalies *and* birth complications who develop later behavior disorders, but there is no firm support for this possibility. The results obtained by Firestone et al. suggest that the use of minor physical anomalies as markers of hyperactivity or other behavior disorders would be of little value, since the number of false positives in any one family would be high.

In a longitudinal follow-up of 136 infants with high and low anomaly scores selected from a large newborn screening population, Rapoport and her associates (Burg, Hart, Quinn, & Rapoport, 1978; Burg, Rapoport, Bartley, Quinn, & Timmins, 1980; Quinn, Renfield, Burg, & Rapoport, 1977; Rapoport et al., 1979) investigated the possibility that high anomaly scores in infancy would predict hyperactivity in the early preschool years. The examiners who subsequently assessed the children were blind to the newborn anomaly scores. These scores were found to be reliable and stable over time and to correlate with infant irritability at one year of age. In the high anomaly group there was a positive correlation of both irritability and hyperactivity at one year with either (a) a family history of hyperactivity and/or behavior disorders or (b) a maternal history of pregnancy and obstetrical complications. At age two high anomaly infants were more likely to be difficult, as rated by parent interview and direct observation. However, at age two there was little agreement between cross-situational and cross-temporal behavior ratings, and there were *no* significant predictors of behavior problems based on any newborn or year one measure. These findings suggested that the newborn anomaly score by itself was unlikely to prove clinically useful in predicting hyperactivity or other preschool behavior problems for an unselected population. In the third year of the study parent interviews revealed that infants with high anomaly scores were somewhat more likely to exhibit problem behavior at age three, particularly in the form of hyperactive-impulsive behavior in boys. Preschool teachers' and psychologists' ratings showed no significant relationship to anomaly score, but the methodology here was poor. The psychologists' ratings were carried out in a one-to-one novel setting, which should lower the probability that the child would exhibit hyperactive behavior; and the teachers' ratings were obtained from many teachers in a variety of settings, which made it unclear as to what the effect would be of many different raters in settings that might differ in structure and discipline. Having the psychologist rate the children outside of the classroom eliminated the opportunity of having the teachers' ratings confirmed by an independent observer.

The conclusion to be drawn from the research is that the relationship between minor physical anomalies and problem behavior is a weak one, if indeed any exists at all. Clinical usefulness of this measure as a predictor of problem behavior in general or hyperactivity in particular is limited. However, minor physical anomalies may yet prove to be of value as contributors to the prediction of hyperactivity if combined with other factors such as temperament and parenting variables. As we have pointed out, within an interactionist position the search for predictors on the basis of univariate analysis is unlikely to generate useful clinical information. Werner (1980), Ross (1976), Loney (1980b), and others have noted that powerful relationships that remain undetected with a univariate approach often emerge with multivariate analysis. One interesting speculation raised by Kinsbourne (1979) is that if minor physical anomalies prove to be predictive, some anomalies may be more predictive of the onset of behavior disorder and more contributory to it than others. For example, visible anomalies such as unattractive facial characteristics may elicit negative social reactions, particularly on the part of the parents and later, peers, whereas less visually prominent anomalies may have no such effect.

PREDICTING DRUG RESPONSE IN HYPERACTIVE CHILDREN

In Barkley's (1976) excellent comprehensive review of research on prediction of drug response, which is also the first review on this topic to appear in the literature, he reported that 75 percent of hyperactive children responded positively to stimulant medications, while in the remaining 25 percent the hyperactive symptoms were either unchanged or exacerbated by stimulant drug intervention. The percent of positive responders varies across investigations, but there is general agreement that a substantial number of hyperactive children are positive responders, that is, they do exhibit a short-term favorable response to stimulant medication. However, the fact that as many as 25 percent are nonresponders has underscored the need to identify those variables that discriminate between the two groups. Although serious side effects in those who are changed or exacerbated are not common, there is no reason for complacency on this score. The categories of predictor variables to be considered here are neurological, psychophysiological, ratings and psychological tests, and parental characteristics. The research on these topics has several limitations. It is our opinion that one of the most serious and most common defects has been the high priority given to early publication rather than to cross-validation of the initial findings on another sample. Barkley (1976) has noted several important methodological shortcomings including differences across studies with respect to definitions of hyperactivity, drug regimens, experimental designs, assessment instruments, and criteria of improvement. Loney (1978, p. 167) has attributed a substantial part of the difficulty in identifying the predictors of positive drug (methylphenidate) response to basic differences in the operationalization of *drug response,* with some investigators using observed changes or change scores based on the child's predrug behavior, while others have used reported outcome or outcome measures with the behavior of nonhyperactive peers as a reference standard:

... much of the difficulty in arriving at a settled opinion on the predictors of response to CNS drug treatment has arisen from difficulties in defining response. Some investigators, for example, have used an initial response or *improvement* measure, while others have employed a longer-term response or *outcome* measure. Initial response or improvement tends to be framed in self-relative terms ("He is more attentive than he used to be") or to be measured as a difference between pre- and post-treatment symptom scores. Long-term response or outcome tends to be expressed in terms of severity ("He is quite attentive") or in terms of the hypothetical normal child ("He is as attentive as most") or to be defined as a position on a symptom measure obtained at follow-up. It is one thing if an improved child is one who merely has less of a problem than he used to have and quite another if he is one who has less of a problem than others do. As the work of Weiss and her colleagues has recently suggested, the connection between early response to treatment and condition at follow-up is far from simple or strong.

Neurological Predictors

Finger Twitch Test. One simple measure that appears to predict differential response to stimulant drugs is the finger twitch test (Barcai, 1971). In this procedure the child sits opposite the examiner with his hands hanging between his knees in a normal position and his fingers moderately flexed. The interval between the start of the test and the time of the first brisk twitch of a finger is recorded. Although Barcai (1971) has described the test procedure in considerable detail, there are no reliability and validity data, and the only norms available are for boys aged 10 to 12. In his study the finger twitch appeared in all nonresponders after 25 seconds and, in 18 of 21 positive or equivocal responders, before 25 seconds had elapsed. Rapoport, Quinn, Brabard, Riddle, and Brooks (1974) also reported accurate predictions of drug response with this test. One line of research that merits priority is the establishing of reliability and validity levels, replication of findings, and expansion of the age norms.

In a discussion of this test Barkley (1976, p. 338) commented:

> At first glance, this simple test appears to be associated with motor inhibition and extrapyramidal signs of neurological impairment. A closer look at the instructions to the child also suggests that it may involve that aspect of attention span known as "maintenance of set." However, whether it is the motor or the attentional aspects of this test which underlie its usefulness as a predictor is uncertain at this time.

Soft Signs. Considerable research and clinical attention has been given to the diagnostic and predictive utility of soft signs (Casey, 1977; Ingram, 1973; Safer & Allen, 1976; Varga, 1979). Although some investigators have reported a more favorable drug response in hyperactive children with increased soft signs, particularly when they occur in conjunction with EEG abnormality (e.g., Satterfield, Cantwell, Saul, Lesser & Podosin, 1973), others have found no such association (e.g., Weiss, Minde, Douglas, Werry, & Sykes, 1971). The soft sign controversy is further complicated by Conrad and Insel's (1967) finding that a combination of soft signs and unspecified emotional pathology appeared to predict a poor response to stimulant drugs.

Organic Impairment. The same pattern of equivocal results exists with respect to evidence of organic impairment. When hyperactive children are categorized as organic or nonorganic on the basis of accepted, objective indices of organic impairment, there is evidence of a positive relationship between organicity and drug response (Epstein, Lasagna, Conners, & Rodriguez, 1968; Weiss, Werry, Minde, Douglas, & Sykes, 1968), no organic–nonorganic differences on drug response (Knights & Hinton, 1969), and a negative relationship between organicity and drug response (Rie, Rie, Stewart, & Ambuel, 1976a).

Although the trend in this heterogeneous group of studies suggests that the presence of several different indices of neurological impairment in a hyperactive child may be predictive of favorable drug response, more research is clearly needed before any definitive statements can be made. One problem with many of the studies in which hyperactive children have been assigned to diagnostic categories in order to determine if these categories are predictive of drug response is that there is no report on how reliably children can be classified into the various diagnostic categories. In the absence of this essential information, subsequent analysis becomes meaningless since it rests on a possibly unreliable base. The danger here is that potentially productive avenues of attack may be cut off by falsely negative results. In noting this methodological defect, Cantwell (1978a) has commented that the most that can be said is that diagnostic subgroupings have not been reliably able to predict drug response.

Psychophysiological Predictors

EEG Abnormality. There is no clearcut evidence of a relationship between EEG abnormality in general and drug responsivity (Barkley, 1976), but one EEG measure that has proven useful in differentiating between drug responders and nonresponders is the average evoked response (AER). With the hyperactive child this measure consists of recording the effects on the EEG of presenting various patterns of visual and auditory stimuli. The resultant evoked responses or potentials are averaged over many stimulus trials, and if consistent effects occur, these will accumulate. Exploratory studies have indicated that the AER is well suited to the prediction of clinical drug response because it is sensitive to changes in attentional state and can be dramatically altered with various medications (Halliday, Gnauck, Rosenthal, McKibben, & Callaway, 1980). Halliday and his associates (Halliday, Rosenthal, Naylor, & Callaway, 1976) have demonstrated that AERs can be used to predict clinical response to stimulant medications. In an initial study and then a replication, they showed that certain measures of the visual evoked potential discriminated between hyperactive children who were subsequently judged by their pediatrician to be responders to Ritalin, as compared to hyperactive children who showed poor or marginal response to this drug. Similarly, research on auditory evoked potentials has demonstrated significant differences between drug responders and nonresponders on a cluster of AER measures: drug responders, for example, had higher predrug AER amplitudes, lower recovery of evoked responses, less change in latency and intensity of these responses with age, and greater variability (Buchsbaum & Wender, 1973; Satterfield, Cantwell, Lesser, & Podosin, 1972).

Electropupillogram (EPG). Knopp, Arnold, Andras, and Smeltzer (1973) have reported a method of discriminating between drug responders and nonresponders on the basis of their autonomic arousal levels as inferred from the EPG responses. They measured the changes in dark-adapted pupil diameter in response to light in three subgroups of hyperactive children prior to and following the administration of amphetamines. Fish's (1971) diagnostic system was the basis for assigning the children to the unsocialized aggressive, hyperkinetic, and overanxious reactions to childhood subgroups. The latter group showed generally normal EPGs prior to drug intervention and minimal EPG change during drug treatment. Hyperkinetic subjects showed evidence of overarousal (high predrug electropupillary contractions), whereas the unsocialized aggressive subjects had low electropupillary contractions, which suggested underarousal. During drug treatment both groups changed significantly in moving closer to the mean EPG of normal children. The same pattern of underarousal, followed by treatment with stimulant drugs, leading to a significant increase in EPG level, has been reported by Yoss and Moyers (1971). Taken together these studies suggest that it is the over- and underaroused hyperactive children (with arousal defined in terms of EPG response) who respond to stimulant medication. It follows that the EPG may be useful in predicting response to drug intervention.

Cardiac-Related Measures. Although various cardiac-related measures have been investigated for their discriminant value, only baseline heart rate has distinguished between good and poor drug responders, with good responders having significantly lower levels (Porges, Walter, Korb, & Sprague, 1975). Other cardiac parameters including blood pressure, heart rate variability, pulse rate, and heart rate deceleration were found to have no discriminative validity.

Respiration. An indication of the methodological difficulties in accurately identifying predictors of drug response comes from a study by Barkley and Jackson (1977) in which mean predrug levels of respiration were correlated with degree of improvement on a number of activity level and attention measures obtained during drug treatment. Predrug respiration proved to be positively *or* negatively correlated with improvement on activity level and attention span depending on which measure of these two variables was used. The respiration measure, for example, correlated negatively with wrist and seat movement activity during a televised school program, and positively with improvement in toy change activity during a restricted play period. Clearly, any promising predictors should be subjected to comprehensive empirical scrutiny before their predictive utility can be considered established.

The psychophysiological variables that have discriminated between responders and nonresponders are those related to attention span and, as Barkley (1977a) and Douglas (1972, 1974) have pointed out, these findings are consistent with the fact that the major effect of stimulant medication in the hyperactive child is upon attention span.

One criterion of predictive utility is practicality (Dubey, 1981). The fact that responders and nonresponders can be shown to differ statistically on a complex measure such as the AER may be of considerable theoretical interest but is of little practical value to the pediatrician who typically lacks both the equipment and the expertise needed to obtain such a measure. Of the measures described here, the finger twitch test (Barcai, 1971) appears to be ideal in terms of the criterion of practicality. A battery of such measures, complete with standardization and normative data, would represent a major contribution to the management domain.

General Evaluations

Ratings. Clinician, parent, and teacher ratings have been inconsistent as predictors of differential drug responsiveness in hyperactive children. Of the three, clinicians' ratings have proven to be the most useful. Barcai (1971) was able to predict favorable and unfavorable drug response with impressive accuracy when he combined his finger twitch test with clinicians' ratings of personality characterisics assessed during a psychiatric interview. Favorable drug responders were more active and less able in terms of planning ability, language skills, ability to abstract, imagination, sense of perspective, and acceptance of social rules. When Zahn, Abate, Little, and Wender (1975) rated hyperactive children on attentiveness, anxiety, and tendency to act out, they found that poor drug response was associated with higher scores on anxiety and acting out. These results were consistent with Fish's (1971) report that hyperactive children in her unsocialized aggressive and overanxious reaction of childhood categories tended to be poor responders, as well as with Conrad and Insel's (1967) report of a link between poor drug response and primary emotional pathology, and the model proposed by Loney (1980b) of the role of aggression in outcome. Although clinicians' ratings have proven to be of predictive value in the foregoing and other (Butter & Lapierre, 1974) studies, several investigators (e.g., Rapoport et al., 1974) have not confirmed these relationships. The same pattern of inconsistent results is apparent in studies of teacher ratings. Schleifer et al. (1975) assigned hyperactive preschool children to extreme, moderate, and low activity groups on the basis of teacher ratings on an unidentified 3-point activity scale with no reported reliability or validity data. Extreme hyperactive children showed more improvement than those in the other two groups. But other investigators have not found teacher ratings to be useful in predicting drug response (e.g., Hoffman, Engelhardt, Margolis, Polizos, Waizer, & Rosenfeld, 1974; Rie et al., 1976a). In the case of parent ratings the bulk of evidence is against their utility in predicting drug response (Barkley, 1976; Rapoport, Abramson, Alexander, & Lott, 1971; Rie et al. 1976; Werry & Sprague, 1974; Zahn et al. 1975). As Barkley (1976) has noted, one major difficulty in rating scale studies is the lack of empirical proof that the scales do assess the constructs that they purport to assess. The fact that activity rating scales often do not correlate with objective observations of activity level (and hence lack validity) raises questions about the criteria that adults, particularly parents, use in reporting behavioral improvement in hyperactive children as a function of drug intervention.

Psychological Tests. The prediction of drug response with standardized psychological tests has for the most part proven disappointing. Commonly used tests such as the Wide Range Achievement Test, Bender Visual Motor Gestalt, Illinois Test of Psycholinguistic Ability, and the Wechsler Intelligence Scale for Children, yield inconsistent results in prediction of drug response. The psychological variables such as reaction time, and tests such as the Kagan Matching Familiar Figures Test and Porteus Mazes, that are the most sensitive indicators of drug response are for the most part related to attention span (Barkley, 1976). In a study of the predictive utility of attention span indices Barkley (1976) measured the effect of drug intervention on a variety of indices of attention and activity level. His results showed that the higher the predrug activity level the greater the improvement in activity behavior with drugs. However, the more significant result related to attention span: the more inattentive the hyperactive child was initially, the greater his improvement in attention span and reduction in activity level during drug treatment. This finding suggests that attentional indices are useful in the prediction of drug responsiveness. Ferguson and Trites' (1980) data were less supportive of this relationship. In a double-blind crossover trial with three medication periods, each of which was three weeks long, and a test battery with a preponderance of attention measures, only one of eight attention variables was found to differentiate between responders and nonresponders. The most interesting finding in terms of predictors was that the drug responders had higher minor physical anomaly scores. In view of the simplicity and speed with which such scores can be computed, this finding is one that clinicians could readily validate. Swanson and Kinsbourne (1976) have developed a laboratory learning test based on a paired-associate task that they have used successfully with more than 150 children in predicting medication response. The paired-associate learning paradigm was chosen because proficiency in associative learning is closely related to school success, particularly in the elementary grades. This predictive test requires a laboratory setting and a full school day to administer.

Parental Characteristics

Inconsistent and often contradictory results have been reported concerning the relationship between drug response and various aspects of parental influence such as the parent–child relationship, parental attitudes towards drug intervention, and psychiatric status of the parents. Some investigators (Conrad & Insel, 1967; Loney, Comly, & Simon, 1975; Paxton, 1972; Weiss, Minde, Douglas, Werry, & Sykes, 1971) have found that a favorable response to drugs is associated with good parent-child relationships, while others (Werry, Weiss, Douglas, & Martin, 1966) have reported that neither the mother–child relationship nor the overall climate of the home were related to drug response. In the study of preschool hyperactive children by Schleifer and his associates (Schleifer, Weiss, Cohen, Elman, Cvejic, & Kruger, 1975) the fact that true hyperactives exhibited a more favorable response than did situational hyperactives, and had poorer relationships with their mothers, has been interpreted by Barkley (1976) as evidence against the importance of a good parent–child relationship to drug response. We disagree with this interpretation. The fact that the severity of the hyperactivity was greater in the true than in the situational group means that severity of hyperactivity could contribute to the variation in response to stimulants (Loney, Prinz, Mishalow, & Joad, 1978). Knobel (1962) has emphasized the differential effects of medication-accepting and medication-rejecting households and has suggested on the basis of clinical experience that a positive parental attitude to stimulant medication is likely to facilitate positive drug response. Although this belief has considerable face validity, there are no supporting empirical data. On the basis of his own family studies of hyperactive children, Cantwell (Bellak, 1979) reported preliminary clinical evidence that children with a positive family history of hyperactivity in a first-degree relative showed a favorable response to stimulants, whereas those in the antisocial spectrum parent group did less well. This clinical observation is consistent with Conrad and Insel's (1967) finding that a group of hyperactive children with at least one grossly deviant or socially incompetent parent had significantly fewer good responders to stimulants than a group without such parents. However, according to Cantwell (1978a), Satterfield found that drug response was unrelated to the presence of psychopathology in either first or second degree relatives. Lastly, there was no evidence of parental predictors of drug response in a study by Loney, Prinz, Mishalow, and Joad (1978). Instead the independent variables that predicted drug response were perinatal complications, age at referral, and severity of hyperactivity. This study underscores the informational value of multivariate methods in the study of responses, such as drug response, that are likely to have multiple determinants. Unlike the ordinary two-variable linear correlation, that is, the Pearson r, the multiple regression analysis used here allowed the investigators to specify the relative importance of each of the independent variables in terms of the specific amount of variance in the criterion variable for which it independently accounts. In this analysis severity of hyperactivity was a much less important predictor of drug response than either of the other two variables.

Overall, the results of this substantial body of research confirm Sroufe's (1975) conclusion in his landmark review of the stimulant medications that no basis exists for either predicting whether a specific hyperactive child will benefit from drug intervention or determining which medication will be most effective. This conclusion has been reiterated by Varga (1979) and also by Cantwell (1978a, p. 253) in a major paper on stimulant medications:

> In summary, while it is clear that not all hyperactive children do respond positively to central nervous system medication, there is precious little research evidence supporting which variables are most important in determining treatment response. The diagnostic heterogeneity of the patients used in various studies, differences in the definition of and measurement of criteria of positive response, and differences in design of the various studies, make comparison of the same factors between studies virtually impossible. In an *individual* child it is nearly impossible to decide definitively prior to treatment whether or not he will respond.

In terms of possible research directions, one potentially profitable area would be the identification of homogeneous subgroups within the drug responder group and the investigation of predictors or clusters of predictors for these subgroups. Ullman, Barkley, and Brown's (1978) findings are relevant here: when hyperactive children who were responders were measured on a series of activity and attentional problems, there were no indications that these children were more homogeneous with respect to behavioral symptoms than the hyperactive population in general. Another direction concerns the possibility of treatment × subject interactions. Research by Whalen and her associates (Bugental, Whalen, & Henker, 1977; Whalen & Henker, 1976) suggests that the causal attribution system of the hyperactive child is a potentially important subject variable. Finally, the finding that measures of attention span and its correlates appear to be the most promising predictors of drug response in hyperactive children (Barkley, 1976) suggests that priority in the search for predictors should be given to further research on the predictive utility of attention-related measures.

PREDICTING OUTCOME IN ADOLESCENCE

The hyperactive adolescent is at risk for school failure, emotional difficulties, poor peer relationships, and trouble with the law (Hechtman, Weiss, Finklestein, Wener, & Benn, 1976; Huessy, Metoyer, & Townsend, 1974; Mendelson, Johnson, & Stewart, 1971; Milich & Loney, 1979a) regardless of whether he has undergone stimulant medication treatment or behavioral intervention. Although stimulant medication may have effectively modified the primary symptomatology of hyperactivity in the middle childhood years, there is a growing body of evidence that attests to the fact that neither treatment with stimulant medication nor the nature of the child's response to the medication is systematically related to outcome in adolescence (Blouin, Bornstein, & Trites, 1978; Minde, Weiss, & Mendelson, 1972; Weiss, Kruger, Danielson, & Elman, 1975). The failure to find a relationship between drug intervention and outcome in adolescence has dismayed and puzzled investigators and has caused them to seek out new directions in the search for predictors. On the basis of follow-up studies by others and extensive research of their own, Loney and her colleagues have successfully demonstrated the predictive utility of childhood aggression, a symptom that traditionally has been categorized as secondary, or resultant, in the primary–secondary grouping of hyperactive symptomatology. In follow-up studies over the past decade, measures of aggression at referral and aggression-related variables such as family pathology have been clearly associated with outcome in adolescence (Milich & Loney, 1979a). Representative of these studies was that of Weiss, Minde, Werry, Douglas, and Nemeth (1971), in which ratings of childhood aggression and family pathology, punitive child-rearing practices, poor mother–child relationships, and poor parental adjustment at the time of referral were significantly related to antisocial aggression in adolescence. Research by Loney and her associates (e.g., Kramer & Loney, 1978; Langhorne & Loney, 1979; Loney, Kramer, & Milich, 1981; Loney, Langhorne, & Paternite, 1978; Paternite & Loney, 1980) has provided impressive evidence of a relationship between aggression at referral and outcome in adolescence. The significance of this finding is enhanced by the fact that there is only a minimal relationship between hyperactive symptomatology at referral and adolescent outcome. The starting point for their focus on childhood aggression as a predictor was a factor analytic study of the primary and secondary symptomatology at referral of 135 hyperactive boys (Loney et al., 1978). This single-source principal axis factor analysis yielded two relatively independent symptom dimensions: (a) a Hyperactivity factor encompassing hyperactivity, inattention, and judgment deficits, and accounting for 23.4 percent of the factor variance; and (b) an Aggression factor encompassing interpersonal aggression, negative affect, and control deficits, accounting for 44.6 percent of the factor variance. Loney et al. (1978) described the lack of overlap between these two symptom factors as "striking." A hyperactive boy with higher scores on the

Hyperactivity factor was described as more impulsive, demanding of attention, restless, and overactive. His peers are more unaccepting of him and his father is rated as less loving towards him. He displays more visual-motor difficulties in psychometric testing, and he responds better to central nervous system stimulant drug treatment. A hyperactive boy with higher scores on the Aggression factor was seen as more destructive, defiant, and inconsiderate. He is younger at referral and has fewer neurological signs. His family is of lower socioeconomic status, his parents are rated as less loving toward him, and his mother as more lax toward him. These findings on the independence of the hyperactivity and aggression dimensions have since been replicated and validated (Milich, Loney, & Landau, 1981).

The next step was to conduct a series of multiple regression analyses (Loney, Langhorne, Paternite, Whaley-Klahn, Blair-Broeker, & Hacker, 1976) to determine whether the Hyperactivity and Aggression factors and other measures at referral would predict symptoms at follow-up in adolescence. The predictors making the greatest contribution to symptom variation at follow-up were the Aggression factor, socioeconomic status (SES), and father autonomy-to-control, that is, hyperactive boys who at referral were more aggressive, lower SES, and had less controlling fathers tended to have a more unsatisfactory outcome in terms of severity of symptoms in adolescence as rated by their mothers and psychologists. The Hyperactivity factor was *not* a significant predictor of adolescent outcome. A further analysis of these data (Paternite & Loney, 1980) showed that aggression at referral was the single best predictor of aggressive and hyperactive symptomatology at follow-up, whereas hyperactivity at referral contributed significantly to only one of the regression analyses, academic achievement. Further support for the importance of childhood aggression to adolescent outcome comes from the following findings. Aggression at referral and not hyperactivity, as has commonly been stated, predicted self-esteem deficits in adolescence (Langhorne & Loney, 1979). Aggression at referral combined with ecological (urban settings) and familial (size of family, parenting variables) measures predicted antisocial aggression in adolescence (Kramer & Loney, 1978); ecological variables and childhood aggression also predicted adolescent hyperactivity. Childhood hyperactivity was predictive of academic performance, but a better predictor of later academic functioning was childhood achievement (Loney et al., 1981).

Treatment response was also found to be a predictor of outcome in adolescence. A favorable response to stimulant medication in childhood was associated with less negative affect, higher achievement scores although there were still marked academic deficits, and a lower incidence of illegal drugs at adolescent follow-up. No association was found between treatment response and later hyperactivity symptoms (Loney et al., 1981).

In a discussion of the predictive utility of childhood aggression for adolescent outcome, Milich and Loney (1979a, p. 109) emphasize that their findings should not be interpreted as evidence that aggression is the only significant predictor of outcome for this population. Rather, the identification of significant predictors would appear to depend upon the specific outcome measures one is interested in predicting ... both hyperactivity and aggressive symptomatology, as well as drug response, achievement measures, and parenting and environmental variables ... may all make significant contributions to the prediction of adolescent outcome, depending upon the specific outcome measures one is interested in predicting.

The potential of these findings makes independent replication mandatory, as Loney (1980b) has noted, but there appears to be little doubt that aggression at referral makes a significant contribution to the prediction of adolescent outcome for the hyperactive child.

The next step planned in the Loney series is the identification of adolescent predictors of adult behavior. A preliminary report on this topic has been presented by Weiss and her colleagues (Hechtman, Weiss, Perlman, & Amsel, 1980). They have followed their adolescent group into early adulthood and from adolescence data have reported some predictors of a group of outcomes in adulthood (emotional adjustment, peer relationships, academic accomplishment, police involvement, car accidents, and nonmedical use of drugs). From a predictive viewpoint their findings can be summarized as follows: Aggression was related to almost every outcome measure including academic accomplishment, and continued to be an important predictor but always in conjunction with other variables. Antisocial behavior and hyperactivity were relatively unimportant. Hyperactivity, for example, no longer contributed to school achievement as it had in adolescence (Loney et al., 1981; Weiss et al., 1971). Family parameters, particularly mental health of family members and emotional climate in the home, and Peterson–Quay Behavior Problem Checklist scores were strong contributors to several adult outcome variables including emotional adjustment, peer relationships, encounters with the law, and nonmedical use of drugs. A more comprehensive analysis of the predictive potential of their adolescence measures is currently underway.

One possibility that researchers seeking predictors should be alert to is the idea that simple, easily identifiable predictors may be present but unnoticed. In the last decade the search for predictors of behavioral and medical disorders has involved increasingly complex and costly procedures. Chedd (1981), for example, has recently developed a predictive procedure for spinal bifida that begins with a prenatal blood test of the alphafetoprotein level and continues, for those pregnant women with reported high levels of this protein, with a repeat blood test, ultrasound testing, amniocentesis, repeat ultrasound and amniocentesis, and further biochemical analysis of the amniotic fluid. The whole procedure requires skilled technicians, costs hundreds of dollars, and involves at least five clinic visits. Although complexity of procedure is unavoidable in instances such as this, it is important that investigators not focus so completely on advanced technology and complex approaches that they ignore the possibility that simple predictors may exist. In the literature on prediction there are a surprising number of such predictors. For example, there is general agreement (Cantwell, 1979; Sleator & Ullman, 1981) that the situational specificity of hyperactive behavior often makes it difficult for the pediatrician to diagnose hyperactivity in the office situation. One characteristic that appears to be predictive of hyperactivity, and one that pediatricians can observe for themselves, is excessive ticklishness as a response to tactile examination of the trunk. This observation was reported by Mofenson, Greensher, and Horowitz (1972) as a characteristic that in combination with a particular history could confirm a diagnosis of hyperactivity. Mofenson et al. (1972, p. 687) stated that "most of our hyperactive children were unable to control this response even though the procedure was explained and they were allowed to place their hand on top of the examiner's hand during the abdominal palpation." Although there is no empirical evidence of the predictive validity of excessive ticklishness, a number of pediatricians have subsequently confirmed this relationship to us and, more importantly from a predictive viewpoint, their chart records have shown that this ticklishness was present even early in the preschool years. If future research replicates this finding, a very simple predictor of hyperactivity may have been identified.

There are many other examples of simple, potentially valuable predictors. In a study of adolescents with grand mal epilepsy (Hodgman, McAnarney, Myers, & Iker, 1979) the best predictor of successful adjustment and self-responsibility at home and in social functioning was whether the child was in the appropriate grade for his age. In the initial search for gifted children, Terman and his associates (Terman & Merrill, 1926) reported that a highly accurate predictor of giftedness was being the youngest child in the class. Numerous studies have confirmed that the best predictor of adult adjustment is peer ratings in childhood (Milich & Landau, 1981). Rayburn and McKean (1980) have reported that an excellent predictor of a change in fetal well-being is an increase or decrease in rate of fetal kicks, a measure that the mother can easily provide. And as a final example, Oster (1980) has reported that an early predictor of pancreatic cancer, a cancer that is notably difficult to diagnose in the early stages, may be intractable hiccups, that is, hiccups occurring 20 to 40 times per minute with consequent difficulty in breathing and eating.

CHAPTER 6

Drug Therapy

The use of drugs to quiet restless children is not a recent phenomenon. The last of the great Greek physicians, Galen, prescribed opium for restless, colicky infants; medicinal blends containing substantial amounts of alcohol have been used for centuries to sedate irritable infants; and bromides and barbiturates were used extensively for chronic restlessness in the late nineteenth century (Goodman & Gilman, 1975). However, the central nervous system stimulants are a product of twentieth-century technology. Although they were first introduced for use in children with behavioral and learning problems in the 1930s (Bradley, 1937; Molitch & Eccles, 1937), reports of their efficacy attracted little clinical and research attention during the subsequent two decades. By the early 1960s the wonder drugs were an established part of the American scene, and antibiotics were correctly credited with having the potential to save more lives in a decade than had been lost in World War II. There was now a climate of readiness for drug solutions to children's behavior disorders, an attitude of receptivity that had not existed in 1937. By the late 1960s both the amphetamines and methylphenidate, which had been introduced in the late 1950s (Zimmerman & Burgemeister, 1958), were being used with indiscriminate enthusiasm, and in the process became the subject of considerable controversy and debate.

With the Omaha and other reports (Hentoff, 1972; Maynard, 1970) that as many as 10 percent of all elementary school children were being given stimulant medication for behavior disorders and learning difficulties, the drug controversy erupted and escalated despite subsequent statements that the reportedly high drug treatment prevalence rates were in error. The protagonists engaged in a series of sharp criticisms and firm rebuttals, symposia were organized, professional groups made position statements, textbooks and books for the layman abounded, and inevitably the mass media entered the fray, giving an inordinate amount of coverage to the topic in general and lawsuits in particular. The controversy and concern further intensified with the first reports that hyperactivity was not a time-limited disorder, but instead appeared to be a chronic and possibly lifelong condition. The lack of consensus among the different factions can be attributed in part to the conflicting results from the inadequate and unsystematic research that characterized the 1960s and much of the first half of the 1970s. Although the issues of the early 1970s appeared to be both diverse and multitudinous, in fact they reflected two major concerns (Werry, 1977, p. 446):

> (1) that some of the drugs used are undesirable or downright dangerous, (2) that doctors are putting creative, bored, dissenting, oppressed, or otherwise rightfully troublesome children into chemical straitjackets.

In the early 1970s reactions to drug treatment tended towards unqualified extremes of approval and disapproval:

> To those who have seen the results of such treatment (stimulant medication) in minimal brain dysfunction children ... the present limited use of drug therapy is as upsetting as it is unbelievable.... It would not be hard to argue that in many instances psychotherapy of children with this syndrome virtually constitutes malpractice ... stimulant drug therapy ... is the treatment of choice ... withholding it represents an injury to the patient and his family. (Wender, 1971, p. 130)

> I have never prescribed stimulants for these patients, and I never will.... Stimulants merely mask the symptoms without curing the disease ... the hyperactive child's problem can almost always be identified and treated if the physician is willing to take the time and trouble ... (Walker, 1974, p. 43)

During the late 1970s and currently, in the early 1980s, the trend has been towards an increasing skepticism concerning the benefits of drug treatment as the initial breakthrough status attributed to the stimulants has failed to hold up in the face of empirical data. Although the polarity of views remains, the extremes of the early 1970s have been tempered by a scholarly caution coupled with scientific restraint:

> ... while concentration may be improved (with the stimulants) decreased interest in the affective reactions to the environment may cancel out the short-term effects thus making long-term gains from drug therapy essentially nil. (Barkley, 1977, p. 157)

> ... we do not know the long-term consequences of learning to view oneself as a person who needs medication to cope with everyday situations that other people can manage on their own. (Henker & Whalen, 1980b, p. 165)

> Drugs should never be regarded as definitive treatment in themselves ... drug treatment should be seen as *synergistic*, and not in competition with other treatment (p. 448).... At the moment most drug therapy is fumbling empiricism, but there are many hopeful signs that a more rational approach may ultimately be possible. (Werry, 1977, p. 462)

In this chapter we will first discuss the current status of the drug treatment of hyperactive children. The primary emphasis is on the clinical facts, empirical findings, and practical considerations relevant to the use of the central nervous system stimulants. Then we will consider the antimedication group's position that the stimulants are dangerous and are being misused, and that the problem of hyperactivity would be better handled by other, nonpharmacological modes of intervention. Finally, we will discuss some potentially valuable directions for future research. No attempt will be made here to provide an exhaustive review of the voluminous literature on the drug treatment of hyperactive children. For the reader who is interested in such comprehensive coverage, Werry (1978b) has edited an excellent text on pediatric psychopharmacology that contains concise discussions of the basic principles of using behavior modifying drugs with children as well as review chapters on individual drugs. This text should be mandatory reading for anyone seriously interested in the psychopharmacotherapy research aspects of hyperactivity. Several other summaries of different aspects of drug treatment are also available in the literature. Allen and Safer (1979), for example, have presented a risk benefit analysis of the long-term effects of stimulant therapy; Barkley (1977) has provided a comprehensive review of stimulant drug research, as well as a review (Barkley, 1976) of prediction of drug response; Cantwell (1978a) has an interesting chapter on the use of stimulants with hyperactive children and has also collaborated with Carlson (Cantwell & Carlson, 1978) on a critical review of these drugs; Cohen (1979) has edited a text on the psychopharmacology of the hyperactive child, and this topic has also been given comprehensive coverage by Gadow (1979); Sprague and Ullman (1981) have contributed a fine chapter on psychoactive drugs and child management, including a discussion of recent litigation; Sroufe (1975) has written an excellent critical review; Werry (1976, 1977) has discussed medication for hyperactive children; and Gadow and Loney (1981) and Whalen and Henker (1980a) have produced comprehensive texts with an emphasis on different facets of drug treatment.

THERAPEUTIC REGIMENS FOR STIMULANT DRUGS

The three basic groups of medication that have been used to treat the hyperactive child are the central nervous system stimulants, tricyclic antidepressants, and antipsychotic drugs. The central nervous system stimulants to be discussed here include the amphetamines, particularly dextroamphetamine (Dexedrine); methylphenidate (Ritalin), magnesium pemoline (Cylert), and caffeine. The stimulants have been found to be most effective, and of these, methylphenidate and the amphetamines are by far the most widely used. Deanol (Deaner) is a stimulant that is infrequently used with hyperactive children and consequently will not be discussed here. For the reader interested in this stimulant, Conners (1973c) and Lewis and Lewis (1977) have evaluated the research on it. It is important to keep the prevalence of stimulant use in perspective. Although reports in the mass media of the early 1970s (Hentoff, 1972; Maynard, 1970) have suggested that as many as 10 percent of all elementary school children were being given stimulant medication for behavior disorders and learning difficulties, the results of a series of recent surveys have indicated that drug treatment prevalence rates are generally between 1 and 2 percent of the elementary school population, that is, between 235,000 and 465,000 elementary school children (Bosco & Robin, 1980; Conway, 1976; Krager, Safer, & Earhart, 1979; Lambert, Sandoval, & Sassone, 1978). In a critical and comprehensive review of the prevalence of drug treatment for hyperactivity and other behavior disorders, Gadow (1981) has noted that the prevalence surveys differ markedly in sampling methodology, subject populations, and data analysis procedures, but are similar in respect to the absence of validity checks of their prevalence data (the Bosco and Robin study being the lone exception) and the absence of attempted checks on the amount of under- or overreporting of stimulant usage.

The tricyclic antidepressant that has been used is imipramine (Tofranil), and the antipsychotics are thioridazine (Mellaril), chlorpromazine (Thorazine), and haloperidol (Haldol). Neither the tricyclics nor the antipsychotics, either alone or in combination, have been found to be as effective as the stimulants are with the average hyperactive child. Of the two groups, the tricyclics are generally the next drugs of choice for children who do not respond to the stimulants (Cantwell, 1978a). We will begin with a discussion of the therapeutic regimens for methylphenidate and the amphetamines with school-age hyperactive children. The use of stimulants with adolescents and adults, a comparatively recent and consequently less well-understood development, will be discussed later in the chapter, as will the dubious practice of using drugs with preschool children.

Methylphenidate

Methylphenidate is less potent than the amphetamines. Potency is defined as the amount of a drug that must be administered to obtain a particular response. Although it is often prescribed as if it were approximately half as potent as dextroamphetamine on a weight basis, a direct comparison (Sprague & Sleator, 1975) of the effects of the two stimulants on a laboratory test of learning showed that methylphenidate was more than half as potent as dextroamphetamine. Wender (1971) recommends a daily dosage range of from 20 to 100 mg of methylphenidate, whereas Lytton and Knobel (1958) have used up to 200 mg per day with some hyperactive children. Schain and Reynard (1975) have reported drug success with dosages ranging from 5 to 60 mg per day for elementary school children, with single doses being used for many of the children. An interesting finding in their study was that overweight children did not respond well to methylphenidate, even though the dosage was equivalent to that in children who were categorized as drug successes. Gross and Wilson (1974) state that the dosage requirement can be reduced by half if liquid methylphenidate is used. The foregoing recommendations are for standardized or average dosage procedures. Sprague and Sleator (1973) recommend that dosage be titrated individually, beginning with small doses and gradually increasing them until a satisfactory reduction occurs in the hyperactivity, or side effects appear that are of sufficient severity to warrant no further increase in medication. With both standarized and individually titrated dosages, the general practice is to gradually increase the dosage level until the hyperactive child's mother reports satisfactory results. Sleator and von Neumann (1974) have deplored this practice on the basis of empirical evidence that parents are insensitive to variations in dosage as well as to medication-placebo differences, and have urged pediatricians to base dosage decisions on more precise evaluative information, preferably obtained from multiple sources. Sprague and Sleator (1976) recommend dosage determination on an mg/kg basis, whereas Kinsbourne and Swanson (1979) contend that as children get older and heavier they require smaller, not larger, dosages. They have developed a micromethod for measuring methylphenidate to investigate the possibility that better gastrointestinal absorption may allow older children to achieve effective serum levels with smaller dosages (Soldin, Hill, Chan, Swanson, & Hill, 1979).

Dose Response Curves. Individually titrated dosages of stimulants are unquestionably preferable to the standardized procedures. Another refinement that is sufficiently well documented to merit clinical attention is the empirically established dose-response curve data. The dose-response curve refers to the changes that may occur in the target behavior as a function of the amount of stimulant drug administered. As the dose is increased there is usually a greater effect on different response systems to a point of maximal response, and after that point is reached for a specific response system, further increases in the amount of drug ingested have no positive effect, and in fact may cause the response to diminish in efficacy. An example of this phenomenon occurred in a study (Sprague, Werry, & Davis, 1969) using a memory recognition test in which the child's task was to identify from a series of pictures those that he had previously been shown. Figure 6.1 shows that dose-response curves may be linear and curvilinear: the *reaction time curve* was linearly related to dosage level, but the *accuracy of responding curve* was greatest at 0.20 and 0.30 mg/kg of methylphenidate with a marked diminution of accuracy at 0.40 mg/kg. More recent research by Sprague and his colleagues (Sprague & Sleator, 1976, 1977; Werry & Sprague, 1974) has demonstrated that for methylphenidate optimal dosage levels differed for different target behaviors, that is, learning and behavior were differentially sensitive to dosage changes: some *cognitive* behaviors had a curvilinear relationship to dosage (e.g., optimal performance was obtained at 0.3 mg/kg, but deterioration set in with higher dosages in the 1.0 mg/kg range); but *social problem* behaviors showed a monotonic relationship with optimal performance at 1.0 mg/kg. The dilemma for the clinician lies in deciding on dosage priorities, for while cognitive performance is of major importance to classroom functioning, social behavior must also be considered. The 0.3 mg/kg dosage for cognitive tasks would be approximately 10 mg of methylphenidate per day for an average 9-year-old boy, a dosage substantially lower than that commonly used in clinical practice. This discrepancy suggests that the failure to document a stimulant drug-academic achievement gain may be simply due to many hyperactive children being overmedicated in terms of classroom performance.

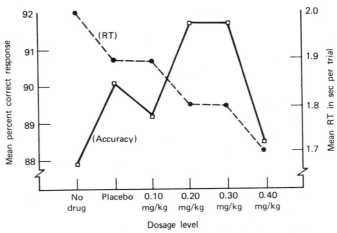

Figure 6.1 Dose-Response Curves of Methylphenidate for Speed and Accuracy of Responding. Reprinted, by permission, from Sprague, R. L., Werry, J., & Davis, K. Psychotropic drug effects on learning and activity level of children. Paper presented at the Gatlinburg Conference on Research and Theory in Mental Retardation, 1969.

Working along the same lines as Sprague and his colleagues, Swanson, Kinsbourne, Roberts, and Zucker (1978) have conducted laboratory-based time-response analyses of individual hyperactive children's response to stimulants, using paired-associate learning as the task. A particularly interesting feature of these investigations is the recording of behavior descriptions along with the learning data. Figure 6.2 shows clearly the problems the clinician faces in setting a dosage level that optimizes both cognitive performance and social behavior.

The fact that the peak effect of methylphenidate on cognitive performance occurs between one and two hours after administration with effects lasting for about four hours (Swanson et al., 1978) has caused pediatricians to conclude that only a few children can be satisfactorily maintained on a single morning dose of methylphenidate, with most children requiring a dose in the morning and again at noon. However, in a comparison of single and multiple doses of methylphenidate and dextroamphetamine, Safer and Allen (1973) found a single standardized morning dose of 20 mg of methylphenidate to be as effective for schoolday use as multiple dosage forms of dextroamphetamine. Whitehouse, Shah, and Palmer (1980) reported that a 20 mg sustained release form of methylphenidate given once daily was as effective in all respects as

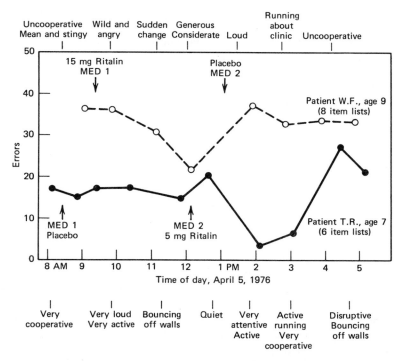

Figure 6.2 Comparison of Two Patients' Responses to Ritalin Administration. Reprinted by permission from Kinsbourne, M., & Swanson, J. J. Models of hyperactivity: Implications for diagnosis and treatment. In R. L. Trites (Ed.), *Hyperactivity in children*. Copyright 1979, University Park Press, Baltimore.

the standard form of methylphenidate, that is, 10 mg twice daily. A single dose has the advantage of an appreciable reduction in the cost of medication; more important, the child is spared the embarrassment of being singled out for medication by school personnel. That being on medication can be a source of embarrassment is illustrated by the following excerpt from the response of an 8-year-old boy to the question, What would you like most?

Just one thing, I would like to only take these medications at home where no other kids know. I am calling them medications because ever since last year when we all had to write poems about real-life things I hate the word Pill. Last year my teacher was always saying, "Did you take your pill, David?" and pretty soon the other kids started saying it and then that dumb Susan Neilson wrote her poem on me and this is the poem. I heard it a million times already:

David Hill
Did you take the pill
That makes you work
And keeps you still?
Take your pill, Hill.

And in baseball when I swing out and I almost always do the kids all yelled it. Sometimes I wish I could go to another school and start over. And once I wished that Susan Neilson would have to take pills and then she was away with some sickness and when she came back she did have to take pills and she had them in a little pink thing like my mother has powder in and all the girls thought it was cute and darling and no one ever said mean jokes about *her* taking her pill. I was real mad when everyone was just sort of interested in her pills.

Dextroamphetamine

Dextroamphetamine may be administered in tablet form or in a sustained-release capsule with a duration of action of six to 18 hours. Tablets have the advantage of allowing greater flexibility and accuracy in maintaining optimum dosage, but have two disadvantages: a precipitous drop-off effect occurs when the medication wears off, and the child is more aware of being on medication particularly if the tablets are administered by school personnel. The sustained-release capsule has a less precipitous drop-off effect, and usually only a single daily dose is required. The appropriate dosage for dextroamphetamine and the other central nervous stimulants is a matter of contention, with clinical dosages frequently being based on subjective opinion rather than empirical fact. Wender (1971) suggests a beginning dose of 5 mg of dextroamphetamine before breakfast, at lunch, and again after school if necessary, but emphasizes, as does Solomons (1973), that many hyperactive children can tolerate much higher dosages, with 20 mg per day being considered the median effective dose. Other clinicians (Gross & Wilson, 1974; Pincus & Glaser, 1966) have advocated lower doses of this drug. Dextroamphetamine has an advantage over methylphenidate in that it is more robust in the face of gastric juices, whereas methylphenidate is destroyed by gastric acidity and must be given at least 30 minutes before meals. Dextroamphetamine does not have this restriction.

Stimulants for Adolescents and Adults. There is general consensus among researchers and clinicians that hyperactive adolescents (Cantwell, 1979a; Mac-Kay, Beck, & Taylor, 1973; Safer & Allen, 1975b) as well as adults (Arnold, 1979; Mann & Greenspan, 1976; Wender, 1979; Wender, Reimherr, & Wood, 1981) can benefit markedly from stimulant medications; for some adults, imipramine has proven satisfactory. There are many similarities between the drug effects on children and those on adolescents and adults; for example, both groups experience similar direct effects as well as similar minor and major side effects, with the exception in the latter case of suppression of growth in stature. A major difference between the drug regimens of the two groups is the extreme variabilities in dosage that have been reported as effective with adolescents, and particularly with adults. In fact any summary statement of dosage with the adolescent and adult hyperactives is impossible at this time.

However, there are excellent general guidelines for drug management with adolescents (Cantwell, 1979a) and adults (Arnold, 1979) and some interesting data on adult drug responses in a report by Huessy, Cohen, Blair, and Rood (1979). The optimum drug treatment for these older hyperactives is a research area destined for marked expansion in the early 1980s.

Stimulants for Preschool Children. The foregoing therapeutic regimens refer to school-aged hyperactive children. There is increasing dissent among both clinicians and researchers concerning how early in the life cycle stimulant medications can be safely used. Some physicians do use these medications with infants and young children (Nichamin, 1972), even though their use in the preschool years has not been approved by the Food and Drug Administration. Wender (1971) considers the amphetamines to be much less effective in preschool children, and sets the trial dosage for these children at 2.5 mg twice a day. The treatment schedule used by Gross and Wilson (1974) was 2.5 mg per day up to age four. The overall weight of empirical evidence is against the use of stimulants for the preschool hyperactive child. In a comparison of the effects of methylphenidate and placebo on the psychological, motor, and cognitive test performance of preschool hyperactive children, and on ratings of them by teachers and pediatricians, Conners (1973b) concluded that the children's overt behavior showed considerably less response to drug treatment than that which typically occurs in school-age children. On a mean dosage of 11.8 mg of methylphenidate per day the side effects were minimal, with no differences between groups. Schleifer, Weiss, Cohen, Elman, Cvejic, and Kruger (1975), using individually titrated dosages, also reported methylphenidate to be relatively ineffective with the preschool child. Although it reduced the level of activity exhibited by 3- and 4-year-old children at home, there was no evidence of improvement in their nursery school behavior or psychometric test performance. Significant overall improvement, that is, improvement in behavior plus an absence of side effects or only minimal side effects, occurred in only three of the 28 children in the drug treatment condition. A mean dose of 5 mg of methylphenidate in the morning and at noon often had a negative effect on mood, resulted in solitary play and poor peer relationships, and was associated with insomnia and anorexia. Zara (1973) reported that 4-year-olds who were on medication and who had shown a positive response to it were less competent verbally in an experimental learning situation than the same-age hyperactive controls who had never been on medication. In addition, those on medication were characterized by a cognitive inflexibility not seen in the control children.

The practice of administering stimulants to young preschool children and occasionally infants is not a common one, but neither can it be described as rare. The following report (Hughes & Brewin, 1979, p. 113) by the mother of a boy who was diagnosed by a child psychiatrist as hyperactive at 11 months of age and put on methylphenidate, describes stimulant-induced side effects of a severity that pediatricians have assured us is not uncommon in very young children:

The drug seemed to calm him down but he suffered severe side effects ... one was suicidal tendencies ... he also had a loss of appetite and insomnia and he mutilated his hands and fingers. The drug made him so nervous that he kept picking on his nails and cuticles. His skin was torn to his knuckles ... (when he was five) he used to ask me for the pills in the morning, he got into such a habit. He'd say, "I feel so awful when I take them, I wish I never have to take them. I will do anything to not have to take these pills anymore."

When I stopped giving them, my son went through periods of depression, anxiety, sleeplessness. Then he would sleep all day. He wouldn't get up and get dressed. He would stay in his pajamas all day and not even wash himself. He was extremely unhappy and had pains in his stomach. Some doctors say there are no withdrawal symptoms from Ritalin.... If what my son went through is not withdrawal, I don't know what it is. It reminds me of heroin withdrawal on a milder level.

STIMULANT DRUG EFFECTS

The results of stimulant regimens can be categorized into *direct intended effects, side effects* that are unexpected and unrelated to the intended results, *interactive effects* of both a pharmacological and psychological nature, and *emanative effects*. The latter category has been suggested by Whalen and Henker (1976, 1980b), and refers to the cognitive and social results of medication and treatment programs for the hyperactive child and others in his environment. Although there is general consensus about some of the effects of stimulants, others are so controversial and researched that they merit the status of issues. Because the purpose of this section is to provide an overall picture of stimulant drug effects on hyperactive children, coverage of the controversial effects will be limited here to a brief statement of the opposing views, followed by a detailed discussion in the section on issues.

Direct Effects

Generalized Response to Stimulants

There is empirical support for a generalized overall improvement in cognitive and behavior symptoms in about two-thirds (Kinsbourne & Swanson, 1979) to three-quarters (Barkley, 1977) of the hyperactive children who are given a trial of stimulant medication. Clinicians usually set the positive response level at about 70 percent with the qualification that allowance must be made for idiosyncratic specificity, that is, the fact that many children will respond well, but not to the first stimulant or psychoactive drug administered (Knopp, Arnold, Andras, & Smeltzer, 1973; Weiss, 1975). A 2-week trial period should be allowed before deciding whether to continue with the medication or terminate it. Wender (1971) has suggested that the delayed positive response may be due to the occurrence of a metabolic change during the period between initial administration of the medication and onset of a positive response. One possible explanation offered (Wender, 1971, p. 101) for the mechanism of drug action in the delayed positive response is that of

> drug-induced production of a false neurotransmitter. The theoretical model . . . is that the chronic administration of amphetamine might result in the production of a neurohormone(s) which does not normally occur, which in turn would interfere with or react with the neurotransmitters customarily present in the particular child.

Of the group who respond favorably to stimulants, one-third to one-half experience an immediate and marked positive response that Fish (1971) has described as so dramatic and rapid that only a short trial is needed to confirm the efficacy of the drug. The remainder of this group experience a moderate response. The foregoing categories of positive and moderate improvement refer to a generalized, overall improvement in cognitive and behavioral symptoms. The possibility that the response to stimulant medication may be hierarchical in nature has been suggested by Porges, Walter, Korb, and Sprague (1975, p. 732):

> . . . although attention and behavioral hyperactivity may be influenced by methylphenidate the response affected may be a function of the individual's deficit. . . . Influences on attentional behavior may precede influences on social behavior; or, if attention is adequate, social behavior may be influenced.

A neutral response with no reaction other than minimal side effects occurs in some children, whereas in others three kinds of negative responses occur: The symptoms are exacerbated, and this effect does not diminish with increased or reduced dosage but disappears gradually over a 48-hour period when the medication is discontinued; or the child becomes withdrawn and silent with a marked deterioration in his social relations, or he develops an acute psychotic reaction, which generally disappears with the withdrawal of medication. Occasionally a child exhibits immediate and dramatic improvement only to develop a rapid tolerance, a phenomenon called tachyplaxis. In this condition the child responds only temporarily to increased dosage and usually must be withdrawn from medication, although sometimes a different medication proves satisfactory (Gross & Wilson, 1974).

Specific Short-Term Effects

The evidence from studies regarded as methodologically sound is that the stimulants have the most consistent positive effects on the cluster of cognitive and social behaviors perceived by parents and teachers as disruptive, impulsive, and socially inappropriate. There is no firm evidence, however, that stimulants improve performance on intelligence and achievement tests (Barkley,

1977; Rie, Rie, Stewart, & Ambuel, 1976a, 1976b); this latter topic is a matter of dispute and will be discussed in the Issues section. There is general improvement in the ability to self-regulate behavior in accord with a variety of situational demands, particularly in structured and semistructured settings (Barkley, 1977; Conners & Werry, 1979; Gittelman-Klein & Klein, 1975). There is also improvement in the quality of social interactions with parents (Barkley & Cunningham, 1979; Humphries, Kinsbourne, & Swanson, 1978), and teachers and peers (Collins, Whalen, & Henker, 1980; Henker & Whalen, 1980b). Although there is a calmness about the hyperactive child that is often interpreted as a decreased activity level effect, particularly in structured situations, the increased calm may be, as Henker and Whalen (1980a, p. 324) suggest, "a side effect of enhanced focal attention; when the ongoing situationally appropriate task consumes a child's attention, atypical motoric patterns, impulsive acts, and disruptive manoeuvers may diminish naturally." There is consistent evidence, particularly from the McGill studies, of increased ability to focus and sustain attention, respond promptly and accurately, and inhibit impulsive and extraneous responses (Douglas, 1972, 1974, 1980; Humphries, Swanson, Kinsbourne, & Yiu, 1980); and also evidence of marked improvements in learning, particularly associative learning, and memory (Barkley, 1977; Cantwell & Carlson, 1978; Werry & Aman, 1975; Werry & Sprague, 1974). Comprehensive reviews of the short-term effects of stimulants on a wide variety of specific tasks are contained in Barkley (1977), Cantwell and Carlson (1978), and Conners and Werry (1979). There is no firm evidence for *long-term* gains in academic, cognitive, social, or other psychological functioning with stimulants (Barkley, 1977; Cantwell & Carlson, 1978; Whalen & Henker, 1980a).

Side Effects

Side effects are actions or effects of drugs other than those intended. They can be categorized in terms of *desirability* as positive or negative, with some of the negative effects being of a severity that justifies discontinuation of the medication; and in terms of *duration*, as short-term or long-term. The potential side effects of the stimulants listed in the *Physician's Desk Reference* are numerous and may occur in almost every part of the body. However, the small number of published reports of significant side effects suggests that these effects are relatively uncommon (Cantwell & Carlson, 1978). Side effects do not occur in all children. When they do occur, they generally increase proportionately with an increase in dosage (Cantwell & Carlson, 1978).

Short-Term Mild Side Effects

The most frequent short-term side effects of the stimulants are anorexia and insomnia, both of which are usually of short duration and occur more frequently with the amphetamines than with methylphenidate. A common side effect that is particularly distressing to parents is the "amphetamine look," a sunken-cheeked, sallow, dark shadows under the eyes look that Solomons (1971) calls the "panda effect." Although it is not considered to be of any physiological importance, it may do some psychological harm as evidenced by the following statement from a six-year-old boy with a marked amphetamine look:

> I would like not to take those pills. I do not think those pills are good. Ladies say to my mom, "Why is he so *pale*? Doesn't he get enough sleep?" and my mom hates that and she says,"He's on medication," and they all look like I'm a new animal in the zoo and then real quick they start talking about some other things but they all keep looking at me in a real funny way and I don't feel good when they do.

Other short-term side effects of the stimulants that are less often reported include sadness, depression, fearfulness, social withdrawal, sleepiness, headaches, nail biting, stomach upset, and weight loss. It should be noted that weight loss often seems to be unrelated to appetite, since slowing of weight growth has been reported when no anorexia was present (Gross & Wilson, 1974; Safer & Allen, 1973).

The few empirical investigations that have been conducted on the sleep effects of stimulants all suggest that these drugs have little effect other than insomnia. In an investigation of the effects of stimulants on rapid eye movement (REM) in children, Feinberg, Hibi, Braun, Cavness, Westerman, and Small (1974) reported that dosages of amphetamine sufficient to produce clinical improvement did not substantially reduce the percentage of REM in spite of some increase in the amount of sleep preceding the first REM period (REM latency). Nor was there any elevation (REM rebound) in the percentage of REM on withdrawal of the drug even though REM onset occurred earlier. Furthermore, research by Haig, Schroeder, and Schroeder (1974) has shown that methylphenidate has little effect on the quality of sleep, even with large dosages and with administration close to bedtime. Sleep latency and REM latency were the only measures affected, and both were well below the levels indicative of sleep pathology.

Often the stimulant medications are given only in the morning and afternoon, the rationale for this procedure being that this dosage schedule will prevent sleep disturbances, particularly insomnia. Kinsbourne (1973) has questioned this procedure on the grounds that insomnia is not a stimulant effect but is a stimulant withdrawal effect. His argument is that by evening the medication effects have long since worn off, the child has returned to his hyperactive base state, and because of the rebound accentuation of his hyperactivity may be in a worse state than before medication, particularly if he is on amphetamines, which have a more marked rebound effect than methylphenidate. Kinsbourne reasons that the child should therefore find it easier to go to sleep if given a stimulant late enough in the day so that its period of effect overlaps bedtime; if he awakens during the night, giving him a stimulant should help him to go back to sleep.

Short-Term Severe Side Effects

It is generally believed that neither the amphetamines nor methylphenidate is characterized by a high incidence of immediate severe side effects. Evidence of the low incidence of such effects comes from a long-term study of minimal brain dysfunction in 1056 children in which the mean duration of contact was 30 months (Gross & Wilson, 1974). Only four instances of side effects severe enough to warrant discontinuation of the medication occurred in the children treated with methylphenidate ($n=377$), and only 16 instances in those treated with dextroamphetamine ($n=371$). However, there has been an increasing number of reports in the literature of problems such as drug-associated psychosis (Ney, 1967), hallucinosis (Lucas & Weiss, 1971), and grand mal seizure (Chamberlain, 1974). Greenberg, McMahon, and Deem (1974) have described significant personality deterioration in five of 26 children treated with relatively low dosages of dextroamphetamine. Although the symptoms subsided with discontinuation of the drug, the cases presented emphasize the need for careful observation for such reactions.

A serious although rare side effect of the three stimulants, dextroamphetamine, methylphenidate, and pemoline, and one tricyclic antidepressant, imipramine, is the possibility of the development of Gilles de la Tourette syndrome or the exacerbation of an existing case. Of the three stimulants, methylphenidate is the one most frequently associated with this complication. In some cases tics occur, but the child does not develop the classic Tourette syndrome. In other cases a full-blown Tourette syndrome develops (Bremness & Sverd, 1979; Sleator, 1980) with multiple vocal tics, such as repetitious throat clearing, coughing, snorting, sudden screams, and other similar noises, and motor tics. The latter group start with eye blinking and progress to a variety of quick involuntary movement. Repetitious, involuntary utterances of obscene words occurs, but is not invariably present (Shapiro, Shapiro, Bruun, and Sweet, 1978). Sometimes there is a family history, but in many cases of methylphenidate-induced Tourette syndrome there is no reported personal or family history of tics. Symptoms sometimes disappear with the discontinuation of methylphenidate, but sometimes other treatment, such as haloperidol therapy, may be required (Golden, 1977). There is some dissent as to whether the stimulants, particularly methylphenidate, cause Tourette syndrome (Bremness & Sverd, 1979; Golden, 1977; Shapiro et al., 1978). Nonetheless, pediatricians who prescribe stimulants should be aware that if there is a history of tics in patients and their families, the use of stimulants may precipitate or heighten this disorder.

Long-Term Side Effects

The outcomes of concern here are growth suppression, drug use and abuse, cardiovascular effects, and blood dyscrasias. The first three are controversial issues, with the weight of the data leaning towards a temporary suppression of growth in weight and height, no firm evidence of increased potential for drug abuse, and no immediate cause for concern regarding cardiovascular effects. The research on these topics will be discussed in the section on issues. The remaining possibility, that of stimulant-induced blood dyscrasias, remains unresolved. In 1971 Wender noted that there were no reports of blood dyscrasias occurring as a function of long-term amphetamine administration. However, a case-control study (Newell & Henderson, 1973) did demonstrate a possible link between Hodgkin's disease and the use of amphetamines. When the responses to an interview questionnaire of 100 patients with existing diagnosed Hodgkin's disease were compared with those of an equal number of controls matched for age, sex, race, and socioeconomic status, 19 of the 100 Hodgkin's disease patients had taken amphetamines for at least two months within two years of the onset of their Hodgkin's disease, as compared to three among the 100 controls (relative risk = 6.33, $p<.01$). Newell and Henderson emphasize that this finding is a preliminary one and must be replicated; nevertheless, the possibility of such a link suggests the need for investigations of bone-marrow changes, and particularly the importance of long-term follow-up studies. Another possibility is that the link is not between Hodgkin's disease and the amphetamines, but rather between Hodgkin's and the relative social isolation often associated with hyperactivity that in turn tends to decrease early exposure to infectious agents (Gutensohn & Cole, 1981). Recent research points to childhood as the period in which the risk of development of Hodgkin's disease is to a large extent established, with increased risk being associated with a number of social factors, one of which is relative social isolation and consequent protection from infectious disease exposure in early childhood. Although the excess risk associated with this social isolation-exposure factor is small, it merits consideration.

Interaction Effects

Pharmacological Interaction Effects

Drug interaction occurs when one pharmacologic agent alters the therapeutic or toxic effects of another pharmacologic agent. The action of certain classes of drugs seems to be affected by the concurrent administration of stimulants. Methylphenidate, for example, increases the blood levels of tricyclic antidepressants, which are sometimes used concurrently with the stimulants and thus may potentiate their clinical effect (Cantwell & Carlson, 1978); and one antipsychotic, thioridazine, is reported to enhance the effect of methylphenidate in hyperactive children (Gittelman-Klein, Klein, Abikoff, Katz, Gloisten, & Kates, 1976). Fischer and Wilson (1971) have cautioned that methylphenidate inhibits certain drug-metabolizing enzymes of the liver, thus causing a prolongation of the half-life of such drugs as phenobarbital, dilantin, mysoline, and imipramine, all of which may be used concurrently with the stimulants; as a result, therapeutic doses of these drugs can be elevated to toxic level. The possibility of morbidity from such a combination is high, according to Fischer and Wilson (1971), who note that there have been several reports of ataxia in patients who were simultaneously being treated with dilantin and methylphenidate. Interaction effects between the stimulants and nonprescription medication have also been reported. Huestis and Arnold (1974) described a case of possible antagonism of amphetamine, as a result of the concurrent ingestion of a decongestant-antihistamine compound, in which a hyperactive boy with no known allergy manifested an excellent response to levoamphetamine except when he took cold capsules; during these periods the amphetamine was ineffective. As soon as the cold capsules were discontinued the boy returned to his previous level of improved behavior. Taken together, the findings on short-term, long-term, and interaction side effects suggest that the practice of allowing children to continue on stimulant medication unmonitored for long periods is negligent and potentially dangerous.

Psychological Interaction Effects

There is general consensus in the medical domain that the outcome of intervention may be enhanced by a favorable patient-treatment match in conditions that allow such treatment options. Although it has not been stated in these explicit terms physicians generally agree that patients who are high on personal causality, that is, take responsibility for outcomes, function better on self-regulatory treatment, whereas for those low on this dimension an externally supervised treatment regimen is indicated. In the first research on this subject variable with hyperactive children Bugental, Whalen, and Henker (1977) studied the interaction between children's causal attribution systems (degree of personal responsibility for school success or failure) and two different intervention procedures: self-control training or social reinforcement for task attention. Congruence in the attribution-intervention match was associated with better outcome than noncongruence, the congruent combinations being high personal causality and self-control training, and low personal causality and social reinforcement. Although this study was limited in scope and findings, it points to the potential importance of the effect of the causal attribution system of the hyperactive child on his subsequent response to treatment. One potentially valuable direction for research would be to compare the maintenance of stimulant-improved behaviors *after drug withdrawal,* for example, in drug holidays, in two groups of hyperactive children—those who attribute their improved behavior solely to the drug and those who partially or totally attribute stimulant-induced changes to themselves. For an interesting critique on research on this topic with nonclinical adult subjects see Grimm (1980).

Emanative Effects

Whalen and Henker (1976, 1980b) define emanative effects as the sociocognitive sequelae of drug intervention for the child who knows he is on drugs and for important individuals in his social environments who are also aware of this fact. The existence of emanative effects is consistent with an interactionist viewpoint. The effects include such variables as the message that the medication has for the child and others, and the possibility of a shift from self-to drug-reliance as a function of the efficacy and duration of drug treatment. Examples of this latter phenomenon are contained in an intriguing discussion (Whalen & Henker, 1980b, pp. 26–36) of self-perceived competence and drug dependence within the context of recent research and verbatim comments from hyperactive children. Emanative effects have pervasive consequences, with immediate as well as long-term impact. They relate to a wide range of behaviors and beliefs, such as how the child explains being on medication to himself and others, the effect of medication on his self-perceptions and causal attributions, and how others' perceptions are altered by their knowledge that the child is on drugs.

A common sequence in the life of the unmedicated child is frustration by peers → uncontrollable crying and upset → embarrassment and discomfort. When the child is put on medication, he frequently is assured that such behaviors will no longer be a problem, and consequently he is perplexed and confused when he experiences the side effect feelings of sadness, depression, and irritability despite his dramatically improved behavior and concomitant positive social reinforcement. In this situation one major emanative effect is likely to be bewilderment, as the child's psychological world is thrown into disarray by events that are dissonant with his expectations and beliefs. Similarly, many hyperactive children view peer rejection as exclusively hyperactivity-related, and are troubled when the sharp reduction in hyperactive behavior is not immediately accompanied by peer acceptance. To avoid or at least minimize the problems of ascribing positive outcomes solely to medication and ignoring the contributory role of developing new competencies, Whalen and Henker (1980b, pp. 31–32) suggest that a self-instructional training program designed to increase the child's capacity for self-control and improve his perception of personal causation should precede the onset of the stimulant regimen. These emanative effects could be further decreased by giving the child a simple, accurate, and specific explanation of what can and cannot be expected from stimulants.

In Whalen and Henker's (1980b) approach to the treatment of the hyperactive child whose intervention program includes a drug regimen, emanative effects are considered to be an integral part of the treatment program. These effects have the potential to interfere with the child's progress, and therefore the pediatrician must assume responsibility for identifying them and then periodically assessing their effects on the child and his significant others. The complexity of this task is considerable; there is no question, in this treatment framework, that it is essential.

In our approach to drug treatment of the hyperactive child we have consistently advocated, as a general principle, that only the parents and pediatrician know that the child is to be put on drugs; that the child, his siblings, relatives, peers, teachers, neighbors, and all others not be told of this aspect of his treatment. This controversial opinion is discussed at length in Chapter 10, but it is relevant here because the problem of emanative effects would be largely nonexistent if this principle were adhered to. Under the circumstances that we advocate, the parents would be the only source of such effects, and the fact that they had decided on not telling their child that he was to be on medication would suggest that their behavior would likely be consonant with this decision and reflect their concern for the child's well-being. Feasibility is not a major problem: we know of six cases in which it has been accomplished for two or more years, with substantial parental effort but no apparent cost to the children, who have been spared labeling by teachers, teasing by peers about medication, and the all too common fear that their effective functioning might be pill-dependent. Those who argue that keeping such information from the child is dishonest would do well to consider that the basic tenet of medicine, *primum non nocere*, is as relevant to the behavior disorders as it is to medical diseases. A curious dichotomy of values is suggested when no censure is attached to the withholding of information in the interest of a patient's well-being, yet withholding information contributing to the cluster of difficulties associated with emanative effects would be condemned as dishonest.

Of the stimulant drug effects the emanative effects (Whalen & Henker, 1976, 1980b) have great immediate potential for psychological damage to the hyperactive child. Because few pediatricians are in agreement with us on our principle of drug intervention, which requires that only the parents and pediatrician know that the child is on drugs, the large majority of hyperactive children on medication may experience some emanative effects. Under these circumstances, one profitable line of research would involve devising procedures to minimize these effects.

From all accounts, for example, the hyperactive child known to be on drugs is frequently subjected to merciless teasing (e.g., Cantwell, 1979; Collins, Whalen, & Henker, 1980; Robin & Bosco, 1980; Ross & Ross, 1976), and yet there is no suggestion in guidelines for treatment that the child could be taught to cope with this source of misery. In the past five years we have developed highly individualized training programs for children of normal intelligence, the mentally retarded, and one hyperactive boy, for all of whom being teased was a major problem. In each case the child was interviewed, and the specific kinds of teasing were identified and then incorporated into a training program in which the child was taught how to cope, that is, what to do and say when teased. Emphasis was on general principles (for example, the teaser is essentially a bully, and if the child stands up to him instead of running away or crying, the teaser will back down and look for a new target) and specific behaviors such as letting the teaser known who is in charge (for example, when other children tease you, don't try to make them stop. Instead keep asking them to repeat it; when they finally refuse to continue, tell them how many times they have said it and that you want them to say it more times after lunch). The programs were spectacularly successful. Teasing in all cases came to an abrupt halt; in several cases children used their own program to help their friends cope with teasing; and the programs were used with two primary classes. The most interesting outcome was the brevity of use of the coping techniques. In a large number of cases, once the child knew how to cope with teasing, the teasing stopped *before* the child could put the program into action. Teachers and parents, in attempting to account for this phenomenon, commented that "he had a whole different demeanor the first day he was going to do it." " she seemed to have a confidence that she never had before," "the very day she was going to really use the program the other girls stopped teasing her," and "the other boy teased him but he defused him in one day and he never had any more trouble." As these comments indicate, this approach to handling the teasing problem also served to bolster the children's self-confidence and self-esteem. Other problems attributable to emanative effects would lend themselves to this approach.

ISSUES RELATED TO STIMULANT TREATMENT

Issue: Drugs Are Dangerous or Undesirable

All drugs are potentially dangerous. In the early 1970s the stimulants were often condemned as such (Werry, 1977), but this blanket charge usually failed to make the necessary distinction between the dangers of misuse and the dangers associated with acceptable therapeutic practice. The potential for the misuse of the stimulants in the treatment of hyperactivity is considerable, with physicians, parents, and school personnel all sharing in responsibility for such misuse. The hyperactive child is defenseless in this situation unless at least one of these decision makers takes a firm, critical, and resistant stand against automatic and blanket administration of the stimulants as the sole form of intervention. Physicians generally do not adhere to the guidelines for the use of stimulants. For example, the use of drug response as a diagnostic method is totally outdated yet quite widespread. At one private clinic in California children who are referred for "school problems" are routinely prescribed a trial dose of stimulant medication *before* they come to the clinic, the rationale being that "it saves time for everybody" if the pediatrician knows if the child is hyperactive before he first sees him. Careful monitoring and follow-up of the

hyperactive child on stimulants is the exception (Solomons, 1973). Many physicians allow parents to juggle dosage at their own discretion and often base
repeated increments on parental reports alone, despite the notably unreliable
nature of such reports (Sleator & von Neumann, 1974). The dangers associated with misuse clearly call for action but do not justify the abolition of stimulant therapy. As Werry (1977, p. 463) has noted:

> While it is indisputably true that some doctors do, and always will, misprescribe
> or overprescribe psychotropic drugs in children, this is no more an argument
> against such treatment when properly indicated and supervised than it is against
> any useful yet overprescribed treatment such as penicillin or Vitamin B12.

Parental contribution to drug misuse is formidable. Parents often pressure pediatricians to prescribe "the drug solution," and once the child is progressing
satisfactorily on drugs, typically show little interest in forms of intervention
that require effort on their part (Schaefer, Palkes, & Stewart, 1974). The third
facet of the misuse problem concerns coercion by school personnel in initiating intervention. The Office of Child Development report (1971, p. 27) stated:

> Under no circumstances should any attempt be made to coerce parents to accept
> any particular treatment. . . . It is proper for school personnel to inform parents
> of a child's behavior problems, but members of the school staff should not di-
> rectly diagnose the hyperkinetic disturbance or prescribe treatment.

Yet many parents are directly or indirectly coerced into accepting a period of
trial medication for their children (Grinspoon & Singer, 1973; Stewart &
Olds, 1973). Parents often receive ultimatums from the school authorities that
countermand the recommendations of the child's pediatrician. One California
mother, for example, was pressured for four years to put her son on medication, even though two pediatricians supported her antimedication stand
(Hunsinger, 1970). Another mother reported that every parent with a child
believed to be hyperactive was referred to the same pediatrician "because that
doctor knows what the school wants" (Grinspoon & Singer, 1973, p. 518). An
elementary school teacher pointed out three active 8-year-old boys in her class
in September to one of the authors and said, "I'll have those three on medication by Thanksgiving or they won't be in this class." In November all three
boys were on medication. When asked how she had accomplished it, she re-
plied smugly that "it took a bit of pressure."
    Two other aspects of the misuse problem warrant a brief mention. Expe-
rienced investigators (Arnold, 1979) have expressed concern that drug addicts
may seize the opportunity to pose as hyperactive and obtain amphetamines
more easily and inexpensively than would otherwise be possible. Doctors now
recognize that hyperactivity may continue into adulthood, and some are only
too willing to abdicate responsibility for careful validation of the patient's
complaint. This form of misuse is a distinct possibility, and although on an

infinitely smaller scale, it has its parallel in the wholesale prescription of Valium. The other form that misuse may take evolves from the fact that many hyperactive children have freedom of access to their medication, with some adjusting their own dosage. For classmates, the medication-induced change in behavior in the hyperactive child is both astonishing and enticing. Nonhyperactive children sometimes plead for "those pills that make you get better grades." It is a short step from this point to that of the hyperactive child selling his pills, an all too common happening at the elementary school level (Schrag & Divoky, 1975).

The charges associated with the acceptable medical use of drugs center around the possibility of illicit drug use and abuse as a result of stimulant therapy, stimulant-induced suppression of growth, and effects on cardiovascular functioning.

Drug Abuse

Throughout the 1970s there was an increasing expression of concern in the pediatric domain of parents, educators, clinicians, and researchers that treatment with stimulants or other medication may predispose the hyperactive child to alcoholism and/or drug abuse. This concern is a rational one in view of a conglomeration of related facts. Habituation to almost any drug as well as to the use of drugs is a frequent occurrence. Many adolescents and young adults take stimulants for the euphoric reaction. Goyer, Davis, and Rapoport (1979), for example, described the case of a hyperactive child who was prescribed methylphenidate in Grade Six and two years later was reported to be ingesting pills far in excess of the prescribed rate in order to get "higher." For many hyperactive adolescents stimulants in childhood were the first good thing that had happened to them and they were rewarded explicitly and implicitly for taking drugs (Collins, Whalen, & Henker, 1980; Whalen & Henker, 1980b). The hyperactive adolescent is characterized by low self-esteem, poor school functioning, and a strong desire to be one of the peer group, all of which make him a likely candidate for possible drug abuse. In this sense he could be viewed as at risk for drug abuse (Jessor & Jessor, 1977; Kandel, 1978; Loney, 1980c). Strongly contradicting the likelihood of drug misuse have been the reports of Beck, Langford, MacKay, and Sum (1975) and Collins et al. (1980) that the stigma associated with being on stimulants was so strong that many hyperactive children said that they never wanted to see another drug. Before considering the contribution that empirical investigations have made to this issue, it should be noted that speculation about a possible association between hyperactivity and drug abuse is limited to that group of hyperactive children who are not aggressive. It is already an established fact that aggression and delinquent behavior are precursors of both alcohol and drug use (Kandel, 1978; Robins, 1966) and hyperactive children who overlap these categories join these high risk groups.

Much of the research is methodologically inadequate, limited, or invalid. Many of the retrospective studies also depend on a retrospective diagnosis of hyperactivity, a behavior disorder that was not formally recognized at the time in question (e.g., Cantwell, 1972; Tarter, McBride, Buonpane, & Schneider, 1977). Often the essential distinction between drug or alcohol use and abuse is omitted (Morrison, 1980a; Offord, Sullivan, & Abrams, 1979). Inadequate subject selection is another problem. Many studies involve specialized samples of hyperactive subjects, such as psychiatric patients (Morrison, 1980a) and adoptees (Goodwin, Schulsinger, Hermansen, Guze, & Winokur, 1975), which limits the generality of the data, and preselect nonhyperactive controls who are problem free and therefore also not representative of nonhyperactive groups in general (Ackerman, Dykman, & Peters, 1977; Weiss, Hechtman, Perlman, Hopkins, & Wener, 1979). Some studies use subjects who are too young to have had opportunities for a representative amount of experience with drugs and alcohol (Blouin, Bornstein, & Trites, 1978). Other studies omit the use of control groups and also fail to provide normative data (Laufer, 1971; Mendelson, Johnson, & Stewart, 1971; Satterfield, Satterfield, & Cantwell, 1980). Usually no attempt is made to separate out the hyperactive-aggressive subjects from the hyperactive-nonaggressive ones, so that when a link is reported between hyperactivity and drug and alcohol use, it is impossible to isolate the contribution made by the aggression variable from that of the hyperactivity variable (Kandel, 1978; Loney, 1980c; Loney, Kramer, & Milich, 1981; Robins, 1966).

Information from a small group of the more adequate studies suggests that hyperactive adolescents and young adults are not particularly more prone to engage in drug and alcohol use than their nonhyperactive counterparts, and when trends do occur they generally are in the direction of increased use of alcohol (Kramer & Loney, 1981). Two studies from the longitudinal research series of Weiss and her associates (Hechtman, Weiss, & Perlman, 1979; Weiss, Hechtman, Perlman, Hopkins, & Wener, 1979) suggest that hyperactive adolescents and young adults do not differ from their nonhyperactive peers in either alcohol or drug use. There was some evidence that hyperactive adolescents were more likely to engage in long-term use of nonmedical drugs, immoderate use of alcohol, and use of marijuana and hallucinogens, whereas the nonhyperactive controls began using alcohol earlier and, in one study (Weiss et al., 1979), were more often using hallucinogens. These minimal differences were of interest because the research design enhanced the possibility that differences would be obtained: the controls were selected to exclude behavior and learning problems and so represented a more rarified group. The significance of these minimal differences, however, is limited by the fact that the most frequently prescribed drug for the hyperactive group was a nonstimulant, chlorpromazine. Henker, Whalen, Bugental, and Barker (1981) also found no differences when they compared a small group of hyperactive junior high school students, who had been treated with methylphenidate, with a large group of nondrug-treated classmates. The responses to anonymous group questionnaires showed that the drug-treated group did not differ from their peer controls in frequency of use of common, primarily nonprescription medicine, alcohol, or illicit drugs such as cocaine, heroin, and the hallucinogens. The notable features in this study were the validity and reliability checks: the names of two nonexistent drugs were inserted in the questionnaires with only two subjects claiming to have used these substances, and 21 subjects were interviewed, with no systematic differences between their interviews and questionnaire data. However, essential descriptive data were omitted: no evidence was provided that the groups were equal on IQ, socioeconomic status, and other demographic variables; and no information was provided concerning the severity of hyperactivity.

In an anterospective interview and anonymous questionnaire study of adolescents who had been diagnosed as hyperactive and treated with methylphenidate, Gadow and Sprague (1980) found only occasional and minimal differences between the hyperactive group and nonhyperactive controls: more of the hyperactive subjects expressed a preference for marijuana and had tried cigarettes, whereas more of the nonhyperactive controls preferred alcohol, but the two groups did not differ in their use of drugs and alcohol. There was some evidence that the groups were also comparable on availability of drugs and alcohol and attitudes toward them. Similar findings have been reported by Kramer and Loney (1980) who have pointed out that the subjects in their study, as well as those of Gadow and Sprague (1980) and Henker et al. (1981), were not far into the drug experimentation period. Further evidence against a stimulant treatment-substance use link comes from examinations by Kramer and Loney (1981) of data concerning use of stimulants for hyperactivity, amount of use, and response to stimulants. Neither use of medication nor duration of treatment was associated with subsequent drug use in hyperactive adolescents, in fact, there was some suggestion that a positive response to methylphenidate was associated with a lower probability of drug (Loney, Kramer, & Milich, 1981) and alcohol use (Blouin et al., 1978).

Although research on a possible stimulant-substance use link is riddled with methodological weaknesses and other difficulties, it appears that at the moment there is no reason for concern about an increased probability of later drug abuse in hyperactive children on stimulant medications. In the absence of definitive data, an attitude of vigilance should be maintained and long-term follow-ups with impeccable methodology conducted.

Growth Suppression

Prior to 1970 it was known that the initial period of stimulant drug usage was associated with a transient weight loss that appeared to be secondary to central appetite suppression, but it was assumed that tolerance to the drug-induced effect on weight developed over a period of several months and that the long-term use of stimulant drugs had no lasting effect on growth. In the early 1970s this complacency was shattered by Safer and his associates (Safer &

Allen, 1973; Safer, Allen, & Barr, 1972), who reported significant growth retardation in height and weight in children whose periods on stimulant regimens averaged three years. The effects were even more pronounced for dextroamphetamine; for methylphenidate there were no growth suppression effects in children whose daily dose did not exceed 20 mg. Concern in the medical community about the possible stimulant drug-growth suppression link was reflected in an editorial in which Eisenberg (1972) urged that no hyperactive child be given stimulants without an accompanying careful monitoring of growth. In a continuation of their initial research, Safer, Allen, and Barr (1975) next reported that hyperactive children whose medication was terminated at the beginning of summer subsequently grew in height and weight at a significantly greater rate than those whose medication was continued throughout the summer months. The growth rebounds associated with a discontinuation of medication ranged from 15 to 68 percent above the age-expected increment, with greater gains following discontinuance of amphetamine treatment than methylphenidate treatment, and the rebounds were generally proportional to the degree of growth suppression. These more reassuring findings did little to quell either public or professional concern, and the reaction to the Safer et al. studies was an outpouring of conflicting findings in the form of prospective and retrospective studies, reports at professional meetings, and clinical reports, as well as observations supporting the greater negative effects of the amphetamines as compared to methylphenidate (Beck, Langford, MacKay, & Sum, 1975; Gross, 1976; Gross & Wilson, 1974; McNutt, Ballard, Boileau, Sprague, & von Neumann, 1976; McNutt, Boileau, & Cohen, 1977; Quinn & Rapoport, 1975; Rie et al., 1976a; Sachar, 1977; Weiss, Kruger, Danielson, & Elman, 1975). Sprague (1977) has criticized the methodology of the Safer team and asserted that there is no evidence of growth suppression with standardized procudures. Cohen (1975) has pointed out the errors implicit in the utilization of data that are age dependent, that is, basing the judgment concerning limited versus optimal growth on chronological age, when in fact, as Oettinger (1975) has reported, the children studied could easily vary markedly in the common indices of physiological age.

A recent review of the growth suppression issue by the Pediatric Advisory Subcommittee of the Food and Drug Administration (Roche, Lipman, Overall, & Hung, 1979) noted a wide range of methodological rigor in the research and clinical reports surveyed. Measures of growth in some studies (e.g., Safer & Allen, 1973; Safer et al., 1972) were obtained from yearly or semiannual school chart records, a data source of high potential for inaccuracy in view of the fact that many schools have upper-level students measure and record heights and weights for the younger children. In other studies, notably those of the Illinois group (McNutt et al., 1976, 1977) the measurement procedures were meticulous. In the Illinois studies each child was assigned a pair of shorts for the duration of the study; the measurement procedure included removing objects from the shorts' pockets, and taking posturination multiple readings on an extremely sensitive scale until two readings within 25 grams of each other were obtained. With height, efforts were made to control for the amount of hair on the head and the angle of the measuring rod touching the head; a stadiometer was used to control for variance in how hard the child pushed his head, buttocks, and heels against the wall (Sprague, 1978, p. 199).

Roche et al. (1979) found that the methods of estimating possible growth suppression also varied in rigor. For comparison purposes some investigators used matched, untreated normal controls or untreated hyperactive controls, but without random assignment. Some (e.g., Gross, 1976) used percentile growth norms such as the Iowa City Norms (Nelson, 1950), which are based on data collected 40 years ago from relatively small groups; others (e.g., Puig-Antich, Greenhill, Sassin, & Sachar, 1978) used the British growth velocity charts (Tanner, Whitehouse, & Takaishi, 1966), although the rates of growth of British children in certain age periods differ from those of American children (Roche et al., 1980). Many of the studies surveyed failed to provide adequate information regarding drug dosages, duration of treatment, or age and other relevant subject information. The most methodologically sophisticated study in the growth suppression literature (Kalachnik, Sprague, Sleator, Cohen, & Ullman, 1981) studied the growth suppression effects of methylphenidate in children under 13. Their subjects (all of whom were boys except for two girls) were 26 hyperactive children receiving methylphenidate, eight hyperactive nonmedicated children, and 25 nonmedicated normal controls. The Roche-Wainer-Thissen Adult Stature Prediction Formula (1975) was used to predict adult stature prior to methylphenidate treatment and again after each of the three years of treatment. Dosage variables analyzed were total mg per day, mg/kg/day, and duration of treatment. No significant differences were found between the medicated hyperactive children and the other two groups on any of the growth variables. The investigators concluded that growth (stature) suppression does not occur in boys under 13 years of age with methylphenidate doses of up to 0.8 mg/kg/day for one or two years, and up to 0.6 mg/kg/day for three years.

Roche et al. (1979, p. 849) concluded that despite methodological weaknesses in many of the studies and reports on growth suppression, taken together, the studies provide reasonable evidence that stimulant medications, particularly at high-normal dosage levels, result in a moderate suppression of growth in weight. The evidence for a concurrent minor suppression of growth in stature is less certain, and there is no evidence as yet that early growth suppression continues to be evident in adulthood, although for this latter point what evidence there is is based only on small groups. It is important to remember that the Roche et al. conclusions are based on preadolescent studies. The effects of stimulants on adolescent growth have only recently been documented (Hechtman, Weiss, & Perlman, 1978; Loney et al., 1981), with the data pointing toward a significant relationship between stimulant dosage and final height. The effects of stimulants on fetal development in the young pregnant adolescent on stimulant therapy are a matter of conjecture. There is, however, increasing interest in the research domain in the accuracy of the measurement and prediction of growth in stature and weight (e.g., Kalachnik et al., 1981; Loney, Whaley-Klahn, Ponto, & Adney, 1981) as well as in the mechanisms that alone or in combination could lead to growth retardation. These include decreased food intake resulting from the anorexic drug effect, hypothalamic-pituitary inhibition of growth hormone secretion, diminished production of somatomedin, and direct inhibition by stimulants of cartilage and bone development in the growing child (e.g., Aarskog, Fevang, Kløve, Støa, & Thorsen, 1977; Dickinson, Lee, Ringdahl, Schedewie, Kilgore, & Elders, 1979; Greenhill, Puig-Antich, Sassin, & Sachar, 1977).

Cardiovascular Effects

Small but significant increments in systolic and diastolic blood pressure and/or pulse rate with the amphetamines and methylphenidate have been reported in most studies of cardiovascular functioning (Arnold, Wender, McCloskey, & Snyder, 1972; Epstein, Lasagna, Conners, & Rodriguez, 1968; Knights & Hinton, 1969; Rie et al., 1976a, 1976b), the two exceptions being the studies of Bradley (1950) with d-amphetamine and Conners, Taylor, Meo, Kurtz, and Fournier (1972) with d-amphetamine and pemoline. The causal relationship between doses of methylphenidate (20 mg) and increased heart rate (10 to 15 beats per minute) has focused attention on the question of whether tolerance develops to these methylphenidate-induced heart-rate increases. Allen and Safer (1979) have reported that tolerance does develop within two to five months after beginning medication, and these results have confirmed those of Weiss, Kruger, Danielson, and Elman (1975). No electrocardiogram abnormalities have been noted in relation to long-term methylphenidate therapy (Rapoport, Quinn, Bradbard, Riddle, & Brooks, 1974; Weiss et al., 1975), and no changes in basal cardiac function while off medication have been reported for hyperactive children on methylphenidate therapy (Safer & Allen, 1975b; Weiss et al., 1975). However, mild, consistent resting and exercise heart rate and blood pressure increases following long-term methylphenidate therapy have been documented in the best controlled studies (Ballard, Boileau, Sleator, Massey, and Sprague, 1976; Boileau, Ballard, Sprague, Sleator, and Massey, 1976), which suggests that further research into the heart rate response to methylphenidate must be conducted before these cardiovascular effects can be regarded as transitory effects of little significance.

Now that stimulant drug intervention is being used through adolescence and into early adulthood, it should soon be possible to study the long-term effects of the reported heart rate and blood pressure increases and to determine the extent to which these increases persist. The fact that the changes that have been reported were more pronounced with increased dosage, and that dosage tends to decrease with age starting in adolescence, suggests that these cardiovascular changes may disappear with age.

Issue: Stimulant Therapy Is a Chemical Straitjacket

The medication-nonmedication issue continues to be a controversial one. Opponents of medication charge that children who should not be on stimulants are treated with them, and point to the well-documented instances of blatant and negligent misuse. Walker (1974) has provided impressive examples of children inaccurately diagnosed as hyperactive, when in fact the etiology of their troublesome behavior covered a wide range of medical problems such as pinworm infestation, cardiac problems, and calcium deficiency, none of which is stimulant-responsive. Similarly, the Taft case (Bruck, 1976) represented one of many instances of coercion by school personnel resulting in excessive stimulant therapy for children whose classroom difficulties stemmed from causes other than hyperactivity. A second major point of opposition is the contention that as a form of treatment for the hyperactive child, the effects of medication are unnecessarily restrictive, that the child is put into a chemical straitjacket, and his behavior elicits descriptors such as "robot," "zombie," "sleepwalker," "in a trance," and "as if he was hypnotized." Support for the excessive restriction criticism comes largely from observations of the extraordinary and not totally desirable concentration of the medicated child. Fowlie (1973) described how her son concentrated on a puzzle with a single-mindedness that was unique for him; Wender (1971) reported the astonishment and delight of the parents whose daughter had to be literally pried loose from her homework; and Robertson (1978) reported a teacher's account of a hyperactive child's classroom behavior in which the child, despite several interesting interruptions in the classroom, looked neither to the left or right but worked steadily and systematically on his assignments and had to be reminded of recess. The degree of drug-induced change is difficult for some parents to tolerate, as Robin and Bosco (1981, p. 89a) report in their interview project:

> My mom says she wanted to quit because ... you're too quiet and stuff, and I don't want you and I don't like you like this. (Interviewer: Were you glad that she said that?) No, because I like being quiet.

The unnecessary restriction imposed on the child's behavior by medication also is reflected in the child's state of reduced affect. Rie (1975) described this phenomenon as an "affectless, humorless, and apathetic demeanor" and noted that in a double-blind study of primary grade children, those on methylphenidate could be distinguished without error from the controls solely on the basis of this diminished affect. In a discussion of this drug effect Rie (1975, p. 788) stated:

> The implications of children developing for any period of time with substantially diminished affective arousal may be considerable. At the least, those whose emotional status is a major determinant of their hyperactivity and related problems are inaccessible, under this condition, to any mode of intervention that seeks to

alter their characteristic affective responses, simply because the responses fail to occur. It remains to be determined whether children treated continuously for prolonged periods of time are able to develop age-adequate patterns of emotional adaptation.

In rebutting the straitjacket claim, experienced clinicians such as Gittelman-Klein (1975) believe that far from being a controlled robot, the medicated child has more freedom than when unmedicated because he is able to choose to respond to internal and external stimuli and is no longer bombarded by stimulation. Gittelman-Klein (1975) acknowledges that medication is used to control certain negative aspects of the hyperactive child's behavior, but equates this control to that exercised in the pursuit of other therapeutic medical goals such as vaccines, surgery, and medication for sedative reasons. Her argument is that all therapeutic endeavors aim for some kind of control, and that stimulant drugs properly used control behaviors that are damaging to the child.

Proponents of medication as the optimal form of treatment point to the unequivocal evidence that the medicated hyperactive child functions better in dyadic interactions, such as mother–child (Barkley & Cunningham, 1979; Humphries, Kinsbourne, & Swanson, 1978) and peer interactions (Cantwell, 1979; Henker & Whalen, 1980b; Whalen, Henker, Collins, McAuliffe, & Vaux, 1979), as well as in classroom settings, both socially (Whalen, Henker, Collins, Finck, & Dotemoto, 1979; Whalen, Henker, & Dotemoto, 1981) where he is indistinguishable in many respects from his nonhyperactive peers, and on cognitive tasks (Douglas, 1974, 1980). In the studies by Whalen and her associates one important outcome of medication was the normalization of hyperactive children's classroom behavior and teacher-student interchanges. Support for medication-related changes comes from the interview protocol of Henker and Whalen (1980b, p. 152) in which an 11-year-old girl comments as follows:

C: I wasn't at all—I didn't at all have hardly any friends. I only had two, and that was it. And last year I didn't take it [the medication] in the afternoon, but the last time I saw my doctor he said, "Why don't you have her start taking it in the afternoon?" And then since I've been doing that I've gotten about 20 more friends.

I: How can you tell when you forget to take Ritalin?

C: When I can tell that I'm not concentrating in school. Like she'll [the teacher] give us a half hour to do a math page, like there's about 20 problems, and I'll get about 6 done in 20 minutes, a half hour. But if I take it, I can get them all done in 10 minutes, 20 minutes, and have 10 minutes free.

It is our opinion that the chemical straitjacket view of the medicated hyperactive child derives from overmedication. It is a common observation among clinicians that for some hyperactive children the standardized dosages advocated by experienced clinicians (e.g., Gross & Wilson, 1974; Wender, 1971) as well as the American Academy of Pediatrics (1975) are well above the optimal dosage for overall functioning. At the peak response point such overdosed children do resemble controlled robots. (To document this opinion dose-response curves for variables such as imperviousness to interruption and quality of affect should be developed.) The overmedication is also responsible for the contrast effect, a second cause of the straitjacket view. The impact upon the observers of a rapid, dramatic, positive change in the hyperactive child's behavior is often in the shock range. Parents and teachers are incredulous and the child himself is often overwhelmed by the stimulant-induced changes and appears in a somewhat dazed state. Clinicians have frequently told us that complaints that the child is in a trance, a zombie, and the like, are almost invariably associated with dramatic and immediate responses, and these complaints are made in the first few days or weeks of stimulant therapy before the parents and the child have adjusted to his changed behavior patterns.

Issue: Stimulant Effects on Classroom Achievement

The two main sources of data on the short-term effects (six months or less) of stimulant medications on academic achievement are teacher and parent reports and ratings, and objective measures of academic achievement such as standardized tests. Conclusions based on these data sources concerning stimulant drug effects are notable for their within-source consistency and between-source differences. Teachers and parents view improved academic achievement as one of the major outcomes of the stimulant medication regimen (Arnold, Wender, McCloskey, & Snyder, 1972; Conners, Eisenberg, & Barcai, 1967; Rapoport et al., 1974; Rie et al., 1976a, 1976b; Schain & Reynard, 1975; Sleator, von Neumann, & Sprague, 1974; Sprague, Barnes, & Werry, 1970), whereas more objective measures of academic achievement either fail completely to corroborate these reported gains (Blacklidge & Ekblad, 1971; Christensen, 1975; Conrad, Dworkin, Shai, & Tobiessen, 1971; Rie et al., 1976a, 1976b; Werry & Sprague, 1974) or report transitory gains that dissipate over a relatively short period of time (Gittelman-Klein & Klein, 1976). It should be noted that in the studies using objective measures of academic achievement, the duration of drug treatment (e.g., in the Christensen study, two weeks) was too short to provide a fair test of academic gains, because the achievement tests used as the dependent variables provide too gross a measure of achievement. Tests such as the Wide Range Achievement Test (WRAT) have too few items at each year level to reflect the small amount of improvement that could be expected to occur in two or three weeks (Barkley & Cunningham, 1978; Sprague & Berger, 1980). The point here is that refined conditions for the independent variables require refined measures for the dependent variables.

In considering these differences it is important to remember that teachers and parents tend to attribute the hyperactive child's academic difficul-

no show

ties to his hyperactive behavior and thus believe that stopping the behavior will mean an end to academic difficulties. At the kindergarten level there is some basis for this belief, because the child does not as yet have the deficit in basic skills that is likely to exist after several years in school without intervention or other help. At this one point in the child's school career drugs can help set in motion a sequence that leads to academic achievement: drugs $\rightarrow$ reduced activity and increased attention $\rightarrow$ improved academic achievement. Although kindergarten is probably the only time at which this sequence does occur, teachers and parents of children at other grade levels believe that the often dramatic drug-induced improvement in hyperactive behavior will be accompanied by academic improvement, and this expectation colors their assessment of the child's actual progress. Generally teachers feel that there is very little that they can do for the typical unmedicated hyperactive child in the classroom and consequently they spend a minimum of time on him. According to parental and child reports, teachers increase the amount of time and help given once the child is on drugs, so some classwork-related improvement may be visible to the teacher and parent but not be measured by objective testing. In addition, the improvement in hyperactivity-related behavior that occurs with drugs lends itself to a halo effect on the teacher's view of the child, with a consequent improvement in grades, conduct ratings, and other assessments. One eight-year-old boy reported that he wanted to start stimulants because "as soon as you get on pills your grades go way up." A check with the child's teacher confirmed this observation for seven of the eight medicated hyperactive children in the class.

Empirical findings supporting the teacher–parent objective tests differences were obtained in a careful comparison of the effects of methylphenidate and placebo on a group of primary grade children, most of whom were hyperactive or learning disabled (Rie et al., 1976a). In a double-blind, counterbalanced design, each treatment condition was maintained for 12 weeks. Although the classroom teachers and parents rated the medicated children as exhibiting gains in school achievement, improvement occurred on only one subtest, Word Analysis, of the six subtests on the Iowa Test of Basic Skills, and on only the Auditory Association subtest of the Illinois Test of Psycholinguistic Abilities. The Comprehension subtests scores of the WISC decreased under medication, the only WISC-related difference that occurred. In commenting on the significant discrepancy between teacher and parent reports, and objective measures, Rie et al. (1976a) concluded that classroom teachers' and parents' assessments of achievement are not reliable and may be influenced by more obvious behavior changes such as reductions in activity level. A second study (Rie et al., 1976b) in effect replicated these findings. Rie et al. noted that methylphenidate not only failed to result in academic achievement gains, it also had the potential to mask or confound learning problems because the child was perceived by his teachers and parents to be performing more effectively on academic tasks, when in fact he had deficits in essential achievement-related skills. Sprague and Berger (1980) have contended that the dosage level of 0.8 mg/kg of methylphenidate in the Rie et al. studies (1976a, 1976b) was sufficiently high to produce drug-induced *suppression* of learning performance.

In a comprehensive review of the effects of stimulant medication on academic achievement, Barkley and Cunningham (1978) surveyed 17 short-term studies that varied markedly in methodological rigor and procedural approach. Of the 52 dependent achievement measures used in this body of research, 43 were not significantly improved by stimulant medication and, where drug effects were noted, they were "scattered and inconsistent." These findings led Barkley and Cunningham to attribute such gains that were reported to attentional and other test-skill variables rather than to improved achievement skills per se, and to conclude that in the overwhelming majority of short-term studies, the stimulants produce little improvement in academic performance. Long-term follow-up studies have also generally failed to demonstrate drug-related achievement gains in childhood as well as adolescence (e.g., Huessy, Metoyer, & Townsend, 1974; Mendelson, Johnson, & Stewart, 1971; Milich & Loney, 1979a; Minde, Weiss, & Mendelson, 1972; Weiss, Minde, Douglas, Werry, & Sykes, 1971). In one 5-year follow-up there was evidence of reading improvement in boys who had responded positively to methylphenidate (Loney, 1978). Instances of academic deterioration have also been reported (Riddle & Rapoport, 1976).

Speculation about why there is no association between drug-related reduction of hyperactive behavior and improvements in academic achievement provides no real insight into the problem. Barkley and Cunningham (1978, p. 90) suggest that the age of treatment onset may be a factor, but a "more likely possibility is that stimulant medications are simply unable to influence those etiologic variables which create, or contribute to, the hyperactive child's academic difficulties." Cantwell and Carlson (1978, p. 185) believe that the evidence to date neither proves nor disproves a drug-academic achievement effect because "a proper study evaluating the effects of stimulants on actual academic achievement in the classroom has not been carried out." They go on to describe the methodological difficulties inherent in such a study, particularly that of singling out the effect of the stimulants from the combination of other factors, such as a variety of other concurrent treatments, that could affect the child's academic achievement. Aman (1978) also stresses the methodological problems, many of which should be of concern in any drug study. Sprague and Berger (1980) attribute the failure to demonstrate a positive drug effect on achievement to the insensitivity of the assessment procedures coupled with inappropriate drug dosages, rather than to a lack of stimulant effect on achievement. They have collected single-subject arithmetic test data from an ongoing study that support their contention concerning the importance of dosage level: greater accuracy and shorter latency of response was demonstrated with 0.3 mg/kg of methylphenidate in comparison to either 1.0 mg/kg or placebo.

The fact is that the academic achievement problem requires a refinement of approach that generally is ignored when interest is on crude discriminations, such as drug versus nondrug use, with correspondingly crude standards of subject selection, control of independent variables, and evaluation tools. To resolve this issue, careful single-subject studies such as that of Sprague and Berger (1980) reported above should be conducted. Only when substantive individual data have been collected will group studies be justifiable. The academic achievement issue poses a confrontation that advocates of drug usage, for the most part, have sidestepped while continuing to assert the need for further work and to reiterate the belief that drugs constitute the treatment of choice.

State-Dependent Learning

Sprague and Berger (1980, p. 180) believe that the most rapid progress in the understanding of drug effects on different aspects of children's disorders could be achieved with an integration of animal and human clinical research. With respect to the effects of stimulants on achievement, one possibility that must be carefully studied is that state-dependent learning is a factor in the hyperactive child's achievement difficulties. State-dependent learning means that a response learned under the influence of a particular drug may recur with maximum strength only when that drug condition is reinstated (Overton, 1968). The assumption underlying this phenomenon is that if a specific drug was present during the initial acquisition of a response, later absence of the drug would constitute a novel stimulus environment and the previously learned response would not occur. If state-dependency could be demonstrated to occur in hyperactive children, this finding would have potentially serious implications for pediatric psychopharmacology because it would mean that unmedicated hyperactive children might lose an indeterminate amount of what they had learned while on medication. This phenomenon has been the subject of extensive infrahuman investigations (e.g., Barrett, Leith, & Ray, 1972) but has attracted surprisingly little research attention at the human level. We will describe briefly the limited research on the possibility of state-dependent effects in hyperactive children. Aman and Sprague (1974) tested a group of hyperactive children using methylphenidate and dextroamphetamine on three different learning tasks: short-term memory, paired-associate learning, and fine motor performance on a maze task. Each child learned the tasks under one condition and was then tested for retention 48 hours later under each of the drug conditions, that is methylphenidate, dextroamphetamine, and placebo. The results showed no evidence of either drug-related facilitation of learning or state-dependent learning, that is, there was no interaction between the drug condition for the learning session and that used in retention. In fact, some transfer data were in the direction contrary to what state-dependent learning would predict. Swanson and Kinsbourne (1975) interpreted the failure of Aman and Sprague to demonstrate stimulant-related state-dependent learning to the lack of evidence of drug-related facilitation of the initial learning. According to their reasoning, state-dependency occurs *only* on tasks for which stimulants facilitate the initial learning. In addition, Aman and Sprague (1974) failed to establish that their hyperactive subjects were positive drug responders, a serious flaw in a study of state-dependency.

In the first of a series of studies, Swanson and Kinsbourne (1976) used a paired-associate task to investigate state-dependent learning in hyperactive children who were drug responsive and nonhyperactive children, all from the same learning clinic. On the first day of the two-day study the children learned a paired-associate task in two states: drug (methylphenidate) and placebo, and on the second day they were tested for relearning of each class of learned material in both states. The results differed for the two groups. The hyperactive children exhibited drug-related facilitation of the learning task on the first day, that is, they were significantly better in the drug condition than they were on the placebo. The nonhyperactive group made more errors in the drug than in the placebo condition. On the second day the hyperactive children demonstrated "symmetrical state-dependency learning," that is, during relearning in the drug state they made more errors on items originally learned in the placebo state (the learning and relearning states were different) than on items originally learned in the drug state (where the learning and relearning states were the same). A similar state-dependency effect was observed in the placebo test condition, with more errors made on items originally learned in the drug (different) than in the placebo (same) state. The best learning occurred when the initial learning and relearning were both accomplished in the drug state; the worst learning occurred when the initial learning was in the drug state and relearning was in the placebo state. This latter situation resulted in poorer performance than that which occurred when learning and relearning both took place under placebo conditions. The nonhyperactive group failed to demonstrate state-dependency learning, a result that was consistent with Swanson and Kinsbourne's contention that drug-related facilitation of initial learning is essential to the demonstration of state-dependency. Additional evidence in support of a state-dependency effect comes from a study (Fisher, 1978) of the effects of d-amphetamine and placebo on a selective attention task. Hyperactive boys who were given placebo prior to each of the two training sessions showed a substantial practice effect in the second session, whereas boys in the drug-placebo and placebo-drug conditions showed no improvement.

The findings on state-dependent learning have led Kinsbourne and Swanson (1979) to conclude that longer-lasting drug regimens with agents such as pemoline are essential if learning and other improvements in performance are to endure. However, two research directions must be explored before possibly hazardous around-the-clock drug regimens are accepted as the optimal mode of management. First, the presence or absence of state-dependent effects associated with each of the major types of learning tasks of childhood must be identified empirically (Keogh & Barkett, 1980). Such research would require, as Whalen and Henker (1980b) have noted, that types of tasks, subject characteristics, dosage levels, and temporal dimensions be varied systematically. Nonpharmacological interventions that can disrupt state-dependent learning in experimental paradigms should next be identified and then translated into classroom procedures, for example, state-dependent effects can be offset by prompting aids (Swanson, Eich, & Kinsbourne, 1978). With these steps in mind, consider the predominant learning task in the elementary school curriculum, the associative learning task, which is known to be susceptible to the state-dependency effect (Swanson & Kinsbourne, 1976). Procedures that facilitate associative learning and retention may also then prove to be of use in overcoming state-dependency effects. For example, there is unequivocal evidence that: (a) associative learning and retention can be facilitated through the use of verbal mediational strategies; (b) young children of normal and below-normal intelligence readily acquire these strategies; and (c) mediational strategies presented in diverse training contexts result in long-term retention and transfer of the strategies, with a consequent marked improvement on a variety of associative learning tasks (Ross & Ross, 1973; Ross, Ross, & Downing, 1973). If the use of verbal mediational strategies could be shown to successfully bridge the change-of-state effect that occurs with associative learning (Swanson & Kinsbourne, 1976), then these strategies should be taught in the classroom. This approach to the problems presented by state dependency offers two important advantages: it provides a parsimonious alternative to the use of long-lasting drug agents, and it would equip the child with a self-management skill that, in addition to facilitating initial associative learning and retention, would enhance the child's self-esteem by giving him a sense of being in control.

In using the paired-associate paradigm to demonstrate state-dependent effects, we offer one methodological suggestion. Children of normal and below-normal intelligence often spontaneously generate covert mnemonic strategies to facilitate paired-associate learning, relearning, and recall. The use of such strategies could confound state-dependent effects and distort the meaning of the findings. It is our opinion that the validity of the findings in paired-associate research is in jeopardy unless every effort is made (e.g., postexperimental interviews) to determine whether the use of such strategies has contributed systematically to outcome.

Although the specific components of the drug (or nondrug) state that are critical to the state-dependent effect in hyperactive children have never been identified, it has commonly been supposed that in one state a particular pattern of cognitive activity is present, and that a change of state comprises a novel cognitive complex, making the retrieval of previously learned responses more difficult than it would be with the original complex. Recent research by Bower (1981) with college students has identified a radically different component of the state-dependent phenomenon, namely, *mood*. In a series of studies of the influence of emotions on memory, Bower used hypnotic suggestion to induce fairly strong moods of either happiness or sadness. On learning tasks and other measures the subjects exhibited mood-state-dependent memory, that is, their level of recall was superior under mood-congruent (same mood during original learning and recall) as compared to mood-incongruent conditions. The implications of these findings for hyperactive children are potentially profound. Extreme fluctuations of mood are a salient characteristic of the hyperactive child and stimulant-induced sad or depressive moods (Rie et al., 1976a, 1976b) are a matter of considerable concern to parents. Indeed many parents are unwilling to maintain their hyperactive children on medication because they consider the resultant mood changes repugnant (Robin & Bosco, 1981). The mood-congruity effect demonstrated by Bower (1981) is consistent with the fluctuations in performance characteristic of the unmedicated hyperactive child as well as his temporal variations in performance while on medication, for example, accomplishment of a school task in the morning peak drug-effect period and the inability to do the identical task for homework. We are not proposing a simple cause-and-effect relationship between mood and performance in the hyperactive child. Such an explanation would be inconsistent with the interactionist viewpoint of this text as well as naive in the light of the complexity of the hyperactive child. Instead we are suggesting that the hyperactive child's well-documented fluctuations in mood could be one contributor to his erratic performance in the unmedicated state as well as across states, and as such opens up several avenues for investigative attention. What would be the effects, for example, of systematic variations of drug state and induced mood on the paired-associate learning of hyperactive children using the Swanson and Kinsbourne (1978) task, that is, is mood a more powerful determinant of state-dependent learning in the hyperactive child than medication? If mood fluctuations disrupt performance in the hyperactive child, can they be brought under conscious control by self-instruction? Could stimulus factors (Henker & Whalen, 1980a) be used in the classroom to maintain mood stability over the school day? Are the well-documented disruptive effects of some schedules of reinforcement (Douglas, 1980a) primarily a function of the resultant changes in mood?

Issue: Stimulant Therapy Versus Behavior Intervention

Although there is unequivocal evidence of the efficacy of short-term drug intervention in the treatment of the hyperactive child, evidence of long-term benefits has failed to materialize. This failure, combined with concern over the safety of long-term stimulant administration with respect to linear growth and cardiac functioning and the potential for drug dependency and abuse, has caused researchers to focus on empirical tests of alternative forms of intervention, particularly the behavioral techniques. For an interesting critical account of the shift from stimulants-only to stimulants versus behavior intervention see O'Leary (1980). The behavioral techniques have proven to be effective with children labeled as hyperactive who are institutionalized or have irreversible conditions that permit a crucial test of behavior intervention (e.g., Doubros & Daniels, 1966; Pihl, 1967); they are also effective with nonclinical children in regular and special education classrooms who exhibit relatively mild manifestations of the cluster of behaviors associated with hyperactivity (Becker, Madsen, Arnold, & Thomas, 1967; Kent & O'Leary, 1976), and with hyperactive children in school settings (O'Leary, Pelham, Rosenbaum, & Price, 1976; Rosenbaum, O'Leary, & Jacob, 1975). In the latter studies the finding that the changes in behavior, as measured by the Conners scales, were similar in magnitude to those reported in drug studies, coupled with reports from single-subject and small-group studies that contingency management techniques were as effective as drug therapy in controlling behavior and were significantly more effective in improving academic performance (Ayllon, Layman, & Kandel, 1975; Pelham, 1977; Stableford, Butz, Hasazi, Leitenberg, & Peyser, 1976), has led to a number of studies of the relative efficacy of drug and behavior intervention for hyperactive children.

In the first of these Gittelman-Klein and her associates (Gittelman-Klein, Klein, Abikoff, Katz, Gloisten, & Kates, 1976; Gittelman-Klein, Abikoff, Pollack, Klein, Katz, & Mattes, 1980) compared the efficacy of methylphenidate and behavior modification in an 8-week combined school and home therapy program for 34 hyperactive children aged six to 12. The children, all of whom were reported to be hyperactive in school and to have behavior difficulties at home, were rated by their teachers and parents and then randomly assigned to the following conditions: methylphenidate only, methylphenidate with behavior therapy, and drug placebo with behavior therapy. Methylphenidate dosage was individualized and was increased throughout the study on the basis of teacher and parent reports. A behavior therapy program was implemented in the home with parent training, and in the school. After eight weeks the three intervention procedures were evaluated using teacher ratings of hyperactivity; global ratings of overall improvement by psychiatrists, teachers, and mothers; and independent blind classroom observations. All three treatment conditions resulted in significant clinical improvement, with the methylphenidate-behavior therapy and the methylphenidate-only groups proving to be more effective than the drug placebo-behavior therapy group, but not differing themselves on any measure. The investigators concluded cautiously that at this interim point in their long-term study stimulant medication was the most effective treatment for hyperactivity, and that it was significantly superior to behavior therapy alone. In the second part of the study (Gittelman-Klein et al., 1980) 27 additional children completed treatment. The results from the additional sample were consistent with the interim report, that is, stimulant therapy alone or in combination with behavior therapy was significantly more effective than behavior therapy alone.

This conclusion is a highly debatable one in view of the obvious methodological weaknesses in the asymmetrical three-group design, and other procedural shortcomings and omissions. It is almost impossible to assess the efficacy of the behavior therapy in the absence of four additional treatment conditions, namely, no treatment, drug placebo-attention, drug placebo only, and behavior therapy only groups. With respect to this design deficiency, Loney, Weissenburger, Woolson, and Lichty (1979, p. 135) have noted that

> the change from baseline to follow-up in the group that received behavior therapy plus drug placebo cannot be confidently isolated as (1) a drug placebo effect, (2) a behavioral placebo effect, (3) a genuine behavioral therapy effect, or (4) some combination of the three. Because such an attribution cannot be made, it is possible that the behavioral treatment was merely ineffectively delivered and that the study therefore does not constitute a proper test of drug versus behavior treatments.

Other methodological shortcomings pointed out by Mash and Dalby (1979, p. 186) concerning the first study (Gittelman-Klein et al., 1976) are applicable to the second study as well:

> The findings . . . must be considered in light of the facts that the subjects were "severely" disruptive and were treated with fairly large doses of stimulant medication, and the study was conducted over a short time period with no follow-up, does not include information regarding preintervention medication status, and provides no direct information about possible behavior changes in the home. In addition, it is not clear whether methylphenidate dosage was similar across the two drug conditions (this is not reported), nor is it clear whether the amount and quality of behavior therapy received was equivalent across the two groups receiving this treatment. For example, the number of contact hours with the therapists in each condition is not reported, nor is it evident that the therapist(s) were the same or different in the two behavioral treatment conditions. All of these factors create potentially serious problems in this study.

An important omission in both parts of the study was the failure to establish the drug response status of all subjects prior to treatment. If drug responders and nonresponders were differentially represented in the treatment conditions this information should have been included.

Similar criticisms apply to the study by Wolraich, Drummond, Salomon, O'Brien, and Sivage (1978), in which the effects of methylphenidate alone and in combination with behavior modification procedures were compared, the dependent variables being measures of classroom behavior, academic performance, and teacher ratings on the Conners Abbreviated Teacher Rating Scale. Using a half-day laboratory classroom in a baseline-treatment-reversal design, the 26 hyperactive children (who comprised the entire class) were studied for six weeks, with each sector of the design in effect for two weeks. Under double-blind conditions, half the children were placed on 0.3 mg/kg of methylphenidate and the remaining half were placed on placebo for the entire program. No child had been on a drug regimen in the six months prior to the study, but no information was given concerning their drug response status. The classroom program consisted of a group period in which immediate teacher reinforcement of the children was possible, and an individual work period during which immediate teacher reinforcement could not occur. In the group period, behavior modification caused a significant decrease in the target behaviors (nonattending, out-of-seat, inappropriate vocalizations, and peer interaction). Medication caused a decrease in fidgeting, a nontarget behavior, but had no other effects during the group period. During the individual period the results were reversed, with no significant effects with the modification procedures, but significant reductions with medication for all behaviors except out-of-seat and fidgeting. Behavior modification alone resulted in significant improvement on the two academic measures, a finding that is consistent with other research (Ayllon, Layman, & Kandel, 1975). There were no significant effects for either drugs alone or in combination with behavior modification-drug interactions, that is, neither treatment procedure enhanced or diminished the other. Wolraich et al. (1978) concluded that stimulant drugs may be the preferred procedure if the only goal is the reduction of undesirable behavior, whereas behavior modification may be the treatment of choice where academic improvement is the goal.

Here again the criticisms of no follow-up and failure to determine whether the subjects were all drug responders undermine the significance of the results, as does the failure to use enough groups so that a firm statement can be made about the relative efficacy of the treatments *in this situation*. It is quite possible, for example, that the effect of the sudden change in teacher behavior could have been a powerful independent variable.

Of the three studies on this topic, the one by Loney, Weissenburger, Woolson, and Lichty (1979) is the most limited in terms of goals and best from a design viewpoint. Loney et al. compared the short-term effects of methylphenidate and teacher behavior counseling concerning classroom management skills on the on-task behavior of hyperactive boys from six to 12 years of age, and selected overactive, average, and model classmates. The rationale offered for the inclusion of this somewhat diverse group of classmates was that the true effects of treatment may depend on relative rather than absolute standards of behavior change. Loney et al. (1979) have noted that they do not consider classmates to be an ideal untreated control group, but at the same time they regard them as essential for valid comparison. In this study drug dosage was individually titrated, with parental report being the criterion for adjusting dosage. Significant improvement occurred in both the drug-treated and behaviorally treated groups, with no significant differences between them. In the drug-treated group, however, the hyperactive children's on-task behavior after intervention was no longer significantly different from that of their average and model classmates, whereas in the behaviorally treated group on-task behavior remained significantly worse.

The behavioral treatment effects "spilled over" to the overactive classmates, a phenomenon that we would ascribe to either a modeling effect (Bandura, 1969) or generalization of the teacher training to objects (in this case, the overactive child), most like the target object (the hyperactive child), so that there was also a significant improvement in these children as well as a trend towards significance in the average classmates. With careful controls it would be possible to determine the source of the spillover. This issue is of more than academic interest because spillover could become a useful tool for classroom management. A check could be made to determine whether the hyperactive children and also the spillover recipients maintained their gains in behavior. On the face of it one would expect the hyperactive group's retention scores to be the superior. But these children were under external (i.e., teacher) control, whereas the spillover group were vicarious observers who presumably covertly verbalized events to themselves and with this mediational behavior consolidated the new learning into their behavior repertoire. If this reasoning is correct, the spillovers might show greater long-term gains even when statistical allowances are made for initial differences in the target behavior.

In a three-month study with 24 kindergarten children, Cohen, Sullivan, Minde, Novak, and Helwig (1981) compared the relative effectiveness of drug treatment (methylphenidate), cognitive behavior modification, the two treatments combined, and no treatment. Neither the posttreatment assessment nor the long-term follow-up one year later provided any evidence that any one of the treatments studied was more effective than any other of the treatments or of no treatment at all. In considering the methodological weaknesses and other shortcomings apparent in this study, it is difficult to see how Cohen et al. justified this misuse of the children's time, not to speak of the investigative effort involved. The groups were insufficient in number and size for adequate comparisons to be made; the subjects were not identified prior to treatment as drug responders, and in any case their age would suggest that other independent variables be selected rather than drugs. There is some evidence that methylphenidate is far less effective with 5-year-old children than with older children (Conners, 1975b; Schleifer, Weiss, Cohen, Elman, Cvejic, & Kruger, 1975). The other independent variable, cognitive training, was similarly haphazardly selected. The investigators themselves expressed doubts about the suitability of the training for children who for the most part were unable to independently generate the problem-solving strategies that Douglas (1980) considers essential for optimum treatment-related benefits.

Mash and Dalby (1979, p. 186) believe that the question concerning the relative efficacy of drugs and behavioral treatment is too global in scope:

> Medication is not a unitary treatment and behavior therapy is even more diverse. What is needed are empirical statements re the effectiveness and/or relative effectiveness of specific medication regimens or specific behavior therapy interventions, for specific children, with specific behaviors, in particular situations.

An outstanding example of such an approach has been provided by Conners and Wells (1979) in a case study of a seven-year-old boy who was referred for his excessive activity level and academic achievement problems, as well as verbal and physical aggression and other deviant behavior. Contributing to his problems were some neurological difficulties, physical anomalies, and auditory skill deficits, capped by a poor home situation. Although his Verbal IQ on the WISC-R was 98 and his Performance IQ 77, in all basic academic performance areas he was functioning at a kindergarten level. Conners and Wells (1979) used an *A, B, BC, C* single-case design to assess the effects of stimulants alone and in combination with a self-control classroom training program. A baseline (*A*) was established, then stimulants alone (*B*) were followed by stimulants combined with the self-control training (*BC*), the last step being placebo combined with the self-control training (*C*). In the baseline phase (see Figure 6.3) inappropriate gross motor behavior and inappropriate noise and vocalizations averaged 35 and 25 percent respectively. School behavior improved markedly, but out-of-school behavior deteriorated with the introduction of Ritalin so Dexedrine was substituted. For most of the *B* phase gross motor behavior and inappropriate vocalizations decreased; however, the

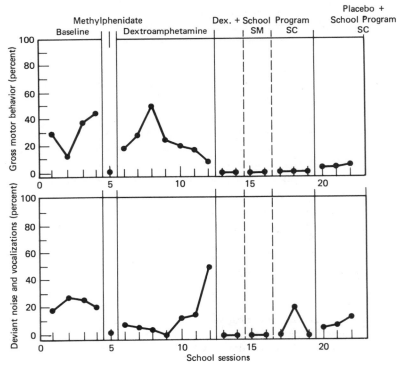

Figure 6.3 Gross Motor and Deviant Vocalications for Patient Tommy. Reprinted, by permission, from Conners, C. K., & Wells, K. C. Method and theory for psychopharmacology with children. In R. L. Trites (Ed.), *Hyperactivity in children.* Copyright 1979, University Park Press, Baltimore.

greatest improvement occurred in phase *BC,* with both sets of behavior decreasing to close to zero levels and then maintaining this position in phase *C* when Dexedrine was withdrawn. As can be seen from Figure 6.4, similar improvements occurred with on-task behavior, and concomitant decreases were observed as well in off-task behavior. The results of this study provide strong support for the approach advocated above by Mash and Dalby (1979) to the drugs versus behavioral intervention issue. It would appear that careful studies of individual hyperactive children, permitting a range in situational specificity, should *precede* the small-group approach to such issues. Of particular note is the flexibility possible in the treatment regimen with the use of single-subject methodology. The study also points to the fact that because drug effects cannot be understood in isolation from the context in which they occur, in this case the self-control classroom training, it is essential that the context lend itself to careful analysis.

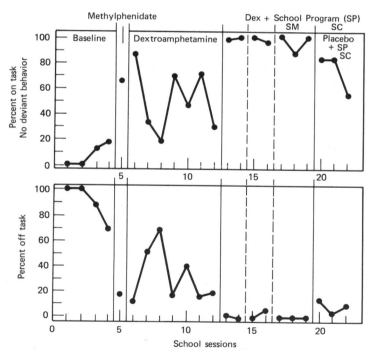

Figure 6.4   Patient Tommy's On-Task Behavior. (Methylphenidate improves classroom behavior, but is withdrawn because of disruptive effects on ward behavior. Dexedrine plus self-monitoring and self-control produce maximal improvement in the classroom.) Reprinted, by permission, from Conners, C. K., & Wells, K. C. Method and theory for psychopharmacology with children. In R. L. Trites (Ed.), *Hyperactivity in children.* Copyright 1979, University Park Press, Baltimore.

Issue: The Paradoxical Effect of Stimulants

A long-standing controversy in the hyperactivity literature has concerned the paradoxical quality of the stimulant drug response. Since Bradley (1937) first expressed surprise that a drug (benzedrine) with a stimulating effect on adults had a sedating effect on children, the weight of opinion in the literature has supported the concept of the response as paradoxical, whereas the weight of fact has questioned the validity and accuracy of the descriptor *paradoxical.* Kornetsky (1970) has specified two objections to this descriptor. A true paradoxical effect of stimulants upon the central nervous system would consist of an inhibitory effect on the activity level of the overaroused child and a disinhibitory effect on the child who is either underaroused or in a normal state of arousal; there is a paucity of support for such an effect, the only instance being a study of pupillary contraction (Knopp, Arnold, Andras, & Smeltzer, 1973). Also the stimulant effects could accurately be described as paradoxical only if they were calming or sedative in the pharmacological sense, and again there is no evidence that this is the case. The stimulants give the impression that a calming effect has occurred, but as Werry and Sprague (1970) have pointed out, the actual change in the hyperactive child's behavior is to more appropriate and better integrated responses in settings characterized by high demands for compliance. Furthermore, evidence against the validity of the paradoxical effect of stimulants comes from research findings from a variety of subject groups that contradict the assumption that the stimulants act selectively only in the hyperactive child. The data have accumulated from studies in which normal children (Shetty, 1971), nonhyperactive children with other behavior disorders (e.g., Gittelman-Klein & Klein, 1976; Steinberg, Troshinsky, & Steinberg, 1971), and normal adults (Weiss & Laties, 1962) were given doses of stimulants comparable to those used with the hyperactive children; in each case these groups reacted as hyperactive children do with increased alertness, decreased motoric responses, and more focused activity. Until recently, Shetty's (1971) study of photic responses was the only one in the hyperactivity literature in which both normal and hyperactive children were given stimulants, with both groups exhibiting the same favorable drug response in the form of increased alpha activity. Recent research by Rapoport and her colleagues (Rapoport, Buchsbaum, Zahn, Weingartner, Ludlow, & Mikkelsen, 1978) has provided further support for the similarity of effect position by demonstrating that on a variety of tasks consistently proven to be drug sensitive with hyperactive children, the stimulants produce the same decrease in motor activity and enhancement of learning and performance in normal children as they do in hyperactive children. Although there are some data that suggest opposite drug responses in hyperactive and normal children on specific laboratory-based tasks (Swanson & Kinsbourne, 1976, 1978), the consensus of experts (e.g., Sprague & Berger, 1980, p. 174) is that the paradoxical issue has been closed by the findings of Rapoport et al. (1978) and that stimulants have similar effects on hyperactive and normal children.

OTHER DRUGS USED IN TREATMENT

Central Nervous System Stimulants

Although the amphetamines and methylphenidate are by far the most widely used drugs with hyperactive children, two other central nervous system stimulants, caffeine and magnesium pemoline (Cylert), have attracted clinical and research attention and will be briefly discussed here.

Caffeine

Caffeine is one of the xanthines, which are among the oldest central nervous system stimulants known to man. It is the only psychoactive drug that is legally available without prescription, and is found in coffee, teas, colas, chocolate, and cocoa. It is not considered addictive in the sense that narcotics are (Goodman & Gilman, 1975). A therapeutic dose of caffeine for a child is from 100 to 150 mg, and in terms of central nervous system potency 150 mg of caffeine is equal to 6 mg of dextroamphetamine. The absorption of caffeine administered orally occurs rapidly and peak blood levels are usually reached within an hour after ingestion. The most common behavioral effects of a therapeutic dose are an increase in attention and well-being, a slowing of the development of boredom, and a general increase in mental and motor efficiency. When tolerance occurs, it is low grade and does not seem to be a problem.

The first evidence that caffeine might be an effective alternative to dextroamphetamine and methylphenidate in the treatment of hyperactive children came from a pilot study by Schnackenberg (1973) of the clinical effects of caffeine on 11 methylphenidate responders whose medication was discontinued because of annoying side effects. In this open-design study, teacher ratings on the Rating Scale for Hyperkinesis (Davids, 1971) were obtained while the children were on methylphenidate, during a drug holiday period, and again while they were receiving a total daily dose of 250 to 300 mg of caffeine in the form of one cup of coffee at breakfast and a second cup at lunch. The two stimulants had similar behavioral effects, but caffeine, in addition, had none of the undesirable side effects that had been evident with methylphenidate.

In subsequent investigations clinical support for the efficacy of caffeine in the management of hyperactive children came from Harvey (1978) and Fras (1974). In addition, Reichard and Elder (1977) found that 200 mg of caffeine resulted in an increase in accuracy on a choice reaction time task, and a decrease in lapses of attention. Further empirical support came from a double-blind crossover study (Firestone, Poitras-Wright, & Douglas, 1978) in which a dosage of 300 mg a day resulted in significant improvement on ratings of classroom and home behavior, and in impulsive responding in a reaction time task. However, in a second double-blind crossover study (Firestone, Davey, Goodman, & Peters, 1978) comparing the effects of daily dosages of 500 mg caffeine, 300 mg caffeine, and 20 mg of methylphenidate, each for a three-week period, no significant improvement occurred in the caffeine conditions as rated by teachers and mothers, or on tests of impulsivity and motor control, but significant improvement did occur in the methylphenidate condition. Consistently negative findings have been obtained in other carefully controlled investigations. Garfinkel, Webster, and Sloman (1975) found no caffeine effects, but the dosages used were approximately half those used by Schnackenberg. Huestis, Arnold, and Smeltzer (1975), however, used dosages equal to those of Schnackenberg and reported that caffeine did not differ significantly from placebo but was significantly less effective than either methylphenidate or dextroamphetamine. Conners (1975a) used a double-blind crossover design with children who had previously demonstrated positive responses to stimulant medications and found no caffeine-placebo differences of either a positive or negative nature on hyperactivity-related performance deficits. The dosages in this study ranged from 140 mg to 200 mg, given twice daily. Negative findings for the efficacy of caffeine have also been reported by Arnold, Christopher, Huestis, and Smeltzer (1978a).

In a discussion of the contradictory findings on the clinical use of caffeine with hyperactive children, Conners (1979c) raised the possibility that the failure to demonstrate positive behavior change could be due to the fact that the amounts of caffeine that have been used may be only marginally active or even completely inactive at the central level. As a test of this possibility Conners (1979c) conducted an experiment to determine whether dose-related changes attributable to caffeine could be detected in central (evoked response) and behavioral (vigilance and activity level) functions that are known to be sensitive to central nervous system stimulants in hyperactive children. In this experiment hyperactive children who were positive responders to central nervous system stimulants were administered placebo, low caffeine, and high caffeine in counterbalanced order one hour prior to obtaining double-blind measures of visual evoked response, alpha time, vigilance, and activity level. Although there was a significant effect on evoked response, indicating that there were clear central effects, the behavioral effects were marginal. There was a tendency for attention and activity level to be affected in a dose-related manner, but not to a statistically significant degree. Conners (1979c) concluded that although caffeine is clearly centrally active, it does not show the congruence between behavioral and central effects that other stimulants, namely, the amphetamines and methylphenidate, have shown. This study would appear to demonstrate conclusively that caffeine cannot be regarded as equal in efficacy to these stimulants in the management of hyperactivity. However, in cases in which the central nervous system stimulants must be discontinued because of moderate to severe side effects, caffeine may be a viable alternative.

Pemoline

Pemoline (Cylert) is a relatively mild central nervous system stimulant that was first studied clinically in Germany in 1956. It is an oxazolidine and is chemically different from either methylphenidate or the amphetamines (Cantwell & Carlson, 1978). Over the years it has been used in this country in the treatment of senility, anxiety, depression, and schizophrenia, and is also reported to have significant antifatigue and performance-enhancing properties in studies with adults and animals. Pemoline has also been used in the management of hyperactivity, but not as extensively as the other stimulants. A single daily dose of 25 to 100 mg of pemoline given in the morning was reported by Knights and Viets (1973) as sufficient to maintain satisfactory behavior. The onset of effectiveness was found to be slower than that of some of the other central nervous system stimulants with maximum therapeutic effect not being apparent for three to four weeks, and it also had a longer half-life, of 12 hours compared to 4 hours for the other stimulants (Conners, Taylor, Meo, Kurtz, & Fournier, 1972; Page, Bernstein, Janicki, & Michelli, 1974). This relatively long duration of action offers important advantages over dextroamphetamine and methylphenidate: it eliminates the social stigma and logistic difficulties often encountered when children must take midday medication at school, and it prolongs the beneficial drug effects on behavior well into the postschool hours. Side effects range from mild to more serious, with the mild side effects being generally similar to those of the other stimulants (insomnia, headaches, anorexia, stomach ache, mild depression, drowsiness, dizziness, and nausea) (Cylert Monograph, 1975). However, a major difference between pemoline and the more commonly used central nervous system stimulants is its long duration of psychostimulant activity without sympathomimetic cardiovascular effects. Changes in heart rate and blood pressure appear to be less marked than those reported with the other stimulants (Page et al., 1974). In addition, pemoline, unlike the amphetamines, has not proven addictive in monkeys (Plotnikoff, 1971). The more serious side effects include growth retardation (Dickinson, Lee, Ringdahl, Schedewie, Kilgore, & Elders, 1979) and weight loss, both of which appear to return to normal after three to six months (Page et al., 1974). With prolonged administration another more serious but also reversible potential effect is elevation of liver enzymes, which necessitates the withdrawal of medication and periodic checks on liver enzyme level (Cylert Monograph, 1975).

Although the research to date on the efficacy of this stimulant for hyperactivity has been limited, the direct effects of pemoline appear to be similar in kind, although slightly less effective than those of the amphetamines and methylphenidate (Cantwell & Carlson, 1978; Dykman, McGrew, & Ackerman, 1974). Preliminary clinical studies suggested that pemoline effected improvement in general behavior and school performance, particularly on tasks involving short-term memory, and facilitated attentiveness to school tasks (Conners et al., 1972; Page et al., 1974). Millichap (1973) reported that pemoline alleviated hyperactivity and was associated with increased scores on the Performance Scale of the WISC. Knights and Viets (1973) found that almost all of the children showed improvements in mood and communication skills, in addition to marked improvement in behavior and school performance. They also reported very few side effects. According to Barkley (1977) the percent of positive response is similar to that reported for the stimulants: in two studies involving 105 hyperactive children treated with pemoline, 73 percent of the children improved, and in the remaining group the behavior either remained unchanged or worsened. In a carefully executed double-blind comparison of pemoline, methylphenidate, and placebo, Conners and Taylor (1980) obtained measures of home and school behavior, achievement, cognitive functioning, and global clinical status at four temporal points: baseline, midtreatment, end of treatment, and posttreatment, with the latter comparison being made after a two-week washout period. Both drugs produced approximately similar degrees of improvement in all areas except the achievement measures, where there was a trend towards pemoline being slightly less effective overall. On the global ratings 90 percent of the subjects on methylphenidate and 88 percent of those on pemoline were improved, as compared to 34 percent of the placebo group. The placebo figure is particularly interesting, and adds to the validity of the increasing investigative attention being paid to the analysis of supposedly "simple" placebo effects. Also of interest was the finding that improvement, particularly as rated by parents, persisted during the 2-week washout period for children receiving pemoline, but not for those on methylphenidate. This finding suggests that pemoline, a slow starter, may also have long-acting effects when the drug is withdrawn. Experimenters whose designs involve intraindividual rotation of a series of different drugs over a period of time should ensure that the design accommodates this characteristic where pemoline is involved. Data reported by Dykman, McGrew, Harris, Peters, and Ackerman (1976) indicated that, in terms of average group performance, methylphenidate was more effective then pemoline on a variety of measures including teacher ratings and Continuous Performance Test scores. However, when individual rather than group scores were examined, it appeared that pemoline was the superior drug for *some* children.

Despite its positive features, pemoline has not been widely used to treat hyperactivity, although the Food and Drug Administration did approve its use with children (Cylert Monograph, 1975). The reasons for the relatively low usage may be related to the delayed onset effect and the consequent less dramatic improvement. Pemoline is available only in liquid form, which pediatricians and parents regard as less convenient, and it is more costly than the other stimulants. In most studies, pemoline has not proven to be quite as effective as the more widely used of the stimulants. In addition, experienced clinicians (e.g., Cantwell, 1979) feel that as a general rule an established drug that has been in use for a significant period of time should be prescribed before a newer drug, unless there is overwhelming evidence of the latter's clinical superiority.

Tricyclic Antidepressants

The tricyclics are chemically somewhat similar to the phenothiazines and share some of their properties. Included in this group are imipramine (Tofranil), amitriptyline (Elavil), and desipramine (Pertofran), with imipramine being the most widely used with hyperactive children. The tricyclics are of some value in the management of hyperactivity in that they reduce activity level, decrease misbehavior, and have a stimulant-like effect on vigilance (by increasing it) and impulsivity (by decreasing it). However, these effects are less predictable and less striking than those achieved with the stimulants. Imipramine has been reported to be effective in from 45 to 85 percent of cases, depending on the dosage used (Cantwell, 1978a). At one time relatively high doses (14 mg/kg per day) were considered to be safe for children. The prevalence and severity of side effects, which *medically* were considered insufficient to arouse concern, consisted primarily of effects such as drowsiness, weight loss, stomach aches, irritability, nausea, mild depression, and sweating (Greenberg, Yellin, Spring, & Metcalf, 1975; Rapoport, Mikkelsen, & Werry, 1978; Rapoport, Quinn, Bradbard, Riddle, & Brooks, 1974), with some clinical support for a reduction of side effects with divided doses. In the past decade, however, there has been increasing evidence of vulnerability of children to the tricyclics, especially with the high doses that were frequently being used. It has now been unequivocally established that these doses can produce serious side effects including seizures (Brown, Winsberg, Bialer, & Press, 1973; Petti & Campbell, 1975) and cardiotoxicity (Martin & Zaug, 1975; Winsberg, Goldstein, Yepes, & Perel, 1975), with one reported instance of sudden death in a 6-year-old girl following a bedtime dose of 14 mg/kg for school phobia (Saraf, Klein, Gittelman-Klein, & Groff, 1974). The usual starting dosage now with the hyperactive child is around 1 mg/kg, with an upper daily dose limit of 5 mg/kg (Hayes, Panitch, & Barker, 1975). If the drug is effective and if the appropriate dosage is prescribed, an improvement in response becomes evident the next day (Cantwell, 1978).

The tricyclic antidepressants are useful in the management of some hyperactive children. For example, Werry, Aman, and Diamond (1980) conducted a crossover study with 30 hyperactive children using 0.4 mg/kg methylphenidate as a standard in comparison with two doses of imipramine (1 mg/kg and 2 mg/kg), and demonstrated positive effects of imipramine on learning, motor performance, and social behavior. However, the fact that they have the potential to be life-threatening requires particular caution and makes mandatory continual medical surveillance in their usage. The Food and Drug Administration, which has specified 5 mg/kg daily as the maximum allowable clinical dose of imipramine in children, advises electrocardiogram monitoring as this level is reached (Rapoport & Mikkelsen, 1978).

Antipsychotics

The antipsychotics are classified by their chemical structure into five groups, those of interest here being the phenothiazines and the butyrophenones. The phenothiazines were first used around 1950 and have since become the best understood and most widely used of the antipsychotics (Winsberg & Yepes, 1978). Those that have occasionally proven effective in the treatment of hyperactive children are thioridazine (Mellaril) and chlorpromazine (Thorazine).

Most commonly used of the butyrophenones is haloperidol (Haldol), which has been reported as effective in modifying the target symptoms of hyperactivity and aggressivity (Ayd, 1972; Werry, Aman, & Lampen, 1976). These two groups of antipsychotics do sometimes prove effective in the treatment of hyperactive children (e.g., Gittelman-Klein, Klein, Katz, Saraf, & Pollack, 1976; Werry, Weiss, Douglas, & Martin, 1966), but in terms of comparative frequency of use they fall far behind the central nervous system stimulants. They have a wide range of side effects such as drowsiness, blurring of vision, dry mouth, stomach aches, irritability, excitability, depression, enuresis, and increased appetite (Gittelman-Klein et al., 1976), and carry some risk of depressing higher central nervous system functions such as attention and cognition (Werry & Aman, 1975). The average daily dosages of chlorpromazine and thioridazine for children are 3 to 6 mg/kg; the dosages of haloperidol are 0.1 to 0.3 mg/kg (Winsberg & Yepes, 1978). In one of the most careful studies to date, Werry et al., (1976) found haloperidol to be as clinically effective as methylphenidate at a low dosage of 0.025 mg/kg. However, when the dose was increased to 0.05 mg/kg, there was a marked increase in minor side effects and some depression of cognitive functioning. Despite this negative effect, haloperidol was the drug of choice, in both dosages, for parents in this study, and in the low dosage for psychiatrists in it. Teachers preferred methylphenidate.

CATALYTIC DEVELOPMENTS

In any field of scientific endeavor, advances or developments can be categorized in terms of breadth of impact, a concept referring to their potential for diversity rather than to magnitude of importance. Some advances are self-contained by virtue of the boundaries set by the research topic itself; others, with fewer such boundaries, have the potential to generate many new directions of research and clinical activity, and consequently to redirect the focus of established investigative areas. Several developments of the past five years fit readily into the latter category and may prove to be catalysts in the pursuit of knowledge concerning the psychotropic drugs of relevance to hyperactivity. One such event is the sudden influx of a substantial number of hyperactive adults into a hitherto almost exclusively pediatric domain. Another is the renaissance in medicine and the behavioral sciences of the placebo as a potential therapeutic agent in its own right. A third is the dispensing of the misconception that stimulants act selectively only in the hyperactive child. We will briefly discuss the implications of each of these developments for progress in the understanding of drug therapy in hyperactivity.

Hyperactive Adults

The finding in the mid-1970s that hyperactivity is not time limited to either childhood or adolescence but may persist with changing symptomatology into young adulthood has precipitated a need for appropriate treatment regimens for these adult patients, who differ in important respects from hyperactive adolescents and children. The response of the clinical and research establishments to this challenge has been impressive. In 1978, when the existence of substantial numbers of hyperactive adults had barely been documented, Bellak (1979) convened a conference on hyperactivity in adulthood that culminated in an excellent and comprehensive text, a feature of which was the inclusion of stimulating informal discussions by the participants, in addition to the presentation of formal papers. Among the participants in this landmark conference were L. Eugene Arnold, Barry Borland, Jonathan Cole, Donald Gallant, Peter Hartocollis, Hans Huessy, and Paul Wender. In the research domain there is already a cluster of well-designed studies on the successful use of drug treatment with small groups of hyperactive adults (Mann & Greenspan, 1976; Wender, Reimherr, & Wood, 1981; Wood, Reimherr, Wender, & Johnson, 1976) that are notable for their detailed discussions of individual cases, acknowledgment of the heterogeneity of hyperactive adults and emphasis on it, and concern for accuracy in interpreting treatment effects. For example, Wood et al. (1976) refuted the possibility that hyperactivity in adults could be a residual of childhood learning, and Wender et al. (1981) then replicated the Wood et al. (1976) study, substituting pemoline for the methylphenidate used in the earlier study because of concern that the findings might have been a methylphenidate-induced euphoriant effect as easily achieved with substances such as alcohol or heroin.

The major impact of this small but unusually superior body of literature on hyperactivity in adulthood lies in the clinical questions and research problems that have been delineated. It is clear, for example, that the heterogeneity of hyperactive adults will require that diagnostic criteria more restrictive than those used to date be formulated (Cole, 1980). Detailed and explicit reports from hyperactive adults have raised, among other interesting questions, the possibility that the emotional lability of childhood, a symptom viewed as relatively unimportant in hyperactive children, may in fact be a precursor of adult depression. Although drug dosage is problematic, the bulk of opinion leans towards a diminishing dosage with increasing age; adding weight to this view is the anecdotal evidence of a potential for addiction. One intriguing characteristic of the hyperactive adult group is noncompliance even to effective drug regimens. This problem is becoming increasingly common in adults in general, but in the case of hyperactive adults Preis and Huessy (1979) attribute it to a basic reluctance and inability to cope with the flood of stimulant-induced emotions that are new to the hyperactive adult. These topics as areas of research focus have considerable potential in relation to the diagnosis and treatment of adult hyperactivity; they may also cast new light on the arena of childhood hyperactivity.

The Placebo Potential

The placebo has long been taken for granted as a clinical and research tool. Clinicians have used it as a measure of untreated baseline effects (Werry, 1977), to determine if medication can be discontinued, and to prevent self-fulfilling prophecies in parents (Kløve, 1978; O'Leary & Borkovec, 1978; Sleator, von Neumann, & Sprague, 1974); researchers have depended on placebo controls in double-blind procedures and have shown considerable ingenuity in efforts to ensure the credibility of placebo conditions. Swanson, Kinsbourne, Roberts, and Zucker (1978) used identical gelatin casings for methylphenidate and placebo capsules in order to eliminate a slight difference in taste; the Nutrition Foundation prepared seemingly identical challenge and control cookies for Feingold diet research (Swanson & Kinsbourne, 1980a), and Loney and Milich (1978) developed a credible placebo tape for their studies of operant behavior intervention. Despite these instances of concern about credibility, rarely is any interest shown in establishing the validity of double-blind procedures; when such checks are made the results are disheartening. Physicians conducting drug assessment accurately distinguished between medication and placebo 74 percent of the time in one study (Werry & Sprague, 1974) and from 80 to 100 percent in another (Weiss, Minde, Douglas, Werry, & Sykes, 1971). Furthermore, in an unnerving number of instances parents, teachers, and hyperactive children are able to identify the placebo condition, and consequently the validity of placebo-controlled double-blind data becomes suspect. In specific instances this breaking the blind phenomenon can be attributed to factors such as subtle behavior cues on the part of the investigator or clinician, inadequate placebos (Blumenthal, Burke, & Shapiro, 1974), and other variables amenable to control. Some investigators have speculated that the possibility of two sets of effects in the subject on medication (direct and side effects) makes breaking the blind a fairly easy accomplishment even for the relatively unsophisticated observer. Routh (1978, p. 24) has proposed an ingenious solution that would eliminate one of these sets of potential cues, namely, replacing the totally inactive placebo with one that mimics the stimulants' side effects. This suggestion warrants research attention.

The first empirical test of the credibility of the placebo with hyperactive children has been conducted by Henker, Whalen and Collins (1979) within the context of a classroom research program. The major placebo-related concerns were, first, to determine whether nonmedical observers were as able as physicians in detecting placebos, and second, to compare ratings made by observers who were unaware that a medication study was in progress (triple-blind conditions) with those of observers who knew the general design of the study (double-blind conditions) and could be expected to be alert to medication-related changes. A study in which a substantial number of observers is unaware that a research project is in progress is a rarity, and is a measure of the skill, particularly in respect to the concern for validity, that is characteristic of Whalen, Henker, and their colleagues. The patterns of ratings for double-blind and triple-blind raters were identical, which could imply that positive stimulant effects are not attributable to rater sensitization concerning the purpose of the study. It could also mean that the double-blind raters were more highly trained than is often the case on research projects. A subgroup of the double-blind observers who were asked to *guess* the children's medication status were correct more often than would be expected on the basis of chance, averaging a 66 percent accuracy rate. Henker et al. concluded that in this instance medication guesses were based on direct effects, such as cognitive performance and social behavior, because there was no opportunity for the observers to see evidence of the most common side effects such as anorexia and insomnia. This conclusion is questionable, because less common side effects, such as irritability and tearfulness, could have influenced their guesses. Further research on the topic of clues in breaking the blind would have clinical as well as methodological value. One topic that should be investigated is the hyperactive child's ability to accurately distinguish between active medication and placebo. In a study by Dalby, Kapelus, Swanson, Kinsbourne, and Roberts (1978) hyperactive children's predictions were no better than chance. Yet interview data (Henker & Whalen, 1980b) suggest that hyperactive children do recognize differences between the medicated and nonmedicated state.

In the past decade the medical status of the placebo has changed from that of a lightly regarded psychological prop to a potential treatment tool (Bok, 1974; Vogel, Goodwin, & Goodwin, 1980). The possibility that the placebo could play a therapeutic role in the management of hyperactivity merits serious research attention. Two rather disparate facts are pertinent here: one is that as many as 40 percent of untreated hyperactive children respond favorably to a trial of placebo (Werry, 1977); the other is that medical research on pain and other topics has demonstrated conclusively that the placebo is an authentic therapeutic agent capable of altering body chemistry. In some pain patients, for example, the use of a placebo triggers the brain to release pain-fighting chemicals called endorphins, with a consequent suppression of pain. The fact that the placebo-induced benefits disappear immediately following the injection of nalaxone (a substance known to block the action of morphine and related agents), coupled with other placebo responders-nonresponders differences, suggests that the placebo has, in a sense, "tricked" the brain into producing endorphins (Levine, 1978). The question that we are raising is: What biochemical differences, if any, distinguish between hyperactive children who respond favorably to placebo and those who do not? If differences are present, could these naturally occurring substances be of therapeutic value in hyperactivity?

Animal Models and the Paradoxical Issue

The Rapoport et al. (1978) demonstration that the response to stimulants is not paradoxical has important implications for several spheres of clinical and research activity. The data firmly refute the validity of attaching diagnostic significance to a positive drug response. They also suggest that biochemical abnormalities such as dopamine depletion (Shaywitz, Yager, & Klopper, 1976) are not essential for explaining stimulant effects in hyperactive children, although the possibility remains that such abnormalities do exist. Some problems are created for the Shaywitz et al. dopamine depletion model; this model has focused on similarities of stimulant effects in hyperactive children and dopamine-depleted rats, with stimulants reducing hyperactivity in both groups; it has also focused on nonhyperactive children and normal developing rats, with stimulants exacerbating activity level in the rats just as the paradoxical response effect prior to the Rapoport et al. demonstration would have predicted for normal human subjects.

The newly demonstrated diversity of effects in the Rapoport et al. study underscores the importance of the caveat (Sprague & Berger, 1980, p. 171) that if the purpose of an animal model is to serve as a research tool for understanding some of the basic mechanisms of the disorder and its treatments, then it is essential that the model share common salient features of that disorder. Animal models of hyperactivity, for example, should reflect in some manner characteristics such as attentional deficits, impulsivity, and aggressiveness, in addition to hyperactivity. The Shaywitz et al. model and other models such as the Silbergeld model of lead-induced hyperactivity (Silbergeld & Goldberg, 1973, 1974) have tended to focus primarily on activity level. These models could absorb the discrepancies in human-nonhuman activity level responses to stimulants *only* if similarities across the human-animal groups could be demonstrated in other hyperactivity-related behaviors. This restrictive condition greatly limits their applicability as functioning models. A valid animal model of several behavioral aspects of hyperactivity is within the realm of possibility, however. With a septal lesion procedure Gorenstein and Newman (1980) have produced a syndrome in animals that bears a fundamental resemblance across several important dimensions of psychological functioning to human disinhibitory psychopathology. These dimensions include avoidance learning, anticipation of noxious events, inhibition of appetitive responding, stimulation seeking, and mediation of temporal intervals.

Although the findings of Rapoport et al. (1978) that normal and hyperactive children respond similarly to stimulants creates problems for animal models, the similarities in their two groups' responses may also facilitate the development of such models. As Sprague and Berger (1980) have noted, the similarities in stimulant response of hyperactive and nonhyperactive children suggest that it may be possible to derive animal models that use *normal* rather than brain-damaged animals.

CHAPTER 7

Psychotherapy

Psychotherapy is a nonspecific descriptor for a diverse group of techniques that are designed to facilitate the individual's acceptance of his behavior, as well as to modify or eliminate behavior that is creating interpersonal difficulties, is potentially harmful to the individual or others, or deviates markedly from accepted social and ethical norms. The term *psychotherapy* is generally limited to therapeutic procedures that have been developed or implemented by a professionally trained person such as a psychiatrist or psychologist; it conveys no information about the severity of the maladaptive behavior, the duration or intensity of the treatment process, or the theoretical background and affiliation of the therapist (Kovel, 1976). Included under this heading are such diverse treatment procedures as psychoanalysis, hypnosis, operant conditioning, modeling, biofeedback, paradoxical intervention, and psychodrama (Robitscher, 1980).

Two fundamentally different approaches, traditional psychotherapy and behavior therapy, have dominated the field of psychotherapy. The differences between the two approaches center around their conceptualizations of the nature of man and his problems, which in turn determine the therapeutic processes used, the agents of change, and the nature of the therapist–client relationship (Karasu, 1977). *Traditional psychotherapy* is based on a psychoanalytic or medical model that embraces the disease concept of behavior abnormalities (Engel, 1977). According to this concept, abnormalities of behavior are symptoms of an underlying psychic disturbance or neurosis. The therapist's task is to identify the underlying cause of the behavior and modify or eliminate the behavior by effecting changes in the intrapsychic organization of the individual through the restructuring of some of his internal mediating processes. Central to the disease concept is the assumption that long-term benefits from treatment can only be achieved if the individual gains some understanding of the psychic forces that underlie his maladaptive behavior. Hence the development of insight is considered to be of critical importance to outcome.

Behavior therapy can be distinguished from the traditional psychotherapies by its emphasis on observable phenomena in guiding diagnosis and treatment, rather than on inferred processes. Birk (1978) attributes this difference to the fact that the behavior therapies have evolved from the ideas and methods of three major research traditions: the work of Wolpe (1958), Lazarus (1971), and Rachman (e.g., Rachman, Hodgson, & Marks, 1971) with its emphasis on counterconditioning strategies in treatment; the research on operant conditioning of Skinner and his associates (Lindsley & Skinner, 1954; Skinner, 1953) with its insistence on analysis and contingency control of the clinical situation; and the less well known but very important contribution of a group at the Maudsley Hospital headed by Shapiro (1961) and his colleague Isaac Marks (1976) which emphasized the value of the single-subject study of treatment. All behavior therapies have a number of characteristics in common. They all emphasize current behavior problems and attach little importance to the client's history and family background; concepts such as insight are viewed as unnecessary, as are the use of labels and diagnostic categories; observable phenomena are the major focus in the evaluation of intervention; and the goal is a short treatment period (Bandura, 1969; Bergin & Garfield, 1971; Mash & Dalby, 1979). At the same time, the behavior therapies differ on several major dimensions, including the extent to which they reflect a learning theory approach, the amount of training required for their effective use, the degree of involvement of agents of socialization such as parents, and duration of treatment.

In the first half of this century the proponents of these two conceptually different approaches to the modification of behavior were polarized, with each faction strongly rejecting the viewpoint of the other. Traditional psychotherapy was firmly entrenched and its advocates were scornful of the sporadic and unsuccessful attempts of behavior therapists to put therapeutic procedures on a more objective base. However, the next two decades saw a sustained attack on traditional psychotherapy. Concomitantly, a series of publications such as Eyesenck's (1960) text, *Behavior therapy and the neuroses,* and empirical demonstrations of reinforcement and other procedures for effecting behavior change strengthened the position of behavior therapy. Rotter (1954) outlined a therapeutic approach that incorporated many of the procedures and viewpoints that were to appear later in contemporary behavior therapy, including self-reinforcement and the differential reinforcement of related operants, as well as the need to consider client cognitions and to extrapolate from empirical findings to the treatment situation.

By the late 1960s behavior therapy had become an accepted and important area of psychotherapy, one reason being the development of therapeutic approaches that proved effective with behavior problems that previously had defied treatment. In the 1970s a task force appointed by the American Psychiatric Association evaluated the achievements and potential of the behavioral approach. Its report, *Behavior therapy in psychiatry* (1973), concluded that behavior therapy had much to offer informed clinicians in the service of modern clinical and social psychiatry (Birk, 1978). New models of behavior influence were proposed, which served to expand the scope and applicability of behavior therapy. The unidirectional theory of control (Skinner, 1969) was replaced by one stressing bidirectional influences (Bandura, 1974), and more emphasis was placed on the role of cognition and regulatory processes in effecting behavior change (Meichenbaum, 1977).

Concomitantly, the polarization lessened as members of both groups began to acknowledge the validity of some of the criticisms leveled against them. Traditional psychotherapists became more outspoken about the misuses of existing techniques and weaknesses in treatment as well as training methods (e.g., Abramowitz, 1976; Engel, 1977; Robitscher, 1980); behavioral therapists expressed increasingly sharp criticism of shortcomings, misuses, and limitations of the paradigm of behavioral intervention (Mash & Dalby, 1979; McNamara, 1980). For the first time, there was sporadic speculation on the possibility of an integration of traditional psychotherapy and behavior therapy (Wachtel, 1977). A rapprochement is occurring, for example, in the domain of family therapy (Allmond, Buckman, & Gofman, 1979; Framo, 1979; Patterson, 1971; Weakland, 1979; Werry, 1979). However, the great majority of clinicians see little prospect of genuine integration (e.g., Levis, 1970; Sloane, Staples, Cristal, Yorkston, & Whipple, 1975). As a result, there continues to be a wide range of therapeutic approaches to the modification of behavior problems. From this range we will briefly describe a representative group of methods relevant to the treatment of hyperactivity; relevance is defined here as having proven effective in treating hyperactivity, or clearly having the potential to do so.

TRADITIONAL THERAPIES

Individual Psychotherapy

The potential of individual or, for that matter, group or family psychotherapy for the treatment of hyperactivity has received little recognition in the hyperactivity literature. Some authors (e.g., Casey, 1977; Renshaw, 1974) omit any mention of psychotherapy in the treatment regime, while others (Gross & Wilson, 1974; Werry, 1968; Werry & Sprague, 1970) mention it only briefly or with reservations (Levitt, 1971; Prout, 1977; Stewart & Olds, 1973; Wender, 1971). The downgrading of psychotherapy as a useful form of intervention in hyperactivity has a historical as well as a current base. In 1957, and again in 1963, Levitt published extensive reviews showing that psychotherapy as practiced in child guidance or psychiatric clinics was not effective in the treatment of any kind of psychopathology in children; in 1961 Eisenberg, Gilbert, Cytryn, and Molling published a methodologically weak study suggesting that hyperactive children do not benefit from therapeutic intervention. Despite the many valid criticisms of these two sets of work, they formed the cornerstone for the antipsychotherapy position. At the present time, the short-term efficacy of stimulant medication and behavior modification has further convinced many clinicians that psychotherapy is not essential in the treatment program despite the fact that secondary symptoms are almost always present even with an optimum response to the drug regimen.

A second group (Cantwell, 1979; Gardner, 1975; Safer & Allen, 1976; Satterfield, Cantwell, & Satterfield, 1979) advocates psychotherapeutic treatment as an essential adjunct to other forms of intervention. Whereas these latter forms, primarily stimulant medication, focus on the primary symptoms that make life miserable for the child, psychotherapy here is concerned with the secondary symptoms such as poor self-esteem, feelings of depression, and problems in peer interaction. Some within this group see hyperactivity as a basic problem with an emotional overlay (Cornwall & Freeman, 1980). The emotional components manifested in the child's conception of himself and his world interact with the behavioral problem, so that there are two major aspects to be treated, the hyperactivity itself and the emotional problem, and this latter problem is best treated with psychotherapy. Several respected investigators have emphasized the salient role of emotional factors as causes or effects in childhood hyperactivity and have noted that these factors are often overlooked or underestimated in the diagnostic and treatment processes (e.g., Chess, 1960; Childers, 1935; Cornwall & Freeman, 1980). A small subgroup assigns the emotional aspect greater importance: Miller (1978a) regards hyperactivity as primarily an emotional problem, and, more extremely, Sandberg, Rutter, and Taylor (1978) and Shaffer and Greenhill (1979) believe that all of the so-called hyperactivity symptoms can be symptoms of purely emotional disorders, thus questioning the existence of hyperactivity per se.

The belief that psychotherapy should be an integral part of treatment for the hyperactive child has evolved from clinical observation as well as empirical investigation. Hyperactivity often continues to be a problem into adulthood (Borland & Heckman, 1976; Weiss & Hechtman, 1979; Wood, Reimherr, Wender, & Johnson, 1976) and, if left untreated, can lead to serious social and psychiatric problems which may be more difficult to correct than the primary symptoms; as Cantwell (1979) has pointed out, early psychotherapy may minimize hard-to-treat sequelae. The hyperactive child often causes marital and family disharmony (Barkley, 1978) which may be minimized or averted by therapeutic intervention. On the empirical front, it has been established that drugs and behavior modification procedures do not have positive long-term effects on either academic or social functioning (Barkley, 1978; Loney, 1980a), so that without the help of psychotherapy the child is left to muddle along as best as he can in the face of an escalating mass of problems.

Although many hyperactive children are referred to child psychotherapists, there are few articles in the hyperactivity literature on the treatment of these children. Anderson (1970) has described in some detail a therapeutic-learning program that deals concurrently with the emotional problems and the child's behavior and learning disorders. The program, which is essentially an Adlerian approach, is based on the assumption that substantial attention must be focused on the emotional component of the problem for intervention to be successful. According to this viewpoint repeated negative experiences in the

child's major social environments cause him to develop compensatory mechanisms such as incompetency, negative-attention-getting behavior, power, and
revenge, all of which are based on exploitation and directed towards useless
goals. The child finds he can gain both position and status through his learning disorder, and his behavior in any therapeutic program reflects these useless goals. The hyperactive child learns to use his restlessness to gain attention
and avoid work assignments and, as a result, resists intervention designed to
teach him more desirable response patterns that would result in a loss of
status.

One of the more prolific contributors to the literature on psychotherapy for
the hyperactive child is Gardner (1975) whose approach relies primarily on
the child gaining a greater appreciation of reality rather than on working towards the development of insight. To this end he uses reality confrontation
and appeal to conscious control, sometimes by means of dramatization of the
therapeutic communications. The therapeutic message may be presented or
reiterated in the form of audio and video tape recordings or as allegorical
communication at the primary process level. Gardner's (1974) conviction that
the child may be more receptive to the therapist's communications when these
are transmitted allegorically, rather than conveyed in undisguised form, led to
the development of his Mutual Story Telling technique. In this technique the
therapist elicits a self-created story from the child, surmises its psychologically
dynamic meaning, decides which elements are pathological manifestations,
and then uses the same characters in a similar setting to tell the child a story
of his own in which he introduces more adaptive resolutions of the issues in
the child's story. The child's verbal output plays an important role in this
technique, as does the therapist's ability to reconstruct the child's conflicts
and problems in a more therapeutic way.

Freeman and Cornwall (1980) have reported the successful treatment of
children having various manifestations of hyperactivity with long-term insight-oriented psychotherapy and, in two cases, with psychoanalysis. In each
of the five cases reported, the effect of this intervention was to relieve the
emotional distress and, in so doing, to reduce the importance and impact of
the hyperactivity rather than to modify the hyperactivity directly. The following is a brief summary of one of the five cases (Freeman & Cornwall, 1980,
pp. 708–709.).

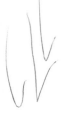

Case 4. John A. Fowler, M.D., in an unpublished manuscript, described Kent, a
boy who had been thoroughly evaluated and diagnosed at age nine as having the
hyperkinetic syndrome and treated for a year successfully with dextroamphetamine. Kent entered analysis when he was 12. Although he was still hyperactive,
impulsive, distractible, and excitable, the emphasis had shifted to his possessive-
ness of his mother, teasing his sisters and peers, overt rivalry with his father,
conscious sexual conflicts, and temper outbursts, all accompanied by inner turmoil, anxiety, and guilt. The interview material clearly showed the interaction
between the traumatic life experiences, ego development, and biologically deter-

mined hyperactivity. Specifically, the hyperactivity related to two distinct levels of conflict. At the age of nine, Kent was still trying to deal with the frightening death of a younger sister from a chronic illness when he was 33 months old. He felt guilty and afraid over this traumatic loss, both as it affected him from his own observations of the death scene, and from the effect it had on his relationship with his parents during the sister's illness and after her death. The other conflicts that became involved in the hyperactivity were of an oedipal nature, with the erotic wish for his mother, and rivalry with and fear of his father. They involved his relationships with all of the important family members. The analytic work did not in itself appreciably change Kent's level of activity, but his activity became more directed and purposeful. He had resolved most of his major conflicts, was relatively free of symptoms, and was developing well as a teenager, with age-appropriate interests, goals, and relationships.*

Group Psychotherapy

For the hyperactive child, group psychotherapy can provide important additional benefits of an interpersonal nature not available in the individual therapy situation. When the two forms of treatment are combined, they make a powerful combination. The group psychotherapy situation provides a peer group that is a reasonably close approximation of a real-life peer group, but one that in addition meets some of the specific needs of the hyperactive child. As such, it is an ideal context for effecting behavioral change. Often this group is the first same-age peer group to offer social psychological acceptance to the child, and sometimes friendships extend beyond the group sessions. Most therapy groups are formed along selective lines of similarity of age, sex, and problem. Seeing that there are other children like him with the same problems has several important effects on the hyperactive child. It alleviates the feelings of loneliness and isolation that so often beset him. For the first time he sees other children exhibiting the same kinds of behavior that in the past have resulted in his being reprimanded and derogated, and this low-threat self-confrontation experience helps him to see himself as others in his own environment—his parents, teachers, siblings, peers—see him. Often he comes to realize just how annoying, disruptive, and inappropriate some of his behavior is. [In this connection, Waxer (1977) recommends having videotape feedback of these sequences.] At the same time, the group situation, with its relatively uncritical audience and the presence of a skilled mediator, provides optimum conditions for practicing newly acquired interaction skills. It is no wonder that when the time comes to leave the group many parents report that their child is desolated, saying, "They're the only friends I've ever had."

*From Freeman, D. F., and Cornwall, T. P. Hyperactivity and neurosis. *American Journal of Orthopsychiatry*, 1980, *50* (1), 704–711. Reprinted, with permission, from the *American Journal of Orthopsychiatry*. Copyright 1980 by the American Orthopsychiatric Association, Inc.

In the typical group therapy configuration one or more therapists treat six to eight hyperactive children simultaneously. The most frequent meeting pattern is two one-hour meetings a week, with an average of about 20 meetings. Usually there are no additions to the group after the first meeting because of the possible disruptive effect of introducing new members into an established group, and no visitors are permitted. At first a therapy group is bound together only by their common meeting place and their relationship to the therapist; peer relationships are usually nonexistent. An important task for the therapist is to foster rewarding peer relationships, because the therapy experience will be of little value to the children if the group is not important to its members (Yalom, 1975). A good therapist will support the children's efforts to become acquainted and, ideally, to make friends, and help them to identify the reasons for their difficulties in relating to each other. At the same time he will intervene when necessary to protect members from destructive attacks, clarify attitudes and feelings, and maintain an emotional climate that will encourage spontaneous comments by the group (Slavson & Schiffer, 1974). The most favorable outcomes and the fewest dropouts occur in groups in which the therapist maintains a delicate balance between the amount of authority he exercises and the structure and stimulation he provides. Also important is the therapist's skill in moving the dialogue along (Grunebaum & Solomon, 1980).

Although there are several excellent review articles (Abramowitz, 1976; Meissner & Nicholi, 1978; Wodarski, Feldman, & Flax, 1974) and texts (Garfield & Bergin, 1978; Slavson & Schiffer, 1974; Wolberg, Aronson, & Wolberg, 1977; Yalom, 1975) on group psychotherapy with children, relatively few studies on this technique have been published since Slavson (1943) first introduced it as a method for treating children. Among published studies empirical data are rare and, in the case of group psychotherapy with hyperactive children, almost nonexistent. In her review of the efficacy of this technique with children, Abramowitz (1976) reports one study by Barcai and Robinson (1969) in which hyperactive preadolescent children in a conventional group therapy situation were compared to those in an art activity group. On the basis of teacher evaluations the subjects in group therapy were judged to be more improved.

Wright and McKenzie (1973) have presented an interesting and detailed account of discussion group therapy for five 10- and 11-year-old hyperactive boys in a residential treatment center. The course of development from an aggregate of five boys, through the emergence of interpersonal conflict to a true, fairly harmonious peer group, is described in detail for each of the 30 sessions. The rationale for discussion rather than activity for this particular group was that discussion is more likely to avoid overstimulation, and more emphasis can be placed on the interpretation of group feelings and processes. No outcome measures were used but there appears to be little doubt that the boys benefited markedly from the therapeutic experience. The following quote gives some of the flavor of the sessions (Wright & McKenzie, 1973, p. 3):

The therapists began the first session by telling the group it would be a talking group this year and every one was to remain seated. As the session progressed, the children gradually became wild and hyperactive, knocking chairs over, screaming and hitting, and totally disregarding the initial instructions. Since it was impossible to get the attention of the group, each member was asked individually what he would do to make it a talking group. Their suggestions were quickly put together in the form of: "The group decided to take turns talking but Jack is talking out of turn, what does the group want to do about that?" Immediate silence followed each time this technique was used. Finally the group was able to continue the talking without total disruption. . . . Another technique was the reinforcement of suggestions; for example, Peter suggested that to maintain order we use the system of raising our hands and when the hands went up the mouths would go shut. . . . All the children agreed except Jack. The therapist singled out Jack by saying, "Everyone is putting their hand up and look! There is one person not with the group. Robert, how do you feel about Jack not being in the group?" This method quickly brought about control. None of the children wanted to be the object of disapproval of their peers. Later, during the first session one member began fighting, but the therapist immediately interrupted it by saying, "Now we have one member of the group starting to fight, after the group voted against that."

The last half of the session the group discussed having a treat at the end of each session. They discussed other topics such as persons who steal and persons who tell lies. Some wanted to have a photography club and they all wanted to listen to the tape at the end of the session. The later part of the session was orderly and conducive for discussion.*

Family Therapy

Family therapy represents a new way of approaching the problem behavior of the individual child in that the object of therapy is the family rather than the child. As a result, a basic redefinition of the therapeutic task is required (Kovel, 1976). In this framework the family is viewed as a small, powerful, intricate, interdependent, dynamic, social interaction system with its own unique set of myths, rules, and communication networks as well as problems. When this system is ignored treatment is likely to be undermined because the family tends not only to resist changes in individual members but also to prescribe members' behavior to adapt to the needs of the system (Framo, 1979; Watzlawick, Weakland, & Fisch, 1974). Symptoms seen as puzzling in individual psychotherapy take on new meaning when they are considered within the context of the family (Framo, 1979) because in the former case, only a part of the total problem is visible; often the basis for what appears to be solely the child's problem exists at least subclinically in one or more other family mem-

*Reprinted by permission from Wright, L. S., and McKenzie, C. D. A talking group therapy for hyperactive 11 year old boys. *Devereux Schools Forum*, 1973, *8* (1), 1–24. Copyright 1972, The Devereux Foundation. *Forum*, Vol. 8, No. 1, Winter 1973.

bers and has been projected onto the child, who then serves as the scapegoat and becomes the symptom bearer of a family-wide disturbance. The basic premise underlying family therapy is that the family is a central force in maintaining or exacerbating behavior disorders such as hyperactivity (Cantwell, 1979), and consequently the best way to help the child is to help the whole family.

The therapist's task of analyzing the patterns of interaction within the family, identifying those processes that are causing or exacerbating the child's behavior problems, and determining how to change them is greatly facilitated by using the family therapy technique of bringing the entire family together in interviews with the therapist. This technique provides a wealth of information: the therapist can observe firsthand the reciprocal effects of the child's behavior problem and the family's pattern of response to it and can arrive at a tentative estimate of the family's motivation and capacity for change. Over a series of sessions seeing the family as a group is particularly useful for identifying the nonverbal communications such as derogation, pity, or dislike, which heighten the child's problems. Secondary gains that the child's symptoms provide for other members of the family, and for the child himself, also become apparent in the family sessions (Cantwell, 1979). One tendency noted by McDermott and Char (1974) is that the child's involvement may be somewhat superficial in that his symptoms are understood only from clichés and myths that avoid the complexity and multicausality of the behavior disorder. To counteract this tendency the therapist must elicit active and specific involvement from the child. One technique for achieving this goal (Villeneuve, 1979) consists of periodically including in family sessions concrete modes of expression and action-promoting procedures such as psychodrama that are perceived by the child as play or as similar to his daily activities. This technique, which is based on a developmental as well as a social system model, also helps the adults to see that they share the responsibility for change with their children. The utility of this technique is apparent in the following excerpt from a case study by Diller and Gofman (1981, p. 10):

> On one occasion the family was asked to draw together on the same large piece of paper, each using their own colored crayon. No other instructions were given for this family drawing. Jon's inability to control himself and his parents' lack of limit setting resulted in Jon literally invading Karen's [mother] and Harry's [older brother] spaces and drawing over their pictures. In a dramatic moment, Harry burst into tears and his parents realized they had done nothing to support Harry against Jon's invasions of his space, literally and metaphorically, a situation that occurred repeatedly at home. Karen was most affected and acted on her new understanding of the need for clearer boundaries. She began separating and setting limits for Jon more effectively.

For the hyperactive child, family therapy is often the optimum form of group therapy because it directly involves the group to which the child most urgently needs to adapt, that is, his own family. It is particularly effective in families in which the child's problem behavior is jeopardizing marital or family harmony. It encourages more mature relationships within the family, often in the form of greater individual freedom coexisting harmoniously with interdependence among the family group. Criticisms of this approach range from the extreme view applied to all therapies that any therapy is likely to have long-term effects on the participants (Hadley & Strupp, 1976; Werry, 1979) to the more manageable points concerning failure to document generality and duration of effects, comparative efficacy, and cost; and lack of a unifying theoretical base (Masten, 1979; McDermott & Harrison, 1977; Werry, 1979). Several critical review articles have appeared (Breunlin & Breunlin, 1979; Gurman & Kniskern, 1978; Masten, 1979; Schomer, 1978), as well as an excellent text for the clinican (Allmond et al., 1979). Evidence of increasing acceptance of this therapeutic approach by other schools of therapeutic thought comes from the partial resolution (Malone, 1979) of the polarization that has characterized the relationship between child psychiatry and family therapy (McDermott & Char, 1974) and from signs of increasing interest on the part of behavior therapists in family therapy (Patterson, 1971; Werry, 1979). The general consensus is that family therapy is as effective as the individual therapies and entails fewer risks (Fox, 1976; Framo, 1979; Gurman & Kniskern, 1978; Malone, 1979; Skynner, 1976).

Brief Therapy

Brief therapy is concerned with the resolution of present problems and has been described by Bellak and Small (1965) as a concentration on target symptoms. From the first of what usually is a therapeutic course of 15 or fewer sessions, this approach works toward direct, specific, and concrete goals. The criteria for the justification of brief therapy, the particular kind of client who is best suited to this short-term intervention technique, and contraindications for it have all received considerable attention in the literature from therapists representing a variety of schools of thought (Barten, 1971; Bellak & Small, 1965; Boileau, 1958; Clarkin, Frances, & Moodie, 1979; Eisenberg, 1975; Freudenberger, 1971; Meissner & Nicholi, 1978; Waxer, 1977).

A brief therapy procedure that focuses on present observable behavioral interaction and uses intervention to change the ongoing system has been developed by Weakland and his associates (Watzlawick, Weakland, & Fisch, 1974; Weakland, Fisch, Watzlawick, & Bodin, 1974) and used successfully with hyperactive children. Treatment is limited to 10 sessions and a 3-month follow-up. In this model the client's problem is viewed as a social phenomenon that reflects some dysfunction within the system of interaction and is best treated by effecting some change in that system. The two elements involved here are the observable behavior, and how it is labeled and judged by the patient or others involved with him. All behavior is viewed as being primarily maintained and structured by interaction between people, especially in the family system, but also in other systems, such as the school for children and work situations for adults. Within this view the question "What is wrong with a particular individual?" is largely irrelevant, as is the search for the root cause of the problem, which presumes a linear idea of causality that is not relevant in this approach. Problems are regarded primarily as outcomes of everyday difficulties, usually involving adaptation to an ordinary life change or transition, which have been mishandled by the parties involved. Mishandling may range from ignoring or denying difficulties on which action should be taken to attempts to actively resolve difficulties that need not or cannot be resolved, with a wide area in between where action is needed but the wrong kind is taken. When such ordinary difficulties are handled badly, things tend to snowball. Bad handling increases the difficulty, soon relabeled as a "problem," then is usually followed by more of the same inappropriate handling, leading to exacerbation or spread of the difficulty, so that originally minor or common life difficulties may readily lead on to serious symptomatology.

Accordingly, the central question in this approach is "What kinds of behavior in the ongoing system of interaction are functioning to maintain the behavior seen as constituting the problem?" The resolution of problems is seen as primarily requiring a change of the problem-maintaining behavior so that this destructive spiraling effect is interrupted. The general treatment procedure stems directly from these basic principles. First, the therapist inquires about the main problem or presenting complaint and attempts to get a clear statement of this in terms of specific concrete behavior. He next inquires about what the patient and others who are involved are doing to try to handle the problem, because these efforts are most likely to comprise the behaviors central to maintaining the problem. Then those who are involved are asked to state their *minimum* goal for the treatment, that is, what observable behavioral change would signify some success in the treatment. This important question is a difficult one for most patients, but change can be most easily effected if the goal is clearly stated and, though significant, is small. If a small but definite change is made in a major but seemingly hopeless problem, this is likely to initiate a beneficial circular effect and lead on to more progress, whereas pursuing vague or global goals is apt to lead only to uncertainty and frustration.

From the outset an attempt is made through attentive observation and listening to grasp each client's "language," the ideas and values that are central to him, because the therapist must perceive and make use of existing motivations and beliefs if he is to change behavior that the patient already considers is right and logical. When all these inquiries and observations have been made, the therapist plans a treatment strategy based on his own summarization of the problem. He concisely formulates the main presenting problem, identifies the behaviors that are central in maintaining it, decides on a goal of treatment, and estimates what concrete behavior would be the best sign of positive change. In general, the therapist will want to prevent the occurrence of the behavior seen as crucial to maintaining the problem, and often does this by substituting opposite behavior. This latter step is generally accomplished by reframing or redefining the problem situation in such a way that the original motives and beliefs of the persons involved will now lead to very different behavior. The following example (Weakland & Fisch, 1975) illustrates this brief therapy procedure with two boys aged 11 and 13 who had been diagnosed as hyperactive and who had both been on one or more medications for several years.

The basic core of procedures used were first, to define precisely the problem that had occasioned referral; next, to use the views and needs of the complainants (the parents) to redefine the whole problem situation and place the now exaggerated problem in a more realistic perspective, then to modify or eliminate the ineffective coping methods of the complainants; and finally, to implement new effective strategies of management of the children. The problem in this case was not the behavior of the boys but rather the parental evaluation of this behavior. The parents were showing exaggerated concern about their sons' misbehavior, which included disruptive classroom behavior, threats as well as one actual incident of aggression to the parents, poor academic performance, and disciplinary problems at home. None of these activities was viewed by the therapists as really serious. The parents' attempts to control their sons had escalated from verbal warning and harassment and repeated medical examinations to more extreme measures such as round-the-clock surveillance, with the reluctant cooperation of school personnel, finally culminating in the voluntary placement of the younger son in the care of juvenile probation authorities who were opposed to this action but were unable legally to refuse the placement. At this point the parents sought professional help.

The problem was largely resolved in 10 sessions by pursuing three lines of attack. First, to reassure the parents that the therapists did indeed appreciate the gravity of the situation a variant of paradoxical intervention was used, with the therapist suggesting that the parents were in fact minimizing the problem. This strategy had the effect of making the parents feel that at last someone finally understood their difficulties and they relaxed enough to agree to bring the younger son home. This move was justified to the parents as a way of establishing exactly how bad things were. Concomitantly, the therapist asked the parents to discontinue the boys' medications for a week and instructed the boys to "be themselves" for the next week. The week went far better than the parents had hoped and medication was permanently discontinued. Next, both parents, but particularly the father, were required to be firmer with the boys. The father was urged to use physical force as necessary to reassure the boys that he was strong enough to protect them should the need arise. Finally, the mother's belief that she had certain powers of extrasensory communication with her sons was capitalized on with the suggestion that this unusual power could be used to control the boys far more effectively than mere words, injunctions, nagging, and the like. As a result, the mother became more confident and less anxious, and was less of a chronic irritant to her sons. A 3-month follow-up showed that both boys had improved at home and school and, more important, the parents had begun to show a healthy interest in their own spheres of activity. Their social life, for example, had changed from what Weakland and Fisch described as "house arrest," due to their feeling that the boys required constant surveillance, to outside activities with friends.

Paradoxical Intervention

Therapists from a diverse group of clinical schools (e.g., Erickson, 1958; Fay, 1978; Gerz, 1966; Haley, 1963; Stampfl & Levis, 1967; Weakland, 1979) have used an intriguing therapeutic technique called paradoxical intervention. It is included here because it is particularly effective in eliminating some of the hyperactive child's most troubling problems, in terms of their visibility (Hare-Mustin, 1975, 1976). With this technique, the child is required to exhibit his misbehavior, to exaggerate it and become more proficient in it, rather than to eliminate it from his behavior repertoire. A frequent result of this manoeuver is the rapid disappearance of the behavior problem. The rationale for paradoxical intervention has been summarized as follows: The more a child tries to change his behavior, the more he is activating the processes that serve to maintain the behavior. The situation is exacerbated by family members or teachers who respond in error-activated ways whenever the specific misbehavior occurs. Even when the parents or teacher seek professional help, this often fails to resolve the problem because the family is able to induct the therapist into its patterns of interaction and communication and by doing so, renders the therapist ineffective in making change (Hare-Mustin, 1976). With paradoxical intervention the child is required to work actively at preserving the misbehavior, to practice it, and attempt to become more proficient at it. In effect, the therapist helps the child to bring under voluntary control a pattern of response that has been largely involuntary. At the same time, the therapist's matter-of-fact attitude serves to reduce the anxiety of the child and his parents concerning the misbehavior.

The efficacy of paradoxical intervention has been well documented in clinical reports (Gerz, 1966, Hare-Mustin, 1975, 1976; Raskin & Klein, 1976; Weakland & Fisch, 1975), but has only occasionally been evaluated empirically despite the theoretical and practical interest evoked by this technique. The reasons offered as explanations of its efficacy vary considerably, as Raskin and Klein (1976) have pointed out in their excellent review of the paradoxical intervention treatment, rationale, and controversies. Most commonly advanced are the following explanations. Within Hullian learning theory terms, massed practice of the misbehavior results in a buildup of response inhibition (a construct analogous to a form of psychological fatigue) that exceeds the strength of the response and results in its cessation. In this theory spontaneous recovery does occur; however, if the child performs the assignment as directed, frequent repetitions of the task performance–inhibition sequence make way for opportunities for other behavioral options such as the acquisition of more adaptive responses. Various explanations center around aspects of the scheduling of the misbehavior by the therapist. One idea is that this scheduling imposes a strain on the behavior by evoking it in a whole variety of stimulus settings, thereby weakening it. Because the value of the misbehavior lies in the control that the child is able to exert on others, prescribing it for a specific time and place undercuts this value. Further lessening of the satisfaction–reward occurs because much of the affect is missing when the misbehavior is unemotionally scheduled for a specific time and place. In addition, having it occur because the therapist requires it makes it into a different behavior and this, coupled with the tendency to resist the therapist, creates confusion by disrupting the child's usual pattern of behavior. The result is that the way is left open for new perceptions and positive changes to occur. Another explanation holds that scheduling the misbehavior serves to redefine it so that it becomes a form of treatment rather than a symptom. Once the child has implicitly agreed (through willingness to perform the misbehavior) that the therapist can make the behavior occur, he has committed himself to the possibility that the therapist can eradicate the misbehavior (Haley, 1963). The above explanations are not mutually exclusive but rather describe different facets of the complex paradoxical intervention situation. Consider them in relation to the following case report and also note the objective detachment of the therapist:

Peter, aged seven, had violent fits of temper whenever he could not have what he wanted. His well-meaning but incompetent parents acceded to all his demands but finally sought professional help when the situation became intolerable. Their therapist pointed out that the fits of temper were distressing, in part, because of their unpredictability so the first task would be to schedule them. In the first week, Peter was told that he could have as many temper outbursts as he wished but only between two and five o'clock in the afternnon, his worst time for such outbursts. In the second week, the temper hours were the same, but now a temper place, the second floor of the house, was specified. If Peter was out during the temper hours, he was to wait until he got home to have an outburst in the temper place. By the third week the frequency of the temper outbursts had diminished markedly. However, the therapist showed some displeasure at this reduction and instructed the baffled parents to see that Peter had at least one temper outburst a day, even if it meant calling him away from his playmates. At this point Peter rebelled and refused to come at "temper time." Therapy was discontinued for him and child-rearing counseling was started with the parents. Subsequent long-term checks showed only occasional temper outbursts.

We attribute the effectiveness of paradoxical intervention in part to the perspective that it provides for the child, and one that previously has been unavailable to him. This approach shows the child and his family the problem behavior at its worst and, in the process, provides them with a psychological baseline that specifies the degree of change that must occur for the particular behavior to become acceptable. Videotaping is of great value in this situation, but is not essential to it. We frequently have noticed that the child who is instructed to be as hyperactive as he can subsequently reacts with surprise that the behavior was not worse. One implication of this reaction is that social input coupled with the duration of the behavior has resulted in the child viewing his problem as insurmountable and disproportionately awful, an attitude that would discourage active attempts to improve. An example of this phenomenon is contained in the following comment by a 9-year-old hyperactive boy who had just viewed his own "worst tantrum ever" on videotape:

> I thought, "Man, this guy [pediatric resident] must be a real green apple [beginner], he says "Let me *see* a tantrum" like I've got measles or a cut finger or something to show him. So I tell him I do not just turn on a tantrum like an electric light and he goes like, "Just act like you're so mad you can hardly speak." And then, Jesus, I did get mad, like this is *so stupid* and I started and had the worst ever tantrum and he just sits there looking at me. Man! what a weirdo this guy is. And when I'd run right down to ground he says real polite-like am I all finished and then he puts on the TV monitor and I get so mad I'm red hot because *the way I act isn't all that bad.* It's no more badder than Max when he loses or Stevie when his bike got run over or Chris when the umpire gives a bad line call or Mrs. Ortona when we forgot to dump the paste and there was a real sicky smell. So why am *I* coming to a doctor and not them? Like the way people dial in [react] to me when I get mad has got me thinking I'm hopeless or something like those cancer kids on TV—like nothing can be done at all. All the time I thought my tantrums are like Gruesome Giant on a mad kick and I'm really not that bad. I'm really just like them ... and this guy [pediatric resident] says, "Is that the best you can do? Let's try that again," and I felt like killing him but I just did it again.

Transactional Analysis

Transactional Analysis (TA) is a system of individual and social psychiatry developed by Berne (1961, 1964, 1972). It has been described (Woollams & Brown, 1979) as a theory of intrapsychic and interpersonal behavior, a point of view about people, and a set of techniques to help people understand and change their behavior.

Underlying TA is the basic assumption that the great majority of infants are *OK*, that is, they have the potential to live effectively and in harmony with themselves and others. In the child's transactions with socialization agents, he receives two kinds of messages: *counter injunctions* from important adults are usually verbal and instruct him on how to be a success in life, and *injunctions* provide verbal and nonverbal interference with normal psychological growth and development. On the basis of these transactions a personal life plan (script) is written and the child, and later the adult he becomes, lives out the script in a way that verifies the impressions he has formed of himself. Whether the child reaches his potential is determined to a considerable extent by the early parent-child relationship. When the transactions between a child and his significant others, such as parents, siblings, teachers, and peers, are predominantly positive (positive strokes), the result is a happy, confident child who functions harmoniously with others (I'm OK–You're OK). An excess of negative transactions (negative strokes) is likely to produce a child who is lacking in self-esteem, the result being that he sees himself as unworthy and others as generally superior (I'm Not OK–You're OK). The other two basic attitudinal positions here are: I'm Not OK–You're Not OK, and I'm OK–You're Not OK.

In the case of the hyperactive child, his social interactions (transactions) with his parents and later with his teachers are predominantly negative (negative strokes) and show him that he is Not OK. He usually receives many injunctions that serve to heighten his sense of inferiority. The child soon acquires a view of his worth in comparison to that of other people described in TA as the I'm Not OK–You're OK position. When the Not OK position is strongly established, the hyperactive child is caught in a downward spiral of events, reactions from others, and feelings about himself that exacerbate his problems. The goal of treatment is to help the child shift from the I'm Not OK–You're OK position, which summarized all of his negative feelings about himself, to the I'm OK–You're OK position before permanent damage is done. An assumption in TA treatment is that the child is capable of understanding the rationale of TA, since he is actively involved in the resolution of his problems, and taking considerable responsibility for his behavior. The child works on a contract for personal change, and the therapist, who could be a teacher or parent, uses the TA frame of reference to facilitate the desired changes. The following excerpts from an interview by Wolf (1977, pp. 176–178) show how one teacher applied TA to the management of hyperactive children:

Interviewer: How do you use TA with hyperactive kids?

Respondent: By the students knowing that I respect them and that they are OK. For example, Charlie, my most hyperactive student, will now sit in his chair for five minutes before moving about. It used to be only two minutes. He would stand on his chair, climb up on the desk, or crawl under his seat. I invited him to do something very physical. Now he goes out and runs around the track in the school yard and comes back in and is able to sit for five minutes and get a lot done in those five minutes. Then it's OK for him to go out and run around again . . .

Interviewer: How have you used the TA concept of permission in working with Charlie?

Respondent: At first he was running around the classroom disturbing the other students. I told him our contract was that he, as with the other students, couldn't disturb the learning of others, and if he wanted to run, he had my permission to run on the track. He doesn't run in the classroom any more or act up in disruptive ways and receive negative strokes from me or the students . . .

Interviewer: Do you work with the hyperactive kids in terms of what ego state they are in while being hyperactive?

Respondent: Not at first. It's not useful for them until they can control themselves. Usually hyperactive kids have been told it's not OK to be hyperactive. It's not OK to be you. My attitude is they are OK people wherever they are and it's OK to be themselves.

Interviewer: Does that increase hyperactivity?

Respondent: At first it does.

Interviewer: For how long?

Respondent: Two weeks usually. Then the students themselves learn that they do have power over themselves. It's like, "Wow! If I choose to be quiet five minutes, why don't I choose ten? Is it really necessary to run around the track forty times a day?"

. . . . Interviewer: What else do you do with the hyperactive kid from a TA frame of reference?

Respondent: Give them lots of positive strokes, especially in the classroom setting. They have not gotten positive strokes or they wouldn't have been labeled hyperactive. If parents or teachers think the child is just full of old nick and are really cute in their activity, they are not hyperactive.

Interviewer: That is, they are not labeled hyperactive.

Respondent: Yes. When they are not cute they are labeled hyperactive and they are not given positive strokes . . .*

The following case history (Edwards, 1979, pp. 61–62) illustrates how TA was used within an interdisciplinary approach with a 10-year-old boy. Note how in the course of everyday events the parents generated and maintained hyperactivity by poor parenting practices.

Toni, a ten year old boy, had been diagnosed as hyperactive when he was four years old. The problem identification stage revealed that Toni had many previously undiagnosed allergies. His mother had over-protected him from birth. Wanting to be the "perfect" mother, she had anticipated his every need and by the time he was two years old she was "overwhelmed" by his "temper" which

*From Wolf, C. W. Transaction analysis and the management of hyperactivity. In M. J. Fine (Ed.), *Principles and techniques of intervention with hyperactive children*, 1977. Courtesy of Charles C. Thomas, Publisher, Springfield, IL.

she "couldn't handle." His father saw Toni's high level of activity, temper and school problems as a sign of a "real boy." The father had acted this way himself as a child and thought his wife should swat Toni more often as his mother had done. Educational evaluation revealed minor perceptual motor difficulties and learning difficulties such as difficulty following instructions, concentrating, selecting appropriate stimuli and organizing thoughts.

Treatment began immediately to desensitize Toni to his many allergies. Family therapy identified and reversed the negative stroking patterns. Parents resolved basic script issues of parental inadequacy. Once mother gave up her "Don't Think" injunction, she was able to set limits, expect Toni to think, and deal potently with his anger. When father recognized and resolved his own "not OK" life position and injunction not to trust, he could support his wife and the school in their expectations for his son. Toni needed and got permission from his parents and the therapist to feel and to think about his feelings to solve problems. He began to identify his feelings and to think about consequences of his behavior and cue himself to the teacher's expectations by anticipating what would happen.... Finally, he began to define what kind of person he wanted to be and model his behavior after this idea.... The school set up a special minimum stimulation environment where Toni could begin to organize stimuli ... and correct his early learning deficits.*

A follow-up report (Edwards, 1981) showed that Toni continued to function effectively both at home (despite his parents' divorce) and at school, where previously he had been at the point of expulsion.

We have discussed TA in some detail here because it has received considerable attention as an individual or group therapeutic approach as well as a behavior management procedure for parents and teachers. However, in our opinion its shortcomings far outweigh its value. It contributes little that is new or of value either to current therapeutic thought or to parental and classroom management procedures. The elaborate superstructure of terminology describes (a) antecedents and consequents that are consistent with other theoretical and applied approaches to socialization, such as those of Thomas and Chess (1977), Bell and Harper (1977), and Patterson (1971), and (b) specific procedures such as contracts, self-reinforcement, and self-instruction, which have been carefully delineated and effectively used by other behavior theorists and therapists (Bandura, 1969; Daniels, 1973; Mash & Dalby, 1979; Meichenbaum, 1978). There is no firm empirical support for the TA approach; it has not been subjected to empirical test as have some other classroom and family management procedures. Although its application to understanding children with problems has been discussed in several texts (Babcock & Keepers, 1976; Harris, 1969; James, 1973) that document in detail the dynamics of the various problems and difficulties of the children, these descriptions fail to include clear and precise descriptions of the specific

*Reprinted by permission from Edwards, S. A. Hyperactivity as passive behavior. *Transactional Analysis Journal,* 1979, *9* (1), 60–62.

course of action that interested adults could follow. It is difficult to see what advantage accrues to parents from advice such as (Harris, 1969, p. 189): "The parents of a youngster who is having difficulty in school . . . must always keep in mind the primary influence of the NOT OK. The rule is "When in doubt, stroke." The theory and language of TA are stated to be understandable to an 8-year-old child, and books on TA have been published for preschool and primary-grade children (Freed, 1971, 1973). However, the use of common referents, such as "game" and "racket," with completely different meanings from those in common usage, is likely to be confusing to a child, as are the destructive associations that are likely to ensue with the TA concept of Parent. In this connection we have serious doubts about the feasibility, value, and effects of presenting the Parent–Adult–Child concept to children with problems and expecting them to be able to "easily respond to the imageries of plugging in the Adult and turning off the frightened Child or the accusing Parent as one would a TV set" (Harris, 1969, p. 203).

BEHAVIORAL INTERVENTION

Operant Conditioning

One of the major behavior therapy techniques, operant conditioning, uses reinforcement procedures to remedy behavior deficits, eliminate maladaptive behaviors that are maintained by their rewarding consequences, and strengthen existing patterns of behavior. The design used in most operant conditioning studies is the *ABAB* procedure; in others, only the first two steps, *AB*, are used. In the four-step procedure the frequency of the problem behavior in naturalistic settings is established in the *baseline period*, (A); then in the *reinforcement period*, (B), the behavior is eliminated with the systematic use of reinforcement procedures; in the *nonreinforcement period*, (A), there is a return to the baseline conditions, that is, the reinforcement procedures are omitted and the behavior is reinstated; and finally in the *return to reinforcement period*, (B), the behavior is eliminated again with reinforcement procedures.

Allen, Henke, Harris, Baer, and Reynolds (1967) used the *ABAB* procedure to increase the attention span of a 4-year-old hyperactive boy in a preschool setting who moved constantly from one activity to another. Concomitant with the frequent changes in activity were short periods of attending. In the baseline period, *A*, the child was observed for 21 successive 50-minute periods of free play (usually two a day) to determine the actual frequency of activity changes, the contexts in which they occurred, and the reactions of the teachers and other adults. In the reinforcement period, *B*, the goal was to increase the duration of time spent on any one activity by making social reinforcement, in the form of teacher attention, contingent on continuous attention of one minute to an activity. This procedure continued for seven 50-minute periods, at which time attending behavior had markedly increased. The nonreinforcement period, *A*, was a reversal stage designed to determine if the crucial factor in modifying the attending behavior was indeed adult social reinforcement. In this stage teacher attention was delivered on the same random noncontingent basis used during the baseline period. In the return to reinforcement period, *B*, the social reinforcement procedures used in the second stage were reinstated, but with one change: the criterion for teacher attention was raised to two minutes of continuous attending. Duration of attending behavior again increased. Thus, by varying the social consequences, the child's attending behavior was successfully extended, shortened, and then further extended. The supporting observational data are shown in Figure 7.1.

In reinstating the *A* stage to demonstrate that the maladaptive behavior has been controlled by environmental contingencies, the *ABAB* design frequently is criticized for giving priority to scientific goals at the expense of therapeutic goals. Critics question the effect on the child of returning his behavior to its original undesirable form and also question the effectiveness of the method if the behavior returns so readily to its undesirable baseline frequency. In rebuttal, it is unlikely that the child is harmed by this experience.

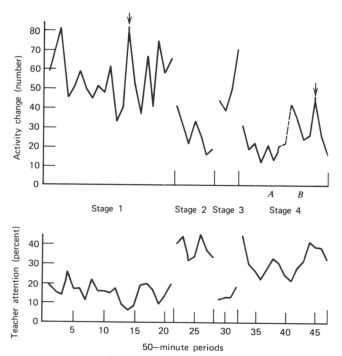

Figure 7.1 Activity changes of subject over the four stages. From Allen, K. E., Henke, L. B., Harris, F. R., Baer, D. M., & Reynolds, N. J. Control of hyperactivity by social reinforcement of attending behavior. *Journal of Educational Psychology*, 1967, *58*, 231–237. Copyright 1967 by the American Psychological Association. Reprinted by permission.

After several days of experiencing reinforcement he is reminded of how much less enjoyable his experiences are when he exhibits the undesirable responses. In addition, the *ABAB* design constitutes a dramatic demonstration to the parent, teacher, or peer that his behavior is influencing the subject's behavior. This kind of feedback is in itself a reinforcer of change in the key environmental figures (Bandura, 1969).

A second criticism concerns the reliance on reinforcement procedures, particularly those involving tangible rewards, on the grounds that such rewards constitute a form of bribery. Good behavior should be rewarding in itself, and the child who is frequently rewarded will soon be unwilling to perform in the absence of reward. In rebuttal, behavior is strongly influenced by its consequences and the use of appropriate incentives has proven to be an effective method for the establishment of new responses, particularly when the new response must replace a well-established maladaptive response. With skillful use, reinforcement procedures can be used to effect changes in several kinds of social behavior and can also facilitate the acquisition of self-evaluative and self-reinforcement systems. Furthermore, a behavior modification program represents a continuum of psychological experiences in which the reinforcement regulating behavior gradually changes so that the original reinforcers can be expected to differ markedly from the stimulus events that ultimately serve to reinforce and control the behavior.

Bandura (1969) has specified four conditions that are essential for the successful use of operant conditioning, the first being the selection of a reinforcer that maintains the child's responsiveness over a relatively long period of time.

The second condition is that the reinforcement be made contingent on the occurrence of the desired behavior and occur immediately following the emission of the response. The need for immediacy is particularly relevant for hyperactive children because their verbal capacity is often limited and consequently they cannot effectively mediate either a delay or an inconsistency in reinforcement.

The third condition concerns the need to find a reliable way of eliciting the desired behavior, because if the behavior seldom occurs, it is unlikely to be strengthened through association with a new reinforcer (Bandura, 1969). If the hyperactive child already has the desirable response in his behavioral repertoire but exhibits the response infrequently, environmental stimulation must be used to elicit it so that it can be strengthened by reinforcement.

The final condition concerns the maintenance of the behavior following the termination of the reinforcement. To maintain the behavior the reinforcement system must be altered during the course of treatment. The following procedural principles can facilitate the transition from reinforcement to no reinforcement (Bandura, 1969). The frequency and magnitude of reinforcement should be reduced as soon as the response patterns are established with continuous reinforcement. The schedule should change to intermittent reinforcement (a schedule that is extremely resistant to extinction) with a concomitant increase in the amount of work required for reinforcement. The locus of reinforcement should change. As adult reinforcement is reduced, for example, the child should be enjoying increased reward from peers. The point here is that when treatment is successful the behavior will be maintained by rewards from the child's own social environment and from the self-reinforcement following the internalization of standards. The form of reinforcement should change. Initially, a combination of tangible rewards and social approval is likely to be most effective. As the behavior is established, tangible rewards gradually can be dropped as social rewards increase. Intrinsic satisfaction will also become reinforcing. In applying these principles, caution should be used in changing the pattern of reinforcement because there is some evidence that hyperactive children are overresponsive to rewards and unusually sensitive to the withdrawal of reward (Douglas, 1980; Parry & Douglas, 1976).

Several single-subject studies have proven the efficacy of operant conditioning for the modification of hyperactive behavior in young children (Allen et al., 1967; Backman, Ferguson, & Trites, 1980; Barnard & Collar, 1973; Daniels, 1973; Frazier & Schneider, 1975; Pihl, 1967; Williams, 1959). The use of operant conditioning in single-subject studies or studies with a small number of subjects has two important advantages: the reinforcement procedure can be designed precisely for the problems and environment of individual children (e.g., Frazier & Schneider, 1975; O'Leary, Pelham, Rosenbaum, & Price, 1976), and typically there is close and detailed surveillance, which results in the identification of undesirable side effects that might pass unnoticed in a larger group.

Behavioral Intervention in the Home

Of interest here are those studies in which the home is the only locus of intervention, with the parents having been trained in the use of behavior modification techniques. In a carefully conducted single-subject study Frazier and Schneider (1975) taught the parents of a 3-year-old hyperactive boy how to use reinforcement procedures to eliminate his high level of inappropriate activity during and after meals. The child's activity level was above the 98th percentile for his age. It was assessed by independent parent ratings on the Werry–Weiss–Peters Activity Scale (Werry, 1968) and by psychologists' behavioral observations of the child under restrictive and free play conditions. To establish baseline levels the parents were taught to record the boy's misbehavior using behavioral categories set up by two psychologists and covering the half-hour period after dinner and a time interval during dinner. Next, a behavior shaping program was instigated for the after dinner period, with social reinforcement for appropriate behavior and three minutes of time-out with restraint in a darkened room for misbehavior. One week later a similar program was started during dinner. The rate of inappropriate behavior decreased steadily and remained at a low level for several weeks during which period two reliability checks were made. Midway through the program the child's behavior had improved enough to allow him to move from a high chair to a regular chair and to eat in a restaurant for the first time in his life.

Another example of the efficacy of training parents as therapists is a study by Barnard and Collar (1973) in which a mother appealed in desperation to a school nurse for help with her 8-year-old daughter who was hyperactive, aggressive, markedly uncooperative, easily frustrated, and excessively attention seeking. Discussion with the mother indicated that the child's disruptive behaviors were being maintained by their attention-getting value. Frustration and tantrums usually resulted from some disciplinary measure, and the tantrum then served as a reason for attention from the mother in the form of argument and verbal persuasion. The mother was instructed in the methods of behavior management and data collection procedures, and she proceeded to gather baseline data over a 6-day period on the following behaviors: mother's positive comments to the child, mother's negative comments to the child, child's positive comments to the mother and other members of the family, child's negative comments to the mother and other members of the family, and the child's aggression. The baseline data in Figure 7.2 shows a high correlation between the mother's and child's comments in the positive and negative categories. Next the mother was instructed in a time-out procedure and in management programs to modify the child's negative comments. The graphic results show clearly that there was a marked reduction in negative comments and marked gains in positive verbal interactions. The relatively high frequency of positive mother–child interaction in the latter part of the 6-week period suggests many more periods of agreement than disagreement. The study is notable for the fact that it was monitored by a school nurse and effectively carried out by a mother with no previous experience with reinforcement procedures. Further support for the use of parents as behavior modifiers comes from a diverse group of studies. Williams (1959) trained parents to discontinue providing social reinforcers for their child's temper tantrums; Daniels (1973) used a combination of behavior modification techniques for increasing attending behavior and decreasing hyperactivity in a 6-year-old boy: the parents were instructed in the use of a conditioning procedure for the child and, because they were quite overactive themselves, were also instructed to model an acceptable level of activity; Hall and Broden (1967) taught parents how to use operant conditioning procedures to modify hyperactive behavior.

A unique approach to training of parents as therapists involves the use of residence units. Wiltz and Gordon (1974) proposed that the ideal parental training situation should combine feedback, modeling, and instructional materials *in the child's natural environment*. To test the efficacy of this proposal these investigators had the entire family of a 9-year-old hyperactive aggressive boy live in a three-bedroom experimental apartment for five consecutive days. During this period the father went to work in the daytime and the mother was home all day. Both parents were observed and given extensive training in behavior recording and control. A marked improvement occurred in the child's deviant behavior. The family then returned home, maintained contact by tele-

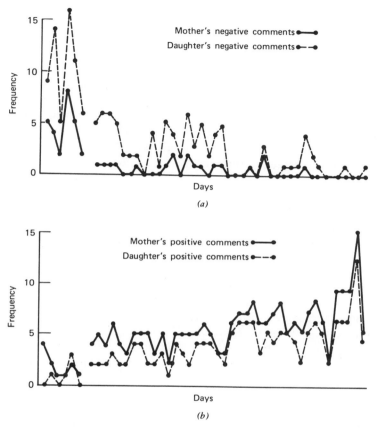

Figure 7.2 (a) Correlation between Mother's and Child's Negative Comments, and (b) Correlation between Mother's and Child's Positive Comments. Reprinted, by permission, from Barnard, K., & Collar, B. S. Early diagnosis, interpretation, and intervention: A commentary on the nurese's role. *Annals of the New York Academy of Sciences*, 1973, *205*, 373–382.

phone, and recorded the child's behavior for 30 days. The results showed significant reductions in deviant behavior. Although the procedure sounds time consuming, in fact the *total* professional time spent by the two investigators on all phases of the study was 33 hours.

Several studies (e.g., Dubey, Kaufman, & O'Leary, 1977; Furman & Feighner, 1973; Tams & Eyberg, 1976) have reported the use of group counseling with parents in which reinforcement procedures are discussed and the parents work at modifying specific target behavior. Using specific parent–child interaction patterns as the basis of training, Eyberg and Matarazzo (1980) compared didactic group training of parents in these patterns with individual parent training. The group training involved lectures, discussion, assigned readings, and recording of the child's home behavior; the individual training involved the use of modeling, practice in real-life situations, immediate feed-back, reinforcement, and further practice. The 29 children, aged four to nine years, were divided with their mothers into didactic group treatment, individual mother–child interaction training, and controls. After five training sessions there was marked improvement in the individually trained mothers and their children in the laboratory situation, but no significant changes in the other two groups. However, mothers in all three groups reported improvements in home management, which in view of the nontreatment accorded the controls is a surprising finding for this group. The investigators tentatively attributed the superiority of the individual training to the use of immediate feedback, reinforcement, and further practice accorded the mothers in the preliminary training.

The successful use of behavior modification procedures in all of the above samples was achieved with relatively small investments of professional time, a feature that in itself is a strong endorsement for the use of parents as therapists. In addition, there is great continuity between the "treatment" and the child's ongoing daily routine because the intervention occurs in the naturalistic setting of the home, with its many opportunities for practicing the new responses. However, the greatest advantage of training parents in behavior modification techniques concerns the long-term effects on the parent–child relationship. With the use of these techniques the parent comes to see that he is often the one who has been maintaining the child's misbehavior. When he sees how the situation improves as a result of changes in responses he makes to the child's misbehavior, the whole situation improves markedly. The parent feels a mastery of the situation and at the same time recognizes his contribution to it. Once the parent grasps the principles guiding the responses he should make, only occasional professional help should be needed. For the reader who wishes to pursue this topic, there are several excellent comprehensive reviews of the theoretical, empirical, and ethical aspects of training parents as behavior therapists for their own children (e.g., Berkowitz & Graziano, 1972; Reisinger, Ora, & Frangia, 1976).

Behavioral Intervention in the Home and School

When intervention is initiated at school, maximum benefits will result only if there is continuity between the new school demands and the child's behavior at home, and this can best be achieved by actively involving the parents. Representative of a home and school study is one by O'Leary and his associates (O'Leary et al., 1976) in which a 10-week home-based reinforcement program was used to increase prosocial behavior and improve academic performance in hyperactive elementary school boys of average intelligence. The presence of hyperactivity was established through teacher ratings on the Conners Abbreviated Teacher Rating Scale, parent ratings on the Werry–Weiss–Peters Activity Scale, independent validation of the teacher ratings, and comparisons with randomly selected same-age peers. Following random assignment of subjects to treatment and control groups, the nine boys in the treatment group partici- pated in a home-based reinforcement program having the following character- istics: (a) classroom objectives were specified for each child every day; (b) social reinforcement was given for efforts to achieve these objectives; (c) end- of-day evaluations of the child's behavior relevant to the specified objectives were made by his teacher; (d) a daily report card was sent home to the par- ents reporting the child's progress; and (e) both daily and weekly rewards were given by the parents. The daily objectives included such behaviors as completing academic assignments, helping classmates, refraining from aggres- sive behavior, and finishing homework. Care and ingenuity were used in se- lecting high motivation daily rewards, such as 30 minutes of extra television or a special dessert, as well as appealing weekly rewards such as a fishing trip with the father or dinner at a favorite restaurant. Individual problem behavior ratings decreased sharply with the treatment group showing significant im- provement. The same pattern of change occurred in the teacher ratings on the Conners Scale; the investigators noted that these changes were generally comparable to those usually reported in treatment with stimulant medication.

In comparison to other studies of the use of reinforcement procedures in naturalistic settings, this study was notable for its use of carefully selected individualized reinforcements, establishment of an individualized problem be- havior rating, independent validation of the teacher ratings, inclusion of a hyperactive control group as well as the behavioral comparison with nonhyperactive peers, and the school–home liaison in which the parents acted as reinforcement agents. The value of the study is limited, however, by the failure to present statistics other than probabilities; and a long-term follow-up should have been seen as mandatory.

Behavioral Intervention Combined with Other Treatment Procedures

The approaches to behavior change discussed in the preceding sections have been described as separate and discrete approaches to the problems of the hyperactive child. There is considerable evidence, however, that the efficacy of any one of these procedures can often be enhanced if it is used in conjunction with one or more of the other procedures. If the goal for the hyperactive child is the acquisition of a new response, initially modeling might be the most appropriate way to transmit the new behavior. Once the behavior is acquired, operant conditioning could be used to strengthen it and the results of such intervention could then be more strongly entrenched if some self-evaluative and self-reinforcing training procedures were introduced (Bandura, 1969). Pel- ham (1978) and Stableford, Butz, Hasazi, Leitenberg, and Peyser (1976) have reported cases in which stimulant drugs used concurrently with reinforcement procedures were then gradually withdrawn as the reinforcement procedures proved increasingly effective.

In summary, operant conditioning procedures have been enthusiastical- ly endorsed by proponents as the answer to behavior problems and denounced by critics as superficial techniques that are not fully understood, with at best transient and in some instances detrimental effects. There is some truth in both these viewpoints. When correctly used operant conditioning procedures have proven highly successful with a variety of discrete operants. Sometimes the effects of these procedures are dramatic in terms of amount and speed of improvement and, for reasons that are not fully understood, are accompanied by widespread improvement in the child's general behavior. One major criticism is that the procedures do not get to the underlying cause of the behavior, and the danger is that an untreated cause will manifest itself in some other misbehavior, that is, that symptom substitution will occur. There is no evidence that symptom substitution does occur following the successful modification of an operant, whereas there is some evidence that it does not occur (Bandura, 1969). In some cases operant conditioning is detrimental. We are not referring here to outright abuse or careless use of the procedures but rather to a more subtle kind of misjudgment on the part of the therapist concerning the predispositions of the child being treated. Operant conditioning can promote control of the child from without rather than from within, an outcome that occurs when the child concentrates completely on the therapist and makes no decisions himself, or when the child makes value judgments as to "good" and "bad" behavior solely in terms of response cost to himself (Ney, 1975). Any professional who is contemplating using operant conditioning himself or training nonprofessionals in its use should read Ney's article and also the discussion by Greenspan (1974) of some of the complex issues in the clinical use of the procedures.

The lack of data on the long-term effects of operant conditioning, as well as on transfer and generalization, makes evaluation of the procedures difficult. In 1971 O'Leary and Drabman specified procedures for achieving generalization, but with few exceptions research in the past decade has been limited to short-term studies in single settings. The state of the field would be considerably advanced if situational tests of transfer and generalization, and long-term retention measures, were mandatory for all operant conditioning studies accepted for publication. Where appropriate, measures should also be obtained of the duration and generalization of changes in parents' behavior, since one major goal of a behavior modification procedure should be the transmission of understanding and retention of behavioral principles by parents and other socialization agents (Patterson, 1971).

Operant conditioning is a *potentially* valuable method for controlling and modifying behavior. Its effectiveness for behavior other than discrete operants has not yet been proven, nor has it been shown to be superior to other forms of intervention in immediate outcome, duration of effect, or therapist time. Exaggerated claims, misuse, and abuse have resulted from the apparent simplicity of the method (Stein, 1975). A baseline of information has been established on the use of the procedure with simple behavior problems. What is needed now are systematic investigations of the efficacy of the procedure for complex behavior problems, in addition to the transfer and generalization data discussed above (Patterson, 1971).

Differential Reinforcement of Related Operants

This conditioning procedure is a more complex variation of the standard operant conditioning procedure described in the preceding section. Its goal is to eliminate an undesirable behavior and simultaneously work toward replacing it with a more desirable related response. Note that the elimination or weakening of an undesirable response does not automatically guarantee the occurrence of the desirable related response; the new response must be elicited and strengthened through reinforcement. The crucial difference between the differential reinforcement of related operants and the standard operant conditioning procedure is that in the former paradigm the therapist is actively working on two related but not necessarily reciprocal target behaviors, one that is to be eliminated and one that is to be strengthened or introduced. In the standard operant conditioning procedure, he is usually working on strengthening or weakening a specific behavior or a set of behaviors, but he is not actively and simultaneously trying to strengthen a related behavior. In operant conditioning change may occur in a related behavior, but it is basically a side effect and, because it has not been directly reinforced, the behavior is not as strongly established as it would be with the differential reinforcement procedure. The two conditioning procedures appear to achieve the same result when the elimination of one behavior automatically ensures the emission of another. For example, if all inappropriate out-of-seat behavior in a classroom situation is eliminated, the desirable behavior of remaining in one's seat will occur automatically; however, the strength of the new response would be greater with differential reinforcement as a function of the direct reinforcement used. But the desired behavior does not always automatically occur as a function of the nonoccurrence of the problem behavior; for example, the elimination of impulsive behavior increases the latency of response but does not guarantee that the child will then reflect on the task in the latency period. Usually he must be taught a reflective strategy, and it is in this type of situation that the difference between the two procedures and the superiority of differential reinforcement is clearly demonstrated.

The prerequisites to the use of differential reinforcement are similar to those described earlier for operant conditioning. The behavior that is bringing the child into conflict with his social environment must be clearly defined and its frequency determined; the situations in which this behavior occurs must be identified; the social and nonsocial factors in the environment that elicit and maintain this behavior must be noted; and procedures to elicit and strengthen the desired related behavior must be planned. One phase of the therapeutic strategy concerns the elimination of the problem behavior by removing eliciting cues, such as attention from the peer group, and ensuring that the behavior is not reinforced when it does occur. As in operant conditioning, punishment may be used to diminish the frequency of the problem behavior if the therapist makes sure that the attention aspect of the punishment is not rewarding to the child. Time-out from a reinforcing situation, response cost, and loss of privileges are all likely to be more effective than physical punishment. A good example of the effective use of such procedures is contained in a study by Lovaas and Willis (1975) of the modification of several kinds of problem behavior in a 7-year-old hyperactive boy. The other phase in the differential reinforcement procedure consists of establishing the desired behavior. If this behavior is already a part of the child's behavioral repertoire, than reinforcement procedures are an effective way of strengthening it. However, if the child does not possess or emit the response, modeling procedures should be used to transmit the response. Once the response has been established, the child should be given a variety of situational tests to determine the stability of the response and the extent to which it generalizes to new settings. The extrinsic reinforcers must eventually be withdrawn and in the normal course of events the naturalistic social reinforcement that occurs, coupled with the child's own satisfaction, should maintain the behavior. Better results will accrue, however, if the child is also taught self-evaluative skills, and when these are mastered, self-reinforcement procedures (Bandura, 1969).

Differential reinforcement was used successfully (Ross, 1967) to modify the impulsivity of a 6-year-old hyperactive boy and to facilitate his acquisition of reflective tendencies. The child's problem was not attentional, as he was able to maintain attention; rather it was that his responses in school, games, and choice situations were consistently hasty, impetuous, and lacking in forethought. His parents were concerned that his impulsivity was becoming increasingly costly for him in terms of failure on academic tasks, missed opportunities, and disappointment. The first phase of the procedure was conducted at home and involved a series of choice situations in which the child was punished through negative consequences whenever he responded without thinking. Because he was so quick to respond, he frequently accepted the first alternative offered, without even waiting to hear the second. His parents were instructed to offer him a reasonably attractive opportunity, for example, "Would you like a Coke or . . ." and, when he accepted without waiting to hear the alternative, to give him what was offered. When he was actively engaged with the chosen alternative, they offered the same choice to one of his siblings, all of whom were highly reflective by comparison. The second alternative was always more attractive and consequently was chosen. When the child saw his sibling enjoying the more attractive choice, he was invariably indignant and disappointed. At this point one of his parents explained that he had accepted without stopping to think and the consequence was disappointing.

His parents were also instructed to use modeling procedures to enhance these demonstrations on the folly of impulsivity. At intervals one parent would make a hasty choice and complain about the consequences, chastizing himself all the while for not stopping to think. Occasionally the child did spontaneously stop and think, and he received strong positive reinforcement for such action. Sometimes his parents urged him to think, helped him weigh the alternatives, and arranged situations so that when he did act reflectively he received both social and situational reinforcement. In addition to choice situations, small-group games were used in which one adult monitored the game so that impulsive moves could be punished and reflective actions rewarded. With this combination of differential reinforcement and modeling the child became more reflective in the home. As he began to show improvement, school-type games were included in the training program. One particularly effective game was Quiz Program, in which points were given for the best answer, additional points were awarded for the fastest best answer, and points were lost for incorrect or inadequate answers. This procedure constituted a genuine conflict situation for this impulsive child because his tendency was to raise his hand immediately, but when he did he was usually punished. In this game the only other players were his parents and older brother, and the procedure used was for them to model impulsivity with consequent punishment and reflectivity with positive reinforcement, and to demonstrate to him that he could take the time to stop and think and still win. Because of its similarity to the school situation, Quiz Program was used frequently.

When the child demonstrated marked improvement as a function of the home training, his therapist enlisted the cooperation of his teacher and the differential reinforcement procedure was extended to the school situation with considerable success. The child was encouraged to recount his school experiences, and appropriate positive and negative social reinforcement was provided for evidence of reflectivity and impulsivity, respectively. After the procedure had been incorporated into the school routine, the parents were then instructed to use a series of situational tests of the child's ability to respond reflectively, and to compile a weekly score. Within six months of the initiation of the program the child was sufficiently improved so that his teacher described him as a "good thinker."

Self-Control Strategies

Over the past decade dissatisfaction with the failure of reinforcement procedures to produce lasting effects once the reinforcers were removed and to generalize across settings has resulted in a shift towards such cognitively oriented interventions as the self-control processes of self-instruction, self-monitoring, and self-reinforcement. In these processes the child learns to take some responsibility for his own behavior; he becomes an active participant in the behavior change program rather than a passive recipient of the efforts of others. The impetus for the shift to self-control strategies also stems in part from the studies of verbal mediation by the Russian psychologists Luria (1961) and Vygotsky (1962). On the basis of extensive work with children,

Luria (1961) has contended that the critical step in the child's development of voluntary control over his own behavior is the internalization of self-directed verbal commands. He has distinguished three stages by which the initiation and inhibition of voluntary behavior come under verbal control: first, the child's behavior is controlled and directed by the speech of others, usually adults; next, the child begins to use overt speech to regulate his behavior effectively; and finally, covert or inner speech comes to govern his voluntary actions. These stages have provided a useful framework for developing training procedures to help a child to control his own behavior. They have particular relevance for the hyperactive child in view of the well documented finding that this child makes many errors on academic and nonacademic tasks even though he may have the information or skills necessary for a correct response. He responds so quickly that his efforts can best be described as guesses or chance stabs at the task (Keogh & Barkett, 1980).

The procedures first developed for the hyperactive child used social and nonsocial environmental slowing-down devices to delay the hyperactive child's response, and so fit loosely into Luria's first stage. This interpretation of Luria's approach had certain weaknesses: using mechanical devices or strategies imposed by others to delay the child's response is effective only if the increased time interval is used gainfully by the child in a task-relevant manner. Although slowing cognitive tempo may be useful in a new learning situation, once the child is familiar with the task demands continued slow pacing may be detrimental and, as Zivin (1974) has pointed out, may not be important in the reduction of performance error. Dalby, Kinsbourne, Swanson, and Sobol (1977) found that hyperactive children performed best on a learning task when the items to be learned were presented at a brisk pace; in conditions in which longer intervals were available for study, performance deteriorated. These latter results suggest that part of the training package should include instruction in making maximum use of increased time intervals between onset of task and response. Research by Bender (1976), for example, suggested that covert self-instruction taught in conjunction with task-specific strategies resulted in better performance than simply modifying latency of response either by other-imposed devices or with self-regulatory training.

The initial experimental test of a training procedure based on Luria's second stage, the use of overt self-regulatory speech, was conducted by Palkes, Stewart, and Kahana (1968). The subjects were 20 hyperactive elementary school boys of normal intelligence. The treatment condition involved two half-hour sessions on individual training in learning to verbalize self-directed commands, such as "stop," "look," "listen," and "think," before responding to a variety of tasks including matching familiar figures. Subjects in the control condition were required only to perform the same tasks. The Porteus Maze Test Revision Series was used as a pretraining measure of impulsivity, and the Porteus Extension Series was used for the posttraining measure. Posttraining scores for the treatment group on both the Porteus IQ (Porteus Test Quotient) and the Porteus Qualitative Scores were significantly higher than those of the control group. The investigators noted that some of the most striking changes occurred in those error categories that reflect the characteristic work habits of the hyperactive child. The self-directed command training group cut fewer corners, crossed over fewer lines, lifted their pencils less often, and threaded the maze with fewer irregular lines than did the control group. The fact that these test behaviors had not been specifically taught suggests that the children generally were performing more carefully. A second study (Palkes, Stewart, & Freedman, 1971) provided further evidence of the efficacy of this verbal training procedure for hyperactive boys. In this study Palkes et al. compared the efficacy of silently read versus self-directed commands in a pre-posttreatment design using Porteus Maze performance as the dependent variable. The group trained to vocalize commands improved significantly, while the silent readers and a no-treatment control group showed no improvement. The obtained gains in the self-directed command group did not extend to performance two weeks later, which underlines the necessity for adequate repetition of training sessions if a lifelong habit of response is to be modified.

Meichenbaum and Goodman (1971) extended the procedure used by Palkes and her colleagues to encompass the third stage in the development of voluntary control of one's own behavior, the internalization of self-directed verbal commands (Luria, 1961). They developed a treatment program to teach children to use covert self-instructions followed by self-reinforcement. The training in self-instruction was conducted in a one-to-one situation and followed by the same three-stage developmental sequence that Luria (1961) had described. In the first stage, the overt verbalizations of an adult were used to control and direct the child's behavior: the child observed an adult perform a task such as the finger-maze task; as the adult worked, he engaged in explicit self-direction verbalizations. The child then performed the same task with the adult providing step-by-step directions. Note the similarity between this procedure and the modeling with guided participation procedure (Bandura, 1969). In the second stage, the child was instructed to use overtly the same adult verbalizations to guide his performance of the task. In the third and final stage of training, he was instructed to use covertly the verbalizations that the adult had modeled and that he himself had used effectively overtly. Thus within the context of the training situation, the child's covert speech became an effective regulator of his task behavior. The verbalizations initially used by the adult varied with the nature of the task, but in general included questions that encouraged planning, self-encouragement and self-monitoring, strategies for coping with difficulty and failure, and self-reinforcement. The following is an example of the adult's verbalizations on a sensorimotor task, copying line patterns (Meichenbaum & Goodman, 1971, p. 117):

Okay, what is it I have to do? You want me to copy the picture with the different lines. I have to go slow and be careful. Okay, draw the line down, down, good; then to the right, that's it; now down some more and to the left.

Good, I'm doing fine so far. Remember go slow. Now back up again. No, I was supposed to go down. That's okay. Just erase the line carefully . . . Good. Even if I make an error I can go on slowly and carefully. Okay, I have to go down now. Finished. I did it.

The Meichenbaum and Goodman procedure has been used with varying degrees of success in a number of investigations with hyperactive children. It has been used alone to improve self-instruction on academic-type tasks, and in combination with other behavior therapy procedures (Varni, Boyd, & Cataldo, 1978). Representative of this research is a study by Varni and Henker (1979) in which three hyperactive disruptive boys were taught to use the self-regulatory procedures of self-instruction, self-monitoring, and self-reinforcement to improve their academic performance and control their disruptive classroom behavior patterns. Using a well-controlled within-subject design, the boys' behavior and academic performance were monitored in both the clinic and classroom setting. Verbal self-instructional training proved to be effective only with an adult present, and self-monitoring had little effect. However, when self-monitoring was combined with self-reinforcement, first in the clinic setting and then in the classroom, academic performance improved and there was a concomitant reduction in hyperactive behavior. These results suggest that the essential component in the successful use of self-regulatory training may be self-reinforcement. According to social learning theory (Bandura, 1976) self-reinforcement improves performance mainly through its motivational function.

Overall, the results of self-control training with hyperactive children, and also with nonhyperactive children who exhibit similar behaviors such as extreme impulsivity, have been disappointing. Some studies have failed to achieve any positive results (e.g., Burns, 1972), and others have been only partially successful (Douglas, Parry, Marton, & Garson, 1976), while apparently adhering to acceptable standards of research and self-control training procedures. Representative of the latter group is an 8-week study by Barkley, Copeland, and Sivage (1980) of a special classroom for six hyperactive boys, aged seven to 10, in which a package of self-control procedures including self-instruction, self-monitoring, and self-reinforcement was used. A within-subjects reversal design was used and measures of on-task behavior and class misbehavior were recorded. In general, the self-control package was effective in reducing misbehavior and improving task attention during individual seat work, but not during group instruction; academic performance was only minimally improved; activity level remained unchanged; and generalization of treatment effects ranged from minimal to nonexistent. Barkley et al. (1980, p. 86) concluded that a longer intervention period might be needed for academic changes to occur and that

only those self-instructional interventions that have programmed for generalization to the classroom have been successful (Bornstein & Quevillon, 1976;

Kendall & Finch, 1976). An obvious solution to this problem is to utilize the treatment package of self-control measures in the child's regular school classroom, rather than to remove the child for treatment in another setting and have it fail to generalize to that (the regular school) classroom.

It is our opinion that the disappointing results in these studies should be attributed to deficits in the overall training program approach rather than to the more routine aspects of the programs such as length of training or kind of setting. The self-control programs that have been used, such as those of Burns (1972) or Barkley et al. (1980), are far too narrow in content and too situation-specific for generalization to occur. What is needed is a program that instills the *concept* of self-control, which means that the program must incorporate the principles of concept development in the presentation of its content. These principles require that the training be presented in the widest possible variety of everyday tasks and procedures, so that the child's experience of the concept of self-control is from as many different directions and in as many different contexts as is feasible within the restrictions of the training situation. The program, for example, should use live modeling of self-regulation by adults and peers, role play in which the trainee participates, games in which the use of self-control procedures facilitates winning, and vicarious exposure to the successful use of self-regulation (and to the adverse consequences when this procedure is not used) through the use of stories and anecdotal reports, and imagery.

Consider Bornstein and Quevillon's (1976) results and procedures in the light of the above discussion. After several hours of training in self-instruction, three overactive but not hyperactive preschool boys' on-task behavior increased dramatically, the behavior generalized across settings, and the gains were still evident at the 5-month follow-up. The training consisted of intentional training in the use of self-instruction, modeling of correct and incorrect usage of the control procedure by the instructor and the other participants, tangible reinforcement for both correct and fractional responses, prompts, fading, the use of a story context for presenting the procedure, and a wide variety of tasks ranging in difficulty from simple sensorimotor tasks to more complex problem solving situations. Bornstein and Quevillon also used imagery, and because this procedure is extremely effective with young children we will elaborate on its use in self-instructional programs.

Schneider (1978), for example, used a turtle imagery procedure to teach self-control to hyperactive primary school children. In this procedure the turtle image was first presented in a story context, then the children imitated the turtle who withdrew into his shell whenever he felt unable to control his behavior. This role play procedure was followed by relaxation, self-instructional, and problem solving exercises designed to teach self-control. Each child was then trained to imagine a turtle's gait and to say to himself, "I will not go faster than a slow turtle, slow turtle, slow." In three weeks of 15 minutes of training a day the children improved markedly, and this improvement persisted over time. Ross and Ross (1979) used imagery combined with a cluster of other procedures, including self-instruction and self-assessment, with a 9-year-old hyperactive boy who had successfully completed a training program on self-instruction but failed to use his newly acquired skill to regulate his behavior, to the distress of his parents. Knowing that the boy was entranced with sound devices, it was suggested that he be given a tape recorder and required each day to first imagine some of the pitfalls he should try to avoid that day and then record instructions to himself concerning these pitfalls. Later in the day he was to listen to these instructions and evaluate on a scale of one to 10 how well they had worked. He was also asked to discuss his progress in self-instruction and regulation regularly with his psychotherapist. This procedure proved to be both popular and effective with the child, and the parents reported that he was immensely interested in the self-assessment as well as the self-regulatory aspects of this activity. It is apparent from the following verbatim excerpts—the first from his tape, which he took to his psychotherapy session, and the second from his psychotherapy session—that he was using his self-instructional training with skill:

[Tape made earlier by the child as part of training program routine] OK now, Brucie Boy, it is September 25 and three days more and its your birthday, right? Right. And it is 7:13 and not one bad thing has happened today because you're still in bed. Now, let's work this out like scientists do, Brucie, and let's see how long before the whole day self-destructs. OK, *now* it is 7:18 a.m. Let's have a plan so we don't space out like at breakfast yesterday. Now let's go in *real* slow for starts . . .

[Child now talks to therapist, session is routinely taped]

And then I put on my socks but not my shoes and I made my bed real real quiet like I was in enemy-land like Gadflyers and I tiptoed downstairs and at breakfast nothing spilled because I did not reach for anything even when I wanted it real bad—like Mom's jam that she made. And when Zeke Morley yelled names at me on the way to school I did not get mad like I used to do—I did not even *feel* as mad as I mostly do—I just kept whispering over and over, "I don't read you, Fatso, I don't read you, Porkpie," and after a bit he stopped like you said if I would not show how mad I was.

It is clear that self-control deficits are of prime importance in the hierarchy of problems plaguing the hyperactive child. Similarly, there is no question that the development of effective intervention procedures for teaching self-control would benefit the large majority of hyperactive children. Clearly this is an area deserving of intensive research interest. Yet the research results to date are discouragingly similar to those on stimulant medication or operant conditioning: short-term efficacy of limited kinds of self-regulatory training programs and only sporadic evidence of long-term retention and generalization. What we find disheartening is that as each new intervention procedure surfaces, the same cycle seems to be repeated: there is a flurry of research resting on the assumption that *this* intervention will result in across the board benefits for the hyperactive child, and so selection of dependent variables can be made on the basis of a shot-gun approach. This nonproductive trend, already noticeable in the research on self-regulatory training, is well-established in the area of biofeedback training, where an apparently unending procession of doctoral candidates is using biofeedback training for the hyperactive child in conjunction with a remarkable array of outcome variables many of which bear a tenuous link, if any, to biofeedback training.

If self-control training is to be given a fair trial and fully developed, it is essential that researchers become more systematic in their explorations of this procedure. We would like to see an *intrinsic* interest in the training technique, which means extending it step by step without concern for rapid data collection and immediate publication, and a concern in the form of an obligation to see that the children, who supposedly are the reason for the research, benefit in some way from their participation in a study. This latter requirement would also result in a more selective and realistic choice of target behavior. Of relevance here is a comment by Keogh and Barkett (1980, pp. 280–281):

> ... interventions with hyperactive children must differentially address behavioral, psychological, and educational components of their functioning. Several generalizations are warranted. Stimulant medication changes social behaviors in school and sometimes affects selected psychological processes, especially sustained attention and perceptual-motor abilities. Behavior modification techniques have powerful effects on specific social behaviors that characterize hyperactivity. Yet, neither intervention has been shown to transfer over time or setting, to have a generalized positive influence on performance on school tasks, or to have long-term effects on achievement in educational subjects. Cognitive control training, on the other hand, appears to modify impulsive responding and to lead to more effective problem-solving strategies compatible with better performance in school subjects; however, cognitive control training techniques do not necessarily reduce activity levels or socially disruptive behaviors. In short, interventions differ in their relative effects on social behaviors, psychological processes, and educational competence.

Modeling Procedures

There has been a paucity of research on therapeutic modeling procedures with hyperactive children, possibly because the operant conditioning procedures with their established record have taken precedence over less clearly defined therapeutic approaches; or because some of the more highly visible characteristics of hyperactive children, such as a short attention span, distractibility, and a relative lack of verbal ability, do not facilitate observational learning. The latter line of reasoning overlooks other attributes of these children, such as high dependency and a lack of self-esteem, that are known to make observers attentive to the behavior of models (Bandura, 1969) and also disregards evidence that none of their inadequacies constitutes a real obstacle to the effective use of modeling procedures. Therapeutic modeling with a hyperactive child begins on a one-to-one basis, and there is well-documented clinical (Cantwell, 1979; Daniels, 1973; Wender & Wender, 1978) and research support (Carter & Reynolds, 1976; Copeland & Weissbrod, 1980; Spiegel, 1977) for the fact that in such situations the hyperactive child is able to attend for reasonable periods of time. There is also unequivocal evidence that hyperactive children (Palkes et al., 1971; Palkes et al., 1968), nonclinical children of average intelligence (Meichenbaum, 1978), and mentally retarded children (Ross & Ross, 1973; Ross, Ross, & Downing, 1973) can be taught the verbal and imaginal mediational skills needed for observational learning. In addition, hyperactive children are usually very aware of being different and are almost desperately eager to be like their peers. With most of these children the desire to be like others is not diffused and unspecified or vague; usually there are one or two peers whom they would like to emulate, and occasionally they do spontaneously imitate the behavior of a greatly admired peer. The yearnings to be like other children constitute a strong motivational force that should be capitalized on in the therapeutic situation. Its strength is evident in the following excerpts from the answers given by hyperactive children in an outpatient clinic to the question, What would you like most?

> Boy, 8 years, 6 months: What I would like best of all would be to be like Jimmy Marshall. When *he* says the wrong answer the other kids all laugh but not mean laughs and when *he* drops something or knocks things down our teacher says, "Oh, Jimmy," but not being real cross and I would like that most of all.

> Boy, 6 years, 11 months: Anything at all? Like are you maybe going to *do* what I say? Well, I'll tell you. First, I would like it a lot if Mrs. Miller (teacher) would just once in a while, even once in the whole of second grade, say, "Here's a boy who's really moving up fast" to me like she did to Stue and Jackie. . . . And I also would like to do some things good like Elliot [older brother] does right from the start. Elliot hit a baseball right off, and he just catches good, and my dad says, "That boy is a natural," and I would like it if I was natural at something.

Before discussing the few studies on therapeutic modeling with the hyperactive child we should mention the detrimental change in thinking that has occurred in modeling theory. Initially, the learning that occurred in the modeling situation did so in the absence of *any* instruction to observe or attend to the model, or in any way to rehearse or imitate the model's behavior. In experimental applications of modeling theory principles, efforts were made to ensure that the research design met the criteria for observational learning: the child, for example, might be seated at a small table and provided with an interesting activity while at the same time the model engaged in a sequence of behavior within the child's range of vision but in another part of the room. In presenting the task to the child, mention would be made of this other person only to justify his presence in the room. If the child attended to the model and subsequently exhibited some of the model's behavior, he did so on his own initiative. This observational learning was sharply demarcated from intentional training, in which one person, usually the teacher, instructs the child in a learning task and requires that he attend and usually rehearse the task behavior. Over the years the boundary between observational and intentional learning has become increasingly ambiguous as a result of introducing intentional training procedures, such as instructing the child to watch the model, imitate his verbal and nonverbal behavior, and expect reinforcement for exhibiting these behaviors, so that now the studies in this field retain the label of modeling studies but fall more accurately into the realm of traditional intentional training. It is our opinion that this trend has been a destructive one as far as extending the promise that the original modeling theory held for understanding and modifying behavior.

Carter and Reynolds (1976) have reported on modifying disruptive home and classroom behavior in a 9-year-old hyperactive girl who was on medication. The behaviors focused on were loud talking, interruption of the activities of others, and ritualistic idiosyncratic arm movements. Over a 5-day period baseline measures were obtained for these behaviors at home and at school. A token economy program used in both settings resulted in only minimal improvement over a 6-week period, so the intervention program was then redesigned to develop generalized imitation of the child's parents and teacher, and medication was continued for this next phase. The "modeling" procedure consisted of the adult using a verbal instruction, "I want you to do what I'm going to do now," and then rewarding accurate imitation with a token. Subjective reports from the parents and teacher indicated such marked improvement at the end of two weeks that the cued imitation procedure could be discontinued and the token schedule reduced to one token at the end of the school day and another at bedtime. Three weeks later observational data identical to that of the baseline period were collected, confirming the earlier subjective reports of improvement. The child was indistinguishable from other students in the class and continued to show social and academic improvement, despite termination of medication and token reinforcement in follow-up contacts over a 3-month period. The ease with which these behavior changes occurred raises a question about the accuracy of the original diagnosis. One criticism of reinforcement procedures such as the above token system is that once the reward procedure stops, the newly acquired behavior drops out. However, if the behavior has relevance to the child's social environments of home, neighborhood, and school, as was the case in this study, it is highly likely that positive reinforcement from these sources will be forthcoming so that the child will continue to exhibit the new behavior.

Goodwin and Mahoney (1975) used a modeling procedure combined with instruction, practice, and reinforcement, to modify in a game situation the tendency of three 9-year-old hyperactive boys to respond to verbal aggression with physical aggression. Pre- and posttreatment measures were also obtained of the boys' aggressive, destructive, and hyperactive responses in the class-room setting. A baseline of coping response to verbal aggression in the form of teasing was established by having each of the boys in turn stand in a circle while the other two boys, standing outside a larger circle, attempted to incite him to anger by means of verbal taunts or gestures. He was told he could respond in any way he wished and his responses were rated by observers. To ensure strong negative assaults on the part of the teasers, tokens were given for successful inciting and active participation, as well as for just participating in the game. One week later the three boys viewed a videotape of a same-age model in the teasing situation, who remained outwardly calm on being teased and coped with the teasing through covert self-instruction, such as "I won't get mad," which was dubbed in on the tape. They then participated in another taunting session. One week later the boys again saw the videotaped model, but this time the model's coping responses were discussed with an emphasis on their value in handling verbal aggression, and the boys verbally reproduced as many of the model's responses as they could recall, following which they participated in a taunting session. One week later the boys participated in the fourth and final taunting session with no videotape of the model and no dis-cussion of his coping responses. A day later, posttreatment measures were obtained of the boys' disruptive behaviors in the classroom. The results showed that the improvement in coping responses that had occurred in the third taunting session was maintained over the fourth session, and posttreat-ment ratings of disruptive behavior in the classroom also improved, with a reduction in disruptive behavior. In addition to the methodological limitations that Goodwin and Mahoney (1975, p. 202) acknowledge, the procedure of having the boys participate as taunters as well as recipients is a dubious one. Having two boys, both of whom are unknown to the subjects, act as taunters and follow a prescribed script would have controlled for some of the variabili-ty in the procedure. During the taunting session each boy's behavior in the circle was rated as coping versus noncoping, and included in the latter catego-ry were responses defined as "talking back." We have developed successful programs for teaching hyperactive children to cope with teasing, and it is our opinion that by far the most effective response that the child can learn to make is the quick retort that puts the teaser at a punishing disadvantage. To advocate silence, even when accompanied by calmness, is to disregard the re-alities of the peer group jungle.

Self-confrontation is an approach that modifies the behaviors characteristic of hyperactivity by making the child more aware of his behavior and its ef-fects on others. The rationale here is that the more the child knows about his behavior, the more he is in a position to do something about it (Sanborn, Pyke, & Sanborn, 1975). The optimal form of self-confrontation is videotape playback. Where videotape is not available, role play by others, a less power-ful self-confrontation technique, may be used. Verbal confrontation generally has little effect on the hyperactive child, possibly because he has heard it all before so many times or because it fails to convey the picture. Videotape self-modeling was used by Dowrick and Raeburn (1977) to teach a hyperactive 4-year-old boy to engage in self-directed play activity. In this technique a video-tape is made of the subject performing in a model way, in this case, playing independently without exhibiting hyperactive behavior, poor concentration, and incessant demands for attention. Although on medication, this boy was unable to role play the target behavior for a period long enough to be filmed, so video editing was used to piece together a tape of the child engaged in a continuing play activity, apparently by himself. The child was then taken off the medication temporarily in order that a "no treatment" unedited videotape could be made of him left to his own resources. In this tape the measured duration of play was 20 percent, as compared to 95 percent in the edited one. Two sets of baseline data were obtained of the child at play in the playroom; off medication and on medication. While on medication in the next three periods he watched the no-treatment film. Medication was then permanently withdrawn at the beginning of the final two periods during which he saw the no-treatment film followed by the treatment film. Playroom observations, which were made after each of these film showings, were continued for another week without film showings and in follow-ups four and six months later. In the last period (of no medication plus the treatment film) the time spent in self-directed play activity rose to 90 percent, from the baseline figure of under 20 percent, and it subsequently remained at about this level. Note here the value of medication as an adjunct to other kinds of intervention. The authors concluded that with careful editing of videotape self-modeling films, children can rapidly acquire more desirable response patterns from model versions of their own behavior. Thelen, Fry, Fehrenbach, and Frautschi (1979) have pointed out the several advantages of videotape and film modeling over live modeling sequences: availability, economy in terms of money and therapist time, flawless performance through careful editing, multiple models if appropriate, repeated observation, and self-administered treatment sessions.

Spiegel (1977) used self-observation coupled with operant techniques in comparing the relative efficacy of seeing oneself rewarded for exhibiting appropriate classroom behavior versus seeing oneself punished for inappropriate classroom behavior such as inattention, aggression, and overactivity. Baseline data on videotape were collected for five days of two hyperactive boys being rewarded for good behavior in a classroom setting, and of two other hyperactive boys being punished for poor classroom behavior. In the next 15 days each boy saw his own film individually before returning to class, where 10-minute observations of his behavior were made. All four boys showed increases in attending and decreases in aggression and overactivity, with the positive reinforcement pair showing the greater improvement in these behaviors. It was concluded that the combination of techniques used in this study may be an effective therapeutic tool in the classroom setting.

On the basis of the limited research on modeling, it would appear that modeling techniques have potential for intervention with the hyperactive child. The procedures used in the studies reported here all had high attention-directing potential: the children observed adults and children who were familiar to them (Carter & Reynolds, 1976), videotaped self-modeling (Dowrick & Raeburn, 1977), or an interesting film about same-age same-sex children (Goodwin & Mahoney, 1975). In each case the children were able to meet the basic requisite of imitative learning, that is, attending to the stimulus presentation, and this achievement underlines the importance of not downgrading the hyperactive child as consistently unable to attend. As Weiss and Hechtman (1979, p. 1349) have noted, "concentration is not a unitary dimension of personality, but is inseparably linked to motivation and interest in the activity."

Biofeedback

Many clinicians believe that biofeedback has potential for the treatment of the hyperactive child, possibly in the role of an adjunct therapy. Their rationale is as follows. Some hyperactive children are thought to be characterized by increased skeletal muscle tension (Bhatara, Arnold, Lorance, & Gupta, 1979; Braud, 1978). Since hyperactive behavior is believed to be incompatible with a relaxed muscular state (Anderson, 1975; Hughes, Henry, & Hughes, 1980; Johnson, 1976; Mulholland, 1973), a reduction or lessening of the muscular tension in these hyperactive children should be accompanied by a concomitant decrease in their hyperactive behavior. The treatment strategy that has been most widely used with hyperactive children is electromyographic (EMG) feedback training to relax the frontalis muscle in the forehead. With continued EMG training and practice, the hyperactive child can learn to bring under almost maximum conscious control tension in the frontalis muscle. This training is sometimes used in conjunction with controlled progressive (Jacobson, 1938) or autogenic (Schultz & Luthe, 1959) relaxation training. The reasoning underlying this combination is that if the child can become proficient at recognizing the quantitative level of frontalis muscle tension and can learn to reduce that level along with his overall body tension, then when he is required to sit still and focus on a task he will not exhibit hyperactive behavior. Although the feedback displays based on the electrical activity of the striated muscles such as the frontalis are the ones most commonly used, research by Patmon and Murphy (1978) has suggested that another physiological variable, the electrical activity of the cerebral cortex (EEG), may be of greater value. In a comparison of the differential efficacy of EMG and EEG feedback, they reported that increased EEG-frequency biofeedback was the more reliable means of lowering frontalis muscle tension and described the reliability of EMG biofeedback as "unimpressive." Sensorimotor-rhythm conditioning, a laboratory method used for seizure reduction in humans, has also been reported to be successful in controlling hyperactivity in children (Lubar & Shouse, 1976).

At the present time a combination of conflicting results and methodological shortcomings makes it almost impossible to evaluate the claims of therapeutic efficacy of biofeedback for the hyperactive child. The situation is further confounded by a well-documented variance in instrument characteristics (Blanchard & Young, 1974). The biofeedback literature presents conflicting results on a number of key issues. Some investigators (Braud, 1978) report significant differences in EMG muscle tension levels between hyperactive and nonhyperactive subjects prior to treatment, while others (Haight, Jampolsky, & Irvine, 1976) report no differences, a discrepancy that is consistent with subgroups of hyperactive children. In some studies, short-term decreases have occurred in EMG-defined muscle tension levels (Anderson, 1975; Baldwin, Benjamins, Meyers, & Grant, 1978; Bhatara et al., 1979; Braud, 1978; Hampstead, 1977; Hughes et al., 1980; Johnson, 1976), but long-term follow-ups have generally been of little concern. Studies concerned with the efficacy of EMG biofeedback in improving the classroom behavior and cognitive performance of hyperactive children are also characterized by conflicting results. In the school setting, results range all the way from a reduction in hyperactive behavior (Braud, 1978; Hampstead, 1977; Johnson, 1976; Patmon & Murphy, 1978) through no change (Anderson, 1975; Bhatara et al., 1979; Haight et al., 1976) to a significant worsening of classroom behavior (Baldwin et al., 1978). Significant improvement in the cognitive performance of hyperactive children following biofeedback training has been reported by some investigators (Braud, 1978; Braud et al., 1975; Hampstead, 1977) but not others (Johnson, 1976; Patmon & Murphy, 1976).

Biofeedback in combination with environmental contingencies has been used in laboratory and naturalistic settings and it is interesting that, despite the problems inherent in doing research in these settings, the methodology in some of these studies is among the best in research on biofeedback with hyperactive children. Moreland (1977), working in the laboratory setting, used biofeedback combined with reinforcement to modify the hyperactivity of a 4-year-old boy, etiology unknown, who could not sit still throughout even a short television presentation. Moreland used withdrawal of television cartoons to reduce hyperactivity, which was operationally defined by a stabilimeter attached to the child's chair. The subject received continuous visual feedback on his activity level from the control box, and when he became too restless, the cartoons were interrupted. An 8-week period for establishing a baseline followed by an 8-week treatment period consisting of 20 minutes a week training resulted in marked gains that were not maintained over time (Moreland, 1978, personal communication), probably due to parental resistance to having the stabilimeter in the home and to the brevity of the training period. However, the stabilimeter-control box method in this study is an interesting one that warrants further refinement, particularly in selection of reinforcers: there is dubious value in teaching a child that television is a big reward.

Biofeedback combined with reinforcement procedures has been used successfully in several classroom studies. Moore (1977) investigated the efficacy of a combination of behavior modification, using tokens to reinforce sitting and studying, and EMG training with hyperactive first- and second-grade children. Measures included behavioral observations by a trained observer in addition to parent, teacher, and school nurse ratings. A reversal *ABAB* behavioral design was used. The baseline observations, in the *A* conditions, showed increased hyperactivity and decreased academic performance; whereas in the treatment periods, the *B* conditions, hyperactivity decreased and academic performance improved. Schulman and his associates (Schulman, Stevens, Suran, Kupst, & Naughton, 1978) used a combination of biofeedback and operant conditioning to modify the hyperactive behavior of a highly active boy in a classroom setting. They used a biomotometer (Schulman, Stevens, & Kupst, 1977), an electronic device that simultaneously measures activity and provides auditory feedback to the subject, in combination with material reinforcers. In this study, baseline, conditioning, and return to baseline data provided empirical support for the efficacy of this innovative training procedure. Hughes et al. (1980), using biofeedback training in conjunction with social and token reinforcement to increase as well as decrease the frontal EMG levels of children engaged in arithmetic tasks, obtained results suggesting a direct relationship between tension and activity levels.

Several important and unfortunately common methodological shortcomings contribute to the difficulty of evaluating the efficacy of biofeedback training for hyperactivity. Overall, the biofeedback studies to date are characterized by a lack of adequate control groups and control group procedures. Most biofeedback procedures are so striking to the patient that a less striking or worse, a no-treatment control group procedure, becomes totally inadequate; the placebo effect makes useless a baseline of either nontreatment or noncontingent reinforcement. The sample size in almost all of the studies is too small to justify any conclusions about the efficacy of the training procedure. A more rigorous evaluation of the therapeutic efficacy of biofeedback itself is needed. There appears to be a powerful placebo effect which could lead to a totally inaccurate and exaggerated impression of therapeutic effectiveness. Although the combination of biofeedback and other procedures, such as token reinforcement, appears to be a useful one in terms of outcome, it tells us nothing about the efficacy of biofeedback itself because this latter effect is confounded with those of the other intervention procedures. Before the continuing widespread, unevaluated applications of biofeedback currently proliferating in the literature can be justified, systematic investigations are needed to establish that the effect of biofeedback treatment is produced specifically by the biofeedback. It is not clear from the existing research, for example, that biofeedback is superior to relaxation training. Relaxation training may in fact contribute to the alleviation of hyperactivity with much less expenditure of clinician resources and equipment than is required in biofeedback. As Miller (1978b) has pointed out, it is a waste of time to design complex control experiments only to find out that there is no biofeedback effect for which to control.

One research topic that merits serious consideration concerns the important secondary benefits that often accrue from this treatment. Biofeedback, for example, teaches the child that he can control aspects of his own behavior to an astonishing extent. A recent report by Stern and Berrenberg (1977) on this aspect of the treatment reported an increase in the subject's internal locus of control as a result of successful biofeedback training. This finding led Conners (1979b, p. 149) to comment that

> It may well be that one of the most important implications of the striking degree of self-regulation possible with biofeedback is an increase in the child's sense of autonomy and self-sufficiency in a world where his general helplessness is all too frequently fostered by malign environments and a history of inability to control events around him.

A clinical example of this and some of the other phenomena suggested in this discussion is contained in the following statement from a 9-year-old hyperactive boy who was currently undergoing biofeedback training:

> What I would like most of everything is millions of days just like yesterday is what I'd like most. See, I have been going to biofeedback—you know all about how that is, don't you? And my BF lady (I call her that when I tell my mom about it) she says I am one of the best ever at doing biofeedback. It is the first time I ever was that good at anything. I am real good at doing that relaxing and soon I will be able to just sit still and all in school and Miss Katzert will not always be getting mad at me.
>
> Well, now, yesterday we were all ready for church and Lizzie [his sister] said, "What about Stewart, Mother?" in that nasty little icky-sweet voice like what are we going to do about all this mud on the kitchen floor. And all my mom said was, "What about him, Lizzie? He looks all ready to me." And I could tell I'd be extra good all through church, not like last Sunday, and I was. Everytime I started to wriggle I just said, "Now, relax, so the train goes slow, you dummy" [biofeedback visual display used for this child] and when it got to people going up for communion when I usually start getting in trouble I just kept having train-talks to myself and after church my mom gave me a special smile and said, "I was *really* proud of you today, Stu," and my dad said, "That goes for me too, son," and I had this real good feeling. I never had that good a day before in my whole life.

THERAPEUTIC TREATMENT OF CHOICE

Ideally, the pediatrician should be able to recommend the therapeutic treatment of choice for the hyperactive child on the basis of such variables as referral problems, parental attitudes and contribution to the problems, availability of treatment costs, and other pertinent considerations. However, the goal of accurately matching type of therapy to the constellation of problems

presented by the hyperactive child (or any other child with a behavior disorder) requires systematic and specific comparisons of treatments, problems,
and age and type of child, and such multifactorial research has not as yet
been done. In the absence of empirical data on the optimum therapeutic intervention for the hyperactive child, certain general considerations may facilitate
a decision concerning the therapeutic approach to be used. It is important to
distinguish between clearly delineated single-problem behaviors of a social nature, in which a child possesses the requisite behavior in his repertoire, those
problems that occur because of deficiencies in socialization training and therefore present more difficulty in modification, and complex multiple-problem
behavior that includes primary, secondary, and sometimes even subsets of tertiary problems.

By the time most hyperactive children reach the referral stage, it is our
opinion that the problem of hyperactivity has been so complicated and exacerbated by a variety of social and nonsocial factors that it comprises a complex, multiple-problem behavior that must be approached within the
framework of the entire social organization of the child, and consequently
cannot be easily modified by a single therapeutic approach. It is essential to
remember that the cluster of behaviors characteristic of hyperactivity each
constitute a symptom whose underlying cause or combination of causes, must
be effectively treated, whether these are parental mishandling of behavior, or
are school-related, or are due to other factors internal or external to the child.
Discussions of management of the hyperactive child typically advocate multimodality treatment, the major modes being pharmacological, psychotherapeutic, and environmental manipulation. The prognosis is probably excellent
when such multimodality intervention includes multiple forms of psychotherapeutic treatment that involve both parent and child in varying degrees.

Of note here is a 3-year prospective study by Satterfield and his associates
(Satterfield et al., 1979; Satterfield, Satterfield, & Cantwell, 1980) that is the
first prospective long-term study of hyperactive children to systematically
evaluate all subjects from a multidimensional viewpoint, formulate a multimodality treatment program tailored to each child and his family, and then
deliver the indicated treatment within a single clinical setting. In this study
treatment plans included some or all of the following: drug treatment, psychotherapy, and educational therapy, the latter two on both an individual and
group basis for each child; and for the parents, conjoint therapy, family therapy, parent training, and both insight-oriented and supportive group therapy.
Children were accepted for psychotherapy only if the parents agreed to become involved in the treatment process, a requirement that is consistent with
the idea proposed by Allmond et al., (1979) that the *family* is the patient. This
multimodality treatment was associated with unexpectedly good behavioral
and academic outcome for the hyperactive boys who remained in the program
for three years, but not for boys who participated for only one to two years.
Of the boys who dropped out after one or two years, those who were reevalu-
ated at three years had lost the gains that they had made prior to dropping

out, leading Cantwell to conclude (personal communication, 1980a) that consistent and intensive treatment is needed at least for a period longer than two years. At the 3-year follow-up point (Satterfield, Satterfield, & Cantwell, 1981) the group who were still actively participating in the treatment program were farther ahead educationally, demonstrated less antisocial behavior, were rated by their teachers as more attentive and by their parents as better adjusted both at home and at school, and were judged by their parents and psychiatrists to be more improved globally than were children who had dropped out of the program. The outcome data for the 3-year treatment group were also found to be exceptionally good when comparisons were made with the results from other long-term treatment studies. The efficacy of this treatment approach for outcome in late adolescence and early adulthood remains to be determined.

CHAPTER 8

Hyperactivity and the School

In our society going to school represents the major activity of childhood. For 12 formative years the average child spends seven or more hours a day, for approximately 186 days a year, at school. This amount of time is further extended by attendance at preschool, kindergarten, and summer school. For the majority of children the total school experience is the most important socialization force encountered outside of the family (Bronfenbrenner, 1979a; Hartup, 1979); for children who spend a substantial amount of time in day care centers or with babysitters, the socializing impact of the school may equal or even surpass that of the home. The school is a world in miniature, with a set of tasks, assessment procedures, rules, and constraints that parallel to a surprising extent the social, vocational, legal, and competitive demands of the adult world. The inhabitants—principal, teachers, peers, school nurse, librarian, counselor, bus driver, cafeteria workers, and custodian—are in many respects the counterparts of the significant others with whom the child will have to coexist in adulthood.

Although there is general consensus concerning the importance of the school's role in the socialization process, the extent and range of the school's responsibilities are a matter of dispute. Traditionally, the schools have regarded the transmission of the basic academic skills as their primary and in many cases their sole responsibility. During the past two or three decades, however, an increasing demand has arisen from a variety of sources, including parents, press and other media, and medical, legislative, and administrative personnel, for an expanded definition of the school's responsibility. This trend is reflected in philosophic statements of concern for the child (Bronfenbrenner, 1979b; Gross & Gross, 1977; Mnookin, 1978; Young, 1980) as well as in more practical and direct actions such as the demand for accountability on the part of the schools (Hastrop, Mecklenburger, & Wilson, 1973; Lessinger & Tyler, 1971), the increase in private and public litigation for specific school services (e.g., Chapin, 1978; Reutter & Hamilton, 1976; Sprague, 1981; *Wyatt* v. *Stickney*, 1972), and the change in venue of school health programs from the clinic to the school setting (Kappelman, Roberts, Rinaldi, & Cornblath, 1975; Nader, Emmel, & Charney, 1972). Although proponents of increased responsibility have pressed enthusiastically for expansion of the school's role, opponents have angrily denounced such a trend. Nowhere is the polarization on this issue more sharply defined than in the management of the hyperactive child (Browder, 1972; Grinspoon & Singer, 1973; Welsch, 1974), where the crux of the controversy centers on the issue of drug intervention (Jones, Loney, Weissenburger, & Fleischmann, 1975). The catalyst for this controversy was the Omaha incident (Maynard, 1970), aptly entitled by Bosco and Robin (1979) as "the Watergate of hyperactivity." The Omaha incident triggered off a series of investigations in public school systems that focused on issues such as whether teachers were dispensing stimulant medication on their own initiative, whether school personnel were applying undue pressure on parents and pediatricians for drug intervention, and the possibility that unruly children were being drugged solely for classroom peace and teacher convenience (Bosco & Robin, 1979; Gadow, 1981; Grinspoon & Singer, 1973).

A diverse group of events and findings served to sustain the controversy concerning the school's role in the problems of the hyperactive child. Wells (1973) and Bruck (1976) reported litigation concerning unwarranted school pressure to prescribe drugs; accounts of improved outcome of hyperactivity in adulthood supported the implication that the school situation was a poorness of fit (Chess, 1979) situation for the adolescent (Weiss, Hechtman, & Perlman, 1978); a new awareness of children's rights was making itself felt in matters related to schooling (Feshbach & Feshbach, 1978; Weithorn, 1979; Young, 1980); and the mandate of the least restrictive environment imposed by Public Law 94–142, the Education for All Handicapped Children Act (Palfrey, Mervis, & Butler, 1978), caused further reverberations. In addition, the well-documented finding of cross-situational and cross-temporal variability in the hyperactive child's behavior strongly reinforced the position that the environment rather than the child was at fault (Loney, 1980a).

Investigative interest inevitably turned to the quality of the classroom, particularly in relation to the possibility of school-induced hyperactivity (Bax, 1972; Bettelheim, 1973; Cunningham & Barkley, 1978b; Gadow, 1981) and to the alternative of changing the school to fit the child rather than drugging the child to accommodate the school (Silberman, 1970; Young, 1980). With these issues in mind, let us first consider the central figure in this controversy, the hyperactive child, then move on to the role of the school in identifying and treating him, school programs for him, and research contributions to program development.

THE HYPERACTIVE CHILD IN THE CLASSROOM

The diverse group of problems that the hyperactive child presents in the classroom begin to be apparent in the preschool setting (Drash, 1975; Schleifer, Weiss, Cohen, Elman, Cvejic, & Kruger, 1975), are serious enough to trouble and exasperate his teachers in the elementary school years (Campbell, Endman, & Bernfeld, 1977; Minde, Lewin, Weiss, Lavigueur, Douglas, & Sykes, 1971), and they escalate in high school as the hyperactivity-related problems interact with the stresses of adolescence (Milich & Loney, 1979a). Although the majority of clinical referrals of hyperactive children come from school personnel, with the main reason for referral being the problem behavior, it is only in the past five years that systematic attempts have been made to describe the child in the classroom (Klein & Young, 1979). Prior to 1975 information about the hyperactive child in the classroom was curiously one-sided, leading Whalen, Henker, Finck, and Dotemoto (1979, p. 65) to comment that

> little is known about what hyperactive children actually do—the what, when, where, and how of their behavior. Most available data have been obtained through the filter of parents' and teachers' perceptual processes, rather than through direct observations of the children themselves.

In the past five years this imbalance has been partially rectified by findings from an impressive group of systematic investigations of the hyperactive child in both actual and simulated classroom settings. The result has been the accumulation of a body of information of considerable importance in school program planning. The major contribution has come from Whalen and her associates (Henker, Whalen, & Collins, 1979; Whalen, Collins, Henker, Alkus, Adams, & Stapp, 1978; Whalen, Henker, Collins, Finck, & Dotemoto, 1979a; Whalen, Henker, Collins, McAuliffe, & Vaux, 1979b; Whalen, Henker, & Dotemoto, 1980, 1981) in a series of studies that are models of methodological rigor, creativity and ingenuity of design, scholarly restraint in drawing conclusions, sophistication in translating empirical findings into practical applications, and concern for placing the psychological well-being of the subjects ahead of experimental expediency. Other important contributions have come from Campbell and her associates (Campbell, 1976; Campbell, Endman, & Bernfeld, 1977; Campbell & Paulauskas, 1979) and Zentall and his associates (Zentall, 1980; Zentall & Lieb, 1981; Zentall & Shaw, 1981; Zentall & Zentall, 1976; Zentall, Zentall, & Booth, 1978). The effect of the combination of these findings about the interaction between characteristics of the hyperactive child and social and nonsocial classroom factors, existing knowledge of the hyperactive child's academic and cognitive abilities, and theoretical statements (Bell & Harper, 1977; Bronfenbrenner, 1979a) has been to provide a fairly comprehensive composite picture of the hyperactive child in the classroom and school setting.

Effect of Classroom Ecology

Recent research suggests that the unmedicated hyperactive child is a negative force in the classroom, with adverse effects, just as he is in the family (Barkley, 1978). The possibility of a detrimental effect on the ecology of the classroom was first raised by Campbell, Endman, and Bernfeld (1977) when in the course of an observational study they noted that the presence of a hyperactive child seemed to have a generalized negative effect on teacher-pupil interactions. In preschool and at the elementary school level, the hyperactive child is more active and disruptive during classroom activities than are his nonhyperactive peers, and his restlessness and disruptiveness continue into adolescence. He has a shorter attention span, solicits teacher attention at inappropriate times, is more impulsive, and has more frequent energy bursts and spontaneous verbalizations (Buchan, Swap, & Swap, 1977; Klein & Young, 1979; Whalen et al., 1978; Whalen et al., 1979b). It is not surprising, then, that his behavior usurps considerable teacher time, usually in the form of negative sanctions. Although the hyperactive child is not continuously in trouble, as anecdotal accounts would suggest, his dysfunctional behavior is highly conspicuous, as one teacher reported:

> When one of my high active boys knocks something over it disrupts the class temporarily but it's no big deal, whereas Danny's mishaps are almost always a 15-minute restoration job and a topic of conversation for the rest of the school day. If he trips over the waste paper basket, it's not only the contents of the basket that go. He grabs at my desk as he trips, catches the writing pad, pulls everything off so that there is some breakage, and what isn't already ruined he finishes off as he "helps" me clean up.

The effect on the teacher is to make her more intense and controlling in her interactions with the child (Whalen et al., 1981). She singles him out more often, usually for a reprimand, and his presence significantly increases the amount of negative feedback from the teacher to other nonhyperactive children. Campbell et al. (1977) have stated that the hyperactive child generates changes in his behavior settings, which in turn have an impact on his own subsequent behavior. This cycle is set in motion when the child's behavior elicits controlling behavior from the teacher because the hyperactive child is at his best when he is in charge and can dominate the situation. As the teacher becomes more intense and controlling, he becomes more restless and noncompliant so that his behavior deteriorates further, leading to more intensive controlling action on the part of the teacher. It is not surprising, then, that hyperactive boys are well aware of their teachers' disapproval, as Loney, Whaley-Klahn, and Weissenburger (1976) have reported. In their study the responses of hyperactive, high active, and normoactive elementary school boys were obtained on a behaviorally focused school attitude questionnaire called the Teacher Approval–Disapproval Scale (Loney, 1974a) (see Table 4.7 in Chapter 4). The respondents were required to estimate the frequency of certain teacher behaviors toward themselves personally and toward the class as a whole. The hyperactive boys saw themselves as receiving less teacher approval and more disapproval than their normoactive peers for their school work, work habits, and general classroom behavior, and also as being more unhappy in the school situation. However, high active boys reported the most teacher disapproval, a finding that caused Loney et al. to speculate that teachers might have seen them as students who could behave if they wanted to, whereas the hyperactive boys might have been seen as unable to control themselves. An alternative explanation for this finding is that it might reflect the generalized negative effect on teacher-pupil interactions observed by Campbell et al. (1977): the teachers' frustration concerning the disruptive effect of the hyperactive boys' behavior may have been expressed in increased verbal aggression for misbehavior toward the logical displacement targets in the classroom, that is, the high active boys.

The picture that emerges of the hyperactive child's general behavior in the classroom is a curious one in that he appears to be a victim of his own extremes of behavior. Whalen et al. (1979) state that much of his behavior is distinguishable from that of his nonhyperactive peers in terms of style rather than content. He talks too loudly, too fast, and too much, and in addition is too noisy, vigorous, intense, and dominating. The fact that he is at his best when managing a social situation suggests that the dominating behavior might be a coping mechanism in the service of self-pacing, rather than a personality trait. However, when he attracts others with his generally negative-attention-getting antics, he does not know when to stop, and he fails to perceive that continued repetitions of the behavior are inappropriate because the surprise-novelty effect is largely lost after the first response.

Academic Performance

One of the first things that the teacher notices about the hyperactive child, in addition to his behavior problems, is that his academic performance is characterized by great unevenness. This fluctuating school performance pattern is reportedly present in the substantial subgroup of hyperactive children who are also learning disabled (Lambert & Sandoval, 1980) as well as in those who do not qualify for this diagnostic category. In fact, he exhibits the same irregularity in the classroom that he does at home, performing well some days and not others. A number of factors, which other children take in their stride, exert a strong influence on his performance so that on any given classroom task the chances that conditions will be optimal are slight. He functions better, for example, on self-paced rather than teacher-paced tasks (Douglas, 1972), and on straightforward rather than challenging tasks. In the latter case, he is unable to mobilize his resources at all and his behavior falls apart. He has great difficulty learning the ground rules for a new activity and then settling into it (Whalen et al., 1979). This inability to adapt readily to new situational demands is particularly apparent when he is expected to change set, although it is easier for him if the change is from a formal to an informal situation, rather than the reverse (Jacob, O'Leary, & Rosenblad, 1978). Adding to his difficulties is a pervasive inefficiency in such matters as usage of class time and the ability to estimate time (Cappella, Gentile, & Juliano, 1977). The cumulative effect of these characteristics is a significant discrepancy between level of achievement and intellectual potential, a discrepancy that worsens as the child progresses through school with an increasing backlog of unmastered skills.

The reasons for the academic difficulties are not fully understood, and this lack in itself heightens the problem for the teacher. Most teachers find it hard to tolerate a real discrepancy between IQ test scores and school performance, and when such a situation does occur it helps if there is some readily identifiable cause other than their own degree of skill as a teacher. One coping approach is to question the accuracy of the IQ score; a second is to attribute performance deficits to psychological characteristics of the child, such as motivational level.

The IQ Issue

Teachers frequently speculate that the IQ score of the hyperactive child may be spuriously high, in which case there is no performance deficit because the child's achievement level is consistent with his actual (as opposed to his measured) intellectual status. This possibility stems from the fact that the hyperactive child generally performs better in one-to-one situations, so the argument here is that this uncommon situation tends to artificially inflate the IQ score. The whole line of reasoning serves to underline the abysmal lack of understanding on the part of many teachers about the purpose and attributes of carefully constructed IQ tests such as the Stanford-Binet or the WISC.* Conditions should be optimal in the administration of *any* test, and most certainly an IQ test, with its long-range effect on the child's treatment throughout his school years. Furthermore, it is virtually impossible to falsely inflate a score, assuming that the prescribed administration procedures are strictly adhered to, because the calibre of test construction is so high. It is very difficult to guess correctly consistently enough to have a marked effect on the total score. What are the chances, for example, of defining a word that you have never heard of? If anything, the IQ score obtained by the hyperactive child is likely to markedly underestimate his intellectual potential. His well-documented liabilities are likely to have a detrimental effect on his performance in any test situation. With the IQ test, the benefits of one-to-one interaction are greatly offset by the child's short attention span, inability to listen and follow directions, lack of confidence, expectations of failure, and apparent inability to benefit from academic experiences in the way that other children do. This last mentioned point is particularly costly because the typical IQ test has a

---

*It is our experience that a lack of any grasp of the *basic* concepts necessary for an understanding of the meaning of an IQ score and its relationship to a child's performance is far too common among teachers, all of whom should have had a thorough grounding in test theory. In effect, these teachers are manipulating a piece of important and potentially damaging information without the essential prerequisite understanding. It is this kind of basic lack that supports our conviction that the probability is slight that the teacher will be equipped to handle the similarly important and potentially damaging knowledge that a child is to be put on medication for hyperactivity.

large component of school-learned tasks, a not unreasonable characteristic since the original purpose of the IQ test was to predict success in school.

The effects of the hyperactive child's apparent inability to benefit to the fullest from academic experience are, as one might expect, least obvious in the early school years. Neither hyperactive boys (Prinz & Loney, 1974) nor girls (Loney, 1974b) in the primary grades differ in IQ from nonhyperactive controls, but in the upper grades hyperactive children score significantly lower than nonhyperactive controls (Miller, Palkes, & Stewart, 1973; Minde et al., 1971; Palkes & Stewart, 1972), a finding that is consistent with differential benefits from educational training rather than genuine differences in intellectual ability. The Palkes and Stewart data (1972) support this explanation, but it should be pointed out that the conclusion that they drew opposes it. In their study the hyperactive group were well below their nonhyperactive classmates in achievement as well as IQ, so Palkes and Stewart concluded that the hyperactive children *were* learning at a rate commensurate with their IQs, and the gap between their school performance and that of their peers reflected the difference in IQ. In other words, they viewed the IQ scores for the hyperactive children as true IQs and consequently saw the hyperactive group as innately less able than their nonhyperactive peers. We disagree with this conclusion. It is our opinion that the IQ score of an untreated hyperactive child is more a measure of the effects of attributes of hyperactivity on the test score than of actual intellectual ability. However, the Palkes and Stewart conclusion warrants further discussion because it has a certain acceptance among teachers as an explanation for the poor performance of hyperactive children.

The Below-Average Ability Issue

Despite the fact that the hyperactive child is often depicted in the literature as of average or above average intelligence (Cantwell, 1979; Loney, 1980a; Millichap, 1975), some teachers contend that his performance problems occur because he is less able than his nonhyperactive peers. One basis for this contention is that it is uncommon to find hyperactive children who perform at or above grade level (Keogh & Barkett, 1980) which could be interpreted as support for lower than average, but still normal, mental ability in hyperactive children. An alternative explanation is that the more able hyperactive children are, by virtue of their satisfactory school performance, not identified as hyperactive. Both the "behavior equivalents" in the prevalence study of Sandoval, Lambert, and Sassone (1980), as well as the children noted by Jones et al. (1975), who for whatever reason were not referred for hyperactivity even though their behavior was in the hyperactive range, could have been hyperactive children who achieved at a high level and were accepted as normal for this reason. A notable example of this explanation was the case of a 7-year-old extremely hyperactive boy with an IQ of at least 145 (he lost interest in the test before completing it), who was reading at the fifth-grade level on the occasions when he stopped long enough to look at a book, and whose disruptive behavior was dismissed by the teacher as just showing that he was "a real bundle of boy." In the same classroom, a hyperactive boy who was much less able was on stimulant medication as a result of the teacher's complaints about his behavior.

The Motivational Explanation

Another possibility that teachers have advanced is that the hyperactive child has a motivational deficit that is a major factor in his unsatisfactory academic performance. The pattern of irregularity that pervades the child's behavior contributes greatly to the commonsense view that he could do it if he tried. However, several sets of empirical findings argue against a motivational deficit as the *major* factor, although given the child's history of inadequate if not failing performance, motivation undoubtedly contributes to the problem.

In a 5-year follow-up (Weiss et al., 1971) involving cognitive and motor individual testing sessions, psychologists reported that many of the children were overconcerned with accuracy and good performance on the tests almost to the point of obsessiveness, which suggests that in this particular situation the hyperactive child's performance problems may be the result of task-related deficits (Douglas & Peters, 1979; Keogh & Barkett, 1980) rather than a lack of motivation. Hyperactive children in class-competition situations often engage in a kind of ferocious struggle to perform well, but nevertheless fail to do so. In a study on motor speed (Stevens, Stover, & Backus, 1970) one group of hyperactive children and nonhyperactive controls were presented with a multitrial tapping task, a second group was urged after the trial to tap faster, and a third group was offered monetary reward for each increment of speed after the base trial. The results showed that the hyperactive children were slightly faster than the controls in the task-only condition, but when urging or rewards were introduced the nonhyperactive subjects performed faster. Stevens et al. concluded that although the hyperactive children were clearly trying, they were limited by a narrow range of performance speed that was not affected by the presence of incentives. These results are consistent with the finding that hyperactive boys of elementary school age have a narrower range of gross motor speed that nonhyperactive controls (Ross & Ross, 1976, pp. 217–218).

Although these data suggest that in some situations the performance deficit reflects a lack of requisite competencies rather than a motivational deficit, we are still left with the fact that under some circumstances, notably one-to-one situations, the hyperactive child performs as well as his peers of equal mental ability. The hyperactive and nonhyperactive children are similar in *competence*, which is the demonstration of proficiency under ideal task conditions. However, in terms of *performance*, that is, the ability to use skills appropriately and consistently in everyday situations, the hyperactive child is far less able. Well-documented clinical and research evidence supports the fact that the hyperactive child possesses the requisite skills for effective classroom performance on some tasks but does not make consistent use of them, resulting in a marked discrepancy between his overall classroom performance and the level predicted on the basis of his IQ. We offer the following unsubstantiated explanation for this phenomenon, based solely on subjective observations of hyperactive children in naturalistic settings. Level of performance on a specific task is largely determined by the interaction of three factors: the requisite skills and abilities for performance of the task, the cognitive energy of the child (which we envision as a psychological rallying of intellectual forces), and stimulus control factors in the task and its environment. If the attributes of the task are sufficiently powerful—for example, novel, exciting, visually focusing—to mobilize the child's cognitive energy *and* he possesses the requisite task competencies, then he will perform at a level appropriate for his IQ score. It is our opinion that the primary contributor to the poor performance in the classroom is a cognitive energy deficit, an inability to continuously mobilize the intellectual forces needed to perform routine classroom tasks, rather than an unwillingness or a lack of desire to perform. This cognitive energy deficit hypothesis is consistent with the finding that when the hyperactive child has the requisite competencies he generally performs far more effectively in one-to-one situations than on the same task in a group situation. He also attends closely to television programs, movies, and to the passing scene while riding in an automobile for relatively long periods. In these situations his cognitive energy is to a great extent being mobilized for him: in the first case by a compelling adult, and in the others by an attention-directing presentation. This explanation differs markedly from the motivational deficit explanation in its implications for classroom management. It follows that approaches to remediation based on these two constructs would reflect this difference.

Other Explanations

Douglas and her associates (Douglas, 1972, 1974; Douglas, Parry, Martin, & Garson, 1976; Douglas & Peters, 1979) attribute the classroom performance problems of the hyperactive child to cognitive deficits and difficulties, the major determinants being the problems of attention and impulse control that are viewed in their framework as reciprocal aspects of the same process. The picture that emerges from their research on attention in the hyperactive child is indeed complex. It suggests that the child's attentional problems constitute a heterogeneous group of strengths and weaknesses. For example, the child performs as well as his normal peers when he is helped to focus his attention prior to the presentation of the task and is allowed to work at his own rate; he shows evidence of a costly impulsivity of response, and his behavior is characterized by lapses of attention; but he is not more easily distracted than his nonhyperactive peers on *some* tasks. Support for the important role that attentional factors and impulsivity play comes from descriptions of his task-related behavior. Klein and Young (1979) reported that hyperactive children in the primary grades alternated between on-task and off-task behaviors throughout an activity, with the off-task responses including high rates of gross motor activity and disruptive verbalizations. These findings were also consistent with the classroom observations of Campbell et al. (1977) and of Whalen et al. (1978, 1979) in a quasi-naturalistic classroom.

Because the hyperactive child is unable to sustain attention for reasonable periods of time he is often depicted as a daydreamer. In fact, the amount of time that he spends daydreaming is very small (Klein & Young, 1979). Douglas (1972) has suggested that the child tends to be occupied by goals differing from those of the teacher rather than being engaged in random aimless activity such as daydreaming. Support for this idea comes from a study by Baldwin (1976) who reported that hyperactive boys in the elementary grades did not differ from nonhyperactive controls in either length of attention span or number of stimuli attended to. The difference was in the focus of their attention. Hyperactive boys focused on nonacademic stimuli, such as parts of their bodies, while their nonhyperactive peers attended to academic materials and the teacher for a longer span. The costly impulsivity that has so often been described by Douglas and her colleagues is very much in evidence during routine classroom activities. When the class is given an assignment the hyperactive child is often the first to start work because he plunges in before having the complete instructions. He is the first to raise his hand to answer a question, whether he knows the answer or not, and if he is not called upon he is likely to blurt out a usually incorrect answer.

THE ROLE OF THE SCHOOL

The role of the school in identifying and treating the child as hyperactive is an issue that is complicated by justified parental concern (Bruck, 1976) and considerable disapproval on the part of the medical establishment (Browder, 1972; Walker, 1974). The controversy centers on the events in the entire sequence that follows the teacher's first awareness that the child's behavior warrants investigation.

The Teacher's Role

There is no opposition to the role the teacher plays in setting in motion the process that may result in the diagnosis of hyperactivity because generally she is qualified to make a preliminary judgment concerning the child's classroom behavior. She usually has had considerable experience with the range of classroom behavior that approximates the normal, and also has a sizable group of the child's same-age peers as a comparison base for evaluating the intensity and frequency of certain behaviors. In addition, she sees the child for a long period of time each day and in a variety of situations. Given this base, what should happen (Johnson & Prinz, 1976) when a teacher suspects that a child has a problem is as follows: the teacher should document the extent and kind of behavior problem as she sees it in the classroom and school setting by recording the frequency, time of occurrence, and situation in which the disordered behavior occurs; she should then make any changes in the psychological and physical environments that appear to have the potential to modify the behavior. Psychological changes might include changes in the presentation and spacing of tasks, or in allocation and type of positive reinforcement; physical changes might involve separation from peers who instigate the problem behavior or reinforce it, or removal of certain distractions. When the teacher has exhausted her resources with no improvement, she should seek consultation with the school psychologist concerning referral.

The Preferred Referral Procedure. The referral sequence should continue with the school psychologist observing the child in the classroom to confirm that it is the child who is the problem rather than environmental and psychological factors in the classroom. The parents are then notified, a parent-school conference is scheduled, and the child is referred to a pediatrician for formal evaluation. The child may be given a battery of tests at school, and these results, other pertinent school test data, and reports from the teacher describing his classroom behavior would be relayed to the pediatrician. This phase of school participation would then end with selected school personnel meeting with the pediatrician and the rest of his team, at the pediatrician's invitation.

What Often Happens. Once the teacher has noticed the problem behavior she makes the diagnosis of hyperactivity with no input from any professional, and the diagnosis is likely to be dictated as much by personal imperatives as by objective criteria (Werry, 1977). She schedules a meeting with the parents, sometimes with no other school personnel present, and issues an ultimatum concerning action about the child's disordered behavior in the classroom. The ultimatum is virtually always a choice between medication and less desirable class placement. Faced with the specter of segregation and formal labeling of the child, the parents hastily contact their pediatrician or in some cases a pediatrician recommended by the school and known for his readiness to prescribe stimulant medication. Unfortunately, in either case stimulant medication is often prescribed after only a cursory examination of the child or sometimes with no examination. Browder's (1972) belief that the impetus for prescribing stimulant medication frequently is the result of pressures and demands within the school is supported by this verbatim quote from the angry mother of an 8-year-old boy:

> The teacher called us [both parents] in and said either Jimmy goes on medications or else it's special class. She said Wilson Elementary can't handle boys as disruptive and lazy as Jimmy is. We were really astounded because he's been there four years and always got good reports but she said that the Fourth Grade is when MBD gets to cause problems. I asked her who else had looked at Jim-

my, like the school psychologist or the nurse, and she said "Mrs. Morrison, no one knows these children the way I do and Dr. Andrews [psychologist] and the principal *always* agree with my decisions on what goes on in my class." We told her we'd talk to our pediatrician and she wanted us to go to one the school recommended. All the other boys in her class on medication, there are six of them, went to this pediatrician. She couldn't understand our attitude—she said all the other parents had cooperated real nicely as soon as she suggested medication. I don't know how she thinks she knows so much about Jimmy when he's only been in her class for a little over a month.

It is totally inappropriate for a teacher to attempt a diagnosis of hyperactivity. Many teachers are far from knowledgeable about the cluster of behaviors and other attributes that are considered to be diagnostic evidence of hyperactivity (Blunden, Spring, & Greenberg, 1974; Johnson & Prinz, 1976) and they lack the formal training and skill necessary to eliminate conditions that may be present with hyperactivity as a symptom. The symptoms of concern can be related to a variety of etiologies, including medical problems such as chronic illness or neurologic disorders, boredom, frustration, transient anxiety, the more severe behavioral disturbances such as juvenile manic depression, and mental retardation (Walker, 1974). Even within the teacher's sphere of influence, the classroom setting, she often lacks the objectivity and expertise required to identify difficult behavior. Whalen et al. (1979) have distinguished between classrooms that function as *provocation ecologies* by magnifying behavioral differences between hyperactive children and their nonhyperactive peers, and *rarefaction ecologies* that minimize these differences. It would be difficult for a teacher to see that an attribute such as her teaching style might be accelerating the problem or that class membership was causing her to perceive the child's behavior as more of a problem that it actually was (Calhoun, 1975). Werry (1977, p. 447) has specified that in order to make an objective diagnosis there must be a set of explicit rules to follow, the necessary and sufficient criteria must be spelled out including the disqualifying ones by which the diagnosis can be made, and there must be accurate ways of detecting these criteria. He believes that the teacher typically has neither the knowledge nor facility to meet these requirements.

The School's Role in Treatment

Treatment may consist of behavior modification procedures, changes within the regular classroom, individual tutoring or special class placement, drug intervention, or any combination of the above. If behavior modification procedures are to be used it will most likely be the teacher or the psychologist who implements them and assesses their efficacy. For these and all other recommended changes in classroom procedures, it is the teacher's responsibility to put them into effect without stigmatizing the child. These behavioral and environmental interventions are handled competently by teachers and school personnel according to a substantial body of empirical reports (Barkley, 1978; Madsen & Madsen, 1974; McDonald, 1978; Zupnick, 1974). A major reason for this competence is the fact that the role of the classroom teacher and other school personnel in respect to these modes of intervention has been explicitly defined and is not a matter of controversy.

This state of relative harmony does not extend to drug intervention. There is strong disagreement concerning the school's role in prescribing drug treatment for the hyperactive child. Some educators and psychologists (Tobiessen & Karowe, 1969) believe that the school personnel are the logical ones to persuade parents and pediatricians to place hyperactive children on stimulant medication, whereas many physicians and laymen are outraged at the school overstepping the boundaries between education and medicine (e.g., Browder, 1972; Bruck, 1976; Grinspoon & Singer, 1973; Walker, 1974; Welsch, 1974) and have issued strong warnings about the general implications of this school policy as well as the specific dangers of yielding to school pressure to prescribe drugs. Jones et al. (1975, p. 388) have concluded that "many of the problems in defining the appropriate role of the school are due to the assumption that once a child is diagnosed as hyperactive, CNS stimulants should routinely be prescribed."

Drug Treatment

Stimulant medication is the most frequent and often the only treatment procedure used (Barkley, 1978; Cantwell, 1979; Safer & Allen, 1976). In *theory*, the teacher should play an important part in monitoring the child's response to medication. She is in a position to best judge the efficacy of dosage because the child is in school during the peak dosage periods, and her ratings assume prime importance in providing feedback to the pediatrician and parents. The teacher qualified for this role would know what academic and behavioral effects to expect from the medicated child, and what not to expect. She would recognize side effects and know when their significance justified reports of such effects to the pediatrician. All this activity could be carried out with discretion and tact, so that the child would be unaware that he was the focus of unusual scrutiny. In *practice*, most teachers do not begin to approach the level of knowledge and understanding that are prerequisite to the competent handling of this role. For this reason we advocate *not* informing the teacher that a child is on medication. This opinion is consistent with our firm belief that only the parents should know that the child is on medication, and that this restriction is absolutely in the best long-term interests of the child. (For a further discussion of this issue as it relates to the child, see Chapter 10.)

This position does not in any way eliminate the contribution that the teacher should make in keeping the pediatrician informed about the child's behavior. There is unequivocal evidence of the accuracy of teachers' assessments, as well as their sensitivity to minor modifications of dosage under carefully controlled experimental conditions (Sprague & Ullman, 1981). We are not disputing the obvious importance and value of these behavioral data. What we are opposed to is the teacher having knowledge of the drug regimen of the hyperactive child and making decisions concerning it. The teacher's responsibility should be limited to her particular area of expertise, namely, the observation, assessment, and reporting of the hyperactive child's behavior. She should still make notes on his behavior, be alert for any abrupt changes that have no apparent explanation, follow certain evaluation procedures set up by the pediatrician and his team, and have responsibility in managing behavioral and environmental interventions. All of these activities could be conducted in the absence of any knowledge of the medication aspects of the intervention program and without sacrificing either the range or quality of the information and procedures. In the following two case reports (Barkley, 1979, p. 414) note that the teachers' reports of behavior deviating from the norm were *not* dependent on knowing that the children were on medication:

> . . . a 12-year old severely hyperactive boy who was admitted to our hospital for depression, weepiness, agitation, fearful behavior, and extreme social withdrawal. He was felt by the school staff to be manifesting a severe emotional disturbance. Discussion with the family revealed the child to be receiving 100 mg of Ritalin daily—a surprisingly high dose for this thin, spindly child. All of his behavioral and emotional manifestations are now known to be side effects of Ritalin. Once the medication was discontinued, the boy returned to his normally happy, yet hyperactive, state with no sign of emotional symptoms . . . if not recognized, such symptoms or side effects can interfere with adequate social adjustment and academic performance in the school setting.

> Recently, the mother of a hyperactive child receiving Cylert noted that she had received complaints from the boy's teacher of his picking his fingers and toes during class. The boy was said to remove his shoes and socks during classwork to pick at and pinch his toes. The ridicule and teasing from other children did not diminish this child's habits. The mother's surprise, however, was that she had never witnessed such behavior at home, and hence she suspected the accuracy of the teacher's reports. In actuality, the boy was displaying this stereotypic behavior in class about 60 to 90 minutes after receiving a dose of Cylert with it diminishing within 2 to 3 hours thereafter. Decreasing the dose of Cylert resulted in a disappearance of the behavior.

Research on teachers' knowledge and attitudes about stimulant medication supports our view that teachers generally are ill-equipped to handle the potentially damaging-to-the-child information that he is on medication. Teachers usually are not well informed about these drugs, are uncertain about their use and contrary to the stereotypic notion of the teacher as a "pusher" (Rapoport & Repo, 1971) and, quite commendably in view of their reported ignorance, favor a passive role for the teacher in drug usage (Johnson & Prinz, 1976; Robin & Bosco, 1973; Treegoob, 1976). In the Robin and Bosco study, for example, only one-third of the respondents knew that Ritalin (methylphenidate) had side effects, and in the Johnson and Prinz study less than one-sixth of the group were aware of adverse side effects. Furthermore, a study of the involvement of school personnel in the medication process (Okolo, Bartlett, & Shaw, 1978) indicates a lack of communication, not between teacher and pediatrician as might be expected, but rather a within-school problem between school nurse and teacher. The results of this study indicated no systematic feedback of information from teacher to nurse, a critical omission in view of the fact that minimal standards for drug therapy require data collection by teachers in the classroom setting (Neisworth, Kurtz, Ross, & Madle, 1976).

Behavior Intervention

As part of the management program the teacher may be asked to implement some form of behavior intervention in the classroom. The intervention procedures, such as operant conditioning and modeling, are not difficult to use. However, their use requires careful preparation and planning with the teacher because their apparent simplicity is conducive to casual misuse. Before initiating behavior intervention in the classroom, it is essential to obtain a firm commitment to the treatment program from the school personnel because considerable teacher time and effort may be required.

Inherent in this situation is a problem of critical importance to the efficacy of the treatment plan for the hyperactive child. Typically, there is no difficulty in procuring teacher commitment either during the initial treatment planning period or while the program is being set up in the classroom under the direction of the investigator. During this period, which is also the period customarily reported in journal articles, the program is almost invariably successful whether with an individual child (Patterson, Jones, Whittier, & Wright, 1965; Wahler, Sperling, Thomas, Teeter, & Luper, 1970) or with a group of children (Doubros & Daniels, 1966; Rosenbaum, O'Leary, & Jacob, 1975). However, the gains maintained during the investigator-present stage frequently diminish sharply once the investigator leaves the classroom and the teacher is on her own. Brown, Montgomery, and Barclay (1969) have demonstrated unequivocally that the sharp drop in gains is related to the termination of investigator-supplied reinforcement for the teacher, which coincides with the investigator's exit from the classroom as soon as the teacher has been trained to his satisfaction. In the study by Brown et al., positive reinforcement by classroom teachers was used to modify out-of-seat behavior in an educationally retarded 9-year-old boy. In the baseline period the rate of positive reinforcement by the two teachers for in-seat behavior was recorded. For the next six days the teachers reinforced the boy for in-seat behavior and the investigator reinforced the teachers for *their* adherence to the program. In the third phase, the investigator discontinued his social reinforcement of the teachers, and in the fourth and final phase he again reinforced the teachers. The effects of investigator reinforcers on maintenance of teacher reinforcement of in-seat behavior are shown in Figure 8.1. The impact of these variations in teacher behavior on the behavior of the deviant child were consistent with reinforcement theory. The child's rate of out-of-seat behavior was high during baseline, diminished sharply as a function of the teacher's social reinforcement in the second phase, increased markedly concomitantly with the decrease in teacher reinforcement in the third phase, and dropped sharply in the fourth phase; in other words, almost a vertical mirror image of the frequencies shown in Figure 8.1.

The implications of these results for behavior intervention involving teachers are considerable. A sequence that has frequently been noted with behavior intervention in the classroom is a marked, often dramatic improvement in measured behavior as a function of a relatively brief period of intervention of perhaps two or three weeks, followed by a sharp deterioration in the target behavior when follow-up checks are conducted. These latter measures are usually obtained when the program has been the sole responsibility of the teacher for several weeks. The sharp decrease in target behavior improvement is often attributed either to inadequacies in the program or to the child becoming habituated to the reinforcers. The results of Brown et al. (1969) suggest that the

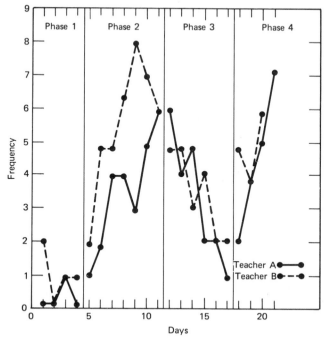

Figure 8.1   Frequency of Social Reinforcers Emitted by Two Teachers under Investigator Present (Phase 2 and 4) and Absent (Phase 3) Conditions. Reprinted, by permission, from Brown, J., Montgomery, R., & Barclay, J. An example of psychologist management of teacher reinforcement procedures in the elementary classroom. *Psychology in the Schools*, 1969, *6*, 336–340.

failure to maintain the initial gains may simply reflect the fact that the teacher has discontinued the program out of disinterest on her part. Instead of regarding the disappointing long-term data in such cases as suggestive of weaknesses in the program format, it may be more accurate to view the data as measures of a back to baseline condition.

Before leaving the topic of the school's role in treatment we will briefly discuss a trend that has occurred in school health programs. During the last decade school health has come to be viewed as directly related to the learning process, and advocates of this viewpoint (Kappelman, Roberts, Rinaldi, & Cornblath, 1975) have urged the redefinition of school health to include the behavior and learning problems of childhood. Furthermore, Kappelman et al. and others (Nader et al., 1972) have recommended that school health programs give these problems top priority. This approach requires a pediatrician with specialized training and expertise about school facilities and educational methods, as well as a multidisciplinary team of educational, psychological, nursing, and other specialists. This team provides on-site diagnosis, makes recommendations for remedial action, conducts some of the remedial work, and follows up each case to evaluate the outcome. School health programs have been operating for some time with considerable success in the Baltimore schools (Kappelman et al., 1975). In describing their effectiveness, Kappelman et al. note an increase in number of referrals over the previous year when no such program was available. Such an increase is open to more than one interpretation. It could mean that teachers are more adept at identifying children who should be referred, with the result that intervention is initiated far sooner than it ordinarily would have been. It could also mean that the presence of the team in the school district has resulted in overreferral. Whatever the reason, in-service training for teachers in the school should be concomitant with such a program so that they maintain perspective on which problems lie appropriately within their own jurisdiction.

SCHOOL PROGRAMS FOR THE HYPERACTIVE CHILD

The first special school programs were developed in private schools after the encephalitis epidemic of 1918 when it became apparent that the behavior sequelae of the epidemic were incompatible with the demands of the regular classroom (Bond & Appel, 1931; Hallahan & Cruickshank, 1973; Kessler, 1980; Strecker & Ebaugh, 1924). One of the best of these was that of the Franklin School of the Pennsylvania Hospital, a residential school program that has been described by Bond and Appel (1931). Prior to World War II, special programs in the public school system were virtually nonexistent, a deficit that reflected the current thinking and economic conditions of the time. Hyperactivity was seen as a medical or at most a disciplinary problem rather than an educational one, and the economic depression had seriously depleted available school funds. Following World War II, a rapid burgeoning of the special education field occurred at all levels of the educational hierarchy, but unfortunately program development did not keep step.

In the case of the hyperactive child, relatively few intervention programs have been developed in the last three decades. Clinicians and educators alike have believed that stimulant medications and behavior modification were sufficiently effective in modifying the behavior problems of the hyperactive child in the classroom. Parents readily accepted drug intervention and so abdicated their role as a potentially powerful source of pressure for special school programs: as soon as hyperactive children are on drugs and apparently functioning adequately, many parents tend to be disinterested in other forms of intervention (Schaefer, Palkes, & Stewart, 1974). More recently, the view of educators that labeling and placement of mildly handicapped children in self-contained special classes is not the most advantageous solution has led to the passing of Public Law 94–142. This law mandates the mainstreaming of almost all children with special learning needs, the rationale being that segregation in special classes deprives the child of important social interaction experiences and exposes him to the stigma associated with special class placement. As a result, the incentive for developing special programs has been largely eliminated because the target population for such programs has been absorbed into the regular classes where presumably regular class programs are being used. We should digress here to point out that in our opinion Public Law 94–142 has had and will continue to have a disastrous effect on the large majority of children who formerly qualified for special education classes. It is naive in the extreme to think that a child with behavioral and academic problems will not be labeled as a misfit merely because he is in a regular classroom; that physical proximity will mean psychological acceptance by his peers; and that the teacher will have the ability, time, and interest to modify the regular curriculum to meet his special needs.

A fundamental characteristic of the first programs developed was the belief that the school should be changed to fit the child, the assumption being that a changed classroom would result in a changed child. Although behavior modifying procedures were included, the major emphasis was on changes in classroom teaching procedures, constraints, and nonsocial environmental conditions. This philosophy of education has its roots in the belief that institutions should be changed to fit the individual, rather than the reverse, and other offshoots are prison reform and concern for individual rights. It has the support of a number of critics (Glasser, 1968; Holt, 1964) who have steadfastly maintained that altering the sedentary nature of the classroom and modifying the rigidity of present school requirements would eliminate many behavioral and achievement problems. The idea that the hyperactive child's school problems are largely a function of unreasonable constraints and demands in the school setting has continued to find support from diverse sources such as post-Omaha critics of the school (Grinspoon & Singer, 1973; Ladd, 1970), parents who are convinced that their children's hyperactivity stems from the pressures of rigid classroom procedures and are greatly impressed by the enthusiastic accounts from advocates of "open" classrooms, experienced clinicians (Bax, 1972; Bettelheim, 1973), and other investigators such as Weiss and Hechtman (1979), and Whalen and her colleagues (Henker & Whalen, 1980a; Whalen et al., 1978, 1979, 1980b), who have documented the power of stimulus control techniques that can be manipulated to either maximize or minimize the differences between hyperactive children and their nonhyperactive peers in the regular classroom.

Of the classroom programs developed since World War II, only a fraction have been subjected to experimental test or at least some form of objective assessment. The lack of systematic research on existing special programs is due to the disinterest that educators traditionally have shown in research of any kind. Programs frequently are established on an intuitive basis rather than on firm empirical evidence of their efficacy. Educational journals show this tendency to intuitive acceptance particularly in the field of special education. Innovative procedures reported as successful by their proponents usually fail to produce the claimed results when they are subjected to objective assessment, in the unlikely event that they are in a form that lends itself to replication. In no other profession concerned with the problems of children is there such a lack of concern for establishing an empirical basis for new management techniques. The programs that have been evaluated can be categorized as follows:

1.   Minimal stimulation programs in which the emphasis is on the reduction of extraneous social and nonsocial environmental stimulation.

2.   Open classrooms with an emphasis on individualized instruction and activity, freedom of movement, flexibility in scheduling, and teacher-pupil decision making.

3.   Parent involvement programs in which educational and psychotherapeutic intervention have been systematically combined to modify the behavior of the parents as well as that of the child.

4.   Short-term intensive training programs designed to equip the child with a specific skill or modify a particular response pattern that is detrimental to his functioning in the classroom.

Minimal Stimulation Programs

In the post-World War II era the first comprehensive classroom program for hyperactive children was developed by Strauss and Lehtinen (1947), who viewed the hyperactive child as brain-injured and considered his central problem to be his distractibility, that is, his unusually high responsivity to environmental stimulation. The fact that in a learning situation he was unable to maintain focus on the central part of a task and was distracted by stimuli that were peripheral to the task context suggested to Strauss and Lehtinen that the child's ability to focus attention would be improved by sharply reducing the number of stimulus elements in the environment. An important feature of their program was a stimulus reduction strategy which required the removal of all visual distractors such as bulletin boards, elimination of patterned parts of the visual field by frosting the lower parts of windows, reduction of auditory stimulation, neutralization of walls and ceilings by painting them in neutral tones, and reduction of social stimulation by requiring teachers to dress inconspicuously and by increasing the space between desks. To further minimize responsivity to extraneous stimulation, the desks of the most distractible children were sometimes placed in corners facing the wall. No stigma was associated with this procedure; both teachers and children viewed it as constructive and helpful, and often the child was the one who decided when he was ready to rejoin the group. The ratio of pupils to teachers was low, in order to increase the amount of individual attention, and lesson activities were designed to provide frequent activity breaks. To Strauss and Lehtinen, the special classroom was much more than just a room with a low pupil: teacher ratio; it was in itself a teaching instrument and they made maximum use of it. The behavioral response of children in these classrooms was described as "immediate," and impressive examples of the changes that occurred were provided (Strauss & Lehtinen, 1947, pp. 132–133):

> Loud talking, running in the room, attacks on other children diminish and often disappear in a matter of days; the formerly unmanageable child becomes quite tractable. A first grade pupil whom the teacher finally refused to keep in her class ran about the room, sang, laughed out loud, removed shoes and stockings, and completely disrupted any organized group activity. After a week behind the screen in the special class, this behavior disappeared so completely that the screen was no longer needed.

The work of Strauss and Lehtinen has been subject to much legitimate criticism particularly in respect to their failure to use adequate statistical procedures in the evaluation of their results, and the lack of rigorous control in the procedures used to diagnose a child as brain injured (e.g., Sarason, 1949). The methodological shortcomings should not, however, detract from recognition of the catalytic effect their work had upon the entire field of special education. Their conception of the problems of the brain-injured child served as a stimulus for research on psychoeducational problems, and the educational procedures they devised provided guidelines for subsequent remediation techniques.

The Cruickshank Experiment

An experimental test of the hypothesis that hyperactivity is precipitated by an excess of environmental stimulation was conducted in four public school classrooms by Cruickshank, Bentzen, Ratzeburg, and Tannhauser (1961). Their subjects were 40 children (37 boys, three girls) who were hyperactive, aggressive, and educationally retarded. Half of the sample had unequivocal evidence of injury to the central nervous system, and the other half had no evidence of central nervous system damage. Each of the four classes had five brain-injured and five nonbrain-injured children. The four groups were matched in terms of relevant age, achievement, medical, and behavioral variables. The mean chronological age was eight years, one month, and the mean IQ was 80.3.

Each classroom had an experienced teacher and a teacher aide. Two of the classes formed the control group and were taught by traditional methods; the other two became the experimental group, using a modification of the Strauss and Lehtinen procedures in a program that incorporated five basic principles:

1. The reduction of environmental space through the use of cubicles.
2. The elimination of nonessential visual and auditory stimulation.
3. A structured approach in lessons, classroom procedures, and nonsocial classroom events with an emphasis on predictability, the initial elimination of choice situations, and the almost complete elimination of failure experiences.
4. The use of attention-directing teaching materials combined with minimal background distraction to focus attention on the task.
5. A multisensory teaching approach with specialized teaching materials.

A pre- and posttest design was used with measures obtained with the Stanford–Binet Form L, Goodenough Intelligence Test, Stanford Achievement Test, Bender–Gestalt, Vineland Scale of Social Maturity, and Syracuse Visual Figure-Background Test. The major finding was that there was no convincing evidence for the efficacy of the minimal stimulation classroom in either the posttest data or the follow-up data collected one year later.

The Cruickshank et al. experiment has come in for considerable criticism concerning the analysis of the test data and the failure to provide information generated by the data. When one or the other group performed better on the pretest no correction for this difference was made on the posttest analysis, which makes it difficult to determine the real meaning of intergroup posttest differences. Considerable emphasis was placed on establishing a balance in each class between children diagnosed as brain-injured and those having no such diagnosis. However, no comparisons were reported on the performance of these subgroups. It would have been of value to determine whether the subgroups were affected differentially by either the experimental or the control procedures. Also, no intercorrelations were computed among the various test measures. Such information would have permitted a comparison between the structure of abilities of the two groups of children and those of normal children, and indicated whether patterns of cognitive abilities were influenced by the two kinds of classroom intervention. It was not until more than a decade later that Hallahan and Cruickshank (1973) acknowledged the limitations of the 1961 study and admitted that there was little empirical support for the efficacy of a stimulus reduction strategy. Despite this crucial lack of essential support, Cruickshank, his associates, and many other educators (e.g., Alabiso,

1972; Kirk, 1972) continued to endorse the reduction of environmental stimulation as a management technique for hyperactive children.

The central assumption of the Strauss and Lehtinen (1947) approach, that is, that task performance will improve and activity decrease with a reduction of environmental stimulation and an increased level of within-task stimulation, received little support from the Cruickshank et al. study and has since been firmly refuted by other empirical investigations, particularly those of the Zentall team. From the latter research it is clear that the locus and level of stimulation interact in diverse ways with the task performance and activity level of the hyperactive child, and that the variable results cannot be accommodated within either the two-factor overarousal formula (Strauss & Lehtinen, 1947) or the underarousal model (Zentall, 1977). Consider the stimulation x task x activity complexities inherent in the following findings. The task performance of hyperactive children improved and their activity level decreased when rock music was presented within the context of a boring sitting task and a routine cancellation task (Zentall & Zentall, 1976). Auditory distractors disrupted the performance of hyperactive children as a function of task complexity, that is, degree of information load, but facilitated performance when the task had been previously practiced (Conners, 1975b). Hyperactive children were more active and performed worse on arithmetic and alphabet tasks (Zentall & Shaw, 1981) and general classroom work (Whalen et al., 1979) under conditions of high rather than low ambient noise. High stimulation (novelty) tasks in low structure (child-directed) settings resulted in increased activity in hyperactive children (Zentall, 1980). Decreased task structure is associated with increased hyperactivity (Zentall & Lieb, 1981). Added within-task stimulation does not facilitate task performance in hyperactive children as Strauss and Lehtinen (1947) believed, but appears to be associated with initially poorer performance, even when the added stimulation is noncompeting (Zentall, Zentall, & Barack, 1978; Zentall et al., 1978). The varied effects of differences in level of stimulation and task difficulty suggest that there is little likelihood that any single set of classroom environmental stimulation conditions will prove to be optimal for the hyperactive child. Many more variables, such as the effect of variations in level of stimulation on use of learning time, remain to be subjected to systematic investigation.

Open Classrooms

Advocates of open classrooms often attribute hyperactive behavior to the demands and constraints of traditional classrooms rather than to factors inherent in the child (Nyquist & Hawes, 1972; Silberman, 1970) and regard these classrooms as cold, authoritarian, rigid, and therefore harmful. The major distinctions between the two approaches center around the number of different activities in progress simultaneously, the extent to which choice and decision making is the child's option, the degree of self-pacing of activities, and the amount of peripheral stimulation in the room (Koester, 1976). Open classrooms are characterized by more freedom of choice and more individualized instruction, with considerable flexibility in scheduling. Options are not predetermined by the teacher and the children have considerable freedom of movement around the classroom as they pursue their individual interests. Advocates of this approach view it as an educational Utopia that is warm, open, flexible, and supportive of creativity and uniqueness; in it, every child is happy and productive (Silberman, 1970).

Although the hypothesis that environmental social and nonsocial factors can cause certain patterns of behavior to be either heightened or played down is consistent with contemporary theoretical viewpoints, there has been surprisingly little interest in an empirical test of it as it applies to the open versus traditional classroom issue. Most of the support for open classrooms is anecdotal in form and is colored by the cultlike enthusiasm of those advocating this philosophy of classroom management. The research that has been reported is characterized by methodological weaknesses limiting the conclusions that can be drawn from the data. Generally, the groups studied have been small, inferior or inadequate dependent measures have been used, and no attempt has been made to systematically investigate the effect of classroom structure on academic competency. Flynn and Rapoport (1976) looked at the behavior of hyperactive children, most of whom were on medication, in open and traditional classes and reported no differences in achievement test scores or activity level across classrooms. However, in subjective assessments teachers in the open classrooms perceived their hyperactive students as less disruptive and less distinguishable in overall behavior from their nonhyperactive peers. Hirst (1976) with a single subject study and Doster (1977) both reported higher activity levels with teacher-specified activities than with child-selected options. Jacob et al. (1978) studied the effects on unmedicated hyperactive boys of formal instruction with teacher specification of a small number of tasks versus informal instruction with free choice and a variety of tasks. Although they reported a significant difference in hyperactivity, which was defined in terms of attention getting, aggression, noncompliance, changing position, daydreaming, and emitting strange vocalizations, they did not regard their results as convincing support for the open classroom because the data lent themselves to several interpretations. Jacob et al. (1978, p. 58) concluded that "until academic achievement data are obtained arguments regarding the desirability for formal and informal settings for hyperactive children are moot."

It is our opinion that the open versus closed classroom issue cannot be satisfactorily resolved with the foregoing kinds of research. What is needed is, first, to specify the attributes of the hyperactive child that must be accommodated in the classroom if he is to perform effectively. For example, he has difficulty changing set, functions better in one-to-one than in group settings, works more effectively under self-paced than other-paced conditions, and responds somewhat unpredictably to certain reinforcement procedures. Which of these attributes are critical for effective classroom functioning and so require accommodation? Next, it would be important to determine the feasibility of incorporating procedures to accommodate these attributes, to decide on the extent to which they *could* be accommodated in either or both types of classroom. The question here concerns the costs to the classroom as a whole (teacher, pupils, pupil progress) of incorporating procedures that accommodate the attributes of the hyperactive child. The experimental test then would require the comparison of classrooms in which the special procedures are operative to the maximum feasible extent. The question that the research should be designed to answer is, Which type of classroom is best for the hyperactive child in terms of (a) achievement, (b) acceptance by the group, and (c) overall effective functioning?

The foregoing approaches to school programs for the hyperactive child were essentially unidirectional, that is, teacher → child, and issue-related, for example, minimal versus normal stimulation or open versus closed classrooms. The next two categories of program are representative of the shift to a bidirectional viewpoint concerning children's problems. The child is made responsible for much of his own behavior, and the focus of teaching is on the child in interaction with his social environments, with an accompanying emphasis on the transmission of social skills. One negative feature of many kinds of school intervention for children with problems is that in most cases the parents, secure in the knowledge that the child has years of schooling ahead, tend to abdicate their responsibility. In the following programs parent involvement is mandatory and a time limit is imposed. The effect of a time limited program is to establish a climate of urgency for the process of behavior change, which is reinforced by the requisite of parent participation. At the same time it also suggests a certain optimism.

Parent-Involvement Programs

The Medical College School Program (MCSP) (Zupnick, 1974) is a treatment-oriented day-school program for 7- to 12-year-old children of normal intelligence but with behavior problems, such as hyperactivity, poor attention span, excessive talkativeness, teasing, and fighting, that are so severe that effective functioning in regular classrooms is out of the question. The program provides a three-pronged attack on the problem of childhood hyperactivity. A structured classroom setting based on behavior modification principles is used to promote behavioral change in the child. To extend the gains achieved through the school program into the family setting, the parents are required to participate in two accompanying kinds of intervention: An insight-oriented therapy group designed to facilitate change in parental behavior and family structure that may be maintaining or exacerbating the child's problems; and a course in the use of behavior modification techniques that teaches the parents how to apply these principles, thus ensuring school-home continuity. Previous attempts to make systematic and simultaneous use of both home and school in modifying behavior problems have focused almost exclusively on the treatment of the child. The MCSP is unique in using psychotherapeutic techniques to bring about change and understanding in the parents, while concurrently instructing them in techniques of contingency management for the child.

Because the main difficulty for children admitted to the MCSP is poor behavioral control, the children are grouped according to their behavior patterns and problems, rather than on the basis of academic standing or chronological age. The classes are divided into three levels, with six children in a class: incoming (Level 1), intermediate (Level 2), and outgoing (Level 3). All children are placed in Level 1 when they enter the program and baselines of their behavioral and academic strengths are determined. As a child progresses he moves to Level 2 and then to Level 3, and is expected to function more independently as he moves from level to level. In Level 3 he is expected to function as he would in a regular classroom with a minimum of individual attention. A point system for good behavior and completion of class assignments is used to determine rate of advancement and daily privileges, with point totals being charted at the end of each period to ensure immediate knowledge of results. Good behavior is defined in terms of specific problems, for example, an excessively talkative child would earn points for being quiet. The maximum number of points possible per day in each category is 50, with the maximum weekly total being 500 points. The number of points earned determines whether a child will participate in the social and free-time reinforcement activities that are built into each day. The total points required to participate in a special activity, as well as the desirability of the activity, increase at each level. In addition to its reinforcement function, the point system also provides an objective method of feedback information to the parents and allows them to set up a reward system in the home contingent on behavior in school. The children are required to reach a specified point level within a designated time period. If they are so badly behaved that they cannot meet this requirement, they are returned to the public school system for more appropriate special class placement. During the one to two academic years that children spend in the program, there is an emphasis on academic advancement as well as behavioral improvement. Upon completion of Level 3, a child is returned to a regular classroom appropriate for his academic level. Children who have completed the program show significant advancement in the core subjects and continue to function effectively in the regular classroom.

The MCSP procedures can best be illustrated with an actual account of one child's program. The case study of Robert (Zupnick, 1974, pp. 81–83) demonstrates how well the program lends itself to carryover in the home and underlines the importance of requiring parents to participate in therapeutic sessions and obtain behavior modification training.

Robert S., a 10-year-old white male, was referred to MCSP because of consistent behavioral disruption in his fourth grade classroom. Examples from the referral report indicate that he was "not able to sit longer than 10–15 minutes; [is] constantly speaking out of turn, disrupts teachers and students; [is] disrespectful to students and teachers; [is] constantly putting things in his mouth." Furthermore, "He reads well but functions below grade level because he will not complete an assignment." At home, according to Mrs. S., "Robert is constantly disrupting all games, talks loudly, yells, throws objects, and uses foul, horrible language. He makes odd noises with his mouth and nose, blinks his eyes and torments the dog. He voids on the bathroom floors on purpose and in general is a disruptive influence in the home." He had previously been labeled emotionally disturbed, hyperactive, and minimally brain damaged, and had been on medication since age four. Upon admission to the program, he was taking upwards of 300 mg of Deaner per day.

Upon entrance into the program, Robert was continually provoking others, engaging in fights, leaving the classroom, and fighting so frequently in the cab, that the driver refused to transport him. He was constantly attempting to manipulate the environment by crying, and asking for his mother. He varied between charming and cursing the adults around him.

In line with the goals of the program, the treatment employed a two-fold approach. At first, Robert was given only minimal work but was provided with strict structure and behavioral guidelines. Classroom disruption resulted in spending "time out" sessions in an isolated carrel in the hallway with a corresponding loss of opportunity to earn points. During this period, there were a number of incidents of flooded toilets and complaints by other children in regard to Robert's teasing and hitting. He had few children with whom he could play or socialize. It soon became apparent, however, that this was Robert's method of "adjusting" to a new situation based upon previous negative experiences. Thus, as he became more acclimated to the setting, structure, and children, he was able to complete longer and more difficult assignments. More importantly, he began to interact in a meaningful fashion with other children. The frequent trips to the bathroom, sniffling, hitting and teasing, all but disappeared. In addition, his medication was gradually decreased so that by the end of the school year it was totally discontinued. Table 3 shows Robert's combined academic and behavioral point totals for his initial two quarters on Level 1. It points out the increase in positive behavior as he progressed through the weeks such that from the sixth week on, he was able to meet the weekly criterion of 350 points.

Table 3. Robert's Level 1 Point Totals

	Weeks								
Quarter 1	1	2	3	4	5	6	7	8	
	250	215	190	327	305	355*	395	355	
	Weeks								
Quarter 2	9	10	11	12	13	14	15	16	17
	360	370	377	411	371	373	382	375	425

*Criterion reached for the first time. At the time of Robert's entrance into the program, the distribution of time within Level 1 was one to two quarters.

Despite Robert's general improvement, he continued to display much difficulty in the area of verbal self-control. He was constantly losing behavioral points for swearing, and quite often the other children would complain about his language—a sure indication that it was well out of hand. Near the end of the final school quarter, a specific program of extinction was designed to reduce this behavior. Every time Robert's teacher or two classmates heard him swear, he was made to stand in a corner of the hall and in a loud voice, repeat the word for a three-minute period. This technique resulted in the rapid reduction and frequency of classroom swearing in a little over a week's time (Table 4).

Table 4.   Robert's Frequency of Classroom Swearing

Days	1*	2	3	4	5	6	7	8	9	10
Frequency	11	10	12	8	5	3	1	3	0	0

*Days 1–3 were baseline days.

Concurrent with Robert's treatment program within the school, Mr. and Mrs. S. were seen on a continuing basis in an effort to produce changes within the home. Initially, their attitudes regarding Robert, and his effect upon the family structure, were discussed. Since he was one of five siblings, it was pointed out that certainly, he was not the sole cause of *all* the fighting and arguing occurring at home. Furthermore, an effort was made to bring Mr. S. back into the family (as an insurance agent, he frequently was conveniently not available in the evenings). Finally, Mrs. S.'s feelings concerning her reluctance to punish Robert, and her habit of immediately defending him in family squabbles, were discussed. She became aware of how these actions fostered Robert's extreme dependency and how they might have arisen in defense against her negative feelings towards him.

Following the initial sessions of insight therapy, specific behavioral plans—designed to extinguish Robert's annoying behaviors at home and school—were discussed and implemented. It had been noted in the classroom that Robert would often work to his minimum—i.e., once his daily points were earned, he would begin to disrupt the other children. To counter this, two simultaneous plans were inaugurated. On the one hand, Mr. and Mrs. S., on their own initiative, hired a local university student as a "Big Brother" for Robert. He visited the home twice weekly and on the weekends. The length of his stay became contingent upon Robert's behavioral points on two successive school days.

Mrs. S. also inaugurated a plan so that when Robert earned his minimum number of daily points he was taken to his favorite local restaurant. What he could order depended upon the number of points earned beyond the minimum. Both plans were inaugurated shortly after Robert began the program, and they began to take effect concurrent with his upward surge of weekly points (Table 3). The visits to the restaurant were quite significant in that the family had stopped taking him to any restaurant because of his "atrocious manner." Furthermore, the frequency of noise-making, blinking, and excessive urination previously noted at home all began to dissipate during the same time period. Other plans designed to regulate Robert's temper tantrums at home and utilizing a time-out procedure were initiated and met with similar success. These tantrums, which involved screaming, banging walls and swearing, decreased in frequency from an average of four to two times per day.*

Short-Term Intensive Programs

Douglas and her colleagues (Douglas, 1980; Douglas, Parry, Marton, & Garson, 1976; Garson, 1977) have developed a three-level cognitive training program based on the findings of their previous empirical investigations. Its purpose was to teach hyperactive boys of elementary school age effective strategies for approaching academic and cognitive tasks and social situations. At the most basic level the goal was to help the child understand the nature of his deficits, their causative relationship to his difficulties, and the proposed ways to help him overcome them. Particular attention was given at this level to the problems caused by failure to attend and impulsivity. At the second level considerable effort was given to making the child aware of his role as a problem solver, and encouraging him to actively assume this role and deal effectively with problems. The child was urged to take charge of his own behavior by monitoring his own work for accuracy. Success was a common occurrence, because tasks were carefully graded for difficulty, and the level of difficulty was increased gradually. Behaviors that interfered with successful task performance were noted and modified. At the third level specific problem-solving strategies were taught that were geared to the child's age and capabilities. The target deficits were an inability to sustain attention and effort, poor impulse control, and problems related to the modulation of alertness and arousal. Many of the strategies at this level focused on carelessness and other kinds of inefficiency such as ineffective use of time, forgetting, and failing to plan. Across all levels there was considerable emphasis on tailoring the training and materials to the individual child and on the use of self-verbalization, particularly in the form of self-instruction, self-monitoring, modeling procedures, and self-reinforcement techniques.

This cognitive training program was tested empirically first by Douglas et al. (1976) and then by Garson (1977), with essentially the same results. In the first and more comprehensive study the experimental group subjects were 18 hyperactive boys in elementary school who participated in two 1-hour sessions a week for a total of 24 sessions spread over a 3-month period. An additional 18 sessions were held, six with the child's classroom teacher and 12 with his parents to discuss the treatment procedures. The control group subjects were 11 hyperactive boys. Pre- and posttests were administered to both groups, the dependent variables being scores on a comprehensive battery of cognitive and

*Reprinted, by permission, from Zupnick, S. A new approach to disturbed children: The Medical College School Program. *Psychiatric Quarterly* (New York State Department of Mental Hygiene), 1974, *48* (1), 76–85.

motor tasks, and teacher ratings. Apart from the testing sessions, the control group subjects received no other attention; their names were merely placed on a waiting list. The results of the posttests showed that the experimental group improved on about half of the dependent measures, and these gains were generally maintained at the time of a 3-month follow-up. Surprisingly, no gains were made on the Conners Teacher Rating Scale. Douglas et al. attributed this failure to the fact that their program stressed the development of inner control processes more than observable behavior, a weak explanation at best, and raised the possibility of a delayed effect. Since further improvement was not demonstrated at the 3-month follow-up this possibility would appear to have little basis. Other suggestions included the idea that the failure of the training program to modify the negative and disruptive behaviors assessed by the Conners scale could indicate a need to combine stimulant medication treatment with the training program. One idea having considerable promise involved using the cognitive training to emphasize to the child the maladaptive consequences of the Conners cluster of behavior: the modeling procedures included in the training program would offer an excellent context for such variants of modeling as role play and self-confrontation with videotaped sequences, and the frequent contacts with the child's teacher could facilitate feedback concerning changes in the Conners target behaviors.

Over the years Douglas and her colleagues at McGill University have built up a solid body of research on the attentional deficits of the hyperactive child. Unlike the large majority of investigators, they have then proceeded to bridge the chasm between research findings and their application by translating their accumulated results into a training program for classroom use. At an even more rarefied level in respect to investigators in general, they have subjected their program to empirical evaluation. Given this commendable background, it is inexplicable that these investigators would weaken the empirical test of what is in effect a culmination of years of research, by permitting a serious methodological flaw in their research design, namely, failure to provide equivalent experience for the control group on certain independent variables known to influence performance regardless of training content. In attempting to justify this unjustifiable procedure, Douglas (1980, p. 313) states that

> Children in the control group were placed on a waiting list and were offered no training during the period covered by the study. We felt that it was unethical and impractical to include an "attention" or "placebo" control group because of the duration of the study and because parents and teachers participated in the training.

A proper test of a new program requires that treatment of the experimental and control groups be identical in all respects other than that of *content* of the new program, that is, the control group should have an equal amount of adult attention and time, under similar conditions of reinforcement, and with activities that are similar in attractiveness and general content to those used by the experimental group, but which offer no training in the specific content of the program being tested; and in this particular case, teacher and parent conferences concerning some aspect of the control children's progress should also be held. Only under these conditions can valid comparisons be made between the control and experimental groups and gains on the latter group's part be interpreted correctly, that is, as gains resulting from exposure to the unique content of the training program.

Before dismissing the above standards as unnecessary and unrealistic or, as Douglas puts it, "unethical and impractical," consider the following experiment (Ross, 1969) in which young mentally retarded children participated in a 2-month training program to increase knowledge of social responses and improve skill in logical reasoning. The experimental group learned social responses using doll play, live models, film slides, and puppets within a practical syllogism framework. The control group had identical time, attention, reinforcement, and media, but with content unrelated to the experimental training. The control group activities did not provide them with content relevant to the test situation but did give them a long period in which there was ample opportunity to develop the same *test-taking skills* that the experimental group were acquiring through participation in the social training. The control group children were required to listen, respond verbally, and offer a variety of responses. They became confident in and accustomed to the question-answer routine with questions presented in a series, by means of different media, and with the expectation on the experimenter's part that they could answer the questions. The attention-response set that they learned was similar to that required for satisfactory behavior in test situations in general. On both the Social Behavior Tests and the Logical Thinking Tests the control group showed significant gains on the pre- versus posttest comparisons ($p<.01$ for the Social, $p<.05$ for the Logical) and these gains were made in the absence of *any* training in the content of the tests. The experimental group made far greater gains ($p<.0005$ on both tests) and consequently, in the light of the control group treatment, these could be attributed to the training program that was being evaluated.

Two other short-term school training programs have been developed. In one of these (Cameron & Robinson, 1980) the goal was to develop a cognitive training program that would promote generalization to classroom behavior and academic tasks. In the training program self-instructional and self-management strategies were taught within the context of visual-perceptual tasks and mathematics activities to three hyperactive elementary school children who were individually trained in 12 half-hour sessions. An important feature of the training program was an emphasis on also teaching the children to monitor the effect of the strategies on their academic achievement. A multiple baseline across individuals design (Baer, Wolf, & Risley, 1968) was used to evaluate the effects of training on on-task behavior and accuracy in mathematics. With this design the stability of the dependent variables is demonstrated by successively introducing subjects to the experimental conditions and showing that behavior changes occur only when the treatment is introduced (Cameron & Robinson, 1980). The results showed a significant improvement in on-task behavior for two of the three children, and in mathematics accuracy for all of them. Increased self-correction in oral reading for all three children suggested that generalization of training had occurred.

The crucial test of the overall efficacy of the Cameron and Robinson training program, a long-term follow-up, was omitted and appears not to be of interest to these investigators. Instead, they report that a second experiment is underway to establish the relative contributions of the self-instructional and reinforcement components used in the first study. This step is clearly premature in view of the small sample size and the relative ease with which short-term gains can be demonstrated. There is little value in determining the relative contribution of the independent variables if their effects may be, at best, only temporary. Furthermore, the training components important over the short term may not continue to be important over the long-term period. In our verbal mediation studies with young retarded children (Ross & Ross, 1978; Ross, Ross, & Downing, 1973) tangible reinforcers were successful in eliciting the initial desired responses, but their appeal diminished as the children's satisfaction with their performance of the task became increasingly important to them. This latter reaction, which involved a sense of accomplishment, satisfaction, and increased self-efficacy, would seem to reflect a mastery factor that is more basic and pervasive than self-reinforcement (Bandura, 1977). The connotations surrounding the statement, *I'm good at this*, are different from those associated with *What a good boy I am* or *How good I am to do this*. One possibility may be that self-reinforcement is an early-stage prerequisite to the development of mastery-related behavior.

In the other short-term training program initially reported on by Varni (1976) and then by Varni and Henker (1979), a well-controlled within-subject design was used to teach three hyperactive elementary school boys to use a self-regulation approach to reading and arithmetic tasks. The training components were self-instruction, self-monitoring, and self-reinforcement, with training being conducted first in the clinic and then the school setting. The verbal self-instruction training proved to be effective only under experimenter-present conditions, and self-monitoring alone had little effect. However, when self-monitoring was combined with self-reinforcement, academic output increased and a reciprocal decrease occurred in hyperactive behaviors. Once again, however, the value of the findings remains in limbo in the absence of long-term follow-up data.

Varni's findings (1976) that verbal self-instruction only worked under adult surveillance and that self-monitoring had little effect paralleled our findings *in the early stages* of the above verbal mediation experiments. However, as the children in these studies came to understand the idea of self-instruction and self-monitoring, that is, when they understood the utility of these techniques, they used them increasingly and self- and other reinforcers dropped out or diminished in relative importance. Before an experimenter moves on to the experimental test and analysis of procedural refinements such as those currently being investigated by Cameron and Robinson (1980), it would be far more productive to repeat and extend the programs to permit the collection of long-term follow-up data. If the effects of the training program are still apparent long after the end of the training period, those children should be interviewed and group discussions conducted in an attempt to identify what the variables are in the children who are still showing improved performance. Information obtained in this way should then be incorporated in a second training program for a new group of hyperactive children, and this cycle repeated until retention is demonstrated in a high proportion of children in some subsequent group. Only when these results are then replicated should the data be accepted for publication.

Rosenbaum and Drabman (1981) have provided a scholarly and comprehensive critical review of research of self-control training in the classroom. This review is notable for its thoughtful consideration of the issues associated with self-control training, including the reliability of self-observation, response maintenance, generalization, and the role of external control in self-control training.

THE OPTIMUM SCHOOL PROGRAM ISSUE

The issue of an optimal school program for the hyperactive child is an ubiquitous one in educational theory and practice. In the space of half a century the pendulum of school placement for the hyperactive child has swung from exclusion and expulsion from school, through the private residential school such as the Franklin School (Bond & Appel, 1931) and its contemporary counterparts, on to a variety of special class arrangements in public school settings, to the current mandate by Public Law (PL) 94–142 of maximum possible inclusion of the hyperactive child in the regular classroom. At the present time PL 94–142 is long on idealism and short on practicality. The goal of regular class placement is a commendable one, but little direction has been provided in the form of concrete advice on the mechanics of integrating the hyperactive child into the regular classroom. Comprehensive pilot studies culminating in an integration blueprint should have preceded nationwide implementation of the law. Until effective integration procedures can be specified the supposedly "least restrictive environment" of the regular class setting, required by PL 94–142, is likely to be a demoralizing experience for the hyperactive child.

School programs for the child with problems can be categorized on a variety of bases, such as teacher-pupil ratio or source of control. Of relevance here is the hypothetical parsimony continuum proposed by Cowen (1973, p. 450) in which the first point would lead to the kind of classroom that would provide a base for an optimal school program for the hyperactive child, and the third and fourth points are representative of programs developed to date for this child:

... one can nevertheless identify a step-stage progression of approaches spanning a hypothetical parsimony continuum. ... It is most parsimonious to engineer settings that optimize adaptation in the first place. Next, approaches that enable teachers to deal effectively with problems *in* the classroom are preferable. Considerably less parsimonious are appeals for assistance from some higher power (within or outside the school, as resources dictate) and environmental manipulations (i.e., changing the child's classroom or school) designed to "manage" him better. Least parsimonious of all are shifts which essentially give up on the child by turning over his education or management to an outside agency. Such steps not only rupture the child's contact with his natural environment, but may also label him irretrievably as a misfit.

The goal of engineering settings that optimize adaptation is by no means an unrealistic one. Within the framework of a small ecosystem model, research by Whalen and her associates (Whalen et al., 1978; Whalen et al., 1979) has demonstrated that classrooms can function as *provocation ecologies* that magnify behavorial differences between unmedicated hyperactive children and their peers, or as *rarefaction ecologies* that minimize such differences. Consider the following minor factors that were likely to disrupt the behavior of the hyperactive children, while leaving that of their nonhyperactive peers relatively unimpaired. Changing set was difficult for the hyperactive child, and a shift from informal activities to formal activities was more difficult than the reverse shift; high ambient noise and difficult tasks resulted in reduced task attention and increased verbal and nonverbal behaviors that could be disruptive; increased familiarity with a task setting often resulted in a deterioration in behavior; the hyperactive child functioned better on self-paced than on other-paced tasks but self-paced tasks often resulted in increased verbalization, social interaction, and high energy episodes. In contrast to these areas of difficulty, low levels of ambient noise and easy-appropriate levels of task difficulty were associated with high task attention, low child-generated noise, and fewer high-energy behaviors. Particularly impressive in this research was the finding that varying some of the ecological parameters of the classroom modified some hyperactive behaviors as effectively as medication had done. Whalen et al. (1979, pp. 79–80) interpret the foregoing findings as evidence of the power of stimulus control techniques in regulating the behavior of the hyperactive child, and point out that many of his classroom difficulties could be accommodated with minor procedural modifications and attitudinal changes on the part of the teacher:

> ... certain distinguishing behaviors are not necessarily dysfunctional and may even be adaptive in some contexts ... verbalization does not necessarily have to interfere with learning and performance. Academic activities could be designed in which interpersonal transactions were functional rather than disruptive, and in such contexts hyperactive boys may show enhanced social and academic performance.

Some teachers function best in quiet, orderly classroom settings. . . . Other teachers . . . thrive in a more complex, flexible, and multidimensional environment. One relatively low-cost and potentially high-yield intervention would be to optimize the match between teacher attitudes and behavioral styles . . . and child characteristics. . . . For child behaviors that are generally dysfunctional *across* situations, sequential intervention programs can be designed which involve (a) a greater proportion of environmental adaptations, initially, followed by (b) progressive demands for behavior change in the child that coincide with increases in the child's cognitive and interpersonal competencies.

The research by Whalen and her colleagues has focused on the functional relationships between the ecology of the classroom and social-behavioral outcome. Although appropriate behavior is essential if learning is to occur, such behavior does not in itself lead to improvement in academic performance. Keogh and Barkett (1980) have emphasized the importance of treating the social-behavioral, psychological, and educational components of hyperactivity as partially independent domains that are affected differentially by intervention procedures and instructional demands. In an excellent analysis of empirical findings on intervention procedures for these three components of hyperactivity, they have been critical of the tendency to assume a causal relationship between the behavior problems of the hyperactive child and his academic performance, and have pointed to the need for identifying the nature of the interactions among the functional components of hyperactivity. Within their schema social and nonsocial interventions that decrease disruptive behavior and enhance educationally relevant psychological processes provide a base for the implementation of techniques that will lead to increased educational competency. Throughout their discussion of the hyperactive child's achievement problems there is consistent recognition of the heterogeneity of the hyperactive child as well as evidence of a concern for a bidirectionality component in intervention procedures. The Keogh and Barkett chapter (1980) should be mandatory reading for any investigator interested in the classroom functioning of the hyperactive child.

An optimal school program for the hyperactive child is within reach and could become a reality if researchers and educators join forces to review the known findings and identify the research gaps in the area of classroom conditions that facilitate effective functioning in the hyperactive child. On the basis of this review, the development of a master plan for conducting the necessary research would then be followed by a series of long-term trials of the resultant school programs in actual and simulated classroom settings. The Whalen model, with its cycle of revisions, modifications, and further trials, should be used in order to develop a set of programs that any interested and reasonably competent teacher could implement. Until these essential preliminaries have been successfully completed, the probability of effectively implementing PL 94–142 on a wide scale is near zero.

CHAPTER 9

Prevention

Traditionally, prevention has been viewed as a unitary process differentiated by its focus on either the group or the individual, and by its point of initiation, either early or late in the developmental sequence of the condition (Mausner & Bahn, 1974). Within this framework, *primary prevention* refers to efforts to forestall illness or dysfunction in major subgroups such as entire kindergarten groups or whole communities. When attention is focused on the individual, with the state of the dysfunction ranging from less advanced to well-established, three categories are described: *early secondary prevention* involves the early identification of evident or incipient dysfunction and the initiation of procedures to keep the condition from becoming more severe; *later secondary prevention* applies this approach to more advanced conditions; and *tertiary prevention* is an intensive attempt to eliminate or reduce the severity of an already well-established dysfunction and minimize its residual effects.

The contemporary viewpoint rejects the inclusion of the latter two stages in the preventive model on the grounds that their aims, methodologies, and programs differ radically from those of primary and early secondary prevention and are more accurately described as management. Thus in this view the term *prevention* includes only primary and ontogenetically early secondary preventive procedures (Cowen, 1973). We concur with this contemporary preventive model and will limit our discussion of the prevention of hyperactivity to a brief discussion of primary and a more extensive coverage of early secondary preventive procedures, thus reflecting the current imbalance of research and development between the two categories.

PRIMARY PREVENTION

In the first half of this century the targets of primary prevention were the acute and chronic diseases, with immunization being the major tool. Since 1950 the picture has changed considerably. Advances in pediatric technology and immunology have effected important changes in both the severity and the prevalence of many of these diseases. Smallpox, for example, has been virtually eliminated. One result has been a shift in interest to the preventive possibilities inherent in the behavioral disorders.

Several rather diverse developments have contributed support to this shift. Our knowledge and understanding of the behavior disorders has undergone a sharp increase in the last 30 years, and most of the research and clinical findings on this topic are a product of this period. Factors related to outcome, particularly those that can be influenced through early intervention, have been a major focus of research and clinical interest. Concomitantly, increasing alarm has been voiced by medical economists (Kristein, Arnold, & Wynder, 1977) about rising mental health costs, and they have urged that high priority be assigned to the federal funding of large-scale prevention programs. Unequivocal empirical support for their position is provided by the well-documented fact that early behavioral dysfunction frequently predisposes to later more serious and costly psychopathology (Robins, 1966). At the same time, the expression of societal concern for the rights of children has intensified and, while this concern is undirected and nonspecific, it does create an atmosphere conducive to change. Contemporary society has become a vocal and demanding force that considers the attainment of health as an inalienable right of every child, equates health to a broader spectrum that includes psychological well-being rather than solely the absence of disease, and consequently expects pediatric preventive care to encompass the entire continuum of growth and development, including the prevention of behavior disorders (Casey, Sharp, & Loda, 1979).

The cumulative effect of this widespread concern has been increased pressure for the development of primary preventive programs that are oriented to the role that influential social environments play in the development of behavior disorders. As an example, consider the rapidly increasing incidence of pregnancies in girls under 16 (Gallas, 1980). The salient negative effect of these pregnancies is their tendency to end in prematurity and to produce low birth weight children, that is, children whose birth weight is less than 5½ pounds or 2500 grams. Low birth weight children, whether premature or full term, have a higher incidence of neurological defects, intellectual impairment, childhood behavior disorders, and other problems than those of normal birth weight (Anastasiow, Everett, O'Shaughnessy, Eggleston, & Eklund, 1978; Field, Hallock, Ting, Dempsey, Dabiri, & Shuman, 1978). In Dunn's (1979) longitudinal study of 500 low birth weight infants, almost half of the 335 children who were still in the study at age 6½ had developed one or more neurological problems. The most common problem, minimal brain dysfunction, occurred three times as often in the low birth weight group as in a normal birth weight control group (Dunn, 1980).

Although the low birth weight infant is clearly at increased risk, the birth weight–risk relationship is not an invariant one because development is not an orderly sequence of efficient causes and inevitable outcomes operating on passive organisms (Sameroff & Chandler, 1975). Instead, there is a complex interplay between the child and his environment which may dissipate or amplify the effects of factors such as low birth weight. There is considerable evidence, for example, that the possible negative effects of low birth weight can be offset to a remarkable degree by the quality of caretaking (Werner, Bierman, French, Simonian, Connor, Smith, & Campbell, 1968). It follows that if younger teenage girls were given intensive training for parenthood prior to pregnancy, this training could result in improvements in the caretaking environment great enough to offset some of the effects of low birth weight of infants born to the young adolescent. Such intervention could also result in improved maternal coping during the early adjustment period, a period that may be of critical importance to the later mother–child relationship (Campbell, 1979a; Gallas, 1980). Further, the contact with health professionals and hospital settings intrinsic to such a program could result in primiparous adolescent mothers, particularly those in inner city settings, seeking out these support settings rather than relying almost entirely on nonprofessional support sources (Badger & Burns, 1980; Zuckerman, Winsmore, & Alpert, 1979). Bronfenbrenner (1974, pp. 60–61) emphasizes the need for training for parenthood and stresses that it must occur within the context of direct rather than vicarious experience:

> It is commonplace among educators to affirm that the task of the school is to prepare the child "for life." There is one role in life the overwhelming majority of all children will ultimately play but for which they are given virtually no concrete preparation. It is parenthood. In cross-cultural observations I have been struck by the American child's relative lack of ease in relating to infants and young children, engaging their interest and enjoying their company. With the important exception of certain minority groups, including blacks, many young people never have experience in extended care of a baby or a young child until they have their own.
>
> A solution to this problem, which speaks as well to the need to give young people in our society genuine and consequential responsibility, is to introduce truly functional courses in human development into the regular school curriculum. These would be distinguished in a number of important ways from units on "family life" as they are now usually taught in junior high school (chiefly to girls who do not plan to go on to college). Now the material is typically presented in vicarious form, that is, through reading or discussion or possibly through role-playing rather than actual role-taking. In contrast, the approach being proposed here would have as its core a responsible and active concern for the lives of young children and their families. Such an experience could be facilitated by locating day-care centers and preschool programs in or near schools so that they could be made an integral part of the curriculum. The older children would work with the younger ones on a regular basis, both at school and in the young children's homes, where they would have an opportunity to become acquainted with the youngsters' families and their circumstances.*

Working within the framework proposed by Bronfenbrenner (1974), and motivated by concern about the burgeoning problems associated with the rap-

*Reprinted by permission from Bronfenbrenner, U. The origins of alienation. *Scientific American*, August 1974, *231*, 53–61.

idly increasing incidence of pregnancies in girls under 16, Anastasiow et al. (1978) have developed a classroom and practicum program to teach seventh and eighth grade students about child growth and development. Included in the program are experiences in hospitals and other child-care centers. Beginning the program in grade seven ensures that the maximum number will be exposed to it; pregnancy usually terminates the young adolescent's education regardless of race or socioeconomic status and thus prevents her from participating in programs in the upper grades (Moore & Waite, 1977). The Anastasiow program has been offered at selected sites across the country, with excellent preliminary results; participating students scored higher than controls on measures of positive attitudes toward and knowledge of normal and handicapped children, child development, and the benefits of hospital care. The approach used clearly has the potential to increase the probability of effective coping with the simultaneous demands of a difficult infant, adolescence, and parenthood. However, the full impact of this program cannot be determined until longitudinal follow-ups assess the students as parents or as those involved in child care. It is a sorry reflection on government priorities that such a follow-up on this program is in jeopardy because of reluctance on the part of the funding agency to continue its support (Anastasiow, 1980).

Primary prevention programs have also been developed for adolescents under 15 years of age who are already pregnant. These adolescents are high medical and social risks (Phipps-Yonas, 1980) and their infants are at increased risk for prenatal mortality, prematurity, and neurological abnormalities. The risks for both members of this dyad increase markedly when the mothers are inner-city, poverty-level, unmarried members of minority groups whose knowledge of health care systems is limited. These young adolescents rarely take advantage of available prenatal medical resources and fail to follow through with well-baby care (Zuckerman et al., 1979). All too often the risks escalate with the rapid subsequent pregnancies that are a common occurrence in this group.

To cope with this increasingly serious problem medical centers across the country have set up primary prevention programs to help young adolescents cope with the demands of pregnancy and motherhood. Representative of these efforts is the Adolescent Parenting Program at the Michael Reese Medical Center (Creedon, 1980) for inner-city, pregnant, black adolescents age 15 and younger who are planning to keep their babies. This weekly discussion group and training program provides continuity of prenatal care for the mother-to-be along with intensive parenting training that is enhanced by excellent role models. Routine and emergency care is readily available for the infant and his development is regularly monitored. Creedon (1980, p. 22) describes this program as "a flexible, multidisciplinary approach that recognizes developmental stages and crises and that provides nurturance and opportunities for physical well-being as well as psychosocial competency." The assumptions are that such a program will have a positive impact on the lifestyle of the pregnant participant and increase the probability that she will maintain contact with the appropriate health care systems. Preliminary results from a one-year study of the project were excellent, with participants functioning more effectively than controls. The crucial test, however, will be long-term outcome for these young mothers and their children.

At the adult level, primary prevention is urgently needed to combat the effects of maternal drinking and smoking during pregnancy. The incidence of the fetal alcohol syndrome coupled with the high prevalence of drinking in young women (Langone & Langone, 1980; Potvin & Lee, 1980) makes it mandatory that intrauterine exposure to alcohol be regarded as a major public health problem. Smith (1979b) has urged the development of programs that foster the concept of mothering from *conception,* as opposed to mothering from *birth.* This concept should be basic to programs at the young adolescent level but, in any event, every pregnant mother should be made aware by her physician of the fact that the alcohol she drinks is alcohol ingested by her fetus; just as she would not allow her infant to drink alcohol after birth, neither would she want him to ingest it before birth. One approach with other hazards to health has been to attach warning labels to the products. In discussing responsibility for such education, Smith (1979a, p. 128) comments as follows:

> At present, the burden of educating the public in this regard falls mainly on the medical community. Recently, the Treasury Department's Bureau of Alcohol, Tobacco, and Firearms decided against a proposal to require a label on alcoholic beverages warning about drinking during pregnancy and possible birth defects; the decision ran contrary to the initial advice of the FDA and the National Institute on Alcoholism and Alcohol Abuse, among others. Instead of the warning label, the Bureau proposes to begin a multimedia educational campaign (funded by the liquor industry), the impact of which is to be measured in polls over the next two years; should the campaign fail significantly to improve public awareness of the dangers of drinking during pregnancy, the Bureau says that it may change its position and require the label. The involvement of the liquor industry in a campaign to educate the public about the adverse effects of ethanol on prenatal development, however, does not impress me as a wise choice.

On the basis of their past record the medical community at the present time does not appear to be coping adequately with their rightful task of educating patients concerning known risks. In discussing the issue of warning labels on alcohol (which he opposes), Etzioni (1978, p. 22) makes the following point:

> ... it seemed unwise to rely on physicians and other health professionals to alert women to the problem, as several commentaries had suggested. The experience with birth-control pills suggests that doctors tend not to pass along such information. The Food and Drug Administration had initially left this matter to doctors, but reluctantly concluded that it had to reach consumers of contraceptive pills more directly. It required that a warning of the risk of blood clots and heart attacks from the pills be inserted in the packages.

Although the etiological role of maternal smoking in hyperactivity is less clearly delineated, there is unequivocal evidence that cigarette smoking during pregnancy has a significant and adverse effect on the well-being of the fetus and newborn infant (Winter, 1980). Of relevance here is the causal relationship between maternal smoking and infant birth weight: infants of smoking mothers have an average birth weight of 200 grams less than the infants of nonsmokers; birth weight decreases as a function of number of cigarettes smoked, and the resultant pattern of retardation in fetal growth is one of decreases in all dimensions customarily measured, that is, body length and head and chest circumference. As Dunn (1979) and others (e.g., Phipps-Yonas, 1980) have pointed out, infants of low birth weight are also at greater risk for behavioral disorders than are those of normal weight. In view of the recent sharp increases in smoking in adolescent girls and young women (Bachman, Johnston, & O'Malley, 1981; Surgeon General's Report on Smoking and Health, 1979), educational programs concerning the prevention of maternal smoking are urgently needed.

Despite significant gains in the past decade, the development and implementation of prevention strategies for the behavior disorders in general and for hyperactivity in particular are still in the embryo stage. Primary preventive action in the area of hyperactivity has been inhibited by the dramatic short-term efficacy of the stimulants, coupled with the firmly entrenched belief that hyperactivity was a time-limited disorder, and the extensive voids in our knowledge of its etiology. Influences of a more general nature include deficiencies in pediatric training for behavioral disorders, federal funding interests being mainly those related to the major medical problems, and the general orientation of this society and its medical establishment to the treatment of disorders rather than to their prevention. The resulting lack of progress in prevention strategies makes early intervention doubly important.

EARLY SECONDARY PREVENTION

Our interest here is on the child who is beginning to exhibit misbehavior routinely or to experience difficulties likely to lead to more serious problems. In this sense, the qualifier *early* refers to the point at which the child's behavior generates heightened parental concern and intensified pediatric attention, rather than to his chronological age. The target of this concern, however, is usually the infant or young preschool child who is characterized by the cluster of symptoms and behavior patterns that are indicative of a child at risk for behavior disorder and possibly hyperactivity. Fouts (1974), for example, has demonstrated the efficacy of a brief early intervention procedure in which mothers of consistently overactive infants were taught to use reinforcement principles to reduce the activity level of their overactive infants long before this behavior could become a serious problem. Early secondary prevention programs have also been used successfully with older children who have been identified as at risk for school maladaptation. For the past 20 years primary-grade children have been screened for early behavioral or academic problems as part of the Primary Mental Health Project (PMHP) developed by Cowen and his associates (Cowen, Trost, Lorion, Dorr, Izzo, and Isaacson, 1975). In this program children who are identified as experiencing difficulties that may later become serious problems work on an individual basis with nonprofessional aides (housewives) who are under professional supervision. Although over the years there has been little systematic evaluation of the PMHP program, it has been reported to be highly successful and, with some modifications, has been implemented in urban and suburban school systems throughout the country (Alden, Rappaport, & Seidman, 1975; Durlak, 1977). The efficacy of the PMHP approach has received empirical support from Rickel, Smith, and Sharp (1979), who developed a preschool program based on it for nonwhite 3- and 4-year-old children from lower income families.

The issue of screening is a controversial one. We are opposed to general screening of a blanket kind whose purpose is to identify children *prior* to school entry whose test scores indicate a disability of some kind that is related to future performance. (The exceptions to this opinion are routine vision and hearing tests.) Almost no test of a psychological or educational nature justifies the confidence that such total dependence on test scores would indicate. Furthermore, many children with various test score abnormalities function successfully with no intervention of any kind. In our opinion it is a dangerous and destructive practice to label such children as problem children in the absence of supporting behavioral data obtained in the school setting. Only *after* a teacher at the kindergarten or primary level has observed the child over a period of time and noted apparent problems should that child be brought to the attention of the appropriate school personnel for a possible evaluation. To assume a one-to-one relationship between test scores and future problems is a gross oversimplification of the situation and an exceedingly naive position to take.

It is essential that the pediatrician be alert to the presence of at-risk behavior patterns and acknowledge their importance. During this period of rapid development and increased vulnerability the pediatrician typically has more contact with the child than any other professional and is the chief decision maker on the question of whether or not to initiate intervention procedures. Too often the pediatrician either fails to see the cumulative importance of the assorted complaints and anxieties concerning her child's behavior that the mother attempts to describe, or dismisses such patterns of behavior with (groundless) assurances that the child will grow out of it. In either case the erroneous implication is that the difficult behavior is merely a normal variant. One serious consequence of this view of the problem is that at an optimal time for preventive intervention the pediatrician fails to initiate immediate action to help the parents cope with the management of their difficult child. In discussing the tendency to assume that difficult infants grow out of it, Berlin (1974, p. 1454) states:

The aphorism of past generations that children "will grow out of their troubles" is not true. Children, especially those with troubles related to biologic rhythms—sleep, feeding, activity rate—discernible in the first year of life, *do not grow out of these problems.* They rather grow *into* them.

Because the at-risk pattern is less clearly defined and differentiated in infancy than in early childhood, we will discuss each age stage separately.

Infancy

The at-risk signs are in the infant's adaptation to the basic functions of sleeping, eating, and style of responding to the environment; patterns of deviation in these functions indicate a disturbance in overall adaptation. The onset of such patterns may occur as early as the first few weeks or months of extrauterine life (Sandoval, Lambert, & Sassone, 1980). Maternity nurses often report that one neonate stands out from the group in the hospital nursery as being unusually difficult in routine caretaking situations. He may be characterized by a disturbance in sleep patterns and by a pervasive restlessness that is expressed in his waking hours as an unusually high level of general motor activity and in his resting periods as an inability to settle down. Empirical evidence of the early onset of these patterns of deviation comes from the excellent longitudinal studies of Thomas and Chess (1977), who identified one difficult behavior pattern characterized by high activity, restlessness, and marked lability of mood that was clearly discernible at the age of two months.

One pattern of deviation that should cause the pediatrician to watch an infant closely is that of restlessness and irritability characterized by a light, uneasy sleep from which the infant can easily be aroused, crying of long duration that appears to be intensified by efforts to comfort him, a wild driven kind of physical activity that continues to a point of exhaustion, startle responses to a variety of mild sensory stimulants, and a tendency to be very easily distracted during feeding. The infant with this pattern seldom smiles at his parents and sometimes seems not to recognize them; he may be friendlier to total strangers. He resists routine caretaking such as being bathed and frequently has tantrums if he is picked up during ongoing physical activity.

Retrospective interviews with parents of hyperactive children (Barnard & Collar, 1973; Loney, Kramer, & Milich, 1981; Rapoport, Quinn, Burg, & Bartley, 1979; Routh, 1978; Stewart, Pitts, Craig, & Dieruf, 1966) have shown that the parents were sometimes aware in early infancy that their child was different, and the differences were similar to those identified by Thomas and Chess (1977). Although retrospective accounts do have well-documented weaknesses (Solomons, 1973), there is reason to believe that a mother would accurately recall her first awareness of her infant being different because of the trauma involved. The following account by a young mother describes her initial reluctance to admit even to herself that her first child's behavior was in any way unusual, followed by her sudden painful acceptance that something was clearly amiss:

> Even when I first had Petie, even on the second day in the hospital I knew *something* was wrong. He acted so different from all the other babies, at feeding time he didn't cry, he *screeched,* and all the nurses looked funny and he was so stiff and he kicked all the time same as he did when I was pregnant. But then I thought it was probably something wrong with how I handled him because I was an only child and I never had much to do with little babies and I thought I wasn't doing a good job and Petie knew it. Then when I got him home he'd have some real bad days so I almost went crazy and some days there were so great I'd think, "What could be wrong with a baby like this? It's all in your mind." And John [her husband] was away a lot so he didn't really know what Petie was like and I never *really* told the pediatrician. I'd say about Petie's bad days but not what it was really like and he'd say that they all have bad days the first year. And I didn't want to know, I know that now, I'd take Petie to the park on good days but on bad days I'd bake and clean and stay in so people wouldn't say anything. And when other babies screamed their lungs out I'd feel good and think that they all do it.
>
> Then, one day my pediatrician was sick and the other doctor saw Petie and we had to wait and Petie was just terrible in the waiting room, the worst he'd ever been. It was *awful.* And when I saw the doctor he sat and asked me all about Petie and I started to tell him *really* how it had been for the whole eight months and all of a sudden right in the middle of telling—I'll never forget it, it was St. Patrick's Day, and there were all of the doctor's certificates on the wall and a whole lot of cute really happy-looking baby pictures that I guess he'd delivered and I was looking at them and all of a sudden I thought, "Petie is *not like them,* he's not like them *at all.* There's *something wrong* with Petie"; and I felt all shaky like getting flu and I felt like yelling and screaming and I thought "What'll I do, there's something wrong with Petie." and I looked at the doctor and I could tell, *he* knew too.

It would be very difficult to specify with certainty the cause of the at-risk behavior pattern; it could be due to brain damage, poor maternal caretaking, temperament, or physical disorder; or it could be a precursor of hyperactivity. We say *precursor* because the age at which hyperactivity can be diagnosed is a matter of dispute. Some investigators (Drash, Stolberg, & Bostow, 1977; Kinsbourne, 1979; Rapoport et al., 1979; Werry, 1968) believe that hyperactivity is apparent late in infancy or the very early preschool years, while others (Cantwell, 1979; Dunn, 1979) contend that no firm diagnosis can be made until later in the preschool years. The issue is one of academic interest, since a specific diagnosis at this time is of no particular value to the infant. What is important is the early recognition of the at-risk situation and the possibility of behavior disorder, and the prompt initiation of intervention procedures to modify the difficult behavior patterns and limit sequelae, particularly those of a psychological nature.

Early Childhood

The general developmental pattern from infancy through early childhood is characterized by increasing differentiation. This trend also applies to the at-risk signs exhibited in infancy and continuing into early childhood. By this time the patterns of deviation will have become so clearly defined and differentiated that the child can be accurately described as at risk for hyperactivity. The trend to increasing differentiation is clear in the following accounts of a child at nine months of age and again at one year, 11 months. The first description was written by the mother as part of the intake procedure when the parents first sought help with their difficult infant; the second account was part of a taped interview with a different pediatrician.

[At nine months] What Mikey most reminds me of is this crazy alarm clock we had when we were children. You could never tell when it would go on, how long it would stay on, or how to turn it off. Mikey cries a lot for no reason at all that I can see and his crying is a really weird-sounding cry. People look astonished when he starts. He's really *resistant* to everything—he sort of clamps his mouth shut when I try to feed him and he spits an awful lot out. He gets stiff when I dress him and he arches his back when I'm trying to bathe him. He wakens a lot in the night and cries or worse still he laughs—a horrible, maniacal laugh. He doesn't go to sleep early either, he rackets round in his crib . . . He seems very, very active to me, he shunts up and down and he's worn out his crib mattress already. He's not a bit lovable but sometimes he'll be quite good right in the middle of a terrible screaming fit. I can't figure him out. I know a baby isn't a machine but there's no system at all to Mikey. I'm terribly disappointed in him. He rarely responds to either of us . . . he never smiles at me . . . Dan and I are both wrecks. We hardly ever get a good night's sleep and we don't enjoy each other as much as we did before Mikey.

Although this infant's behavior at nine months was highly suggestive of an infant at risk for a behavior disorder, no intervention was introduced. The pediatrician attributed the difficult behavior to temperament, suggested that it was normal for new parents to have difficulty adjusting to a first-born infant, offered no suggestions about how the behavior might be modified, and failed to make subsequent checks on the status of the problem despite continuing complaints from the mother. When the couple consulted a second pediatrician the infant was one year, 11 months old. The father reported that the first pediatrician had urged them "to wait until he is a year and a half or two years. You won't believe the change." He added bitterly that he would not have believed that a baby could get so much worse in such a short time. In the following verbatim report note that although the behaviors that the mother describes at one year, 11 months are more clearly defined and differentiated, the basic modalities that she complains about are the same as those that had concerned her when the infant was nine months old, including his lack of sociability. In view of the adaptive value of an infant's sociability in developing early positive attachments (Ambrose, 1969; Stayton, Hogan, & Ainsworth, 1971), this deficit alone is reason for concern.

> [At one year, 11 months] We both find the whole situation intolerable. This child is so unpredictable you can hardly believe it. Neither of us could tell you what he'll do next. He's a real picky eater, a light sleeper, he sometimes cries for hours but he doesn't cry when he bangs into something or falls when you'd expect any child to cry. He has terrible tantrums any time we want him to do something he doesn't want to do. Then right in the middle of one he'll just stop and start jumping around in his crib (it's like a cage, the sides are so high, otherwise he'd be out of it in two minutes) or running round the room. He's a real Jumping Jack, he never stops and looks at anything—it's pick it up throw it down or better still, throw it *at* someone. He's gotten so aggressive—he bites, throws things, kicks, knocks things over, makes horrible sounds but doesn't talk, *not one word,* and he grabs hold of anything he can reach. I can't take him to the store with me. Babysitters can't believe him. One time he was real good the first time a sitter came and the next time he tore her dress grabbing at it and scratched her face. He wears out his clothes in no time at all. I have padded knees in his pants to save him, he falls down so much. And now he seems to do things deliberately like knocking light furniture over. We're tired, disappointed, worried and we're never going to have another child. If our marriage survives Mike it'll be a miracle. And I don't know how he's going to learn to be with other children because he isn't friendly. If I was picking one word for how he is mostly to us and to strangers, I'd say *unsociable.* It's strange because most young children are sort of shy but kind of friendly but Mike isn't at all. He tries to take over other children. He's big, strong, aggressive, and his tantrums are frightening to other children ... Our neighbours call him Mike the Menace and I don't blame them.

The behavior patterns indicative of a young child at risk for hyperactivity differ quantitatively rather than qualitatively from those of his nonclinical peers. Many young preschool children are *at times* overactive, rebellious, easily upset, difficult, given to temper tantrums, distractible, impulsive, and irritable; but they generally do not exhibit these behaviors consistently. However, when an otherwise healthy child exhibits these behaviors to a degree that seriously disrupts the household, has few quiet sunny periods, and generally seems very difficult to manage, the pediatrician should instigate some changes. Even if it becomes clear that the deviations have been blown out of proportion by the parents, are a normal variant, or are the result of a maternal style of caretaking, a problem *does* exist. Its seriousness is one issue, its effect another, and the two are not really related. Minor problems can have a devastating effect on a household and, when this is the case, should be treated with professional respect.

ASSESSMENT PROCEDURE

For optimal monitoring of the well-being of the child, the pediatrician must first gain the basic trust and confidence of the mother. When the pediatrician believes that the child is at risk for hyperactivity, it is of critical importance that such a relationship be firmly established before the assessment procedures are set in motion. The mother must feel that the pediatrician is a firm ally who understands and is genuinely sympathetic about her problem, is ready and qualified to discuss any aspect of it with her, and who receives without censure her sometimes negative confidences about her child. Only then can the pediatrician set in motion the comprehensive multidisciplinary investigation required to confirm the at-risk diagnosis and provide a basis for intervention.

In terms of stimulus input the nonworking mother typically has more information about the child than has any other adult in his environment. Yet relatively few empirical attempts have been made to determine the accuracy of maternal report. Thomas, Chess, and Birch (1968) found mothers in their sample to be quite accurate, whereas Minde, Webb, and Sykes (1968) found little agreement between birth histories and maternal report, and Solomons (1973, p. 335) went so far as to state that

> . . . a history given by parents concerning the behavior and activity level of their child is largely unreliable. Studies show little agreement between the parents, and they are unable to provide objective information concerning the maladaptive behavior of their own children. Not only does their lack of objectivity affect the accuracy of their perceptions, but it may also affect their willingness to report and their honesty in reporting. Compared with fathers, mothers are more defensive, distorting and censoring their information. A mother may describe with chronological precision the onset of a cough, rash, or temperature, or the duration and character of a pain; however, she may color her appraisal of the mental age of her child and the manifestations of his behavior and personality because of her fears of the evaluation and her unrealistic expectations for the child's future.

Although Solomons (1973) attributed the lack of parental agreement to a basic inability to report objectively, coupled with anxiety concerning the outcome of the evaluation, two alternative explanations should be considered. One is that the mother's perception of the extent of the problem is heightened by her increased contact with the child plus a genuine sex difference in perception of the child's behavior. To the mother, a level of activity that is reason for consultation may, to the father, be viewed as the normal exuberance of childhood (Hegeman, 1977). (Empirical support for this explanation could be obtained by having each parent independently rate videotaped sequences of the child's behavior.) The other alternative is that the differences between the parents' accounts are source related (Langhorne, Loney, Paternite, & Bechtoldt, 1976), that is, the parents constitute different social environments and, as a result, their separate descriptions of the child's behavior are characterized by cross-situational variation. This environment-specific explanation has theoretical (Mischel, 1969), empirical (Kenny, Clemmens, Hudson, Lentz, Cicci, & Nair, 1971; Schleifer, Weiss, Cohen, Elman, Cvejic, & Kruger, 1975), and clinical (Cantwell, 1979) support. In the light of this evidence, the pediatrician should evaluate the parental descriptions separately by source rather than interpreting the differences as a sign of invalid or weak patient data. This approach could reveal patterns of behavior systematically related to the child's different social environments; and this information could be helpful in the development of a preventive intervention program.

From a practical viewpoint the pediatrician has certain opportunities to confirm the accuracy of at least some of the mother's information. He can check on previous histories and other records, observe the degree to which the mother–child interaction in the office confirms her reports of her caretaking procedures, and use some repetition of questions. In respect to questioning the mother, Thomas et al. (1968) felt that they obtained accurate responses as a result of the specificity and careful wording of their questions. They recommend that questions be framed in terms of common situations in order to elicit factual descriptions of the child's and mother's behavior in specific situations. In assessing level of activity, for example, the pediatrician might ask: "If you were drying the baby after his bath and you had to get another towel from the other side of the room, would you feel safe in leaving him for a few seconds or would you be afraid that he'd fall off the counter?" "If you are visiting friends and you put the baby down on a blanket on the floor with some toys to play with, would he just stay on or near the blanket or would he wriggle off and be over on the other side of the room in a very short time?"

Keeping in mind the possible idiosyncratic nature of his sources of information and the various means of adapting to them, the pediatrician should proceed with a comprehensive multidisciplinary investigation. In such an evaluation a basic clinical history, physical examination, behavioral assessment, and some psychological testing should be regarded as mandatory.

History

The developmental history obtained from the mother should yield the routine facts that are an integral part of any infant assessment, as well as information that can provide support for the at risk diagnosis. It is important to obtain details about the pregnancy, neonatal and early infancy periods, preschool developmental patterns, medical history, and history of familial disorders. Infants and young children with more than one developmental or familial correlate of hyperactivity are more likely to be hyperactive (Safer, 1973). For example, the probability of hyperactivity in a low birth weight child with alcoholic and low socioeconomic parents is higher than in a low birth weight child alone. The presence of these correlates does not constitute evidence of hyperactivity but it does support such a diagnosis.

Particular attention should be given to stress factors in the prenatal period, such as infectious or viral diseases or other problems. During pregnancy mothers of hyperactive children are more likely to have experienced vaginal bleeding and preeclampsia, a condition characterized by high blood pressure, proteinuria, and swelling (Pasamanick, Rogers, & Lilienfeld, 1956). The birth weight of the hyperactive child is more likely to be below normal and prematurity is more common (Denhoff, 1973; Dunn, 1979; Kløve & Hole, 1979). In the perinatal period respiratory and hemolytic complications also occur more often in the hyperactive child. He is more likely to have had a low Apgar score (Pasamanick et al., 1956) and physical defects at birth than is the nonhyperactive child. In infancy the hyperactive child is more likely to have exhibited extremes of activity, have a history of developmental delay, particularly in reference to speech development (Safer & Allen, 1976; Wender, 1973), sleep and feeding problems, and evidence of brain malfunction such as seizures (Bernstein, Page, & Janicki, 1974). In the preschool period the hyperactive child is more likely to have exhibited the primary or core symptoms of hyperactivity and may have shown evidence of the secondary symptoms, especially learning difficulties. Wherever it is possible to do so, the mother's report of this information should be verified with the birth, obstetrical, and pediatric records.

Both parents should be questioned about familial instances of hyperactivity, other behavior disturbances, and psychiatric disorders in the first or second degree relatives of the child. They should also be asked independently to describe the specific behaviors that have prompted the consultation, their severity and frequency, the extent to which the individual behaviors are situation-specific, and the duration of the problem. The pediatrician must determine the meaning the child's behavior has for the parents, that is, what each parent perceives as the cause of the behavior, what levels they attach to it, whether both have the same labels, and if there is self-blame or mutual blame. He must also obtain information about the coping procedures the parents have used. Sometimes one or both parents have reached a point of frustration that makes them fearful of losing control and harming the child. As a result, the parental responses will have factual and affective components, both of which are likely to be of major importance in reaching a decision about the child.

In pinpointing the primary causation factor in the child's behavior three etiological possibilities should be considered as contributing causes of the problem behavior. These are temperament, social or nonsocial environment, and maternal handling. It is essential to determine through questions, discussion, and observation during the history taking and subsequent physical examination periods if any of these factors plays a role because the same problem behavior could result from any one or a combination of these factors; consequently, the approach used to modify the problem behavior would differ markedly depending on the relative contributions of these factors.

Temperament. The behavior problem may be a function of the child's difficult temperament, that is, his own individual style of responding to the environment. Thomas et al. (1968) have defined three types of temperament ("easy children," "difficult children," and "slow to warm up children") which described 65 percent of the children in their major longitudinal study. These investigators recommend that the pediatrician routinely familiarize himself with the child's temperament to increase the probability of providing the parents with appropriate support and advice on basic caretaking routines. Difficult children, for example, typically overreact to variations in basic routines and changes in the social and nonsocial environment. One young mother reported that her 16-month-old son screamed for almost an hour when she used dark bath towels instead of her customary white ones, and alternately screeched at the top of his lungs and sobbed disconsolately when a new babysitter came. Such strong reactions could be avoided or at least minimized by introducing changes gradually.

A practical instrument for the assessment of temperament is the Infant Temperament Questionnaire (Carey & McDevitt, 1978) which is a simplification of the temperament research interview used by Thomas and his colleagues (Thomas et al., 1968). A Toddler Temperament Questionnaire for 1- to 3-year-old children is in preparation (Fullard, McDevitt, & Carey, 1978).

Social or Nonsocial Environment. The child's behavior could be the result of factors in the social or nonsocial environment that are affecting him negatively. Those to be considered here include such diverse causes as allergy, noxious substances such as lead, noxious forces such as noise and interpersonal tension, and discomfort factors in the child's immediate environment.

Maternal Handling. The difficult behavior could stem from the way that the mother interacts with the child. In considering this possibility the pediatrician should make the following kinds of observations. Is the mother relaxed? If her leg muscles are tense, the child is unlikely to rest peacefully on her knee. Are her movements as she holds him unhurried or are they jerky? While she is doing any caretaking does she carry on a quiet affectionate conversation with him? When does she respond to the child? Does the child appear to be warm and comfortable?

Physical Examination

Although the hyperactive child is usually physically normal, the possibility of a medical disease or condition, such as a progressive or treatable disease of the central nervous system, that presents as hyperactivity must be investigated. It is particularly important to check for hearing loss and to determine whether the child has a history of ear infections. Recent reports (Hersher, 1978; Paradise, 1980) have shown that the frequency of otitis media is significantly increased in hyperactive children; this finding suggests a sequence of hearing loss → school misbehavior → misdiagnosis. A routine neurological examination should always be performed. An examination by a neurologist and the use of specialized neurological tests ordinarily are not required except to rule out seizures, growths, or degenerative brain disease. Clements and Peters (1962) have specified the procedures that should be included in a neurological examination of a child tentatively diagnosed as hyperactive. Descriptions of neurological examination procedures for the detection of soft signs are contained in Close (1973) and Werry, Minde, Guzman, Weiss, Dogan, & Hoy (1972), and a play neurological examination that can be conducted in conjunction with a psychiatric interview of the child is described by Goodman and Sours (1967). The significance of soft signs is a highly controversial issue, with some investigators (Safer & Allen, 1976) attaching diagnostic value to them and others (Varga, 1979) regarding them as of little clinical significance. For excellent brief discussions of the soft sign controversy, see Ingram (1973) and Touwen and Sporrel (1979).

To help determine if the child's physical growth and development and his intellectual development are progressing normally, the pediatrician may decide to assess the developmental status of the child with a test such as the Bayley Infant Scales of Development (Bayley, 1969). The Bayley yields mental, motor, and behavioral scores. One group of items giving a Mental Score measures responses to visual and auditory stimuli, manipulation and play with objects, social interaction responses, discrimination of shapes, simple problem solving, memory, naming objects, understanding prepositions, and having the concept of "one." A second group, giving a Motor Score, measures gross motor abilities such as sitting, standing, walking, and stair climbing, and fine motor coordination such as grasping objects. The third part of the Scales is a behavior rating scale measuring such aspects as the child's emotional and social behavior, activity level, response to objects, attention span, persistence, and endurance. Testing usually is done in several sessions. The Mental and Motor Scales take from 45 to 90 minutes. Excellent standardization procedures have been followed in developing the scales and providing norms. The test reliabilities are satisfactory. The Mental Scale validity coefficient of .57 was determined by correlating the scores of 2-year-old children with their Stanford-Binet scores over the 6-month age overlap of the two tests. There are no validity data on the Motor Scale, but in a study by Berk (1979) the Motor Scale provided the most accurate identification of infants with suspected neurological impairment. The Bayley Scales are widely used for assessing mental and motor developmental status in children. In reviewing them, Collard (1972, pp. 728–729) states:

The value of the Bayley Scales as a research instrument lies in its careful standardization, high reliability, and broad coverage of many aspects of the behavior repertoire of infants. . . . [It is] by far the best measure of infant development available today.

An infant intelligence test such as the Cattell Infant Intelligence Scale may be used to rule out the possibility that the restless or difficult behavior is related to gross behavior abnormality. This test is considered to be a highly satisfactory instrument for infant testing (Anastasi, 1976). It provides an extension of the Stanford-Binet Intelligence Test from 30 months down to two months and gives a mental age (MA) and IQ computed in the same way as the Binet MA and IQ. The test items are grouped into 20 age levels, with five items and one or two alternates at each level. The short time intervals between age levels and the relatively large number of items per level provide a more precise measurement than is usually the case with infant tests. At the youngest level the tasks are largely perceptual (e.g., following a dangling ring with the eyes or looking at a spoon) with a few motor items (e.g., transferring an object from hand to hand). With increasing age, more complex manipulatory tasks are introduced using blocks, formboards, cups, dolls, and other toys, and increasing use is made of verbal functions. At the upper levels the child follows oral instructions with these objects and does more highly verbal tasks such as naming pictures of objects. All of the materials are standardized. There are no time limits and the order of item administration can be modified to suit the child and the testing circumstances. Testing usually requires 20 to 30 minutes. The standardization sample and procedures were satisfactory. Split-half reliability is unsatisfactory only at the 3-month level; other level reliabilities are between .71 and .90. When Cattell IQs were correlated with Stanford-Binet Form L IQs for 3-year-old children in the standardization sample, the reliability coefficient was .87. The predictive correlations of Cattell IQs for children below the age of 12 months and the Stanford–Binet IQs of the same children at age three are little better than chance. However, after the 12-month age level the predictive correlations become increasingly high, ranging from .56 at 12 months to .83 at 30 months (Frankenburg & Dodds, 1967).

Careful attention should be given to the presence of minor physical anomalies such as head circumference out of the normal range, epicanthus, widely spaced eyes, curved fifth finger, no ear lobes, and a wide gap between the first and second toes (Gallant, 1979). A list of these is contained in Table 9.1 along with the scoring weights assigned them by Waldrop, Pedersen, and Bell (1968). The anomalies are not all applicable to all ages. Fine electric hair, for example, does not appear in infancy. One or two of these anomalies are commonly seen in children in the nonclinical population and are of little or no importance. It is the presence of *multiple* minor physical anomalies that may be important. Waldrop and her associates have reported a high incidence of minor physical anomalies in hyperactive boys and have attributed the anomalies and the hyperactive behavior to the same causative factors occurring early in the first trimester of pregnancy (Waldrop et al., 1968). This increased incidence in hyperactive boys has been confirmed by Rapoport, Quinn, and Lamprecht (1974), and was associated in their sample with severity of hyperactivity and with either reported childhood hyperactivity in the father or a history of early obstetrical difficulty in the mother. Perhaps the most compelling evidence for the significance of these anomalies for hyperactivity in

Table 9.1.   List of Anomalies and Scoring Weights

Anomaly	*Weight*
Head—Electric hair:	
Very fine hair that won't comb down	2
Fine hair that is soon awry after combing	1
Two or more whorls	0
Eyes—Epicanthus:	
Where upper and lower lids join the nose, point of union is:	
Deeply covered	2
Partly covered	1
Hypertelorism:	
Approximate distance between tear ducts:	
≥ 1.5 inches	2
$> 1.25 < 1.5$ inches	1
Ears—Low seated:	
Bottom of ears in line with:	
Mouth (or lower)	2
Area between mouth and nose	1
Adherent lobes:	
Lower edges of ears extend:	
Upward and back toward crown of head	2
Straight back toward rear of neck	1
Malformed ears	1
Asymmetrical ears	1
Soft and pliable ears	0
Mouth—High palate:	
Roof of mouth:	
Definitely steepled	2
Flat and narrow at the top	1
Furrowed tongue (one with deep ridges)	1
Smooth–rough spots on tongue	0
Hands—Fifth finger:	
Markedly curved inward toward other fingers	2
Slightly curved inward toward other fingers	1
Single transverse palmar crease	1
Index finger longer than middle finger	0
Feet—Third toe:	
Definitely longer than second tow	2
Appears equal in length to second toe	1
Partial syndactylia of two middle toes	1
Gap between first and second toe (approximately $\geq 1/4$ inch)	1

boys comes from the finding that a high anomaly score in infant boys may be a reliable indicator of an infant who is likely to exhibit hyperactive behavior in the preschool years (Waldrop, Bell, McLaughlin, & Halverson, 1978).

As with all contacts with the parents and child, the pediatrician during the physical examination should validate through direct observation the mother's reports of the child's behavior, particularly those categories of temperament that may show up in the examination setting, and should observe the way the mother interacts with the child.

Evaluation of the Social Environment

A comprehensive evaluation of the child's social environment is mandatory. The rationale for investigating this area is that regardless of the primary cause of the at-risk behavior, there are almost certain to be secondary factors that are maintaining or even exacerbating the behavior; the identification and subsequent modification of some of these factors could result in a significant improvement in the problem behavior. The evaluation procedure provides additional information relevant to developing the prevention strategy, including the positive and negative potential that different members of the family have for participation in the intervention process, the parental philosophy of child rearing, the quality of the mother–child interaction particularly during basic care routines, the tone of the household, the financial status of the family, and relevant information about siblings. In evaluating the child's social environment, the extent of the child's contribution to the behavior problem and to the tenor of the household should not be underestimated. Because the young child is relatively helpless in a number of areas, the tendency is to view him as a somewhat passive recipient who is acted upon by other forces in the environment. In fact there is substantial evidence that even in the early years the child shapes the responses of his caretakers to an astonishing degree (Bell & Harper, 1977). Even the best behaved infant or young child is a powerful and active force in the household who directly and indirectly affects the interpersonal relations of other members of the household. The effect is even more powerful if he is an only child or if he has a difficult temperament. Clinical reports (Aleksandrowicz & Aleksandrowicz, 1975; Barkley, 1978; Brazelton, 1961; Chess, 1979) attest to the fact that the child at risk has the potential to create a network of interpersonal difficulties, such as alienation, negative affect, and tension in the household.

The At-Risk Diagnosis

No absolute guidelines can be given for diagnosing an infant or young child as at risk because at the present time we lack an objective basis, such as a score, for assigning at-risk status to a specific child. What is urgently needed is a scoring system analogous to the optimality score that Kalverboer,

Touwen, and Prechtl (1973) used to provide a global measure of the integrity of the nervous functions in the newborn infant. Lacking this type of tool, the diagnosis must depend in part on the global impression of the child yielded by the various assessment measures. However, if a child is at risk for hyperactivity, one would expect to find some supporting evidence in the history to eliminate a medical, neurological, and intellectual basis for the behavior, and to see sometime during the assessment period some clear-cut demonstrations of the behavior that has prompted the investigation. Since no absolute guidelines are available for the definitive at-risk diagnosis for hyperactivity (or most other behavior disorders), the possibility exists that a child will be incorrectly diagnosed as at risk and started on a preventive intervention program that is unnecessary because his difficulties are transient ones that will disappear spontaneously with time. If the assessment results lean toward an at-risk diagnosis, it is our opinion that the child should be started on a preventive intervention program *presented to the parents as routine changes in caretaking that are likely to be better suited to the child's temperament, without labels or the use of anxiety-arousing terms, and with a matter-of-fact attitude about the difficult behavior of the child.* There is little risk to the child or his parents in the preventive intervention approach to be described here providing the above principles are adhered to. The potential advantages of early preventive intervention far outweigh the disadvantage of false identification, whereas there is a substantial risk in a "wait and see" or "he'll grow out of it" approach.

If the pediatrician has serious doubts about an at-risk diagnosis he should consider postponing a decision. He should reconsider the information obtained during the assessment period and should outline a plan for improving the household situation without mounting a full-scale intervention program. The point here is that as long as the parents think that there is a problem, then there *is* a problem. It is best that the pediatrician work for solutions within the framework of the parents' perception of the problem. By providing a set of changes to be made, the pediatrician is acknowledging that a changeworthy problem exists. The alternative, to tell the parents that no problem exists, will likely alienate the parents and will certainly not help the child. Periodic follow-up checks over some predetermined time interval should accompany these changes, along with any assessments such as psychological tests that may be indicated. With this approach the pediatrician could construct a cumulative risk profile (Field, Hallock, Ting, Dempsey, Dabiri, & Shuman, 1978; Parmelee, Sigman, Kopp, & Haber, 1975) that would lend itself well to an objective review at the end of the specified time interval by other members of the interdisciplinary team.

THE PREVENTIVE STRATEGY

In general outline, the preparation of a preventive program involves the following steps. The pediatrician and a team of professionals coordinate all the available information on the child and his environment and decide what elements in the situation, such as maternal attitudes, factors in the mother–child relationship, and nonsocial factors, should be changed. They decide how best to change them, keeping in mind that the intervention procedures must consist of modifications that would not impose any undue hardships on the parents, seriously disrupt the household, or convey the impression of abnormality in the child. The pediatrician then outlines the preventive program to the parents, familiarizes them with the procedures to be followed, arranges for additional professional help to the parents in carrying out the procedures, and monitors the child's progress just as he would with a pediatric medical problem. Although the specific intervention procedures used in any particular case vary, most prevention programs require procedures that provide psychological support for the mother, instruct the mother in routine caretaking techniques that facilitate the handling of a difficult child, modify the child's behavior, and improve the overall quality of the mother–child relationship.

Psychological Support for the Mother

Mothers of difficult children are frequently characterized by incapacitating feelings of self-blame and guilt that sometimes lead to a disorganizing anxiety. In some cases these feelings are the result of critical and careless comments by harassed husbands, unperceptive relatives, or busy pediatricians implying that the mother has failed in the performance of her responsibility to the infant. The effect is to reduce the mother's already shaky confidence in her ability to care for her child so that the troubled mother–child relationship suffers further deterioration. Particularly in the case of the young infant, the mother must accept that the infant's behavior is to a certain extent independent of her child rearing practices. Where the problem behavior appears to be a function of temperament, the pediatrician should emphasize that this is the child's own style of responding to the environment. The pediatrician and the mother will have to work within it; but, at the same time, changes can be made to improve the situation and professional assistance will be arranged to help the mother in making changes. Two kinds of psychological intervention should be considered: supportive psychotherapy and a discussion group for mothers with difficult children.

Psychotherapy

Supportive psychotherapy (Meissner & Nicholi, 1978) focuses primarily on the patient's present problem and rarely probes into the past. The duration of this form of therapy is determined by the therapeutic goal which, in this case, is to help the mother mobilize her resources to deal effectively and adaptively with her difficult child and also reduce the resultant household tension. Supportive psychotherapy can be of tremendous value to the mother who feels defeated by the combination of her difficult child and her own uncertainty about how to cope. Such a mother often suffers from a debilitating degree of guilt about her ambivalence toward her child or outright dislike of him, and experiences considerable anxiety about the effect of the child on the household. In this therapeutic situation the psychiatrist is reassuring, supportive, and firm. He offers constructive advice, provides helpful information, shows clearly that he is strongly allied with the mother, and emphasizes his availability for help. At the same time the therapist limits the frequency and duration of the mother's visits, a restriction that serves the dual purpose of suggesting that the problem is not an unduly serious one and that the mother can manage for reasonable periods without consultation. With psychiatric help the mother can gain an improved perspective of the problem. At the same time the psychiatrist can identify maternal behavior and attitudes that may be exacerbating the child's patterns of difficult behavior. As the mother increases in confidence and understanding, the psychiatrist should have occasional sessions with both parents present.

Discussion Group

The second kind of psychological support that should be considered is a discussion group for the mothers of children with problems. In most metropolitan areas these groups are conducted regularly by public health agencies, the purpose being to teach mothers ways of interacting with their children that will strengthen the mother–child relationship, provide an opportunity for the exchange of information, and reduce through group interaction the feeling of aloneness that besets almost every mother of a child with a problem. The efficacy of such groups on the participants' morale and in meeting the above-stated goals is well documented (Berlin, 1974); the benefits obtained are consistent with affiliation (Schacter, 1959) and social learning (Bandura, 1969) theories.

The discussion group format provides an opportunity for two kinds of learning: *intentional training* through brief, formal didactic presentations, and *imitative learning* from observation of the group leader and the other participants. In the case of imitative learning, the entering mother is provided with multiple same-age models whom she perceives as similar to herself in age as well as in respect to the type of problem and its accompanying anxieties. Such perceived similarities are known to facilitate imitative learning (Bandura, 1969). On a dimension of competence, the mothers in a discussion group generally would be classed as *coping* rather than as *mastery* models for each other (Thelen, Fry, Fehrenbach, & Frautschi, 1979). Coping models are trying to manage and are experiencing some success, whereas mastery models exhibit exemplary skills and handle the problem of a difficult child with consummate ease. At this stage in the intervention program the uncertain mother needs models who vary in competency, with the majority falling in the coping category. The influence of such models is likely to have both cognitive and affective components, that is, the models demonstrate coping techniques that are helpful to the mother in the effective management of her difficult child, and they transmit attitudes that are likely to be anxiety-reducing for her. Their efficacy is heightened by regular and frequent exposures alternating with periods in which practice of the newly acquired learning can occur. The result is a reciprocal interaction between periods of observation and opportunities for performance that bodes well for increasing competence and confidence in the young uncertain mother. The salutory effects of multiple models are apparent in the following report of a young, inexperienced, and very anxious mother to her pediatrician after several discussion group meetings. Her account demonstrates a particularly beneficial result, the development of a critical but not self-destructive assessment of the problem (Ross, 1973):

> It [the discussion group] changed my whole life. Up till when I joined I just crabbed and crabbed at Cindy. Even when she was born I blamed *her* because she wasn't a boy! And all my girl friends with babies acted sort of funny about her—like supersweet, like she was MR or something—and that made me even crabbier. I think I felt like I'd got stuck with a second-rate baby. Then my pediatrician made me join MDB (Mothers with Difficult Babies) and I could see right off that Cindy was way way better than some of the ones there. And when I saw how the other girls acted to their babies *no matter what was wrong* like one baby was *blind*, I knew I'd been a really hateful mother. Cindy started out real ornery, even my pediatrician says that, but I made her a thousand times worse. Every time she acted up I'd say, "*Now* what's the matter with you?" when I should have said what was the matter with *me*. Why I didn't even call her by name—it was always "the baby" or "you." I didn't even know I did that till one of the girls in MDB asked me didn't I like Cynthia for a name because I never called her that.
>
> After I'd been in MDB a couple of months I said to Steve [her husband], "I guess I've been a terrible mother," and I know that I expected him to say like, "No, you haven't, Hon," but all he said was, "Well, you'll learn. Having a baby doesn't make you a mother," and I felt really ashamed because *he* knew I'd been hateful too . . . About two weeks ago something made me see how much I'd changed with MDB. I was playing a little game with Cindy and right in the middle of it she looked me straight in the eye and she laughed, really *laughed*, and without really thinking, I picked her up and hugged her and I was standing there hugging her and I thought that I'd never ever *wanted* to hug her before and I started to cry. . . .

Arrangements That Facilitate Basic Care Routines

The routine care of a difficult child is a continuing challenge to the parents', particularly the mother's, ingenuity, patience, and strength. However, improvements can almost always be introduced in the handling of specific basic care routines (sleeping, eating, bathing, dressing) that will result in a more harmonious mother–child interaction.

Sleep. If the parents of children at risk were to rank their problem behavior in terms of annoyance value, it is likely that sleep problems would rank highest. Even in normal infants and children sleep problems, such as night waking, are a common source of parental concern (Anders, 1979). The child at risk typically does not go to sleep easily, and when he does, the duration of sleep is much shorter than that of the average child. Research by several investigators (Ambrose, 1969; Barnard & Collar, 1973; Freedman, 1969) has suggested that duration of quiet sleep may be increased through stimulation by rocking. Barnard and Collar (1973) used an isolette rocker that combined periodic horizontal rocking movements with auditory stimulation in the form of heartbeat sounds at approximately 85 decibels. These investigators reported a marked increase in duration of quiet sleep in the premature infants after four weeks in the rocker. Although the rockers used in these studies would probably constitute a major expense for young parents, Stewart and Olds (1973) have suggested that a similar effect can be achieved with a set of four springs that can be attached to the legs of the infant's crib and an electronic gadget that simulates a heartbeat, both of which are available in department stores and are quite inexpensive. The sleep-inducing property of other types of continuous monotonous stimulation, such as continuous white noise, lullaby, and metronome, have also been demonstrated. Several research findings suggest that continuous stimulation can increase the total sleep time as well as the duration of quiet sleep without decreasing the duration of active sleep. This stimulation procedure can also reduce motor activity. For a comprehensive review of the effects of continuous monotonous stimulation on sleep in early infancy see Schmidt (1975).

Waking Restlessness. Research by Van den Daele (1971) has shown that restlessness in young infants and children can often be reduced by introducing specific types of stimulation into the environment. Their findings suggest that *visual stimulation* in the form of patterning as opposed to plain colors, and visual movement such as mobiles, *auditory stimulation* in the form of talking, singing, and recorded music, and *tactual stimulation*, touching and holding, all serve to quiet the restless infant and young child. With respect to tactual intervention, rocking and other forms of vestibular stimulation have been successfully used with hyperactive children (e.g., Bhatara, Clark, Arnold, Gunsett, & Smeltzer, 1981; Henderson, Dahlin, Partridge, & Engelsing, 1973).

When the daytime restlessness takes the form of steady crying that is not terminated by events suggestive of gastrointestinal discomfort, such as being burped, pacifier sucking may serve to quieten the infant. Wolff (1969) has suggested that the pacifier sucking facilitates sleep by serving the protective function of inhibition of diffuse activity. The rationale for this statement is as follows: one prerequisite for sleep is a relative absence of variable stimulation, a condition not met in the motorically active infant because the proprioceptive feedback from his restless movements maintains a state of arousal. Furthermore, restlessness of the degree characteristic of a hyperactive infant tends to maintain itself in the same way that a temper tantrum does. Pacifier sucking inhibits competing motor behaviors including restlessness, thereby interrupting the self-perpetuating cycle of crying and restlessness, and provides the essential conditions for sleep. According to Wolff's (1969) reasoning rocking quieten the wide-awake infant, or facilitates sleep, because it substitutes a constant, rhythmical form of stimulation for the higher arousal proprioceptive stimulation from spontaneous restlessness and crying, and the result is a lowering of the general arousal state.

Bathing. The overactive child typically is very difficult to handle in the bathing situation: he wriggles about, flails his arms, screams his protests, and generally prolongs the bathing period far beyond the time that should be needed. The mother should be shown how to set up the needed materials and impose restraints on the infant so that the bath routine does not leave both participants exhausted. As she sees that changes can bring about improvements, she should be encouraged to devise strategies of her own. One mother reported the following strategy (Copeland, 1971, p. 38):

> Timmy became so active at five months that I began to use my own special "Copeland" method of diapering. I placed him on the carpet or bed, sat beside him, put my legs across him and diapered him as he struggled and squealed. And when he began walking at eight months I soon learned to pin a diaper on him while he was scooting across the floor.

An essential component in any preventive strategy is the provision of some regular child care arrangement that will provide the mother with a breathing space and permit both parents to enjoy outside activities together. In addition, the father should regularly act as babysitter so that he will appreciate the difficulties the mother faces daily and also be able to contribute to the strategy planning sessions. Although his participation in the prevention program is of necessity limited by the demands of work, the mother will be better able to cope with the child if her husband is supportive (Pederson, 1976).

Modifying the Child's Behavior

A major change must usually be made in the parents' behavior management techniques, particularly in their reactions and responses to signs of distress or disruptive behavior in the child. Typically, the mother (or father) responds to crying, screaming, and unrest, partly because the noise is disturbing to her but primarily because she thinks she can remedy the situation. When the baby is quiet she leaves him alone. According to reinforcement principles this behavior pattern will prolong the disruptive behavior and might even increase it, with a concomitant weakening of tendencies to be quiet (Mash, Handy, & Hamerlynck, 1976). But the fact is that with the really difficult child the mother's presence will not stop the screaming and restlessness. In such instances, what both parents need and what the preventive strategy *must* provide is training in behavior management, preferably in the combined behavioral management–discussion group context that has been used successfully with young parents (Cantwell, 1974; Dubey & Kaufman, 1978; Feighner & Feighner, 1974; Mash & Dalby, 1979). With this training both parents will be able to devise sets of planned responses for handling the child's various kinds of difficult behavior. The planned response enables the parent to know in advance what his response will be to a specific behavior of the child. This approach has the effect of making the parent feel in control of the situation and ready to cope with any problems that may arise. It removes much of the negative, overly emotional content from the interaction—the feelings of helplessness, indecision, generalized anger, and lack of control experienced by the parent. An effective planned response for prolonged screaming, for example, is to have the parent check that the child is comfortable and not hungry, thirsty, or wet, provide brief attention and, if he fails to respond, leave him, preferably with the door shut. When the child becomes quiet, the parent should reenter the room and interact positively with him for a reasonable period. In this way he can reward the child's quiet periods and nonreward his restlessness. The parents must be convinced of the efficacy of this procedure. The mother should reassure the neighbors and have available a statement from the pediatrician because the publicity about child abuse has had the commendable effect of increasing the tendency of neighbors and bystanders to call the police when a child sounds as if he is being mistreated.

Williams (1959) has provided an excellent example of the effectiveness of combining reinforcement principles with the planned response procedure in order to modify tantrum behavior. The subject was a 21-month-old boy who had been seriously ill for the first 18 months of life and had required special attention. When he had recovered from his illness he continued to demand attention by screaming and fussing when he was put to bed. The parents were instructed to put him to bed in a leisurely and relaxed fashion, shut the door, and not return no matter how long he screamed and raged. Figure 9.1 shows that the duration of screaming and crying decreased rapidly until, by the tenth day, he no longer fussed. The second extinction series shown in the figure was necessary because a week later, when an aunt put him to bed, he fussed and she reinforced the tantrum behavior by returning to the bedroom and remaining with him until he went to sleep. Following the two extinction series the tantrums ceased. This intervention required no aversive punishment; all that was done was to remove the positive reinforcement of parental attention and proximity when the undesirable behavior occurred. For the researcher or clinician who is interested in the parental use of reinforcement procedures with infants or the development of parent training programs, there is a comprehensive review (Lancioni, 1980) of infant operant conditioning that underscores the efficacy and feasibility of including reinforcement procedures in early intervention strategies.

A major contribution to the prevention armamentarium is an intensive 8-month behavioral treatment program for hyperactive toddlers and preschool children and their parents developed by Drash, Stolberg, and Bostow (1977,

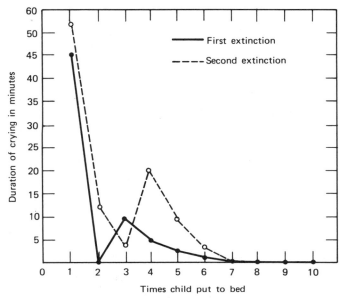

Figure 9.1 Length of Crying in Two Extinction Series as a Function of Successive Occasions of Being Put to Bed. From Williams, C. D. The elimination of tantrum behavior by extinction procedures. *Journal of Abnormal and Social Psychology,* 1959, *59,* 269. Copyright 1959 by the American Psychological Association. Reprinted by permission.

1981). Behavior observations coupled with parent reports established noncompliance, for example, inappropriate responding to verbal directives, as the behavior of primary concern in referrals to this program. These young children had all been diagnosed as hyperactive by referring pediatricians and, prior to intervention, were described by their parents as significantly worse than the average child. The program involved the systematic use of differential reinforcement of compliance, with verbal instruction for the children in both group and individual training settings. In addition, the parents attended weekly 3-hour classes on behavior modification techniques. Pre- and posttraining comparisons were made of changes in child behavior and results of parent instruction; these evaluations involved behavior checklists and true–false and multiple-choice examinations. The results showed that noncompliant behavior was reduced to normal levels and the parents' skill in using differential reinforcement techniques increased to approximately the level of that of trained child behavior specialists.

The results of an ongoing follow-up study (Drash, 1981) using structured telephone interviews and questionnaires are encouraging. The analysis to date shows that 55 percent of the children are functioning adequately in regular classroom settings, 75 percent of the parents reported that they were having no problems or only minor problems, and the same percentage stated that they had continued to use the behavior techniques taught in the original training program.

The Drash et al. program is unique in several respects. It is the first successful modification of hyperactive behavior to be reported in a group of very young children, and its use of noncompliance as the conceptual basis for treatment represents a significant departure from DSM II which was in effect at the time. Later, Barkley (1981) was to echo Drash et al.'s position in his important statement on the rationale for including noncompliance–rule breaking in the primary symptoms of hyperactivity listed in DSM III. It was most unusual to have a long-term follow-up, particularly in the behavior modification arena; also unusual was the low rate of attrition, with 71 of the original 81 children located for the follow-up. The implications of the results of this study are far ranging. It is impressive that a substantial number of young hyperactive children, following training, could function successfully in school and avoid the early school problems experienced by most hyperactive children in the absence of intervention. The value of early preschool intervention is quite apparent and in this form should eliminate any consideration of drug intervention in the preschool years.

Improving the Quality of the Mother–Child Relationship

Even the early interactions of at-risk infants and their mothers are seldom positive social interactions. Instead, they are characterized by a notable lack of positive feeling on the part of both members of the dyad (Field, 1979). If this situation continues unchanged it can have a debilitating effect on the child's psychological development. When early social interactions are characterized by negative affect, the probability is lessened that the child will approach subsequent interactions with positive expectations. It is reasonable, then, that he will probably exhibit avoidance responses which in turn tend to elicit unfavorable reactions from others in his social environment, thus confirming for the child the appropriateness of his avoidance behavior. A pattern may then become established early in life that is a prelude to the social interaction difficulties that are known to cause major problems for the hyperactive child in the school years and that continue to be a handicap throughout young adulthood (Barkley, 1978; Borland & Heckman, 1976; Weiss & Hechtman, 1979). Furthermore, the precursors of cognitive competencies and affective development appear to have their roots in the interpersonal experiences of infancy (Klaus & Kennell, 1976; Sameroff & Chandler, 1975), so an early dyadic relationship that is lacking in positive affect can have a deleterious effect on the child's development in these areas too.

An essential goal of the preventive strategy will be to teach the mother how to interact with her difficult child in a positive, loving manner. Research by Chamberlin (1974, 1975) suggests that this maternal behavior, which he calls positive contact, is related more to situational variables, such as maternal education and number of children in the family, than to parental attitudes. As such, maternal behavior should be quite amenable to change through parental education by pediatricians and other child care workers. It is most important that the mother begin to play with the child. Play will reduce irritability in the child and, more important, will lessen the pervasive feelings of mutual alienation. Game playing during early mother–child interactions also provides a context for learning conversational turn-taking and contingent responsivity (Field, 1979).

One procedure that can be used for both assessment and improvement of the quality of the early mother–child interaction has been described by Bromwich (1976). This intervention model, which was developed by the University of California at Los Angeles (UCLA) Infant Studies Project, is presently being used with considerable success in the UCLA Home Intervention Program. The emphasis in this program is on enhancing the quality of the mother–child interaction. The two major underlying assumptions of this model are that mother–child interaction is a bidirectional process with the behavior of each member affecting the other's responses, and that the prerequisites to maternal warmth and optimum care giving are maternal enjoyment of the difficult child and a feeling of satisfaction about him. The model describes a progression of six levels of maternal behavior. This six-stage schema is similar to Havighurst's (1972) developmental tasks and Sander's (1969) levels of adaptation, in that one level must be established if the next level is to be achieved with reasonable ease.

At the first level the goal is to help the mother have enjoyable interactions with her child even if this enjoyment is limited to brief periods or only to specific dyadic interactions. In subsequent levels the mother must learn to read the child's behavioral cues and respond sensitively to them (Level 2), initiate interactions that set the stage for the development of attachment and the beginning of a system of communication (Level 3), plan experiences that are developmentally appropriate and therefore satisfying (Level 4), initiate new activities that facilitate developmental progress (Level 5), and expand the child's experiences in a way that keeps pace with his changing needs and interests (Level 6).

Although this program is geared to infants below the age of two and their mothers, the maternal behavior described is also of crucial importance for interactions with young preschool children. This program is included here because intervention for a difficult dyadic relationship in the early childhood years should be initiated within the framework of the critical periods hypothesis. If both members of the dyad have failed to acquire the requisite interaction competencies of the infancy period on schedule, they cannot start with competencies appropriate for dyadic interaction at the 3-year level before first mastering the skills of the preceding age levels.

Effective prevention at the early secondary level depends on a multidisciplinary or team effort. The team approach has long been an integral part of intervention in the behavior disorders, and its membership has been generally agreed on. In descriptions of early prevention strategies, however, a crucial omission usually occurs in that the father either does not participate at all or, at best, does so only minimally. Interparental consistency in child rearing methods is usually beneficial to the child under the best of circumstances; it becomes essential when the child is a difficult one and the goal is to make marked changes in his and probably the rest of the family's behavior. The mother desperately needs the active support of her husband in coping with the prevention procedures, yet in most cases little or no provision is made to include him in the procedures. Instead, preventive intervention with a first child takes the form of a two-person strategy for a problem in a three-person system, with little concern for the fact that the third person, that is, the father, is a force with the psychological power to influence or even determine the eventual outcome of the intervention program.

CHAPTER 10

Management

Prior to 1970 hyperactivity was viewed as a transitory disorder of middle childhood and early adolescence with a good prognosis. Supporting this view were clinical reports of diminishing levels of activity with increasing age (Bradley, 1957; Laufer, Denhoff, & Solomons, 1957; Lytton & Knobel, 1958) coupled with the tendency for the problems of hyperactivity to merge with those of adolescence, so that the hyperactive adolescent was far less conspicuous than he had been in middle childhood (Hoy, Weiss, Minde, & Cohen, 1978; Milich & Loney, 1979a; Weiss & Hechtman, 1979). Sporadic reports that all was not well in adolescence (Anderson & Plymate, 1962; Quitkin & Klein, 1969) had little effect on the prevailing belief that hyperactivity was a time-limited, relatively mild neurodevelopmental lag, abnormal only in respect to the age of the child; that in a younger child the same behavior would be normal (Kinsbourne, 1973). Summarizing this view, which was typical of many experienced clinicians, is Eisenberg's statement (1966, p. 593):

> . . . typically hyperkinesis follows a developmental course, diminishing in later childhood and usually disappearing by adolescence. In this it resembles the activity pattern of normal children but displaced chronologically to the right by four to six years.

The view of hyperactivity as a transitory disorder dictated a management strategy geared solely to the immediate problems that had aroused parental concern, the basic strategy being a unimodal one usually consisting of drug or behavioral intervention. This view precluded even a consideration of possible long-term negative consequences and their potentially disastrous effects on later developmental goals.

During the 1970s, prospective and retrospective follow-up data (Allen & Safer, 1979; Borland & Heckman, 1976; Mendelson, Johnson, & Stewart, 1971; Weiss, Hechtman, & Perlman, 1978) and clinical reports (Arnold, 1979; Packer, 1978) made it apparent that hyperactivity is a complex problem with potentially pervasive and long-lasting effects. Cantwell (1978a) urged that for treatment purposes the hyperactive child be considered multiply handicapped and Bosco and Robin (1980, p. 173) referred to hyperactivity as "a chronic, life-blighting condition for children." It was now accepted that hyperactivity could be identified as early as the preschool years and might persist into young adulthood (Bellak, 1979; Campbell, 1976; Cantwell, 1979; Loney, 1980a; Weiss, 1975) and that although the activity level decreases with age, secondary problems of a social, academic, and emotional nature come to the fore that, if left untreated, could result in serious problems in the realm of social functioning (Cantwell, 1979; Milich & Loney, 1979a; Stewart, Mendelson, & Johnson, 1973; Weiss & Hechtman, 1979).

Growing out of these radical changes in the conceptualization of hyperactivity was a heightened interest in evaluating the effectiveness of the established management practices, particularly in respect to the criterion of long-term success. Follow-up data (Blouin, Bornstein, & Trites, 1978; Huessy, Metoyer, & Townsend, 1974; Minde, Weiss, & Mendelson, 1972) showed that neither stimulant medication nor any other intervention procedure aimed at modifying only the immediate problem improved the long-term behavioral, social, or academic outcome. In a survey of these data, Barkley (1978, p. 160) concluded that

> hyperactivity, despite our best treatment efforts, is a life-long disorder, rather than simply one limited to childhood. No longer can we legitimately inform parents to "hang in there" until the child reaches adolescence when the disorder ought to disappear. The fact that it does not *forces us to view treatment from a different perspective* (italics ours) . . . and requires that we approach hyperactivity with the same attitude as we approach developmentally handicapping conditions—as problems to be coped with throughout life rather than to be cured.

Before describing the management strategy that we propose it should be noted that throughout the discussion the emphasis will be on the late preschool and middle childhood years. Early intervention is of critical importance. When hyperactivity has been inadequately treated or has been allowed to go untreated until the early adolescent period, the management problem usually becomes so complex that it moves out of the realm of pediatrics and becomes primarily a psychiatric problem. Proponents of the "wait and see, he'll probably grow out of it" school of pediatric thought should give serious consideration to Cantwell's (1979, p. 69) comments on the importance of early intervention:

> The primary symptoms of . . . [hyperactivity], annoying though they often are to parents and teachers, can usually be treated fairly easily; the secondary problems that develop in the untreated child are often far less easily corrected. These include serious learning difficulties, problems in relating to other children, and consequent lowered self-image and depression. A . . . [hyperactive] child who is not treated until (say) age 12 is a very different child from what he was at school-entering age. At the very least, he is almost certainly one or two grades behind, meaning that even if successfully treated for the . . . [hyperactivity] itself, he will require remedial education—which is often hard to find and even when found is often of indifferent quality. . . . Assuming the child is of normal intelli-

gence—as most . . . [hyperactive] children are—he will know perfectly well what being placed in a remedial class means, and if by any chance he does not, his peers will convey it to him, since they normally refer to it as the "dummy" or "retardo" class. And once a child has acquired a reputation among teachers or peers as a "dummy" or "troublemaker," it takes a lot of living down, even with exemplary behavior. The result can be depression, sometimes culminating in attempted (occasionally successful) suicide. Another serious sequela is frankly delinquent behavior of a kind that brings the child into conflict with the law.*

The social context of the management process, particularly the way in which the three most relevant systems—medical, family, and educational—interact in the identification and treatment of the hyperactive child, has been intensively studied by Robin and Bosco (1976, 1980), who conclude that hyperactive children are not receiving the care that they could receive. In discussing the necessary collaboration among the three systems, they caution that it can occur only when a place is made in the management process for participants from all three systems. Although we concur with Robin and Bosco's general concepts of "making a place" and having a "single integrated support system," we strongly oppose their advocation that the teacher and the child should know that the child is on medication. With this reservation in mind, their concept of "making a place" has particular relevance to effective management (Robin & Bosco, 1980, p. 11):

> To "make a place" for participants in caring for hyperkinetic children means to create those social structures, within medical practices, schools, families and other caretaking organizations, that make participation necessary rather than permissible. It means that the educational plans for the hyperkinetic child are defined as incomplete until the physician's contribution is incorporated. It means that we act on our belief that information from school personnel and parents is essential in understanding the child's problems and solving them. It means that roles of the significant persons in each system are formed to accept and integrate knowledge and information from those in other systems. It means that there is a single integrated support system for the child.

The foundation for the single integrated support system described by Robin and Bosco (1980) is laid in the preliminary stages of the assessment period.

Since the management process is by definition an interdisciplinary effort, the assessment of the child and the interpretation of the results must be made within the context of the child's major environments (Allmond, Buckman, & Gofman, 1979; Weiss & Hechtman, 1979). A tendency to guard against is that of separating the child from his milieu and studying him in isolation in much the same way that a bacteriologist will (rightly) remove an organism from the medium in which it has grown in order to subject it to close and comprehen-

*Excerpted with permission from Cantwell, D. P. The "hyperactive" child. *Hospital Practice,* January 1979, *14* (1), 65–73.

sive examination. The management strategy that we propose is a comprehensive plan of action on an interdisciplinary base. The immediate goal is more effective functioning in the home, school, and neighborhood, and the long-term goal is optimal psychosocial development and educational and vocational progress. The prerequisite to the design and implementation of a management plan is a complete medical, psychoeducational, and behavioral evaluation of the child, including an assessment of his psychological environment, with particular attention to the pervasive effects of his problem behavior. The goal of the evaluation is not merely to arrive at a diagnosis but rather to make a complete assessment of all potentially relevant aspects of the child and his family, with special attention to identifying factors within the child and his environment that may be interacting to maintain his hyperactive behavior. The assumption is that neither characteristics intrinsic to the child nor environmental shortcomings is solely responsible for the problem. This comprehensive evaluation provides a data base that serves the dual purpose of confirming the condition of hyperactivity and providing an objective and rational basis for the development of a management strategy.

For the primary care physician whose task is to arrive at a diagnosis of the school-age referral for hyperactivity, Sleator (1981) has produced a landmark set of guidelines that should be required reading for all pediatricians whose practice includes hyperactive children and for professionals from other disciplines who are participants in the assessment process. Sleator, a highly regarded researcher and an able and experienced physician, has delineated the essential components of the office diagnosis of hyperactivity and urged the elimination of those procedures that do not clearly contribute to the goal of diagnosis. In discussing this parsimonious approach Sleator (1981, in press) states:

> This development probably stems from the realization that the health care system seems well on its way to imposing an intolerable financial burden on our society and, even more important, the realization that more is not necessarily better, as used to be assumed, but may, in fact be worse . . . not only because of the burden of unnecessary time and money expended, but because of the common problem of false positives which may cause severe emotional stress and stimulate further unnecessary procedures with the potential for new false positives.

MEDICAL EXAMINATION

There are two schools of thought concerning the necessity of a complete medical examination in the workup of a management strategy for the hyperactive child. One group favors a complete medical examination (e.g., Blau, 1979; Casey, 1977; Eisenberg, 1966; Safer & Allen, 1976; Sleator, 1981); the other places its confidence in skilled observation coupled with a careful behavioral history (Kenny, Clemmens, Hudson, Lentz, Cicci, & Nair, 1971; Wender, 1971). In a study supporting the latter view, Kenny et al. (1971) evaluated 100 children who were referred for hyperactivity. Each child received a thorough evaluation that included a complete medical and social history, a physical examination, and a neurological evaluation with emphasis on "soft signs." Electroencephalograms (EEGs) were obtained on 78 of the children. Each child was seen by three members of the interdisciplinary evaluation staff who made global judgments of the child's activity level. On the basis of the data, which showed no significant relationship among the neurological examination, EEG, and final diagnosis, these investigators concluded that requirements such as a medical diagnosis, neurological examination, and EEG prior to placement of hyperactive children in special education programs were inappropriate and that "the medical model has, at best, a minimal role to play in the evaluation of hyperactivity."

When this issue was studied in terms of actual medical practice at least one study (Sandoval, Lambert, & Yandell, 1976) showed that a diagnosis of hyperactivity was made primarily on the basis of behavioral indicators and information from the child's personal medical history rather than from data supplied by the physical examination and laboratory tests. The sample of 48 physicians reported that the major diagnostic factor during the physical was the child's general behavior, particularly his emotionality and activity level. The sample were also asked to make judgments about the importance of different diagnostic signs. Table 10.1 categorizes these judgments in terms of their importance in the diagnosis: Column 1 lists signs judged by 80 percent or more to be of considerable importance; Column 2, signs of marginal importance; and Column 3, signs that 50 percent or more rated as being of no diagnostic consequence.

It is our opinion that a complete medical examination is essential, and our management strategy is based on this premise. There are enough unavoidable risks in treating patients without voluntarily adding an unnecessary risk of omission in the form of the cursory examination advocated by Kenny et al. (1971) and others. The fact that the physical and neurological examinations are usually negative does not diminish their importance; they are mandatory in ruling out the possibility of metabolic problems, lead poisoning, and diseases of the central nervous system that may present with hyperactivity as a primary symptom. Some good examples of the failure to initially pursue an intensive medical search for the etiology of hyperactivity in children are contained in an article by Walker (1974), in which he reports several cases of hyperactivity due to medical problems, including an 8-year-old boy with hypoglycemia whose inability to tolerate and assimilate glucose led to hyperactivity which diminished when he was put on a high protein, low carbohydrate diet, and a 9-year-old boy who had been on medication for over two years whose hyperactivity abated as soon as he was treated for a calcium deficiency.

The cases reported by Walker (1974) emphasize the importance of ruling out underlying disease and other conditions that have symptoms in common with hyperactivity, and it is difficult to see how this can be achieved in the absence of a complete medical examination. Although any child who is referred to a pediatrician with complaints of hyperactivity should be entitled to the same complete pediatric study as any other child, he frequently fails to get the complete workup that experienced clinicians (Blau, 1979; Browder, 1972; Cantwell, 1979; Weiss & Hechtman, 1979) feel is mandatory. An all too common sequence is the labeling of a child as hyperactive by school personnel, a hasty and careless confirmation of the diagnosis by a physician, and stimulant treatment of a condition that requires a completely different therapeutic approach (Browder, 1972; Walker, 1974). The pediatrician who diagnoses hyperactivity solely or primarily on the basis of parental and teacher reports should keep in mind that a lack of care in diagnosis constitutes malpractice.

A complete medical examination, including a basic clinical history, complete physical examination with routine laboratory tests, and specialized physiological tests as required, is essential in our management strategy. In addition to the factual data obtained, the examination period provides the pediatrician with an excellent opportunity to assess subjectively relevant aspects of the mother's behavior. The assumption here is that the pediatrician will have already established a comfortable frank relationship with the mother so that in her office visits she no longer alters her parenting style to fit what she sees as the pediatrician's definition of a "good" mother. The mother's perception of the child and his problem are related to long-term outcome. If the mother focuses unduly on the difficulties that the child's behavior is creating for her and her husband, with her main concern being the inconvenience the child is causing her, the pediatrician should initiate a preliminary program to increase her understanding, with particular emphasis on developing a sympathetic imagination about the effect of the problem on the child. Without this empathic base it is unlikely that the mother will be an effective participant in any treatment strategy. Ideally, both parents should recognize and be apprehensive about the disruptive effects of the child's behavior on the family, but at the same time be genuinely concerned about his psychological well-being. Certainly there is increasing clinical evidence of the contribution of the hyperactive child to family disharmony and psychopathology (Barkley, 1978; Diller & Gofman, 1981).

The examination period also provides the pediatrician with firsthand knowledge of one aspect of the child's behavior. In this novel and often intimidating situation the child's behavior may be exemplary and show little resemblance to the disordered behavior that prompted referral (Cantwell, 1979; Loney, 1980a; Werry, 1978a), a phenomenon aptly labeled "the doctor's office effect" (Whalen & Henker, 1980b). Research by Sleator and Ullman (1981) has demonstrated strikingly that only occasionally can the child with a presumptive diagnosis of hyperactivity be accurately diagnosed on the basis of his office behavior. In a study of 95 children brought into their laboratory for workup, only one-fifth of the children, consequently dubbed *obvious hyperac-*

Table 10.1. Physicians' Judgments of Importance of Diagnostic Signs

I. HISTORY: PRESENTING COMPLAINTS AND SYMPTOMATIC BEHAVIOR

A. General Activity Level

IMPORTANT	MARGINAL	NOT IMPORTANT
1. Inability to sit still ª	5. Restlessness in MD's waiting room	10. Spills food often
2. Destructive of toys and furniture ª	6. Talks too much	
3. Overuses, careless with toys, furniture	7. Gets into things	
4. Doesn't play with games; nomadic play	8. Accident prone	
	9. Reckless	

B. Habit Disturbances

1. Inability to delay gratification	3. Irregular sleep pattern	6. Irregular hunger pattern
2. Doesn't complete projects	4. Hard to get to bed	7. Irregular excretion pattern
	5. Adapts slowly to changes in environment	8. Enuresis

C. Interpersonal Attitudes and Behavior

1. Inattentive; doesn't listen	6. Unpredictable show of affection	14. Constant demand for candy, etc.
2. Temper tantrums	7. Can't accept correction	15. Withdraws from new objects or persons
3. Unresponsive to discipline	8. Teases other children	
4. Unusually aggresive in behavior	9. Defiant	
5. Difficulty in obeying commands	10. Doesn't follow directions	
	11. Lies	
	12. Unpopular with peers	
	13. Plays so as to provoke adult intervention	

D. Affect Mood

1. Unable to tolerate frustration ª	2. Irritable	
	3. Negative in mood	

II. PERSONAL MEDICAL HISTORY

A. Prenatal and Perinatal Status, Infancy

1. Early infancy feeding (bottle or breast) problems	4. Extended labor	12. Mother's age at birth
2. Early infancy sleep patterns	5. Fetal distress during labor	13. History of maternal miscarriages
3. Early infancy responsiveness	6. Birth weight	14. Incompatible RH factor
	7. Difficult training for urinary control	15. Over six previous pregnancies
	8. Difficult training for bowel control	16. Operative delivery
	9. Special problems of dependency or anxiety about separation from mother in infancy	17. Infant late in raising head
		18. Late in smiling
		19. Late in turning over
	10. Sleep disturbance in infancy	20. Late in sitting
	11. Withdrawal from affective relating in first two years	21. Late in crawling
		22. Late in walking
		23. Late in talking
		24. Colic of the newborn
		25. Delayed speech development
		26. Night terrors in infancy
		27. Skin disorders in infancy

B. Problems in Later Childhood Development

1. Little capacity for problem-solving in life situations	5. Excessive dependence upon mother	12. Happy and outgoing personality configuration
2. Indications of psychopathology in mother-child relationship	6. Indications of psychopathology in father-child interaction	13. Normal visual acuity
3. Indications of psychopathology in sibling relationships	7. Happy but isolated personality configuration	14. Impression of dexterity
4. Unhappy but taking initiative towards others; may be so intrusive as to antagonize others	8. Unhappy and withdrawn personality configuration	
	9. Provocative and hostile toward others	
	10. Lack of skill in catching a ball	
	11. Awkward use of body skills	

348

Table 10.1 Continued

III. FAMILY HISTORY

IMPORTANT	MARGINAL	NOT IMPORTANT
1. Recognized personality disturbance or learning disability in family [a]	3. Marriage of parents considered unhappy	7. Mental illness present
2. Disagreement in response to patient regarding affection and/or discipline	4. Divorce considered	8. Exceptional intellect and achievement present
	5. Discord in marriage open	9. Child born early in marriage
	6. Discord in marriage covert	10. Open display of affection in marriage
		11. Child born late in marriage with other siblings older
		12. Child close in age to another siblings (9 mo. to 2 yrs.)
		13. Child's birth order position
		14. Convulsive seizures in family
		15. Mental deficiency or mental retardation in family

IV. SCHOOL HISTORY

IMPORTANT	MARGINAL
1. Leaves class without permission	10. Factors suggesting presence of mental retardation
2. History of fights	11. Immature speech
3. Repeated grade in school	12. Problems in articulation (dysarthria)
4. History of discipline problems [a]	
5. Moves from one activity to another in class [a]	
6. Difficulty in learning to read	
7. Current work below grade level	
8. Uneven or irregular academic pert romance	
9. Referral to school psychologist	

V. PHYSICAL EXAMINATION

IMPORTANT	MARGINAL	NOT IMPORTANT
1. Evidence of disturbance in mental status [a]	3. Impaired sensorium	11. Head circumference
2. Disturbed or hyperactive general behavior in exam [a]	4. Cranial nerve #8; hearing and balance	12. Cranial nerve #1; olfactory sense
	5. Major reflexes normal	13. #2 visual acuity and visual fields, pupillary response
	6. Cerebellar damage (problems of coordination, balance, etc.)	14. #3, 4, 6 extra-ocular movements
	7. Sensation (touch, pain position, vibratory, stereognosis)	15. #5 trigeminal nerve impairment
	8. "Soft" neurological signs: asymmetries	16. #7 facial muscle control
	9. "Soft" neurological signs: twirling of self or objects	17. #9 swallowing, gag reflex, deviation of uvula
	10. Toe walking without evidence of contractures	18. #10 voice quality
		19. #11 head rotation, shoulder movement
		20. #12 tongue control and movement
		21. Peripheral nerve damage (weakness, sensory loss, deformity, contractures)

VI. LABORATORY FINDINGS

IMPORTANT	MARGINAL	NOT IMPORTANT
	1. EEG abnormalities—focal or generalized	4. Blood studies—positive findings
	2. EEG abnormalities—"epileptic"	5. Urinalysis—albuminurria; infection; PKU
	3. Abnormal response to hyperventilation or photic stimulation	6. EEG abnormality—slow
		7. EEG abnormality—fast

[a] Majority of physicians judging item "Of Critical Importance"

From Sandoval, J., Lambert, N. M., & Yandell, W. Current medical practice and hyperactive children. *American Journal of Orthopsychiatry*, 1976, 46 (2), 323–334. Copyright © 1976 the American Orthopsychiatric Association, Inc. Reproduced by permission. ▪

tives, exhibited clear evidence of hyperactivity during the office examination. The remaining children, who were diagnosed as hyperactive on the basis of parent and teacher data, showed no evidence of hyperactivity during the doctor's examination. After three or more years of intensive data collection, the two groups did not differ on school grades, teachers' ratings of classroom behavior, amount of stimulant medication prescribed, or duration of drug treatment. In other words, the initial office behavior of this group of hyperactive children had *no* diagnostic or prognostic significance. Sleator and Ullman (1981) concluded that the pediatrician should view historical information from the child's parents and particularly from his teachers as reliable aids in the diagnostic process.

History

The framework for working up the history is a standard clinical one similar to that described in Chapter 9, with particular attention to prenatal events, perinatal history, neonatal and infancy periods, and ages at which developmental milestones occurred (Ingram, 1973). Using this framework as a point of departure, we recommend a wide-ranging creative approach to obtain pertinent information that is available providing the right avenues are explored with astute questions. The etiological role of stress, for example, is often overlooked or underestimated; or a history of otitis media may point to a hearing deficit as a primary factor in the child's hyperactive behavior (Hersher, 1978). In line with this approach is Cantwell's (1975a) recommendation that the developmental history of the child be supplemented with a detailed family history, obtained by a psychiatrist from each parent separately, with information about the family structure and home circumstances, history of illness and psychiatric problems, and interactions and relationships. (Cantwell [1975a] also provides a complete description of the topics that should be covered in diagnostic interviews with the parents and child.) Information should also be obtained about specific individuals in the child's environment who are distressed by his behavior, as well as those who are willing and able to participate in effecting change (Blau, 1979).

Most hyperactive children have a preschool history of the primary symptoms of hyperactivity (Cantwell, 1979; Weiss & Hechtman, 1979), so the child's behavior during this period should be discussed in detail. Of particular relevance to the management strategy is the degree of generality of the hyperactive behavior: is the child unable to control his activity level in any situation even when conditions are optimal, or is his overactivity situation-specific? This distinction between cross-situational and situation-specific overactivity has been noted by several investigators (Loney, 1980b; Schleifer, Weiss, Cohen, Elman, Cvejic, & Kruger, 1975). Age of onset should be determined. Hyperactivity that appears suddenly in the early school years, and in the absence of prior behavioral difficulty, is more likely to be etiologically related to noxious social environmental factors such as inappropriate school placement than is hyperactivity with behavioral antecedents in infancy or the early preschool years. The frequency of accidents, mishaps, and even accidental poisoning should be noted because hyperactive children are more frequently involved in such incidents, particularly in cases of accidental poisoning (Stewart & Olds, 1973; Stewart, Thach, & Freidin, 1970).

Hyperactive children often exhibit learning difficulties in the late preschool and early school years (Safer & Allen, 1976) so the mother's view of the child's school history should also be obtained, to be supplemented later in the investigation with school data including reports from present and previous teachers, cumulative school records, and IQ and achievement test data.

The possibility of misdiagnosis makes it mandatory to assess carefully symptoms and events in the child's history. Appalling examples of grossly inaccurate diagnosis resulting in inappropriate school placement can be found in Levine, Kozak, and Shaiova (1977). Childhood schizophrenia (Huessy, Cohen, Blair, & Rood, 1979), conduct disorders and certain epilepsies (Office of Child Development Conference Report, 1971), antisocial personality (Schuckit, Petrich, & Chiles, 1978), and juvenile manic-depression (White & O'Shanick, 1977) have all been misdiagnosed as hyperactivity.

Physical Examination

The physical examination provides a complete picture of the child's health status, as well as a basis for ruling out the many medical conditions such as hyperthyroidism and allergy which are characterized by behavior similar to that associated with hyperactivity and which may be misdiagnosed as hyperactivity.

A neurological examination, which can be done adequately by any physician willing to take the time to do so, should be conducted to eliminate the possibility of a progressive disease of the central nervous system that may present as hyperactivity. If the child does have major neurological handicaps an examination by a neurologist and the use of specialized tests may be required to rule out seizures, growths, or degenerative brain disease. A routine EEG is *not* justified in the absence of any suspected seizure activity (Casey, 1977; Varga, 1979). In discussing the value of the EEG in the workup of the hyperactive child, Cravens (Schmitt, Martin, Nellhaus, Cravens, Camp, & Jordan, 1973, p. 157) states:

> First, in terms of diagnosis, the normal EEG does not mean that brain damage is absent; nor, reversely, does an abnormal EEG alone mean minimal cerebral dysfunction or minimal brain damage. Diagnosis must depend on the history and physical and neurologic findings—not on the EEG. The specific type of EEG abnormality might be of use to an investigator in neurophysiology but is not useful to the pediatrician dealing with a hyperactive child. Second, with re-

spect to treatment, there is no EEG pattern which either compels or contraindicates a trial of medication.

Both an otological and ophthalmological examination are needed to rule out sensory defects that may be causing or contributing to the child's problem behavior. Defects of vision and hearing are present in a minority of hyperactive children (Stewart, Pitts, Craig, & Dieruf, 1966) and constitute a kind of sensory deprivation that may exacerbate hyperactive tendencies. Level of speech development should also be noted because speech abnormalities and delay are not uncommon in this group (O'Malley & Eisenberg, 1973; Safer & Allen, 1976) and speech therapy may be required.

During the physical examination the number and kind of soft signs should be noted, even though the significance of soft signs, such as strabismus, fine choreiform movements, and right-left confusion, is not known (Weiss & Hechtman, 1979). The pediatrician should also be alert to the presence of the minor physical anomalies discussed in Chapter 9 and listed along with their scoring weights in Table 9.1. Schain (1974) has cautioned that these anomalies may also be a sign of low intelligence and that the slow learner or child of borderline intelligence may react with hyperactive or disruptive behavior to the stress of academic demands that are beyond his ability. The basic management strategy here would be to initiate changes in the school situation rather than introduce intervention procedures such as pharmacotherapy that are aimed directly at the hyperactive behavior.

PSYCHOEDUCATIONAL ASSESSMENT

The goal here is to obtain test assessments and other evaluations concerning all aspects of the hyperactive child's academic and social functioning in the school setting. These latter evaluations include parent, teacher, and peer reports, as well as the child's point of view concerning the problem.

Academic Status

A prerequisite for the management strategy is a report on the current academic status of the child in relation to the educational norms for his age level. Cumulative school standardized test records usually are available but these should be viewed with some skepticism because all too often the test administration procedures deviate from the prescribed instructions, usually to the disadvantage of the child. In the long run it is best to plan on a reassessment of the child's various abilities to be conducted by a member of the management team. In this approach the appropriate tests and assessment procedures can be selected on an individual basis. Too often children who exhibit unacceptable behavior in the school setting are overtested for administrative purposes

(Bax, 1978; Blau, 1979, Garmezy, 1978), with tests casting little light on assets and liabilities (Mercer & Lewis, 1978), and with labeling being the last step in the sequence rather than action on the test results. As a general rule it is useful to begin with an individual intelligence test and a standardized achievement test to rule out the possibility that the child's behavior problem is a reaction to classroom demands far in excess of his capacity. We urge that this testing be performed by a qualified psychometrist. A recent article (Conners, Denhoff, Millichap, & O'Leary, 1978) directed to physicians and proposing that with minimal instruction a physician could administer a variety of tests has elicited a sharp note of criticism from Sleator (1981, in press) concerning the inappropriateness of such a suggestion:

> There is a certain kind of dreadful (but not rare) arrogance in the assumption that doctors can do anything better. This is exemplified in a recent article on hyperactivity addressed to doctors in which one page of instructions is devoted to telling the doctor how to do a WISC, a WRAT, and an assessment of writing and language ability! (Conners et al., 1978).

Intelligence Tests

A large number of individually administered intelligence tests are available. The two most often used are the Stanford-Binet Intelligence Test and the Wechsler Intelligence Scale for Children (WISC).

The Stanford-Binet Intelligence Scale has tests grouped into age levels ranging from Year Two to Superior Adult. The test proceeds by half-year intervals for ages two to five and by yearly intervals for ages five to 14. Each age level from two to 14 contains six tests with one alternative test, all seven being of approximately uniform difficulty. Each child is tested individually over a limited range of age levels suited to his own intellectual level. Testing usually takes 30 to 40 minutes for younger children and an hour or more for older children. There is a wide variety of item content including manipulation of objects and eye-hand coordination, observation and identification of common objects, similarities and differences between sets of objects, commonsense questions, tests of spatial orientation such as maze tracing and paper folding, numerical and memory tests, and many tests employing verbal content such as vocabulary, sentence completion, and proverb interpretation. The technical quality of the standardization procedures is high, with high scale reliability coefficients (.83 to .91 at the preschool levels, and .91 and above for ages six to 13) and criterion-related validity (correlates highly with performance in most academic courses, particularly the predominately verbal ones).

The Wechsler Intelligence Scale for Children (WISC), for ages 5 to 15, provides a verbal score obtained from five subtests (general information, comprehension, arithmetic, similarities, vocabulary) and one alternate (digit span); and a performance score from five subtests (picture completion, picture arrangement, block design, object assembly, coding) and one alternate (mazes). Split-half reliabilities for the Full Scale, Verbal, and Performance Scales are satisfactory (for a sample of 200 7-year-old children, .92, .88, and .86 respectively). The WISC is well standardized, stable over time (scores correlated .77 over a 4-year period), and correlates generally in the .80s with other tests of intelligence (Sattler, 1974).

The Revised Wechsler Intelligence Scale for Children (WISC-R) (Wechsler, 1974) retains much of the WISC along with the following changes: items considered to be unfair, ambiguous, or obsolete have been modified or eliminated; some subtests have been lengthened to improve reliability; the age range has been shifted to 6 to 16 years; verbal and performance subtests are administered in alternating sequence; and nonwhite children are represented in the standardization group in proportion to nonwhite children in the 1970 census. Unlike the earlier WISC, the WISC-R yields mean IQs that are very close to Stanford–Binet IQs (1972 norms) due in part to the improvements in control, administration, and scoring procedures in the WISC-R (Anastasi, 1976). An excellent critical discussion on research on the WISC-R and the issues surrounding intelligence testing is contained in Kaufman (1979).

The Wechsler Preschool and Primary Scale of Intelligence (WPPSI) is a downward extension of the WISC for ages four to $6\frac{1}{2}$. It follows the same format as the WISC, giving a Verbal, Performance, and Full Scale IQ. Three of the 11 subtests (Sentences, Animal House, and Geometric Design) are new. The remainder are adaptations or extensions of WISC subtests. Testing time is 50 to 75 minutes in one to two testing sessions. The standardization procedures were excellent and the reliabilities are satisfactorily high (.92 for the Full Scale after an 11-week interval), but validity data are minimal.

The Goodenough Draw-A-Man Scale is often used for a rapid assessment of intelligence. In this test the child is given a pencil and paper and instructed to "draw a whole man and the best man you can draw. Make all of him." The drawing is scored for detail and complexity. Although the test may appear to be a measure of visual motor coordination, it taps more complex functions. The test score correlates with the Stanford–Binet and the WISC, and correlates highly with social adjustment. It is attractive to children, can be easily administered and scored, and has good reliability. Research by Crowe (1972) has shown that hyperactive boys performed poorly on body image as measured by human figure drawings when compared to normal boys. The differences occurred independently of intelligence. When hyperactive boys were on psychoactive drugs they performed better than hyperactive boys on placebo.

The WISC has been used far more frequently than any of the other tests in this section to make hyperactive–nonhyperactive comparisons, evaluate intervention programs, and measure functions that provide information about areas of academic difficulty in the underachieving hyperactive child of apparently average or above-average intelligence. The fact that the Verbal and Performance IQs of hyperactive children often do not differ from those of nonhyperactive controls (e.g., Douglas, 1974; Keogh, Wetter, McGinty, & Donlon, 1973), together with the finding that hyperactive children typically show more subtest scatter on the WISC (Douglas, 1974), has focused investigative interest on subtest scores. The rationale for this approach is that the summary scores, that is, Verbal and Performance IQs, are often well within the normal range and consequently mask differences that may be of diagnostic and evaluative value. Milich and Loney (1979b) used pattern, factor, and functional analysis procedures in a study of intellectual functioning, as measured by the WISC, of 90 hyperkinetic boys of elementary through high school age. Pattern analysis showed that in comparison to the general population these boys were lower in Verbal IQ, as well as in scores on the Information, Comprehension, Arithmetic, Digit Span, and Coding subtests, and higher on Object Assembly and Similarities. Factor analysis yielded three factors: Verbal Comprehension (Similarities, Vocabulary, and Picture Arrangement), Spatial Organization (Picture Completion, Block Design, and Object Assembly), and Inattention–Distractibility (Information, Arithmetic, Digit Span, and Coding subtests), with the Inattention–Distractibility factor accounting for the major part of the factor variance. For functional analysis, each subject's subtest scores were converted into scores for each of the three factors—Verbal Comprehension, Spatial Organization, and Inattention–Distractibility. Performance on the latter factor was significantly worse than on the other two factors. Milich and Loney (1979b) concluded that use of the three factors, rather than the traditional two factors of Verbal and Performance, in interpreting the WISC performance of the hyperactive child would provide more insight into his academic difficulties. They are not, however, suggesting that the WISC be used as a measure of attention. As Sandoval (1977, p. 312) has noted: "The use of the WISC itself . . . as a measure of attention and concentration is neither appropriate nor justified, considering the availability of other measures."

Achievement Tests

A number of tests have been developed for measuring the child's general educational achievement level in the basic academic subjects. When this type of test is used with children who are entering first grade it is usually called a *readiness test*. For the child who is already in school, the test content becomes more advanced and the term *achievement test* is used.

The Metropolitan Readiness Tests are group tests generally used to measure readiness to enter grade one. Each of the two forms consists of six subtests: word meaning (the child selects from a row of three pictures the one that the examiner names), listening (one or more sentences are used to identify the correct picture in a row), matching, alphabet (the child identifies on the page the letter named by the examiner), numbers (quantitative concepts and simple numerical operations), and copying (geometric forms, numbers, letters). Both the alternate-form and split-half reliabilities are over .90. There is evidence of predictive validity: correlations of end-of-year achievement with test scores ranged from .57 to .67. The test appears to measure abilities believed to be associated with success in early school learning. Standardization procedures were satisfactory. Administration time is 60 minutes, in three sessions.

The SRA Achievement Series and other general achievement batteries (e.g., The California Achievement Tests, the Iowa Tests of Basic Skills) focus on educational skills such as reading, arithmetic, spelling, and language usage; and work-study skills such as map reading. The SRA Achievement Series uses norm-referenced measurement of educational achievement. There are equivalent forms for five levels: Primary 1 (Gr. 1–2), Primary 2 (Gr. 2–4), and three multilevel test forms (Gr. 4–6, 6–8, and 8–9). The items are generally of acceptable quality, but some are too long, some reading items measure opinion as well as comprehension, and some test items are on the same page as practice items. The test is easy to administer but difficult to score. It is recommended that it be given as a power test (no time limit), but giving it as a speed test is permissible. The Kuder–Richardson 20 coefficients are generally in the high .80s but the use of the Kuder–Richardson for a speed test is questionable. No reliability is given for the equivalent forms, a curious omission. Equivalent means are given but no intercorrelations are presented. Also, there are no test–retest correlations. Although the test is designed to measure achievement, no correlations are provided between SRA Achievement scores and other achievement measures, such as batteries or teacher ratings, or other ability measures. However, the standardization data are excellent.

The Wide Range Achievement Test Revised Edition (WRAT) is a timed test with two levels, one for ages five to 11 and the other for ages 12 and over. It gives three scores: spelling, arithmetic, and reading. It is basically an individual test, but there is provision for group administration of some parts. It takes 20 to 30 minutes to administer. It is mentioned here because it is used extensively in experiments evaluating the academic progress of hyperactive children under various treatment conditions (e.g., Conrad, Dworkin, Shai, & Tobiessen, 1971; Denhoff, Hainsworth, & Hainsworth, 1972; Flynn & Rapoport, 1976; Gittelman-Klein & Klein, 1976; Wikler, Dixon, & Parker, 1970) despite significant inadequacies Aman, 1978; Payne, 1974). In a critical review of the WRAT Thorndike (1972, p. 68) concluded that

> This test may have some value in a clinical or research setting in which one is testing individually persons of such diverse ability or background that one cannot tell in advance what level of test would be appropriate, and needs to get a quick estimate of each person's general level of ability and educational background. One would hesitate to recommend it for other purposes.

Tests for Other School-Related Functions

Although many studies of hyperactive children have reported learning difficulties (e.g., Douglas, 1974; Lambert & Sandoval, 1980) the exact nature and reason for these difficulties is often a matter of contention (Keogh, 1971). Although there is no specific test or pattern of test scores that is diagnostic of hyperactivity, the following tests may be useful for the child who is experiencing specific difficulties in school. *Visual perception* can be measured with the Frostig Developmental Test of Visual Perception, *auditory perception* with the Wepman Test of Auditory Discrimination, *language functions* with the Illinois Test of Psycholinguistic Abilities (ITPA), *memory function* with the Benton Visual Recall Test, and *motor function* with the Lincoln–Oseretsky Test.

Behavioral Evaluation

The essential components here are parent, teacher, peer, and self-report data. In tapping each of these sources of information the assessment techniques should identify the child's assets as well as his liabilities. This is contrary to the usual procedure of focusing solely on weaknesses when a child has a behavior problem, at best a negative approach. In addition, significant gaps in the quality of the child's life should be noted (Blau, 1979), the primary targets for change in his behavior repertoire decided on, and priorities assigned to them. Identifying the child's strong points is necessary if the management strategy is to capitalize on them as assets in effecting change. In discussing one of the prime goals of intervention, that of increasing the extent to which the child has social acceptance, Gold (1968) has proposed a competence-deviance hypothesis. In his formulation acceptance is partially determined by the balance between competencies and deviancies, so that the more an individual deviates from the social norm, the more competent he must be in other respects if he is to gain social acceptance. To incorporate this idea in a management strategy requires an accurate assessment of the child's assets.

Parent Reports

Ratings done independently by each parent provide information about their perceptions and tolerance of the child's behavior as well as a basis for making home–school and interparent comparisons. We recommend the Werry–Weiss–Peters Activity Scale (Werry, 1968), which is reproduced in Table 4.5 (see Chapter 4), and either the Conners Parent Questionnaire (Conners, 1970) or the Behavior Problem Checklist (Quay & Peterson, 1967).

Experienced clinicians (Cantwell, 1979; Eisenberg, 1966; Stewart & Olds, 1973) consider a psychiatric interview with each parent to be a primary source of information that is likely to be of inestimable value in planning the intervention procedures. In the interviews, topics such as the meaning the child's problem has for each parent, their coping procedures, and their causal judgments can be explored. Parents often differ markedly in perception of their hyperactive child (Hegeman, 1977) so that their input in the assessment procedure is sometimes superficially dismissed as *unreliable*. However, studies in England (Rutter & Graham, 1968) and in this country (Herjanic & Campbell, 1977; Herjanic, Herjanic, Brown, & Wheatt, 1975) have demonstrated both the validity and reliability of clinical assessments by parents (and also by children). Furthermore, differences between parents in perception of their child are entirely reasonable because the psychological space occupied by the father–child interactions differs from that of the mother–child interactions. To call parental differences unreliable is to assume that there is only one correct view of the child, whereas in fact each facet of the child will be viewed differently by others in his social environment depending on their position in relation to him, just as a view of a mountain varies depending on one's location in relation to it. The parents' views undeniably are subjective and usually unsystematic, but they are based on observations made over extended periods of time. As Weakland, Fisch, Watzlawick, and Bodin (1974) have pointed out, it is essential to grasp the ideas and values that are central to each parent because the therapist must perceive and make use of existing motivations and beliefs if he is to change behavior that the parent already considers is right and logical.

Teacher Reports

The child's teachers should be interviewed to obtain their opinions on the nature of his problem and their assessment of his family. They are likely to be more objective because they have as a frame of reference the behavior of a group of same-age, same-sex children occurring in the same setting, coupled with considerable experience in dealing with parents. The teachers should also complete one of the teacher rating scales, such as the Conners' Teacher Rating Scale or the Conners' Abbreviated Teacher Rating Scale. Teachers' ratings generally have proven to be reasonably reliable and valid measures of a child's current classroom functioning (Chamberlin, 1976; Rapoport, 1980; Rapoport & Benoit, 1975; Ullman, 1978). As is the case with parents' ratings, teachers' ratings serve the dual purpose of providing immediate information of relevance to management, as well as baseline data for subsequent evaluation of the intervention strategies that are used.

Classroom observations of the hyperactive child and one same-sex, normoactive classmate would be of considerable value. As Loney (1980a) points out, the expenditure in time and money would be substantial, but so is the potential payoff of these data. A picture of the teacher in action and of the classroom climate is an additional bonus of inestimable help in evaluating and weighting the teacher report data. Among the excellent classroom observation systems that have been developed are those of Abikoff, Gittelman-Klein, and Klein (1977), Weissenburger and Loney (1977), Whalen,

Collins, Henker, Alkus, Adams, and Stapp (1978), and Vincent, Williams, and Elrod (1977).

Peer Reports

Although the classroom peers of hyperactive children have proven to be accurate in prediction and sensitive in assessment (Campbell & Paulauskas, 1979), it is clear from clinical reports and empirical investigations, particularly follow-up studies, that their potential as valuable informants has not been tapped. There is empirical evidence that peer evaluations are temporally stable across sex of raters and over a wide age range and are surprisingly free of a tendency to respond with prosocial evaluations (Wiggins & Winder, 1961). Furthermore, they have been validated successfully against behavior observations as well as parent, clinician, and teacher ratings (Marsden & Kalter, 1976; Wiggins & Winder, 1961). Peer evaluations of hyperactive children have several strong features: they are obtained in the school, which is the most significant of the social settings that a child encounters outside of the home, and are based on observations made over an extended period of time by multiple same-age children who view the child from a variety of different perspectives (Weintraub, Prinz, & Neale, 1978). To obtain peer opinions the Peer Nomination Inventory developed by Wiggins and Winder (1961) is an effective instrument that supplies several measures including aggression, a characteristic of particular relevance to the diagnosis and prognosis of the hyperactive child (Loney, 1980b). To show the child's place in the social structure, that is, whether he is popular or unpopular, anyone's best or second best friend, and whom he likes and dislikes, sociograms have been used (Mainville & Friedman, 1976).

In *any* of the above procedures involving entry into the classroom setting, it is totally unnecessary to single out a particular child or pinpoint him in any way as the object of an investigation. As a general rule, provide the teacher with the least possible (but accurate) amount of information necessary to explain the presence of the investigator. In classroom observations, for example, the most valid data will be obtained if the teacher is unaware that the hyperactive child is the focus of interest. By having the observer absent from the preliminary management group–teacher meeting, he can appear unrelated to the problem of the child. The observer would be requesting the names of other normoactive children, and observing these children could be the implied reason for his presence, but there is no need to mention the hyperactive child since he has already been identified for the observer. The point of all this circumspection is that it is virtually impossible for even the most cooperative and helpful teacher to be totally unaffected by the presence of a stranger in the classroom whom she knows is watching her interaction with a specific child. Consequently, the information given to the teacher should be kept to a minimum. And for the child's welfare, he should *never* be identified in any way to his classmates as the focus of interest.

Self-Report

The hyperactive child is rarely asked how he feels about his behavioral difficulties despite his strategic position in the social framework of the problem. Loney (1980a, p. 275), in a discussion of ethical considerations inherent to the management of the hyperactive child, has commented that

> another problem is the absence of relevant data from one crucially important person, the child. The hyperactive child has not often been asked, directly or indirectly, whether his or her behavior or other peoples' reactions to it are a source of personal unhappiness.

But Stewart et al. (1973, p. 3) express the more prevalent view of doubt about the validity of self-report data from children:

> Among the many studies of hyperactivity and its treatment there does not seem to be one that is concerned with the thoughts and feelings of the patients themselves. There would be some doubt as to the validity of comments made by school-age children about their behavior and reactions to treatment, but it seems an important field to explore . . .

The criterion of validity is a relative standard rather than an absolute one. The fact that the child's view does not concur with those of his parents, teachers, and peers is not grounds for ignoring it, particularly in the light of the findings on source factors (Langhorne, Loney, Paternite, & Bechtoldt, 1976). The child's feelings and opinions may be valid in terms of *his* perception of the situation. If his perception of the situation is unrealistic, this does not affect the validity of his feelings, but merely indicates that steps should be taken to help him identify the elements in the situation that are important and interpret them correctly. Misconceptions held by the child play a vital part in his whole modus operandi. The only way to identify them is to have extensive discussions with the child himself. Consequently, we strongly advocate that major attention be paid to the child's viewpont. To this end, a child psychiatrist should obtain the child's opinion about the referral complaint, determine if the child sees it as a problem, establish whose problem the child thinks it is, and what the child thinks would improve his whole situation (Sulzbacher, 1975). Often the child recognizes that neither he nor his parents and teachers can control his behavior, and their apparent incompetence, obvious frustration, and anger frighten and puzzle him; sometimes he sees himself as irreversibly defective. The information offered by the child should be viewed as important for itself rather than for the extent to which it is consistent with his parents' and teachers' view of the problem. It is important that the interview be relaxed and nonthreatening; it should establish in the child's eyes that the psychiatrist is aware of the difficulties the problem causes, is sympathetic about the problem, does not blame the child for it, and intends to take ameliorative action.

One outcome of this interview could be a realistic assessment of the extent to which the child might participate actively in the management procedures. The study by Bugental, Whalen, and Henker (1977), discussed earlier, underscored the importance for outcome of a match between the hyperactive child's causal attributions and type of intervention. The child's role in the management strategy might be enhanced by a match between his attributional status and the extent and kind of responsibility assigned to him in the treatment process.

ENVIRONMENTAL ASSESSMENT

The task here is to assess two major facets of the child's psychological ecosystem: relevant etiological social factors and the presence of helpful family and community resources (Eisenberg, 1966). An adequate asessment of these facets requires information from adults in the child's environment. For example, are there social environmental factors, such as family tension, crowding, or a genuinely poor school situation, that might be causing, maintaining, or exacerbating the behavior problem? The identification of such social causes would be based on the team's observations of the parents and other adults who regularly spend a substantial amount of time with the child. The team should decide to what extent, if any, one or both parents and the child's teacher might be contributing to his behavior either directly, through child rearing or classroom practices, or indirectly through mechanisms such as modeling. An assessment should be made of the psychological and financial potential of the family for embarking on a long-term plan of management. The practicality of requiring the family to participate should be established. If the family is to be of no help, this is the time to find out, before incorporating family help into the management program. Do the parents have the time, interest, stamina, and ability to put into action the kinds of intervention that would be recommended? It is important here to assess the school and community resources that would be available, since there is no point in making unrealistic recommendations, such as special individual help, if no such assistance is available.

TREATMENT

When the assessment procedures have been completed the team of investigators will be in a position to make a final decision concerning the diagnosis. It should be apparent from the array of sometimes conflicting data collected that a diagnosis of hyperactivity cannot be made on the basis of any single symptom or test result (Conners, 1975b). Assuming that the original diagnosis of hyperactivity is confirmed at this time, the hyperactive child should be considered a multiply handicapped child who is most likely to benefit from a multimodality treatment approach (Cantwell, 1978a). A program based on this approach should involve some or all of the following components of treatment: psychotherapy, which could include individual therapy, counseling, or participation in peer discussion groups for the child; a similar range of psychotherapeutic options for the parents and other family members, along with training in special behavioral procedures for them to follow at home in handling the child and modifying his behavior; special school arrangements and tutoring for the child; and medication. The empirical basis and conceptual rationale for procedures within each of these major modes of intervention has already been discussed. The purpose of the present discussion is to describe procedures for handling certain steps in the management strategy, make suggestions concerning options within the modes of intervention, and consider certain controversial issues that will confront the pediatrician in the course of directing the management strategy.

Presenting the Diagnosis

It is assumed here that both parents will be involved in the treatment process, thus allowing the pediatrician to deal simultaneously with the child's problem and with family difficulties related to the hyperactivity. There is increasing support for the value of the father being involved in the treatment procedure and assuming some responsibility for the child on a regular basis (Bronfenbrenner, 1979b; Pederson, 1976). While the demands of the father's occupation almost invariably will limit his available time, they should not excuse him from all responsibility. Too often in these cases the father escapes thankfully to work, abdicates all responsibility, has very little understanding of the child's day-to-day problems, and becomes a dead weight that the rest of the family must work around. The first step in implementing the management strategy is to inform the parents that their child is hyperactive, a task that usually falls to the pediatrician. How the pediatrician handles this deceptively simple step will greatly influence the parents' perception of subsequent steps. In the literature on management there is growing recognition of the importance of such interpersonal communications. An increasing number of excellent guidelines have appeared (e.g., Cantwell, 1975a; Katz, Saraf, Gittelman-Klein & Klein, 1975; Wiener, 1977), one of which (Rapoport, 1980), is mandatory reading for every professional involved in the management of the hyperactive child. Since the discussion with the pediatrician will shape the parents' perception of the child's problem to a considerable degree, it is imperative that a careful explanation of the problem precede the use of labels that might arouse anxiety. The explanation must take into account the parents' causal attributions (Rapoport, 1980), which will be known to the pediatrician from the assessment data. The parent who attaches self-blame to the problem and experiences guilt about it or sees the child as defective will re-

quire a different formulation of the diagnosis than the parent who is genuinely concerned but does not view the problem as permanent or in any way
either parent's fault.

The pediatrician should convey a feeling of optimism. Except in extreme
cases of disability and IQ deficit, no prediction can be made with certainty
about how a particular child will grow up. The parents must not come away
believing that the diagnosis of hyperactivity is indicative of permanent difficulties or is a catastrophe. The pediatrician should place the problem of
hyperactivity within the spectrum of childhood diseases and behavior disorders by comparing it to other chronic problems, such as juvenile diabetes,
arthritis, renal disorders that require dialysis, and asthma, and briefly discussing the burden of a child with a serious intellectual or sensory deficit. It is
important to acknowledge that the hyperactive child is difficult and often in-
furiating. At the same time it is essential that the pediatrician help the parents
keep the problem behavior in perspective. This task is more difficult than it
appears because the pediatrician must also combat the cumulative effects on
the parents of the media stereotype of hyperactivity.

At some point, particularly in the lay literature of the past decade, the
hyperactive child has crossed the line from *difficult* to *disaster*. Experienced
science writers (Olds, 1969) have used descriptors such as "tornado" and
"manic"; one psychiatrist equated hyperactivity with predelinquency
(Schrag & Divoky, 1975); *Newsweek* magazine (Clark, 1980) ran a feature
article entitled, "The curse of hyperactivity"; and recently an experienced
clinician (Gittelman, 1979) expounded on interventions that could "rescue
parents." The visibility accruing from such descriptors acts ultimately to the
detriment of the hyperactive child. Inevitably it has a negative effect on his
self-concept, peer relations, progress in school, parental reactions to the diagnosis of hyperactivity, and long-term outcome. The descriptors also create
a set in others: if a child is a recognized disaster, parents immediately become blameless and teachers are not held responsible for the child's lack of
progress. Although the descriptor "like any child but more so" (Allan &
Ornellas, 1977) may not be precisely true, it represents a far more accurate
statement than the currently popular and attention-getting disaster-type labels. It is time for writers on hyperactivity, particularly those whose work
appears in the lay literature, to present the case for the hyperactive child
fairly and in nonsensational terms, and to emphasize as Henker and Whalen
(1980a, pp. 362–363) have done that for many of these children the outlook
is potentially promising:

> But there is also a much brighter side to the picture. The multifaceted prob-
> lem called hyperactivity is a tough but not intractable one. Whether one speaks
> of the 1% to 2% of children who are medically identified and treated or of the
> 5% to 10% who are socially or educationally defined, included are many children
> whose prognosis is one of relative optimism. While some will go on to careers of
> school failure, later delinquency, or adult maladjustment, a great many more will

go on to successfully negotiate the major hurdles of growing up and becoming productive members of society.

In this very important way the outlook for the hyperactive child differs from that for a child with almost any other enduring problem of psychological health. In the last analysis, hyperactivity is just another degree of normality; the potential for change, in either direction, is high. These are challenging children creating, in turn, a challenging area for new interventions and for the continued and conjoint study of both individual development and contextual influences. Because of the potential and the challenge, this area seems an excellent one in which to invest the best of our clinical thinking as well as the necessary time, funding, and effort.

It is likely that more than one meeting will be necessary at this time to ensure that the parents fully understand the problem. Blau (1979) has suggested that providing the parents with a tape recording of the initial session is helpful because it allows the parents to review and discuss the interpretation of the child's problem. Of relevance here is Eisenberg's recommendation (1966, p. 594) that the emphasis in this initial stage should be on

> simple and clear explanations, with due stress on the limits of accuracy of predictive statements; repeated interviews to allow parents time to assimilate the implications of the diagnosis and the opportunity to give vent to their feelings; sensitivity to the almost inevitable tendency for parents to blame themselves; skill in redirecting into constructive channels the energy sapped by self-punitiveness; and knowledgeable guidance in everyday management and long-term planning.

Increasing Parental Competency

The requisite parental competencies for the effective management of the hyperactive child will evolve with the help of the pediatrician, the management plan, and experience. The major task for the parents is to pursue a socialization procedure that is consonant with the needs, problems, and abilities of their hyperactive child. Acquisition of the necessary skills could be markedly facilitated by adherence to two pieces of expert advice which we regard as the best general statements on management in the hyperactivity literature. One is the approach to socialization advocated by Stewart in *Raising a hyperactive child* (Stewart & Olds, 1973); the other is the set of guidelines for living with a hyperactive child developed by Schmitt (1977) and reproduced here in Table 10.2. For the parent interested in more advanced reading, Kilman and Rosenfeld (1980) have produced an excellent guide that emphasizes the understanding of early childhood. Of particular relevance to the socialization of the hyperactive child are their discussions of principles of preventive psychiatry and ways in which society can influence a child's psychosocial development.

Table 10.2   Ten Guidelines for Living with a Hyperactive Child

1. *Accept your child's limitations.* A parent must accept the fact that his child is intrinsically active and energetic and possibly always will be. The hyperactivity is not intentional. A parent should not expect to eliminate the hyperactivity but just to keep it under reasonable control. Any undue criticism or attempts to change the energetic child into a quiet child or "model child" will cause more harm than good. Nothing is more helpful for the hyperactive child than having a tolerant, patient, low-key parent.

2. *Provide outlets for the release of excess energy.* This energy can't be bottled up and stored. These children need daily outside activities such as running, sports, or long walks. A fenced yard helps. In bad weather he needs a recreational room where he can do as he pleases without criticism. If no large room is available, a garage will sometimes suffice. Although the expression of hyperactivity is allowed in these ways, it should not be needlessly encouraged. Adults should not engender roughhousing with these children. Siblings should be forbidden to say "Chase me, chase me" or to instigate other noisy play. Rewarding hyperactive behavior leads to its becoming his main style of interacting with people.

3. *Keep the home existence organized.* Household routines help the hyperactive child accept order. Mealtimes, chores, and bedtime should be kept as consistent as possible. Predictable responses by the parents to daily events help the child become more predictable.

4. *Avoid fatigue in these children.* When they are exhausted, their self-control often breaks down and their hyperactivity becomes worse.

5. *Avoid formal gatherings.* Settings where hyperactivity would be extremely inappropriate and embarrassing should be completely avoided. Examples of this would be church, restaurants, etc. Of lesser importance, the child can forgo some trips to stores and supermarkets to reduce unnecessary friction between the child and parent. After the child develops adequate self-control at home, these situations can gradually be introduced.

6. *Maintain firm discipline.* These children are unquestionably difficult to manage. They need more careful, planned discipline than the average child. Rules should be formulated mainly to prevent harm to himself or others. Aggressive behavior and attention-getting behavior should be not more accepted in the hyperactive child than in the normal child. Unlike the expression of hyperactivity, aggressive behavior should be eliminated. Unnecessary rules should be avoided. These children tolerate fewer rules than the normal child. The family needs a few clear, consistent, important rules, with other rules added at the child's own pace. Parents must avoid being after the child all the time with negative comments like "Don't do this" and "Stop that."

7. *Enforce discipline with nonphysical punishment.* The family must have an "isolation room" or "time-out place" to back up their attempts to enforce rules, if a show of disapproval doesn't work. This room can be the child's bedroom. The child should be sent there to "shape up" and allowed out as soon as he has changed his behavior. Without an isolation room, overall success is unlikely. Physical punishment should be avoided in these children since we want to teach them to be less aggressive, rather than make aggression acceptable. These children need adult models of control and calmness.

8. *Stretch his attention span.* Rewarding nonhyperactive behavior is the key to preparing these children for school. Increased attention span and persistence with tasks can be taught to these children at home. The child can be shown pictures in a book; and, if he is attentive, he can be rewarded with praise and a hug. Next the parent can read stories to him. Coloring of pictures can be encouraged and rewarded. Games of increasing difficulty can gradually be taught to the child, starting with building blocks and progressing eventually to dominoes, card games, and dice games. Matching pictures is an excellent way to build a child's memory and concentration span. The child's toys should not be excessive in number, for this can accentuate his distractibility. They should also be ones that are safe and relatively unbreakable.

9. *Buffer the child against any over-reaction by neighbors.* If he receives a reputation for being a "bad kid," it is important that this doesn't carry over into his home life. At home the attitude that must prevail is that he is a "good child with excess energy." It is extremely impor-

Table 10.2—Continued

tant that his parents don't give up on him. He must always feel accepted by his family. As long as he has this, his self-esteem and self-confidence will survive.

10.   *Periodically get away from it all.* Parents must get away from the hyperactive child often enough to be able to tolerate him. Exposure to some of these children for 24 hours a day would make anyone a wreck. When the father comes home, he should try to look after the child and give his wife a deserved break. A babysitter two afternoons a week and an occasional evening out with her husband can salvage an exhausted mother. A preschool nursery or Head Start class is another option. Parents need a chance to rejuvenate themselves.

Reprinted, by permission, from Schmitt, B. D. (Letter to the Editor) *Pediatrics,* 1977, *60* (3), 387. Copyright, American Academy of Pediatrics 1977.

Psychotherapy for the Family

Parents are often reluctant to enter psychotherapy, although they readily accept that this form of intervention will benefit their hyperactive child. It is essential that they understand and accept that therapeutic intervention with the family is important, for the child as well as for family harmony (Allmond, Buckmann & Gofman, 1979). Familial factors in almost all cases contribute to the hyperactive child's difficulties and exacerbate them. In turn, the presence of a hyperactive child can seriously disrupt the entire family system by provoking marital discord (Barkley, 1978) and causing problems for siblings (Cantwell, 1979). From a practical viewpoint the members of the household need skilled advice on how to cope with the cluster of hyperactive behaviors that has caused them to seek expert help. Although there are a number of books available for managing children's behavior (Gordon, 1972; Patterson, 1971), they are not tailored to the problems of hyperactivity. Without professional help it is exceedingly difficult for untrained persons to look objectively at the family situation, pinpoint the difficulties, and decide on strategies for change that may involve all members of the family. If family disharmony is to be reduced it is likely that changes must be made in the whole system (Allmond et al., 1979; Weakland et al., 1974).

Group therapy and parent discussion groups with a skilled leader have also proven to be effective (Duehn & Mayadas, 1976; Feighner & Feighner, 1974; Mash & Dalby, 1979). The mode of therapy will depend on the parents' needs. What is important is that some kind of skilled therapeutic intervention be provided for the parents for as long as is necessary.

What the Pediatrician Tells the Child

The pediatrician should discuss the child's problems without ever using the terms *brain damage, minimal brain dysfunction,* or other equivalents. The referral symptoms should be presented as temperamental or individual differences, and in concrete terms that young children will readily understand (e.g., comparisons such as race horses vs. farm horses, express trains vs. freight trains, and teachers who are quick-tempered and excitable vs. those who are slow to arouse and generally placid). Next, the pediatrician should show clearly that he is aware of what a problem the child has, and give reassurance that the situation can be improved with everyone working together. If the child is clearly distressed about his difficulties but unable to discuss his anxiety, the pediatrician could use the *third-person technique* of Rothenberg (1972) which often serves as an effective releaser. In this procedure the adult talks about a hypothetical child of the same age and sex as the patient, who experienced anxiety, dismay, despair, and other similar reactions to his school problems, and then asks the patient if he ever felt that way. The pediatrician should then specify the changes that the team is recommending and the role that the child will play in effecting those changes. He must emphasize that he will meet regularly with the child and his parents to discuss progress and problems, and will keep in touch with his teacher.

Psychotherapy for the Child

Individual and group therapy can provide important benefits for the hyperactive child. Many hyperactive children view these therapeutic experiences as havens from the extensive difficulties of their home and school environments. Often it is the first time that the child has had a sympathetic, but objective and skilled, person to talk to who is removed from the major arenas of discord. Regular individual contact with a child psychiatrist or therapist can be of great value for both the emotional support and the perspective that the child gains of his problems. Cornwall and Freeman (1980) have described a case of an 8-year-old boy who responded well to long-term, insight-oriented psychotherapy, and Fowler (Freeman & Cornwall, 1980) has reported the successful analysis of the neurotic factors in a 12-year-old hyperactive boy. In a major prospective study of hyperactive boys ($n = 84$) Satterfield, Cantwell, and Satterfield (1979) used individual and group therapy with notable improvements in the psychosocial adjustment and psychiatric status of the boys.

Group discussions, monitored by a skilled therapist and with same-age hyperactive participants, are also valuable: they reduce the feeling of aloneness, allow the child to see how others cope with problems that invariably arise in the home and school setting, provide a source of acceptance from a same-age peer group, and offer opportunities for activities such as role play, psychodrama, and videotape that allow the child to be assessed and constructively criticized by his peers without him feeling that he is being attacked (Meissner & Nicholi, 1978). Contingency management procedures may also be included in the management strategy, ideally in combination with self-instructional procedures (Meichenbaum, 1977, 1978), and providing that the use of self-instruction is appropriate in the light of such factors as the child's personality attributes and speech competencies. For the parent who is interested in starting with contingency management procedures, Murray (1980) has outlined comprehensive plans for the use of behavioral procedures in the management of older (8 to 13 years) and younger (3 to 7 years) hyperactive children. Beginning with a brief discussion of the use of stimulant medication and the most desirable classroom arrangements, he then offers practical and specific suggestions for initial parent counseling, family assessment, and the analysis of specific behavior problems. Included in the management techniques recommended are positive reinforcement with an emphasis on token economy procedures, extinction procedures, and punishment through isolation. The problems and pitfalls of corporal punishment are delineated as are guidelines to enhance the efficacy of corporal punishment should it be needed.

School Program Modifications

If the array of intervention strategies that is being initiated constitutes the first systematic help that the child has received for his hyperactivity problems, it would be wise to postpone special help in the school setting for several weeks in order to determine if the expected improvement in behavior eliminates the need for school help. For some hyperactive children special help in the school setting will not be needed if the school will show some tolerance and modify some of the regular class demands (and if included in the outside help that the child is receiving is training in coping with the demands of the regular class environment). For others, long-term special help ranging from special tutoring within the class setting to private tutoring in addition to regular school work, moving to a new class, or private school placement, is critically needed. It should be recognized that making any major change in schooling is a serious decision that may result in a whole new set of stresses that could impose limitations on the child's intellectual and social development. Particular thought should be given to intervention that reduces the demands on the child or sets him apart from his peers. As Chess (1972 , pp. 34–35) states:

> As far as possible one would wish to avoid undue reduction of environmental expectations, particularly if the social and educational situation is in fact not a deviant one. Reduction of expectations may actually be limiting a child's opportunities for full choice of social and economic activity in adult life. Of course, if his capacities are genuinely limited then nothing is to be gained by making him face repeated failure and a sense of unworthiness. But if his capacities are adequate, and only his prior experience and training inadequate, then intervention should be designed to remediate the experiential deficit at a pace and in a manner optimum for the child.

An important supplement to most school programs would be extracurricular activities that provide the child with opportunities to capitalize on his assets. Such activities might consist of special coaching in some athletic activity, increased responsibilities at home, or hobbies.

Medication—What to Tell the Parents

If medication is to be part of the management strategy the parents must understand that it is synergistic to the other intervention procedures rather than a substitute for them (Werry, 1977) and that medication alone will not alter long-term prognosis (Satterfield, Cantwell, & Satterfield, 1979). It is particularly important that the pediatrician explain that drug intervention will not make the child more intelligent; if he does better at school it will probably be because he is better able to attend and the teacher feels more positively toward him (unfortunately often a factor in the child's grades regardless of his actual performance). The parents must be reassured that a positive response to drug treatment is not an indication of physiological defect. Recent research (Rapoport, Buchsbaum, Zahn, Weingartner, Ludlow, & Mikkelsen, 1978) suggests that any child is likely to be more attentive and less restless on stimulants. In addition, the pediatrician should make sure that the parents understand why medication is needed, the rationale for medication trials, importance of follow-up checks, use of placebo, necessity of immediately reporting side effects, and importance of not changing dosage without consulting the pediatrician first (Solomons, 1973). Interview protocols from the Robin and Bosco study (1981, p. 89a) indicate that on occasion parents as well as hyperactive children deliberately disregard the prescribed stimulant drug regimen:

> Well, if I'm acting good, she [his mother] doesn't give me as much or doesn't even give it to me.

> Sometime, when I didn't want to take them, like at school, I'd throw them away and not let my mom know about it.

Many parents experience groundless anxiety about the effects of stimulant medication on the hyperactive child. Reports in the media, particularly those since the Omaha incident, appear to have conveyed the impression that stimulant medication is a form of mind control that turns children into zombies. Some of the parents' anxiety can be allayed by specifying the known side effects of medication and also discussing the possibility of iatrogenic drug use. Although there is no conclusive body of evidence for or against the possibility of increased risk of drug abuse or dependence in children treated with stimulant medication, the best evidence available (Henker, Whalen, Bugental, & Barker, 1981; Kramer & Loney, 1980) suggests that there is little cause for concern. On this point the pediatrician should be neither overly reassuring nor alarmist. Instead, he should discuss the precautions that any parent should take to prevent nonmedical use of drugs in older grade school children and young adolescents. He should also emphasize the hyperactive child's need for prosocial satisfaction and the importance of the parents' role in not modeling drug usage for nonmedical purposes (Gorsuch & Butler, 1976).

The Issue of Whether to Tell the Child That He Is on Medication

Most clinicians (e.g, Gardner, 1973; Rapoport, 1980; Stewart & Olds, 1973; Wender, 1971; Werry, 1977) believe that a frank discussion about the child's condition and the purpose of medication is psychologically beneficial. Gardner (1973) has written a book for children with minimal brain dysfunction in which he discusses the medication aspect of treatment. Rapoport (1980, p. 251), who believes that the child should be told that he is on stimulant medication, has criticized Gardner's explanation on the grounds that

> these formulations are premature . . . they fail to allow for the flexibility of explanation that often is appropriate; moreover, such explanations solidify the concept of organic deficit beyond the present stage of scientific agreement.

We strongly disagree with the view that the child should be told that he is being given drugs to control his behavioral problem. It is our opinion that while a small number of children benefit from such candor, the large majority do not, and to accurately predict this outcome is nearly impossible for the pediatrician. In the former group are children who already have had considerable vicarious experience with stimulant medication, expect to be put on stimulants as a result of explicit and implicit information from their family, teachers, and peers, and as a result have a number of misconceptions that can be cleared up only if the child is told that he is to be on medication.

The arguments for telling the child are these: he will feel more secure if he knows exactly where he stands; he can participate effectively in decisions about adjustment of dosage; the knowledge that he is on medication will make him feel more confident with a consequent improvement in performance; the pediatrician can make maximum use of the placebo effect that contributes to drug efficacy (Werry, 1977); the child should always be told the whole truth; and there will be an erosion of his trust in his parents and pediatrician if he is not told and subsequently finds out from other sources. The chances of erosion of trust occurring can be sharply reduced if the parents simply do not tell *anyone* that the child is on medication. This includes siblings, grandparents, other relatives, friends, neighbors, and the child's teacher. The arguments for telling the child's teacher center upon her role as a contributor of information relevant to dosage. It is illogical that the standards for rigorous experimental methodology, which require that raters be naive as to the purpose of the ratings and to the treatment condition of those being rated, should be totally waived in the case of teacher ratings of specific children. It should be possible, for example, to have the teacher rate several children, one of whom is the hyperactive child. In any case all teacher ratings should be obtained without telling the teacher that the child is on stimulant medication; they will be less biased and more objective when the presence of a factor predisposing the child to better behavior is unknown to the teacher. Often the teacher's desire for additional, and in our view, unnecessary information is more related to her psychological needs than to a genuine concern for the child's welfare. Consider the following quote from a teacher interviewed by Robin and Bosco (1980, pp. 3–4):

> This is the first time that I've had a child on Ritalin, and I've had many kids that I guess people would say are hyperactive, like–, and, as I say, maybe the medication has him calmed. To me, he has more of a learning disability. But the thing is, I would like to hear from someone other than his mother that the child is on medication, especially when you receive a child that's on medication when you receive him. I received this child. No one said anything to me about it. The mother told me about the medication. She sees that he has it every school day, but I think the doctor should tell me, or at least get in touch with the nurse and have her pass it on to me, because, like I say, I don't know if it's helping him or what.*

It should be noted that our interpretation of this quotation, as an injury-to-ego statement, is not that of Robin and Bosco (1980, p. 3), who view it as indicating that teachers "feel the deepest personal sense of frustration, even anger, at the inability to work things out," and favor providing the teacher with complete information concerning the child's treatment regimen.

By not telling the teacher, the possibility is eliminated that she will make remarks about his pills, with the result that his peers find out and tease and derogate him. The painful aspects of peer and sibling awareness are apparent in this quote from the Robin and Bosco (1980, pp. 4–5) interview study:

Q: Did you ever talk to your teacher, or parent or doctor about changing anything about your medicine or pills?

A: No. I have no control over it.

Q: Did you ever talk to your parents, or teacher or doctor about stopping the medication or pills?

A: No. If I said that I don't know what they'd say.

Q: Do other children ever say anything to you about the medicine you take?

A: Yes.

---

*This and the following excerpt are reprinted by permission from Robin, S. S., & Bosco, J. J. Creating an Approach for Understanding the Diagnosis and Treatment of Hyperkinetic Children. Paper presented at the Annual Meeting of the American Educational Research Association, Boston, 1980.

Q: What do they say?

A: I don't want to say it.

Q: Do other children treat you unfairly because you take the medication?

A: Yes, some.

Q: What?

A: I don't want to say it. Does this go to my mom or dad?

Q: No.

A: Where does it go to?

Q: Western Michigan University. We've talked to a lot of other boys, and girls too, and this is the way we can learn a lot of things about how you feel about taking the medicine.

A: I feel terrible.

Q: Do other children ever tease you about taking the medicine?

A: Uh-huh.

Q: What do they say or do?

A: They just say mean things. I don't want to say them.

Q: Do your brothers or sisters or parents ever say anything?

A: Not usually.

Q: Do your brothers ever treat you unfairly.?

A: Oh, yes. And they also get beat up.

Q: What do they do?

A: Sometimes, they say "pill freak" and they don't live very long.

Relatively little empirical attention has been given to determining the child's viewpoint about being hyperactive, and only one study (Baxley, Turner, and Greenwold 1978) has attempted to assess the child's opinions concerning his medication regimen. In this study, 26 boys ranging in age from 6 to 16 were interviewed about their knowledge of drug treatment and attitudes toward it. All of the boys were currently on stimulant medication and had been on this regimen for from 6 to 85 months. As a first entry into the arena of viewing the child's opinions as important it is unfortunate that this study is characterized by serious methodological weaknesses. The questionnaire is badly constructed. Consider, for example, the ambiguity in the question "Do you want other people [*other people* are defined in the preceding question as teachers, principal, school nurse, friends] to know that you take medicine?" This wording ignores the possibility that a hyperactive child might not mind the school nurse knowing, but might feel strongly opposed to his friends knowing. The group is too heterogeneous on the important variables of age and length of time on medication to support as small a sample as 26 subjects. For this size sample, reporting percentages, while arithmetically acceptable, is statistically questionable.

The parents should be coached to handle tactless comments from others on the child's appearance, should he have the "amphetamine look," by stating firmly that he has been to the doctor and is fine. However, should the child find out, or at any point ask if the pills he is taking are stimulants, we strongly advocate an immediate and unequivocal affirmative response backed up by a discussion of the function of the pills. There is no reason for an erosion of trust if the parents have in the past shown clearly by their behavior that they act in the child's best interests, and if they answer him truthfully on this question. *We are not advocating lying to the child at any time in this management program.* The pediatrician should discuss with both parents the possibility that the child may raise this question, outline the principles that they should adhere to in their discussion with the child (avoiding, for example, the use of such terms as *brain damage*), and have them rehearse answers with the pediatrician. In view of the pseudo-sophistication of the present elementary school group about such matters, it is essential that both parents have an answer ready so that if they are confronted with the question they can respond truthfully, calmly, and objectively, making no excuses for the fact that the child was not previously informed about the stimulant medication but instead referring to it as "just one part of the whole treatment plan."

In not telling the child that he is on medication (unless he asks), what we are advocating is the withholding of information that may have an immediate and long-term negative effect on the child. We have seen children who have been psychologically devastated by hearing the "whole truth," and adults who were diagnosed as having minimal brain dysfunction as children have told us that it was a long time before they were able to think of themselves as "normal." In two cases adults who were apparently well adjusted in other respects reported that they never were able to forget that they had some brain damage or dysfunction.

The arguments against telling the child are as follows. If the child is told that he is on medication he must be given some explanation, and many children are distressed rather than relieved by the explanations provided. It is difficult to explain to a child that there may be some problem in his central nervous system without having him think that he is defective. Although the child may *say* that he understands, this assurance is frequently unreliable. The child may be in the habit of telling authority figures he understands, particularly when any sort of problem is involved; he has often been rewarded in the past for stating with assurance that he understands something when he does not, and he has learned that the subject will likely be dropped and he will be left in peace as soon as he says he understands. The following excerpt is from a taped interview with a 10-year-old boy who was worried and confused about the explanation that had been given (and who had already bought some "growth beans" from a gimmick health food store):

> My doctor said it was like train switch mistakes in my brain and it would always be like that, like bad connections only with this new medicine it would be O.K. But the medicine might stop me growing so I have to stop it on weekends and in

the vacation so I guess I'll have like a relapse then—that'll be terrible, what will my friends think? I don't know how I can explain all this to people and I specially would like to know like how will I be when I grow up. If I don't get this medicine on weekends what will I be like when I date girls and if I have all these bad connections what will I be good at working at? And if I only grow on weekends I wonder if I'll be real short when I grow up because I really like basketball.

It is particularly important that a diagnosis of hyperactivity not be presented as an illness. Note the anxiety in the following statement (Robin & Bosco, 1981, p. 88):

> I asked the doctor why I was on it (Ritalin), and he goes, "Because you have a disease." And I thought, you know, the flu or some bugs inside of me. That's what I got. And I got scared and everything else.

No matter how carefully the child is told about the possible physiological reasons for his behavior difficulties, it usually is impossible for the parents and pediatrician to counteract other information from sources such as television; when this other input is fear arousing, the child may be uneasy, alarmed, or terrified. Consider the following statement from a 9-year-old boy:

> These pills won't make me be *too* different, will they? See, Dr. Norris says now I'll be the way I want to be—like good in school and not crying in baseball and everything. He says I might even feel different in 30 or 40 minutes. Only I'm a bit scared about this because on TV there was this skittsy (schizophrenic) scientist with supercaps and when you took one you changed to how you wished you were in 30 seconds. And this boy, Richie, who was nine just like me he took one and after a bit he started looking funny, like strange, and he said to his friends, "I don't feel like I'm Richie anymore," and his friends all looked like *What's he talking about?* and then one of them said, "Who's *Richie?* There's no Richie here." And I just wondered if maybe I should start slow like with half a pill. It was real scary that his friends didn't even remember him.

The child may become psychologically dependent on his pills, that is, he may view them as the real controllers of his behavior because he experiences success and reward when he takes them (Whalen & Henker, 1976). Psychological dependence is dangerous because it robs the child of feelings of self-confidence and mastery of his already limited sphere of influence. It can be disastrous for him on occasions when he forgets to take his medication. If the child believes that pills can solve all his problems, parents may have some grounds for their fears about addiction because the child's belief could contribute to the establishment of a predisposition for drug solutions. The following statement was made by an 8-year-old boy who clearly felt that all his school problems would be solved with medication:

> Well see these pills? I just take one and look out—Presto—no more Willie the Big Problem Child now it's gonna be Willie Straight A, Willie the Best Batter. My

mom can hardly believe it but that's what happened when Bobby got on pills only he calls it medication. And now at last I'll show Karen who's the smartest kid in Grade Four. She always gives me those nasty little looks like she says, "*You* should be with the *little* ones." ... We call her Lake Superior because she's always doing the right thing. Well I have these pills and she hasn't so look out, Karen. I'm going to be best at everything and I don't even have to try so now I can watch lots more TV.

The belief that drugs are a complete and infallible solution is not uncommon, especially among younger children. Wender (1971, p. 91) reports one bright 8-year-old boy who referred to his dextroamphetamine as his "magic pills which make me into a good boy and makes everybody like me." His teacher confirmed that the boy felt that he could do no wrong when he was taking his pills. However, Kehne (1974) has suggested that a child's reaction to the drugs making him into a good boy might be one of guilt at a conscious level, that is, "if this drug makes me so *good*, I must otherwise be so *bad*."

Summary of Pediatrician's Discussion with the Child

1.   Discuss the actual problems the child is having.
2.   Describe the problems in terms of individual differences.
3.   Do not use terms such as *brain damage*; do not describe the problem as something wrong with the child's brain; make *no* attempt to give a factual account of hyperactivity.
4.   Convey your understanding that it is a real problem to the child *now*.
5.   Describe the changes in school and home that you are recommending.
6.   Emphasize that you will meet regularly with the child (and his parents) to discuss his progress and problems.
7.   If a prescription for medication has been given to the mother say something like, "I'd like you to take some pills, I've talked to your mother and she knows when to give them to you," and do not discuss the reasons.
8.   If the child asks point blank if he is now on stimulants say "yes" and discuss the reason for them, but make sure the discussion conforms to the points listed in #3.

Monitoring the Management Program

Hyperactivity is a chronic rather than an acute condition and should be treated with the same care as any other chronic pediatric problem. This means that the efficacy of all aspects of treatment must be assessed at regular intervals over the long term to meet the changing needs of the developing child. At the same time, a check should be made that all persons involved are fulfilling their commitments to the treatment program and that the participants have regular opportunities and are encouraged to question, criticize, and suggest modifications of the procedures being used. The child's classroom and social behavior, for example, should be assessed regularly and the teacher's reactions obtained; if stimulant medication has been prescribed and is proving effective, periodic decisions will be required on dosage, scheduling of drug-free trials, and termination of medication; if the child is not responding to stimulant medication the possibility of misdiagnosis must be considered. To ensure that all such evaluations occur at appropriate and regular intervals, a timetable specifying the dates of follow-up should be an integral part of the basic management strategy.

Contrary to what one might expect, a positive and definite improvement in the hyperactivity problem sometimes results in increased family *disharmony*. Consequently, it is essential that a psychiatrist or other qualified professional assess the effect of the child's improvement on the family and work with them on problems that previously had been obscured by the enormity of the hyperactivity problem. Consider the underlying meanings of the following report of a mother of a vastly improved 9-year-old boy:

> You'll never believe this but I kind of miss the *old* Stevie. It was somehow easier or simpler or something when Stevie was the great big problem. I thought—I think we all thought—that Stevie was the *only* problem we had as a family. . . . Well, I can tell you, since Stevie went on drugs *everything's* changed for me. At first I felt like I was in heaven. He was *so* good. But than I began to notice how much my girls bicker and how untidy they are. And lately things my husband does irritate me a lot and when I think back he's always done those things. And Stevie's gotten kind of righteous, he's not nearly as much fun as he was and he's doing so well in school now and the girls don't like it at all. Some days I think I must be going crazy but I've started to think of the time before Stevie got on drugs as the best time we ever had as a family . . .

Cantwell (1979, p. 72) sums up the essence of this problem with the following succinct statement:

> The final stage of follow-up concerns not the child but the family. It not infrequently happens that the (hyperactive) child becomes the focus for other and quite unrelated family problems, because, in effect, he carries around a sign saying "Kick me!" When the parents don't have him to kick around any more, their own negative feelings toward one another may surface directly and create problems. The same is true of siblings . . . a hyperactive brother or sister can be a trial, but may also be a protection, since he (or she) can serve as a lightning rod to draw off parental irritation and anger.

Evaluative Follow-Up

When a period of a year or two has elapsed following the end of the monitoring and treatment period, an evaluative follow-up should be conducted to answer the question, How have things worked out for the child? Having first located the former patient in his current setting and obtained his complete or restricted permission to proceed, ideally, interviews and ratings from those associated with him would be obtained. These likely would be teacher, professor, or employer, peer and parent evaluations, along with measures of the former patient's self-rating and an interview with him. If he is still in a school setting at this time, it might be possible to conduct a second follow-up four or five years after the first one. The data obtained would allow the management team to approximate a validity check on their intervention strategies and to obtain new insights concerning the formal and informal demands and stresses of possible future settings for children with whom they are currently working. The long-term follow-up is by far the best way for the practitioner to assess the efficacy of his case handling.

Although there is general agreement on the need for this type of follow-up in the behavior disorders, the difficulties, methodological problems, costs, and sheer indifference have combined to make long-term follow-ups the exception rather than the rule. In the field of hyperactivity the most notable exception is the monumental series of evaluative long-term studies by Weiss and her associates at McGill University. Although the empirical findings from the Weiss and other prospective longitudinal studies are of undeniable value in assessing outcomes of intervention, their focus has been restricted to a small group of subjects who have been intensively studied over the years in laboratory-type settings. In the absence of *any* supporting data on our part, we raise the possibility that the fact of being intensively studied, over a number of years and with all of the participants seeing themselves as having somewhat serious problems, could exert considerable influence on outcome. What direction that influence might have taken is anybody's guess, but it is likely that it did exist.

The focus of the Weiss studies is different from that being advocated here. Although both are concerned with studying the long-term effectiveness of intervention, our interest is in the thousands of other hyperactive children in more naturalistic settings who are undergoing long-term clinical treatment with varying degrees of success. Information from this vast pool of subjects rarely finds its way into the literature, and when it does it primarily describes the course of the disorder up to or just beyond the point of termination of treatment. Yet the potential is undeniably there to accumulate a data base of specific information, such as the incidence of drug abuse in the hyperactive child, as well as to identify general guidelines for designing more effective management strategies. The storage capacity and rapid retrieval offered by computer systems assures the practicality of such a data pool. An example of the data pool idea is the *case register* procedure (Beiser, 1978) for the evaluation of use of treatment services. A case register is a central file in which cumulative statistical records are maintained for all people with mental disorders in a community. These data show the extent of use of different mental health services and pinpoint overlap and gaps in services. Another such data pool, this one an *at-risk register* for newborn infants, has been proposed by Dunn (1979). Such a register would include low birth weight infants, infants who had brain hemorrhages at birth, and those whose mothers had German measles and other illnesses at critical points in the pregnancy period. With the aid of this register pediatricians would be able to detect and treat defects early in infancy and childhood, follow them intensively, and analyze the outcome. We recognize that a case register approach raises a number of ethical and legal questions concerning the confidentiality of records and the invasion of privacy, but it is our opinion that such problems are not insurmountable.

To accumulate a data base of clinical information on hyperactivity would require that the professionals involved keep adequate records of the whole sequence of diagnosis and management, and track the hyperactive child's progress with diagnostic evaluations at regular intervals throughout adolescence and into early adulthood. These clinical reports would then be evaluated, summarized for professional use, and made available as a pool of data. These data could provide a criteria base for the evaluation of ongoing management strategies in addition to information about the efficacy of multimodality treatment approaches to management. Over the long term the result of such a cooperative effort could be a gradual but steady trend towards nationwide improvement in the management of hyperactivity.

CHAPTER 11

The State of the Art

The past decade has witnessed a remarkable burgeoning of scientific interest in the study of hyperactivity, an interest reflected in the proliferation of conferences, symposia, texts, and research papers on this topic. Over a relatively short period, theoretical developments combined with an outpouring of empirical findings from a variety of experimental disciplines have changed the status of hyperactivity from that of a somewhat obscure, little known problem of middle childhood to one of the most diagnosed, discussed, and researched of the childhood behavior disorders (Douglas, 1976). Although one catalyst for this growth spurt may have been the Omaha incident, its unabated pace must be attributed to more fundamental causes, particularly the widespread concern in the pediatric domain of parents, physicians, and educators about the prevalence of the disorder; the failure of current intervention procedures to successfully modify long-term outcome; the tendency of hyperactivity and its sequelae to persist into adolescence and early adulthood; and most particularly the impressive subgroup of able investigators who have appeared on the hyperactivity research scene in the past five years. Among these are Barkley, Campbell, Cunningham, Dalby, Firestone, Gadow, Henker, Loney, Mash, Milich, Porges, Swanson, Trites, Whalen, and S. Zentall. The cumulative effect of their empirical investigations has been to provide a new perspective and considerably enhance progress in understanding hyperactivity.

In commenting on the recent sharp increase of scientific interest in hyperactivity Sprague (1979, p. 217) stated that

> There is a vast literature on hyperactivity, and it is growing at a cancerous rate.... Although one might normally expect that such a large literature would reflect a major body of empirical knowledge, this is not the case because so many of the studies are methodologically weak, unsophisticated, or blatantly biased.... Such a mass of confusing, contradictory, and misleading literature confounds ... researchers...

We concur with Sprague on all three points. The exponential increase in books, journal articles, and dissertations (see Table 11.1) should have been paralleled by an equally sharp increase in understanding of the field, but this has not been the case. The advances that have occurred in our under-

Table 11.1.   A Comparison of the Number of Articles, Books, Theses, and Chapters on Hyperactivity Published in Three Different Four-Year Periods

Publications	1957–1960	1967–1970	1977–1980
Articles	31	205	676
Books	4	18	29
Theses	3	20	47
Chapters (in general texts, not hyperactivity alone)	7	16	33

Sources: *Books in Print, Index Medicus, Psychological Abstracts, Psychopharmacology Abstracts*, and Winchell, C. A. *The hyperkinetic child* (A bibliography). Westport, CT: Greenwood Press, 1975.

standing of hyperactivity have not been proportional to the expenditure of experimenter time, effort, and money.

Close examination of almost any cluster of studies by topic supports Sprague's evaluation. For example, after Barkley's (1977a) review of 110 studies of stimulant drug research with children, Wolraich (1977) reviewed approximately the same literature but eliminated from his review all studies that did not use a placebo-control and double-blind condition. Of the remaining 62 studies, many failed to conform even to the minimum requirements for valid drug studies specified by Sprague and Werry (1971). In a later review of the effects of stimulant drugs on the specific area of academic performance (Barkley & Cunningham, 1978), of the 17 studies that used objective tests and measures of academic performance as the dependent variables, only five were judged to be well designed and controlled. Similarly, there has been a proliferation of short-term studies of intervention in which the small number of subjects, their availability, and other factors all suggest that, if they had wished to do so, the investigators could have collected data permitting the assessment of generalization of the intervention effects in natural settings or in settings closely approximating the natural environment, and in addition could have carried out long-term follow-ups. Instead, the inclination is to plunge eagerly forward to another of the same kind of study, pausing only to comment briefly on what should have been done or what would be the logical next step if firm conclusions were to be drawn, as if the act of acknowledging methodological shortcomings exonerated the investigator from responsibility for publishing ill-conceived and fragmentary work. The fact is that the value of such work from any point of view—the subjects, other researchers, or progress in the field—is near zero, and in the case of the subjects, no intervention would often have been preferable.

A further point concerning the problem of methodological deficiencies concerns those studies that are incorrectly presented as tests of the findings of other investigations or as replications of other studies. These pseudo-replications are characterized by basic procedural changes that confuse the interpretation of the results: it becomes impossible to determine if the results of the original study are then proven to be wrong by the failure to replicate findings, or if it is the procedural changes that are responsible for the conflicting results. Examples of the pseudo-replication phenomenon include several studies that discounted the report (Schnackenburg, 1975) of the efficacy of coffee with hyperactive children but failed to match either the amount or the substance used in the original study (e.g., Garfinkel, Webster, & Sloman, 1975). In such instances the failure to replicate casts an unfair light on the original study and often does little or nothing to advance knowledge in the area. Another example concerns the finding from a pilot and a main study (Cappella, Gentile, & Juliano, 1977) that hyperative children ($n=37$) of elementary school age were significantly less accurate than their nonhyperactive counterparts ($n=100$) in ability to estimate time intervals ranging from seven to 60 seconds. Differences between estimated and elapsed time increased with the length of the interval. Senior, Towne, and Huessy (1979) described as a *replication* of the Cappella et al. study, one in which six hyperactive children and 135 nonhyperactive controls were tested on ability to estimate a 30-second interval. The finding that the two groups did not differ was interpreted by these investigators as a failure to replicate.

Contributing to the general confusion in the field has been the misinterpretation or distortion, possibly due to sloppy scholarship, of others' data and conclusions. One form which this misuse takes is to interpret research on nonclinical children who have some of the characteristics of hyperactive children, as research on hyperactive children. In a study of mother–child interaction, for example, Humphries, Kinsbourne, and Swanson (1978, p. 19) stated that "Previous studies have revealed the considerable amount of control mothers attempt to exert over their hyperactive children (Bing, 1963; Bee, 1967; Campbell, 1973, 1975)." In fact the Bing study was concerned with parental intrusiveness and the development of nonverbal cognitive abilities, the Bee study was on parent-child interaction and distractibility, and neither study involved hyperactive children or mentioned hyperactivity. Only the Campbell studies were of hyperactive children.

To Sprague's negative descriptors of much of the research on hyperactivity we would add afourth one, *unproductive.* An exorbitant amount of time has been spent on unproductive areas of investigation. We would describe as unproductive continued work in any area in which one or more of the following three conditions prevail:

Substantial evidence already exists that a mode of intervention is ineffective or a line of investigation is fruitless. One example of this kind of unproductive area is the Feingold K-P diet (Feingold, 1975a). There is ample research showing that the Feingold diet does not work for the vast majority of hyperactive children, and there is reason to believe that for many of those who do appear to benefit from it, the crucial factors may be psychological rather than dietary (Conners, 1980; Whalen, 1982). Millions of dollars and uncounted work hours have been poured into what is basically a large number of variations on a single investigative theme (Stare, Whelan, & Sheridan, 1980; Taylor, 1979). The result has been a bewildering array of positive, equivocal, and negative findings that often do not relate systematically to methodological rigor (Conners, 1980). The probability is low that further investigations along the same lines will prove fruitful. Instead, what is needed is a carefully charted empirical attack on a diverse and potentially productive cluster of related research topics, for example: the possibility that preschool children may be the best responders (Harley & Matthews, 1980), the report that the basic daily consumption of additives data may be in error (Sobotka, 1976), the role of sugar consumption in behavior disorders (Prinz, Roberts, & Hantman, 1980), sequential effects of additive–nonadditive treatment conditions (Conners, Goyette, Southwick, Lees, & Andrulonis, 1976; Harley & Matthews, 1980), and factors contributing to breaking the blind (Conners, 1980; Wender, 1980). A valuable research tool for those pursuing these topics is Conners' (1980) concise and objective discussion of the state of the Feingold field.

An example of a more general type of unproductive research is the retrospective study and report. Although there *may* have been some justification for some of the early retrospective studies (e.g., Battle & Lacey, 1972; Stewart, Pitts, Craig, & Dieruf, 1966) when hyperactivity was less well understood, there is now almost no scientific basis for their continued use. Any conclusions from such studies must be so qualified by the acknowledgment of inherent methodological deficiencies, particularly the assumptions underlying the retrospective diagnosis of hyperactivity, as to render the data almost totally useless. The irreversible shortcomings of retrospective data were underscored in a recent critical review of hyperactivity and substance abuse (Kramer & Loney, 1981). Despite additional statistical analyses of the data in the studies reviewed, Kramer and Loney's conclusions were limited (by virtue of the restrictions imposed by retrospective data) to a "suggested" relationship between hyperactivity and substance use that was further qualified by an emphatic statement on the need for verification with follow-up studies. We urge a complete moratorium on the retrospective study of hyperactivity.

The research to a specific point on a topic is so well documented that continued effort that is basically replicative is unproductive. Far too much time has been spent on short-term contingency reinforcement experiments and demonstrations of classroom and home usage. It is abundantly clear that for many hyperactive children (1) contingency reinforcement works on the short-term, (2) its effect diminishes when reinforcement is withdrawn, (3) there is little evidence of generalization, and (4) the benefits gradually disappear (Mash & Dalby, 1979; Mash, Handy, & Hamerlynck, 1976). Yet the field continues to be beset by replications with hair-splitting variations, many of which add insult to injury by substituting public acknowledgment of the inadequacies of their studies ("what should have been done," "our findings are limited because," and "in another study we will") for *prepublication* effort directed towards eliminating known inadequacies. To develop contingency reinforcement further, effort should be directed to the problems of how to handle withdrawal of reinforcement and effect long-term retention and transfer.

The topic is worthwhile but the basic assumptions underlying it are inaccurate or unjustified. An example of *inaccurate* assumptions is the cluster of modeling studies (e.g., Copeland & Weissbrod, 1980) in which the object has been to demonstrate that a child who observes a high-active model will become high-active himself, the idea being that hyperactivity may be a function of observational learning. The faulty assumption in these studies is that excessive activity is an indication of hyperactivity when, in fact, it is inappropriate activity that is one of the indicators of this problem. It is quite reasonable that a high-active model will have a disinhibitory effect on an observer (Bandura, 1969) (or, if the situation is a novel one, that the observer will think that that is how one should behave in it) leading to high activity on the observer's part. But what is needed in these experiments is to begin again, to reformulate the assumptions making sure that they are accurate. An example of *unjustified* assumptions is contained in the rapidly growing body of research on biofeedback. Although experienced clinicians and investigators (Astor, 1977; Blanchard & Young, 1974; Miller, 1978b) are focusing on such problems as what accounts for positive biofeedback effects, and comparisons of the therapeutic value of biofeedback with other currently available forms of intervention, an increasing number of doctoral candidates appears to have seized on biofeedback or relaxation training as the all-purpose intervention strategies. In this latter group of studies the usual format is pretest followed by a short period of biofeedback or relaxation training and then posttest. The dependent variables are hyperactivity or scores on one or more of a bewildering array of standardized tests such as the Wechsler Intelligence Scale for Children—Revised and the Illinois Test of Psycholinguistic Abilities, and other less well-developed measures such as the Observed Behavior Checklist or the Quick Neurological Screening Test. The rationale for the assumptions concerning the effect of biofeedback on the dependent variables in these theses usually ranges from weak to nonexistent, making it difficult to see much justification for conducting the research in the first place. (References for this body of work have been purposely omitted here because it is the thesis chairmen rather than the doctoral candidates who are at fault in this situation.) A perusal of this literature brings to mind Gordon's First Law of Research (Bloch, 1977): "If research is not worth doing at all, it is not worth doing well."

One fact to keep in mind in any discussion of the failure of many studies in the literature to meet an acceptable standard is that *all* of the studies were accepted usually after multiple reader review and subsequent editor approval. Clearly the caliber of such screening is inadequate in many of the established journals in the field. One positive line of action would be to start a new journal, *Hyperactivity*, with an editor who has demonstrated consistently high methodological standards for worthwhile research and is as well a recognized expert on hyperactivity (Robert Sprague immediately comes to mind for this post). Readers having the same propensities would be chosen, and a reader fee levied to discourage the submission of inferior efforts. Such a journal could have a catalytic modeling effect on the field.

METHODOLOGICAL ADVANCES

The foregoing shortcomings in methodology are counteracted to some extent by a scattering of significant methodological advances. Consider, for example, the following areas in which marked progress has been made.

Prevalence

Prior to 1975 accurate prevalence data on hyperactivity were totally lacking, a serious gap in view of the important role of such data in the preventive intervention and management of hyperactivity or, indeed, any behavioral or medical problem. The literature abounded with a range of prevalence estimates that varied with the degree of methodological rigor, diagnostic criteria used, if any, and inclinations of the personnel responsible for providing the data (e.g., Cantwell, 1975a; Feingold, 1975a; Huessy, 1967; Miller, Palkes, & Stewart, 1973; Office of Child Development, 1971). The period since 1975, however, has produced a series of methodologically sophisticated prevalence studies that constitute one of the most impressive advances in the field (Bosco & Robin, 1980; Lambert, Sandoval, & Sassone, 1978; Sprague, Cohen, & Eichlseder, 1977; Trites, 1979a). Two refinements of previous prevalence methodology should be noted. In the study by Lambert et al. (1978) the situational specificity of hyperactivity was acknowledged by the inclusion of relatively independent information from three different agents of identification: parents, teachers, and physicians. The use of different social defining systems thus allowed Lambert et al. to categorize children into groups and to compute prevalence rates on the basis of the social systems data. The Trites (1979a) study contributed an interesting and potentially valuable extension of prevalence methodology by using the SYMAP computer program to analyze the prevalence data. This computer program, which was developed by Sheppard (1973), can be used to produce both a contour map (see Figure 11.1) as well as a two-dimensional map of prevalence. SYMAPS can rapidly specify prevalence in different parts of a city, sex and age differences, and other variables, independent of population density. The existence of definite peaks and valleys makes it a particularly useful tool for demonstrating prevalence to interested adults who lack experience in interpreting frequency data quickly. It would also have great value for epidemiologists, the medical profession, and educators.

Risk Routes

A more recent methodological development with considerable promise, the risk route model, concerns prediction. From the point of view of preventive

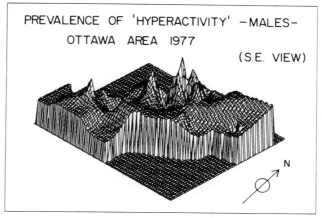

PREVALENCE OF 'HYPERACTIVITY' —MALES—
OTTAWA AREA 1977

(S.E. VIEW)

N

Figure 11.1   Prevalence of "Hyperactivity" in boys in Ottawa area, 1977 (SE view). Reprinted, by permission, from Trites, R. L. Prevalence of hyperactivity in Ottawa, Canada. In R. L. Trites (Ed.), *Hyperactivity in children*. Copyright 1979, University Park Press, Baltimore.

intervention and management it would be a tremendous advantage to be able to predict outcome for infants categorized as difficult (Thomas & Chess, 1977). With existing assessment procedures, however, accurate predication in infancy is virtually impossible, except for the infant with significant damage; when prediction is possible, it usually relates to the group rather than the individual. What is urgently needed is to derive developmental follow-up data that will provide a basis for the prediction of outcome in individual infants who have relatively subtle disorders and deviations. A step towards this goal is the *risk route*, a holistic conceptual model proposed by Aylward and Kenny (1979) that assumes, as does the transactional model of Sameroff (1975), a degree of plasticity inherent in both the child and the environment. A basic premise of this interactional model is that the infant's overall development is the product of three interrelated spheres of influence: medical–biologic, environmental–psychosocial, and behavioral–developmental. The child's course over time can be simultaneously evaluated for each of these spheres. At each evaluation point the spheres of risk are considered to be additive, the rationale for this assumption being that because they are interdependent, they can function in combination to exacerbate risk or foster recovery. As can been seen in Figure 11.2, the risk route for a specific child follows a downward vertical and horizontal progression. At any specific point in time, the risk rating is a function of the interaction between previous effects and current risk indices, that is, the previous overall risk ratings would interact with all three major spheres, and the cumulative effect would then place the infant at a point on the overall continuum that would become the source for the branching of the route at the next evaluation point.

The value of the risk route approach is that patterns or sequences of the three major spheres of influence on good or poor outcome could be identified

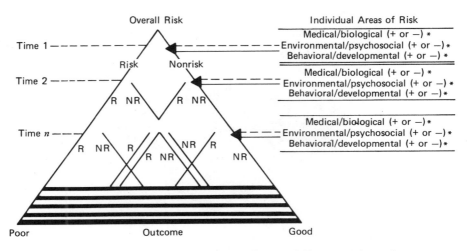

$$\text{overall risk at time 1 (OR-}t_1) = \text{cumulative effect (med/bio}_{t_1} + \text{envir/psychosoc}_{t_1}$$
$$+ \text{ beh/develop}_{t_1})$$
$$\text{overall risk at time 2 (OR-}t_2) = \text{cumulative effect (OR}-_{t_1} \times \text{med/bio}_{t_2} + \text{envir/psychosoc}_{t_2}$$
$$+ \text{ beh/develop}_{t_2})$$
$$\text{overall risk at time n (OR-}t_n) = \text{cumulative effect (OR}-t_1 \times \text{OR}-t_2 \ldots \times \text{OR}-t_{n-1}$$
$$\times \text{ med/bio}_{t_n} + \text{envir/psychosoc}_{t_n} + \text{beh/develop}_{t_n})$$

Figure 11.2   The Concept of Risk Routes.
Reprinted, by permission, from Aylward, G. P., & Kenny, T. J. Developmental follow-up: Inherent problems and a conceptual model. *Journal of Pediatric Psychology*, 1979, *4*(4), 331–343. Plenum Publishing Corporation. Copyright 1979.

and the factors that appear to be influential in development at each evaluation point could be specified. Consider the following example (Aylward & Kenny, 1979, p. 339):

> . . . assume that an infant was initially at biologic risk but was not simultaneously classified as such in the interrelated environmental or behavioral spheres. Further, assume that subsequent evaluations $(t_1 \text{-} t_n)$ in all three spheres also were of a nonrisk nature. If outcome were poor in this infant and in others having the same risk profile, the assumption could be made that this medical/biologic factor is quite influential in development. Reciprocally, if the outcome was good the routes of each sphere subsequent to the initial classification could be evaluated to discriminate which factors may have negated the effects of biologic risk.

The risk route approach provides a relatively simple procedure for the delineation of interaction profiles relevant to outcome that could serve as a model for intervention in subsequent infants with similar profiles. Although, as Aylward and Kenny (1979) acknowledge, the predictive validity of the risk route model must still be dealt with, this graphic approach to outcome appears to have considerable potential both for the monitoring of the individual infant's progress and for research purposes.

Other Methodological Advances

A diverse cluster of techniques has appeared and statements made whose cumulative effect on progress in the field is certain to be influential. Some of these techniques have already been described: one is the response-class matrix of Mash, Terdal, and Anderson (1973), which is an antecedent-consequent system for coding dyadic interactions. Another is the height and weight procedures developed by the Sprague team (e.g., McNutt, Boileau, & Cohen, 1977). Others include work in the field of data analysis: Ross and Klein (1979) have described the O technique, a method for detecting differences in response patterns to drug and placebo. With this method the pre- by posttreatment data matrix is partitioned into drug- and placebo-typical regions as compared to the analysis of covariance procedure of positing a linear relationship between pre- and posttreatment scores and then testing for between-slope or between adjusted posttreatment means differences. In a test (Ross & Klein, 1979) of the O technique and analysis of covariance with ratings of hyperactive children ($n = 155$), the O technique proved to have superior power. In another area Thompson, Kidd, and Weissman (1980) have developed a procedure for the efficient collection and processing of pedigree data that would facilitate family-genetic studies of hyperactivity and other behavior disorders. With their Family Data Form pedigree data are elicited in a way that guarantees that the data will be complete and unambiguous, and they are recorded in a format that allows direct transfer to a computer file. Sprague (1979) and Loney (1981) have contributed excellent papers on methodological considerations in the evaluation of treatments for hyperactivity, and in an editorial comment Cohen (1975) has offered a brief statement on the reference standard for growth studies that should be mandatory reading for researchers in this area. Steinkamp (1981) has pointed to noncompliance with experimental drug regimens as a source of inaccuracy that can be eliminated with some effort on the part of the investigator. She further specifies methods for the periodic measurement of ingestion rate as an essential feature of research methodology and urges that noncompliance rates be routinely included in research reports. Taken together, this heterogeneous group of methodological techniques and statements constitutes a substantial contribution to research on hyperactivity.

Productive Extensions of Existing Knowledge

In addition to the foregoing methodological advances there have been some productive extensions of existing knowledge and technique. We are thinking here of a varied group of topic areas in which continuing and unremitting research and clinical interest, often accompanied by considerable dissent and controversy, has led to refinements which have served both to enhance our understanding of hyperactivity and suggest new directions of investigative interest.

A Broader Definition

An offshoot of the controversy concerning the definition of hyperactivity is an increasing tendency to specify behavioral attributes in hyperactive children that are not among the primary or secondary behaviors most frequently associated with this disorder. The diversity of definitions attests to the pervasive and continuing dissatisfaction with efforts to specify adequately the distinguishing characteristics of hyperactivity. In the past five years the Hyperkinetic Reaction of Childhood (DSM II) has been replaced with the Attention Deficit Disorder With and Without Hyperkinesis (DSM III), and before the ink was dry on this controversial revision, the research of Loney and her colleagues raised the probability of a change in the status of aggression from that of a secondary to a primary component of this behavior disorder. In an excellent critical review of the definition controversy, Barkley (1981) has presented a compelling argument for the inclusion in the cluster of behaviors _rule-governed behavior_ such as the noncompliance of young hyperactive children noted earlier by Drash, Stolberg, and Bostow (1977) as a prominent characteristic.

This trend towards viewing the cluster of behaviors evidenced by hyperactive children as extremely varied, and including many problems not traditionally associated with hyperactivity, has been noted by participants in a symposium on hyperactivity (Wender, 1979), reports by experienced investigators (Huessy, Cohen, Blair, & Rood, 1979; Lambert, 1981), an excellent doctoral dissertation (Salter, 1977), and in parental reports (Gofman, 1979). The obvious dissatisfaction with current definitions and the association with hyperactivity of an increasingly broad range of behavior are indications that the widely used, limited-symptom parent and teacher rating scales for hyperactivity, such as the Conners, Werry–Weiss–Peters, and Davids scales, may be imposing a specific and restricted symptomatology on hyperactivity, with a consequent limiting of the scope of intervention. This possibility merits careful consideration by clinicians as well as researchers.

Self-Confrontation

Another example is a series of extensions of a well established body of empirical findings on modeling procedures with nonhyperactive children. Modeling procedures have been used extensively with children to transmit simple and complex response patterns, and modify a wide range of behavior deficits (Bandura, 1969, 1977). In the course of developing these procedures it was found that perceived similarity to the model (by the observer) facilitated imitative learning, and in a logical extension of this finding, self-confrontation thus becomes the ultimate form of similarity. In addition to its place in modeling theory, self-confrontation is now widely used as an effective therapeutic technique in which the individual is shown samples of his own behavior by means of procedures such as role play with others acting out his responses, or videotaped sequences of himself responding in a particular situation (Feighner & Feighner, 1974; Thelen, Fry, Fehrenback, & Frautschi, 1979). As a therapeutic tool it becomes a form of intentional training, because the individual is instructed to observe the role play or videotape, rather than a pure modeling technique. The success of this tool can be attributed primarily to the considerable attention-directing potential that self-confrontation has for people in general. This characteristic has facilitated its use in modifying a number of specific behavior problems related to hyperactivity (e.g., Bugental, Whalen, & Henker, 1977; Dowrick & Raeburn, 1977; Spiegel, 1977), but it is our opinion that self-confrontation has the potential to make a general and far more important contribution to the management of the hyperactive child. As we see it, the real value of self-confrontation lies in the simplicity and irrefutable nature of this way of conveying to the child how his behavior looks to others. The hyperactive child typically is far less able at accurately judging and reporting on his own performance than are his nonhyperactive peers. Clinicians frequently comment on his tendency to exaggerate self-reports, and teachers and parents often describe him as "untruthful," "a daydreamer," or, as one father scornfully commented, "a real Walter Mitty." A similar interpretation was made by Stewart, Mendelson, and Johnson (1973) of the inaccuracies in the adolescents' reports on acceptance by peers. In their interview study they saw these inaccuracies as evidence that the importance of peer acceptance was such that the adolescents were unable to admit their status of nonacceptance. All of these reactions to the apparent distortions of the hyperactive child are based on the belief that *the child knows the true state of affairs* but, for whatever reason, gives an untrue report. It is our opinion that the child's response is truthful in terms of his perception of the situation—it is his perception that is faulty. On the several occasions when we have used self-confrontation procedures with hyperactive children, they have been genuinely surprised, upset, and horrified at the unequivocal visual evidence of their inappropriate behavior.

The hyperactive child's problem with self-perception derives from his mediational and attentional deficits as well as from his experiential deficits. Certainly, the hyperactive child appears not to benefit from opportunities for incidental learning to the extent that his nonhyperactive peers do. This inability immediately puts him at a tremendous disadvantage in evaluating his own behavior because he lacks the concepts that are gradually built up largely through the process of incidental learning. Using self-confrontation techniques to improve self-evaluation skills would likely also increase the effectiveness of self-instructional procedures, particularly in respect to generalization to other situations. A case in point is the hyperactive child described earlier who only used self-instruction effectively *after* self-confrontation training in listening to and evaluating his own taped self-instruction.

In the absence of any supporting data, it is our opinion that one effect of self-confrontation would be to minimize the disruptive influence that the hyperactive child exerts on his social environment. As such, it justifies an intensive and systematic investigation. As one step, the most commonly occurring inappropriate or ineffective behaviors should be identified and assigned a priority influenced by the nuisance value that they have for the child. As part of the development of self-confrontation programs specific to each of these kinds of behaviors, or possibly to clusters of them, the shock value hazard to the child of self-confrontation should be clearly understood and procedural changes specified for softening the blow of seeing himself as others do. To this end, the sequence least likely to overwhelm the child should also be determined, for example, how much of the fumbling embarrassing behavior of the sort that other children tease him about should he see?

Innovative Approaches

Complementary to the productive extensions are several particularly innovative approaches to the study of hyperactivity. In the first of these, classroom research, there already exists an impressive body of empirical findings. The remaining two—an interbehavior disorder strategy and a neuropeptide treatment approach—are still at earlier levels of empirical development but have considerable potential.

Classroom Ecology Research

Until recently, classroom research in general on the hyperactive child could best be described as pedestrian and unimaginative, with investigators unconcerned with methodological rigor and either unable or disinterested in coping with the obvious difficulties of a naturalistic setting. This state of affairs changed dramatically with the entry into the classroom-research arena of Whalen and her associates with a series of studies within the framework of the small ecosystem model of interactions among behavior, medication, and context in hyperactive children (Collins, Whalen, & Henker, 1980; Henker & Whalen, 1980a; Whalen, Collins, Henker, Alkus, Adams, & Stapp, 1978; Whalen, Henker, Collins, Finck, & Dotemoto, 1979; Whalen, Henker, Dotemoto, 1980, 1981). These studies, at once bold and ambitious in scope, imaginative and innovative in procedure, methodologically sophisticated, and far more comprehensive in the broadest sense than the research of their predecessors, have resulted in new insights on the character and management of the hyperactive child. The potential significance of these insights for the field in general and classroom management of the hyperactive child in particular is profound. The research by Whalen et al. has provided the most comprehensive and best documented picture to date of the hyperactive child in classroom as well as peer interaction contexts, and in so doing has identified previously unknown areas that create a disproportionate amount of difficultly for the hyperactive child. For example, in an ingenious dyadic activity created to investigate how hyperactive children cope with the problems imposed by interdependence with another child, these children were not able to readily adapt to changes in role demands. This inflexibility is a behavior deficit almost guaranteed to cause difficulties for the child, particularly in small-group games. In addition, several well-established beliefs have been firmly refuted. The hyperactive child's difficult behavior, for example, is not continuous but rather is relatively infrequent; problems arise because the behavior, when it occurs, constitutes a highly salient event. The research has also provided unequivocal evidence of the folly and resultant inaccuracy of interpreting differences between unmedicated children and their nonclinical peers independently of classroom and other contexts.

Whalen et al. have demonstrated that the classroom ecology, and presumably that of other settings, can function either as a provocation ecology to maximize differences between unmedicated hyperactive children and their nonhyperactive peers, or as a rarefaction ecology to minimize such differences. One of the most important findings from this phase of their work was that many of the ecological-behavioral relationships were far from simple, with some behaviors showing curvilinear relationships. Disruptions and out-of-seat behavior, for example, were least likely to occur under both highly challenging *and* least challenging conditions. A second major finding here was that varying the ecological parameters of the classroom was as effective as medication for some behaviors. Varying the ecological parameters also provides a welcome alternative to the use of positive reinforcers and is likely to be a more viable procedure.

In terms of impact on the field, perhaps most important of all is the fact that the Whalen et al. studies should serve as a powerful model for other researchers studying the hyperactive child in naturalistic and quasi-naturalistic settings. Throughout this research there is an emphasis on bidirectionality of effect, a feature that is notably lacking in many efforts to study the hyperactive child in naturalistic settings; the experimental designs and statistical analyses are sophisticated and parsimonious; and the classroom observation schedules are more ambitious in scope than any we have seen, with behavior categories that distinguish between content and style and therefore require qualitative judgments which in turn require highly trained observers. Whalen et al. (1979) acknowledged the ensuing difficulties with reliability and have continued to refine their schedules. The difficulties engendered by having observers visible in the classroom have been handled skillfully, and with respect to the acknowledged problems associated with research in the classroom setting, a commendable distinction has been made between methodological rigor and rigidity. In a discussion of the ecological validity of their simulated classroom settings, Whalen et al. (1978) noted that their goal in designing these

research settings was to capture the best of two worlds, the controlled laboratory setting and the naturalistic classroom setting. They have succeeded ably
in their pursuit of this goal.

Interbehavior Disorder Strategy

The primary experimental strategy in hyperactivity research in general and
etiological studies in particular has been the intrabehavior disorder approach,
that is, the intensive study of hyperactive children. Recently, a significant and
potentially productive shift to an interbehavior disorder strategy has occurred
in which the core questions center on such intriguing possibilities as that of
deficits common to different disorders having the same etiological base, and
the identification of the person X environment interactions that result in different outcomes. Porges and his colleagues (Porges, 1980; Porges & Smith,
1980), for example, have hypothesized that there may be a common physiological substrate underlying the defective attention that is a diagnostic characteristic of several clinical pathologies such as learning disabilities,
hyperactivity, mental retardation, childhood autism, and schizophrenia.
Knowledge of this physiological substrate could increase understanding of etiology and enhance the development and efficacy of intervention procedures.
In the same vein, Gorenstein and Newman (1980) have proposed that hyperactivity and several other traditionally separate psychological categories characterized by disinhibition (hysteria, psychopathy, alcoholism) are separate
manifestations of the same genetic diasthesis modified by differential early life
experiences. These innovative etiological approaches call for an interdisciplinary coordination of efforts to identify the common substrate (Porges, 1980)
and diasthesis (Gorenstein & Newman, 1980), as well as the differential modifying of experiential factors that are functionally related to the separate
manifestations.

   These approaches suggest two interwoven lines of research: in the case of
the genetic diasthesis, one starting point should be a search for the mechanism
that mediates the hypothesized genetic vulnerability or propensity for these
disinhibitory disorders. In this search a potentially promising area of study
might be that of the neurotransmitter-related enzymes (Chiong, 1979), because variations in enzyme function, regulation, and structure are responsible
for or are related to many medical and behavior disorders in humans. It is
possible that individual differences in these enzymes could be the mechanism
that mediates genetic vulnerability to the disinhibitory disorders. The second
line of inquiry should focus on the commonalities and differences in child
rearing data across these disorders. A related research question would concern
cultures and subcultures in which hyperactivity is reported to be virtually
nonexistent. Although the possibility of basic enzymatic differences between
children in these cultures and those in which hyperactivity is prevalent seems
unlikely, there may be a proportionally higher prevalence of genetically based
disinhibitory disorders other than hyperactivity in these cultures. As a func-

tion of specific environmental influences, there may be a high prevalence of certain disorders with others being nonexistent *or* the overall prevalence of disinhibitory disorders may be lower in these cultures. It seems most likely that the genetic diasthesis is a universal phenomenon with cross-cultural variability in socialization processes determining the presence or absence of specific disinhibitory disorders within cultures. Empirical data on these questions would have important implications for both preventive intervention and management of hyperactivity.

Neuropeptide Treatment

The possibility that the attentional difficulties of hyperactive children may be ameliorated with injections of a neuropeptide has been suggested by animal research as well as studies of normal populations and clinical groups with attentional difficulties. The compound involved is present in two hormones located in the pituitary gland: adrenocorticotropic (ACTH), and melanocyte-stimulating hormone (MSH). Injections of the ACTH-MSH compound produce the dual effect of improving visual retention and increasing the ability to sustain attention. University students who were injected with the compound, for example, exhibited better retention for brief visual presentations as well as improved attention. When ability to attend was tested using monotonous, repetitive tasks, those who received the compound scored significantly higher than those on placebo. Findings from a number of laboratories including those of Kastin (1981) and Sandman have demonstrated clear influences of a neuropeptide labeled Organon 2766 on attentional and other processes in mental retardates and elderly patients. The research with mental retardates by Sandman and his colleagues (Sandman, George, Walker, & Nolan, 1976; Sandman, Kastin, & Schally, 1981; Walker & Sandman, 1979) is particularly impressive not only for the degree of attentional improvement and for unexpected improvement in communication ability and patterns, but also for the fact that this neuropeptide effect was clearly demonstrated in naturalistic as well as laboratory settings. Proposals for research on this neuropeptide with hyperactive children are currently being reviewed, and one pilot study (Tinklenberg, 1981) is underway. The possibility that Organon 2766 will prove to be effective in the amelioration of the attention deficit of hyperactive children is of particular interest in view of the fact that research with this neuropeptide in 50 laboratories worldwide has not identified *any* short- or long-term negative side effects (Kastin, 1981).

The above methodological advances, productive extensions, and innovative approaches, as well as the major advances discussed in Chapter 1, are representative of the positive aspects of our increased knowledge concerning hyperactivity. While acknowledging that the amount of progress is far less than one would expect on the basis of the investigative effort expended, it is fair to conclude that the field overall has advanced considerably. Or, as Loney (1979) concluded in a recent review of the field, "What do we know? Quite a bit. Where do we go? Onward."

RESEARCH TOPICS JUSTIFYING INVESTIGATION

In the remainder of this chapter we will consider two categories of research topics that justify further intensive investigation. In the first category are topics that have already been the focus of varying degrees of empirical investigative interest in hyperactivity; those in the second category are speculative in that they appear to have relevance to hyperactivity but are not as yet the subject of research in this area.

Topics with an Existing Empirical Base

The Hyperactive Child—An Informational Source

A major informational gap exists in the hyperactivity literature because a valuable and essential source of information, the hyperactive child himself, has been largely ignored. Instead, the primary informants in the natural history studies are parents, teachers, psychiatrists, clinicians, siblings, and peers—everyone but the central figure, the child. Although doubts have been expressed about the validity of response data from school age hyperactive children (e.g., Stewart, Mendelson, & Johnson, 1973), these objections have been refuted by experienced clinicians (Sulzbacher, 1975; Warme, 1980), questionnaire data on hyperactive children's views of the classroom (Loney, Whaley-Klahn, & Weissenburger, 1976), and interview data on hyperactive children's attitudes towards drug intervention (Henker & Whalen 1980b; Robin & Bosco, 1980). In the following quote from the Henker and Whalen study (1980b, p. 160), note the uneasiness expressed by a 10-year-old hyperactive boy concerning the effects of drugs on athletic performance:

> C.:   One time I didn't take Ritalin and I got on my skateboard and Dad timed me and it was about 53 apartments and I went around in 55 seconds and then I took my Ritalin and then he timed me again and it took me about a minute and 30 seconds.
>
> (Later)
>
> C: I was at the Scout Olympics and I didn't take my Ritalin, and I won the running long jump—12 ft.—and I didn't take my Ritalin. And then I took my Ritalin, and that really did it.
>
> I: And what happened?
>
> C: I almost lost—9 ft.

The blind spot concerning the value of the subjective attitudes and opinions of the hyperactive child is surprising in view of the substantial evidence in general medical and behavioral literature relating patient attitudes to outcome of chronic disorders, and the evidence specifically within the hyperactivity domain providing support for the possibility of a hyperactive child × treatment interaction (Bugental, Whalen, & Henker, 1977; Whalen & Henker, 1976). The subjective view is a topic warranting serious study, and the only approach to it is the direct one of providing the hyperactive child with opportunities to express himself and then acknowledging the potential significance of what he has to say.

Behavior Equivalents

One of the most interesting aspects of the prevalence study by Lambert, Sandoval, and Sassone (1980) was their identification of a group of children whose teacher rating scale scores were above the cutoff point for hyperactivity but who were not considered to be hyperactive by any of the three defining agents—parents, teacher, and physician. Lambert et al. labeled these children *behavior equivalents* and other investigators have also noted their presence in the school system (Jones, Loney, Weissenburger, & Fleischmann, 1975). The study of the behavior equivalents offers a new direction for the study of the hyperactive child. If the personal and environmental attributes that enable the behavior equivalents to escape the label *hyperactive* could be identified, attempts could then be made to incorporate these attributes into both the prevention and management strategies for other children. What might these attributes be? One possibility is that the behavior equivalent represents an unusually favorable child × situation interaction. The difficulty with this explanation is that even if the home situation is ideal, the realities of the school situation, with a different teacher at each grade level, make it unlikely that the child would also have an ideal school situation. Another possibility, suggested by Calhoun (1975, p. 198), is that "typicalness" may influence teacher-identification of hyperactivity:

> In (school) settings where even small problems are relatively atypical, referral (teacher identification) may be more likely for relatively unimpaired youngsters; however, where only large deficits are atypical referral may be expected to be seen as appropriate only for children with very major problems.

Here again, this explanation for Lambert et al.'s behavior equivalents rests on the assumption of an unlikely stability, that is, that these children will always be in classes with extremely hyperactive children or with children having other major problems. Neither of these explanations can account adequately for the fact that all three of the defining agents in the Lambert et al. study failed to identify the behavior equivalents as hyperactive. However, the latter possibility may explain a lesser but related finding in this study, namely, that some children moved in and out of the hyperactive group, being designated as hyperactive at some grade levels and not at others. A third possible explanation lies in the competence deviance hypothesis advanced by Gold (1968), that the more deviant an individual is the more competencies he must possess if his deviance is to be accepted, that is, not cause him problems in his various social environments. The child's competencies could be personal attributes as well as environmental features such as wealth and possessions. An example of the former is contained in the description in Chapter 8 of the hyperactive boy with an IQ of 145 who was not seen as hyperactive by his teacher. The competence-deviance hypothesis may also partially account for the imbalance in the ratio of hyperactive boys to hyperactive girls. In a variety of situations, particularly in the elementary school, the behavior of girls is consonant with teacher expectations more often than appears to be the case for boys.

It would be interesting to analyze the data on behavior equivalents in terms of competencies. Whatever the explanation for the success of the behavior equivalent group, they clearly merit intensive further study. One direction that this study might take parallels that of the approach used in the medical phenomenon of *escapees* (Rosenberg, Metzig, & Ast, 1977), a group of adults who are presently the focus of interest in medical research on Huntington's chorea. These individuals are the siblings of patients with Huntington's chorea who have reached the age of 50 without showing any of the symptoms of this genetic-based disease that should have appeared at around ages 35 to 40. The escapee methodology used in the study of this unusual group involves careful comparisons between patients with Huntington's chorea, their children, and the siblings (escapees) of the patients. This methodology is likely to be productive in the development of predictive measures of Huntington's chorea as well as in the management of patients with the disease and those who are at risk for it. The behavior equivalent is also an escapee of sorts, and a modified escapee methodology would appear to be applicable to an investigation of this phenomenon. The behavior equivalents apparently have achieved the goal of prevention and management programs, to function satisfactorily in the various environments, and have the potential capabilities for mastering subsequent developmental tasks. Such an accomplishment merits serious investigative attention. The findings would almost certainly expand the existing knowledge of hyperactivity.

Peer Interaction Problems

A topic justifying intensive work is that of the well-documented peer interaction difficulties that most hyperactive children experience (Campbell & Paulauskas, 1979; Milich & Landau, 1981). Although the immediate relevance of peer problems to the child's poor self-concept and other psychological facets of his development are recognized, and the predictive value of these problems for long-term outcome is established, relatively little attention has been paid to their investigation. Two lines of attack are needed here. One involves the development of programs for modifying the child's immediate ongoing problems with his peers. There is evidence in the form of research results and parent–teacher reports that the hyperactive child rapidly antagonizes new acquaintances (Pelham, 1980). One cluster of behaviors almost guaranteed to annoy other children has been identified (Henker & Whalen, 1980a), but undoubtedly there are others of importance. One approach to the complex problem of program content would be to identify a large pool of such behaviors, assign to each a priority rating based on a subjective assessment of how much each behavior appears to contribute to the child's problems with peers, and develop a multifaceted cluster of intervention procedures for helping the child understand the concept of appropriate behavior for each of these types of interaction. The other line of attack is concerned with causal factors, that is, the reasons underlying the peer problems of the hyperactive child. This area offers a confusing array of theoretical and empirical information. According to Hartup (1976), for example, the prerequisites for adequate peer relations are secure mother–infant attachments followed by early social interaction experiences with same-age peers as a means of learning appropriate behavior controls. However, there is no empirical support for a causal relationship between early peer interaction problems and later peer problems in the school setting, although such a relationship is commonly cited as existing. Nor has an empirical basis been established for a relationship between the child's social status in the group and his peer interactions, one problem here being that the components of social status are a matter of debate.

Topics that would seem to have potential as a source of data include the modeling effect of the classroom teacher on peer acceptance or rejection of the hyperactive child, differences in social skills and other attributes between behavior equivalents (Lambert et al., 1980) and hyperactive children with peer problems, and, in somewhat the same line of thought, differences between hyperactive boys and hyperactive girls. In the case of the latter comparison, there is sporadic evidence (Battle & Lacey, 1972; Prinz & Loney, 1974) of sex differences in the antecedents and concomitants of hyperactivity. The question of differences in peer problems associated with regular versus special class placement also has research potential, and this topic is related to Whalen et al.'s studies of classrooms that maximize the hyperactive child's problems, the specific problem here being that of peer interaction.

Role of Siblings

One area that has been largely ignored on both the clinical and research fronts concerns the role that siblings play in the hyperactive child's life. A start in the direction of determining the effect of the normal sibling on the immediate and long-term functioning of the hyperactive child is the comparison by Mash and Johnston (1981) of sibling interactions in hyperactive and normal children. It is our unsubstantiated opinion that many siblings contribute significantly to the hyperactive child's immediate difficulties, such as his poor self-esteem, and to the duration of the disorder. Most of the siblings of the hyperactive children who we know well are variously unkind, disparaging, hostile, antagonistic, and notably indifferent to the hyperactive child's difficulties. Frequently they deeply resent having a behavior-disordered child in the family and much of this resentment is expressed in a particularly virulent form of teasing designed to upset the hyperactive child. Many of their most spiteful tactics are masked under the guise of prosocial behavior. The antecedents of the clinically well documented sibling hostility should be a topic of empirical investigation. It is likely that a major underlying contributor to the jungle aspect of the sibling–hyperactive child relationship is the implicit approval given to the sibling behavior by the parents. This approval takes such forms as subtle parental modeling of nonverbal antagonistic cues, or failure to put a stop to observed verbal or other direct and indirect attacks on the hyperactive child. Cantwell's (1979) warning that the hyperactive child is often the family scapegoat has considerable nonempirical support. The position in the family of many hyperactive children can best be summed up by the following lines:

Ashes to ashes and clay to clay
If your enemies don't get you
Your own folks may.*

Because of the problem of sibling antagonism, and in the absence of research to the contrary, we are opposed to assigning siblings the role of change agents, a role that teachers and clinicians often advocate. There are undoubtedly some siblings who could perform ably and humanely as change agents, but in the main we believe that it would be cruel and unfair punishment to put most of the hyperactive children that we know under the official jurisdiction of a sibling change agent. Before the possibility of such a step assumes any weight in the intervention strategy, sibling interactions with the hyperactive child should be subjected to intensive but unobtrusive scrutiny in a wide range of situations, and apparently informal chats of a noncritical nature should be conducted. We are not denying that the problems of the hyperactive child cause difficulties on a day-to-day basis for siblings as well as parents. The very unpredictability of this child's behavior would contribute greatly to the household tension and in many ways would be harder to cope with than, for example, the consistent behavior of a mentally retarded child. What we are advocating is that the realities of the hyperactive child-sibling interactions be acknowledged in the planning of intervention strategies, and that the sibling effects be subjected to empirical scrutiny.

*Author unknown.

Attention Deficit

An investigation of the development of understanding of attention with normal children (Miller & Bigi, 1979) appears to have important implications for
hyperactive children. Most of the Grade One children in this study knew that
"paying attention" meant listening. Of 26 hyperactive children in Grades One
through Three to whom we presented Miller and Bigi's preliminary questions
on the meaning of paying attention, only three included listening in their answers. The response most frequently given was some variant of looking alert
such as "sit up straight and look at the teacher." The possibility should be
investigated that the hyperactive child should be taught the meaning of the
concept of attending prior to attention training. It is as though the simple
communication to the hyperactive child of commonplace expectations concerning his behavior is beyond his comprehension, and this failure passes unnoticed by adults perhaps because the simplicity of the communication
induces a set in them that excludes the possibility that the child may not
understand the communication. If this is the case, then preliminary training to
ensure that the child understands the concept being taught should probably
precede all attempts to train the hyperactive child in basic learning skills such
as attending. Oblique reference to this idea occurred in Chapter 7 in the
description of the child whose self-instruction training was not effective until
he acquired skill in self-evaluation which enabled him finally to grasp the concept of stopping and thinking before blurting out answers. This concept came
as a totally new idea to him, although he had undoubtedly been told hundreds
of times to stop and think before answering.

Diagnostic Criteria and Methods

The mandatory procedures for the diagnosis of childhood hyperactivity are
explicit in the criteria of DSM III and have been specified in detail by experienced clinicians (Blau, 1979; Cantwell, 1975a, 1979; Casey, 1977; Eisenberg, 1966; Safer & Allen, 1976; Sleator, 1981). In sharp contrast to the
wealth of detail concerning optimal diagnostic procedures is the paucity of
information about the diagnostic criteria and methods actually used. What
little information is available is not reassuring. A conglomerate of
nonempirical data, including clinical papers, letters to the editor in professional journals and the mass media, and reports from physicians, psychologists, teachers, and parents, suggests that in a substantial number of cases
diagnoses of hyperactivity are based on a single criterion such as drug response, or teacher or parent report. In an empirical investigation of this
topic (Sandoval, Lambert, & Sassone, 1980) the diagnosis of hyperactivity
by physicians rested primarily on behavioral indicators, particularly the
child's emotionality and activity level, and on information from the child's
personal medical history. Some indirect information comes from a study
(Plomin & Foch, 1981) in which children diagnosed as hyperactive by pedia-

tricians were compared to a large unselected sample of nonclinical children on parental ratings on the Conners Symptoms Rating Questionnaire, a battery of laboratory measures of hyperactivity-related behavior, and a set of tests of cognitive ability. The pediatricians' diagnoses of hyperactivity were related to parental ratings and deficits in cognitive abilities, particularly perceptual speed and verbal ability, but *not* to laboratory assessments of activity, attention, and aggression. Plomin and Foch (1981) concluded that these diagnoses of hyperactivity largely reflected deficits in the cognitive skills prerequisite to appropriate self-pacing in school-related tasks.

The criteria and methods used to diagnose hyperactivity merit immediate research attention in the interests of avoiding overdiagnosis and consequent unwarranted treatment as well as of assuring that children described as hyperactive in research studies are, in fact, hyperactive. The diagnosis of hyperactivity by a pediatrician is frequently one criterion for inclusion in research, but there is often no documentation of either the diagnostic criteria used or any direct check on the validity of the diagnosis. Error from diagnostic inaccuracies could take many forms such as increased variability in research results or a falsely inflated picture of the heterogeneity of hyperactivity. The cost of a cycle of such errors to progress in understanding could be, and in all probability already has been, considerable. The first step towards eliminating this source of error would be the documentation and subsequent dissemination of the bases for the diagnosis of hyperactivity in clinical practice. The next step, an insistence on standardization of diagnostic practices and requirements in the clinical and empirical domains, would be the responsibility of the pediatric and research establishments.

Topics of a Speculative Nature

Hibernation Response

Research by Margules (1979) on the hibernation response raises the possibility that an imbalance between two previously unknown branches of the autonomic nervous system, the endorphinergic and endoloxonergic divisions, may be etiologically implicated in hyeractivity. According to Margules' theory, the endorphinergic division stimulates the hunger and overeating patterns characteristic of obesity by releasing peptides, such as beta-endorphins (B-E), which are substances in the pituitary and the brain called opium peptides that produce effects similar to those of opium. The release of B-E produces a sequence of changes that mimics the hibernation response in animals, that is, prefamine hunger → urgent sense of impending danger → overeating → release of insulin → storage of excess calories in adipose tissue. Normally, the effects of the endorphinergic division are counterbalanced by the endoloxonergic branch of the autonomic nervous system. This division notifies the body that there is no shortage of food by releasing hypothetical substances called endoloxones. The effect of these substances is to stimulate activity of all kinds, increase the body's capacity to respond to stimuli, and inhibit the desire for food.

Margules (1979) believes that the two divisions maintain an optimum balance through mutual inhibition. When an imbalance occurs, for reasons not yet identified, endorphinergic dominance can result in obesity and other addictions, whereas endoloxonergic dominance may result in hyperactivity and anorexia. Some evidence for this theory comes from the finding that rats that are genetically prone to obesity have more B-E in their pituitaries than do lean rats. When injected with very small doses of nalaxone, a chemical known to offset the effects of opioids, the obese rats stop eating and drinking but the same dose has no effect on the lean animals. There appears to be an age-related change in the role of both systems, with a shift towards endorphinergic dominance. This shift would be compatible with the tendency of the high level of activity in childhood hyperactivity to diminish somewhat with age. Several of the response patterns associated with endoloxonergic excesses are also typical of the hyperactive child, for example, his atypical activity pattern which presumably is related to an imbalance between arousal and inhibition, his distractibility, and his poor eating habits. The possibility that endoloxonergic excesses may be etiologically implicated in the hyperactivity of a subgroup of these children is an intriguing direction that should be carefully investigated. The finding that peptides have proven effective with a small group of hyperactive children (Butter, Lapierre, Laprade, Firestone, Côté, & Pierre-Louis, 1979; Tiwary, Rosenbloom, Robertson, & Parker, 1975) takes on new significance in the light of Margules' theory.

Environmental Influences on Behavior

Investigations of the effects of variations in the natural low-frequency electrostatic DC fields surrounding the earth and the ratio of positive to negative ions in the air suggest the possibility of creating physical environments that improve behavior. Although each of these areas of research is still in the embryo stage, the possibility that in terms of economic feasibility and practicality the research findings could be adapted to classroom use justifies a brief consideration of their rationale.

Electrostatic Fields. The natural low-frequency electrostatic DC field surrounding the earth is believed by many European scientists to be an important determinant of human behavior and health. There is nonempirical but intriguing support for the effects of this field on human behavior. For example, entering students at the University of Massachusetts typically have scored around the 75th percentile on group intelligence tests. However, one group whose cumulative record was similar in every respect to that of previous groups took the tests during an unusually violent thunderstorm and scored in the 95th percentile, a rise in scores that proponents of the electrostatic theory attributed to the effect of the electrostatic field caused by the storm. This and other examples of the electrostatic theory effect have led proponents to consider the creation of artificial fields to treat different disorders and enhance performance. Unsubstantiated claims have been made that such fields can heal bones, reduce pain, speed reaction time, and reduce deviant behavior in disturbed children. One such artificial field, the Biofield (Smith, 1980), was based on an idea from a Bulgarian nuclear scientist, Cristjo Cristofv, who is known for discovering that high energy explosions can be monitored through electromagnetics, a discovery referred to as the Cristofv effect. Smith's device has been used successfully to quieten race horses who are called stall walkers because they pace continuously about their stalls, a behavior that has serious detrimental effects on their physical and mental well-being. Although American scientists know how to describe and develop the Biofield device, there has been little rigorous research with it. We are proposing that the Biofield might have potential value in the treatment of the hyperactive child. It could easily be subjected to rigorous classroom tests and is relatively inexpensive. If even a subgroup of hyperactive children exhibited improvement further research would be justified in view of the obvious important advantages that a device of this sort would appear to have over drug and behavior therapy interventions.

Negative Ions. There is an optimum ratio of positive to negative ions in the air that can be destroyed by naturally occurring climate changes, for example, winds such as the chinook in the Canadian Rockies, as well as manmade changes such as pollution. When the ratio of positive to negative ions is unduly increased, a subgroup of the population experiences decreased well-being in the form of irritability, sleeplessness, and respiratory distress. Laboratory findings on this phenomenon are both complex and equivocal (Diamond, Connor, Orenberg, Bissell, Yost, & Krueger, 1980); one possibility is that for a subgroup a *decrease* in the proportion of negative ions results in an *increase* in serotonin and a concomitant decrease in well-being. Manufacturers with more concern for sales than human safety have already marketed generators that add negative ions to the air and are claimed to enhance the well-being of some individuals. Diamond (1980) has cautioned that such devices are premature and potentially dangerous because they may also generate excess ozone. However, the possibility that there may be subgroups of hyperactive children whose behavior patterns are in part a function of the ion content of the air merits consideration. We are not thinking here of sporadic climatic or pollutant-related changes in the ion ratio but rather that the ion ratio that is optimum for most children may not be the optimum one for a subgroup of hyperactive children.

Another highly speculative possibility is that the ion ratio is optimum for the hyperactive child in some environments and not others. Negative ions are in short supply in settings where stale air accumulates (Diamond, 1980), a common characteristic of many school classrooms. It is possible that the well-documented home–school variability in the hyperactive child's behavior could reflect differences in ion ratios in the two settings. Oblique support for this possible difference in environment comes from Coleman's (1971) puzzling finding of low peripheral serotonin levels in two hyperactive children in their home setting; the children had close to normal levels and decreased hyperactivity in their temporary placement in a residential research setting, and then the previous low serotonin levels and hyperactivity were reestablished on their return home. The possibility of an ion ratio–hyperactivity link would not be difficult to subject to empirical test and, if confirmed, could have important implications for etiology and management.

This discussion of the state of the art would not be complete without some comments on two distinct and recent trends that augur well for progress in the understanding of hyperactivity. One is the increase in the systematic use and further development of the empirical basis of other investigators' work both within and beyond the field of hyperactivity. For example, modified versions of questionnaires developed for studies of drug use in adolescents in general (Abelson & Fishburne, 1977), as well as for hyperactive adolescents (Henker, Whalen, Bugental, & Barker, 1981), have been used by other investigators (Gadow & Sprague, 1980; Kramer & Loney, 1981). Original data have been reanalyzed for use in subsequent studies of different topics (Kramer & Loney, 1981) and of the same topics, an example of the latter use being the reanalysis of others' multivariate studies by Langhorne, Loney, Paternite, and Bechtoldt (1976), a subsequent critique (Zukow, Zukow, & Bentler, 1978), and further analysis and rebuttal by DeFillipis (1979). On a broader scale, investigators such as Gorenstein and Newman (1980) and Porges (1976) have reached out in their search for etiological commonalities in behavior disorders beyond the boundaries of hyperactivity to the wealth of information that has accumulated in other areas of childhood psychopathology; and Whalen, Henker, and their colleagues, with their small ecosystem model, are forerunners of the rapidly developing convergence of environmental and developmental psychology (Wohlwill, 1980). An integral part of this trend is the readiness and indeed generosity of investigators in making their prepublication work available to others.

The other important trend is the concern on the part of small but influential groups of highly skilled investigators with the refinement of procedures, knowledge, and viewpoints within specific topical areas. The process of systematic refinement is particularly apparent in the area of drug intervention. In the early 1970s the stimulants were for all practical purposes the only available treatment for hyperactivity, and their use was bounded by a limited knowledge of such aspects as dosage and monitoring. Their potential value was not realized, and potential problems were not acknowledged. Instead, most clinicians and researchers assumed a one-dimensional, unthinking, almost primitive approach to drug usage and research that was reminiscent of a comment in another context by Maslow (Millman, 1978): "If the only tool you have is a hammer, then it is very tempting to treat everything as though it were a nail." In less than a decade the refinements of this important mode of intervention have been both diverse and impressive, and include such major developments as the precise specification of dosage for different functions (Sprague & Berger, 1980; Sprague & Sleator, 1977); careful critical discussions of the possibility of stimulant-induced growth retardation (Roche, Lipman, Overall, & Hung, 1979), drug abuse (Kramer & Loney, 1981), and cardiovascular disturbances (Satterfield, Schell, & Barb, 1980); increasing alertness to the placebo properties of drugs as a potential tool in intervention (Werry, 1977); the theoretical statement (Conners & Wells, 1979) on the changes in hyperactivity effected by drug intervention, coupled with Conners' masterly demonstration of the application of this theory to the single-subject experimental methodology; several impressive documentations of medication-related differences in overt behavior in hyperactive children in simulated naturalistic settings (Whalen et al., 1978); the view of stimulants as synergistic (Werry, 1977) and recognition of their potential value for providing a base for other interventions (Mash & Dalby, 1979); and finally, the widespread interest in and concern for the effective use of stimulants with adolescent (Cantwell, 1979) and adult hyperactives (Bellak, 1979).

Epidemiologists who are pushing relentlessly toward the goal of prevention of medical diseases tend to describe progress in terms of centuries. For example, with the conquest of the major infectious diseases the last 100 years have been described as the end of the first epidemiologic revolution, and the next 100 years is seen as the second epidemiologic revolution, the goal being to make similar gains on the chronic disease front (McGinnis, 1980). It is our opinion that in the next decade the impact of the foregoing trends on the understanding of hyperactivity will, in a quiet way, also merit the descriptor *revolution*.

References

Aarskog, D., Fevang, F. Ø., Kløve, H., Støa, K. F., & Thorsen, T. The effect of the stimulant drugs, dextroamphetamine and methylphenidate, on secretion of growth hormone in hyperactive children. *Journal of Pediatrics,* 1977, *90,* 136–139.

Abelson, H., & Fishburne, P. *National survey on drug abuse: 1977. Vol. 2, Methodology.* Rockville, MD: National Institute on Drug Abuse, 1977.

Abikoff, H., Gittelman-Klein, R., & Klein, D. F. Validation of a classroom observation code for hyperactive children. *Journal of Consulting and Clinical Psychology,* 1977, *45,* 772–783.

Abramowitz, C. V. The effectiveness of group psychotherapy with children. *Archives of General Psychiatry,* 1976, *33,* 320–326.

Abrahams, A. L. Delayed and irregular maturation versus minimal brain injury. *Clinical Pediatrics,* 1968, *7,* 344–349.

Achenbach, T. A., & Edelbrock, C. S. The classification of child psychopathology: A review and analysis of empirical efforts. *Psychological Bulletin,* 1978, *85,* 1275–1301.

Ackerman, P. T., Dykman, R. A., & Peters, J. E. Teenage status of hyperactive and nonhyperactive learning disabled boys. *American Journal of Orthopsychiatry,* 1977, *47,* 577–596.

Ahn, H., Prichep, L., John, E. R., Baird, H., Trepitin, M., & Kaye, H. Developmental equations reflect brain dysfunctions. *Science,* 1980, *210,* 1259–1262.

Air Quality Criteria for Lead. Publication No. EPA–600/8–77–017, Environmental Protection Agency, Washington, DC, 1977.

Alabiso, F. Inhibitory functions of attention in reducing hyperactive behavior. *American Journal of Mental Deficiency,* 1972, *77,* 259–282.

Alden, L., Rappaport, J., & Seidman, E. College students as interventionists for primary-grade children. *American Journal of Community Psychology,* 1975, *3,* 261–271.

Aleksandrowicz, M. K., & Aleksandrowicz, D. R. The molding of personality: A newborn's innate characteristics in interaction with parents' personalities. *Child Psychiatry and Human Development,* 1975, *5,* 231–241.

Allan, C., & Ornellas, M. *Like any child but more so.* 16mm film. Master's thesis, Department of Communications, University of California, Berkeley, 1977.

Allen, K. E., Henke, L. B., Harris, F. R., Baer, D. M., & Reynolds, N. J. Control of hyperactivity by social reinforcement of attending behavior. *Journal of Educational Psychology,* 1967, *58,* 231–237.

Allen, R. P., & Safer, D. Long term effects of stimulant therapy for HA children: Risk benefits analysis. In M. J. Cohen (Ed.), *Drugs and the special child.* New York: Gardner Press, 1979.

Allmond, B. W., Buckman, W., & Gofman, H. F. *The family is the patient.* St. Louis: Mosby, 1979.

Aman, M. G. Drugs, learning and the psychotherapies. In J. S. Werry (Ed.), *Pediatric psychopharmacology: The use of behavior modifying drugs in children.* New York: Brunner/Mazel, 1978.

Aman, M. G., & Sprague, R. L. The state-dependent effects of methylphenidate and dextroamphetamine. *Journal of Nervous and Mental Disease,* 1974, *158,* 268–279.

Ambrose, A. (Ed.). *Stimulation in early infancy.* New York: Academic Press, 1969.

American Academy of Pediatrics, Council on Child Health: Medication for hyperkinetic children. *Pediatrics,* 1975, *55,* 560–561.

American Psychiatric Association. *Behavior therapy in psychiatry.* Task Force Report 5. Washington, DC: APA, 1973.

Anastasi, A. *Psychological testing* (4th ed.). New York: MacMillan, 1976.

Anastasiow, N. J. Personal communication, 1980.

Anastasiow, N. J., Everett, M., O'Shaughnessy, T. E., Eggleston, P. J., & Eklund, S. J. Improving teenage attitudes toward children, child handicaps, and hospital settings: A child development curriculum for potential parents. *American Journal of Orthopsychiatry,* 1978, *48,* 663–672.

Anders, T. F. Night-waking in infants during the first year of life. *Pediatrics,* 1979, *63,* 860–864.

Anderson, C. M., & Plymate, H. B. Management of the brain-damaged adolescent. *American Journal of Orthopsychiatry,* 1962, *32,* 492–500.

Anderson, J. A. Electromyographic feedback as a method of reducing hyperkinesis in children. Unpublished doctoral dissertation, Texas Women's University, 1975.

Anderson, R. P. A neuropsychogenic perspective on remediation of learning disabilities. *Journal of Learning Disabilities,* 1970, *3,* 143–148.

Anderson, R. P. Trends in research with hyperactive children. Paper presented at the Southwestern Psychological Association Meeting, Fort Worth, TX, 1977.

Anderson, R. P., Halcomb, C. G., & Doyle, R. B. The measurement of attentional deficits. *Exceptional Children,* 1973, *39,* 534–540.

Arnold, L. E. Philosophy and strategy of medicating adults with minimal brain dysfunction. In L. Bellak (Ed.), *Psychiatric aspects of minimal brain dysfunction in adults.* New York: Grune and Stratton, 1979.

Arnold, L. E., Christopher, J., Huestis, R., & Smeltzer, D. J. Methylphenidate vs. dextroamphetamine vs. caffeine in minimal brain dysfunction. *Archives of General Psychiatry,* 1978a, *35,* 463–473.

Arnold, L. E., Christopher, J., Huestis, R. D., & Smeltzer, D. J. Megavitamins for minimal brain dysfunction. *Journal of the American Medical Association,* 1978b, *240,* 2642–2643.

Arnold, L. E., Wender, P. H., McCloskey, K., & Snyder, S. H. Levoamphetamine and dextroamphetamine: Comparative efficacy in the hyperkinetic syndrome. *Archives of General Psychiatry,* 1972, *27,* 816–822.

Astor, M. H. An introduction to biofeedback. *American Journal of Orthopsychiatry,* 1977, *47,* 615–625.

Aub, J. C., Fairhall, L. T., Minot, A. S., & Resnikoff, P. *Lead poisoning.* Baltimore: Williams and Wilkins, 1926.

Augustine, G. J., & Levitan, H. Neurotransmitter release from a vertebrate neuromuscular synapse affected by food dye. *Science,* 1980, *207,* 1489–1490.

Ault, R. L., Mitchell, C., & Hartmann, D. D. Some methodological problems in reflection-impulsivity research. *Child Development, 1976, 47,* 227–231.

Ayd, F. Haloperidol: Fifteen years of clinical experience. *Diseases of the Nervous System,* 1972, *33,* 459–469.

Ayllon, T., Layman, D., & Kandel, H. J. A behavioral-educational alternative to control of hyperactive children. *Journal of Applied Behavior Analysis,* 1975, *8,* 137–146.

Ayllon, T., & Roberts, M. Eliminating discipline problems by strengthening academic performance. *Journal of Applied Behavior Analysis,* 1974, *7,* 71–76.

Aylward, G. P., & Kenny, T. J. Developmental follow-up: Inherent problems and a conceptual model. *Journal of Pediatric Psychology,* 1979, *4,* 331–343.

Babcock, D., & Keepers, T. *Raising kids OK.* New York: Grove Press, 1976.

Bachman, J. G., Johnston, L. D., & O'Malley, P. M. Smoking, drinking, and drug use among American high school students: Correlates and trends. *American Journal of Public Health,* 1981, *71,* 59–69.

Backman, J. E., Ferguson, H. B., & Trites, R. L. Case study #6. Contingency contracting with a hyperactive boy and his parents. In M. Fine (Ed.), *Intervention with hyperactive children: A case study approach.* Jamaica, NY: Spectrum Publications, 1980.

Badger, E., & Burns, D. Impact of a parent education program on the personal development of teen-age mothers. *Journal of Pediatric Psychology,* 1980, *5,* 415–422.

Baer, D. M., Wolf, M. M., & Risley, T. R. Some current dimensions of applied behavior analysis. *Journal of Applied Behavior Analysis,* 1968, *1,* 91–97.

Bakwin, H., & Bakwin, R. M. *Clinical management of behavior disorders in children.* Philadelphia: Saunders, 1966.

Baldassare, M. *Residential crowding in urban America.* Berkeley, CA: University of California Press, 1979.

Baldwin, B., Benjamins, J., Meyers, R., & Grant, C. EMG biofeedback with hyperactive children. A time series analysis. Paper presented at the Ninth Annual Meeting of the Biofeedback Society of America, Albuquerque, NM, 1978.

Baldwin, M.A. Activity level, attention span, and deviance: Hyperactive boys in the classroom. Unpublished doctoral dissertation, University of Waterloo (Canada), 1976.

Ballard, J. E., Boileau, R. A., Sleator, E. K., Massey, B. H., & Sprague, R. L. Cardiovascular responses of hyperactive children to methylphenidate. *Journal of the American Medical Association,* 1976, *236,* 2870–2874.

Bandura, A. *Principles of behavior modification.* New York: Holt, Rinehart and Winston, 1969.

Bandura, A. Behavior theory and the models of man. *American Psychologist,* 1974, *29,* 859–869.

Bandura, A. Self-reinforcement: Theoretical and methodological considerations. *Behaviorism,* 1976, *4,* 135–155.

Barcai, A. Predicting the response of children with learning disabilities and behavior problems to dextroamphetamine sulphate. *Pediatrics,* 1971, *47,* 73–80.

Barcai, A., & Robinson, E. H. Conventional group therapy with preadolescent children. *International Journal of Group Psychotherapy,* 1969, *19,* 334–335.

Barkley, R. A. Predicting the response of hyperkinetic children to stimulant drugs: A review. *Journal of Abnormal Child Psychology,* 1976, *4,* 327–348.

Barkley, R. A. A review of stimulant drug research with hyperactive children. *Journal of Child Psychology and Psychiatry,* 1977a, *18,* 137–165.

Barkley, R. A. The effects of methylphenidate on various measures of activity level and attention in hyperkinetic children. *Journal of Abnormal Child Psychology,* 1977b, *5,* 351–369.

Barkley, R. A. Recent developments in research on hyperactive children. *Journal of Pediatric Psychology,* 1978, *3,* 158–163.

Barkley, R. A. Stimulant drugs in the classroom. *School Psychology Digest,* 1979, *8,* 412–425.

Barkley, R. A. Specific guidelines for defining hyperactivity in children (Attention Deficit Disorder). In B. Lahey and A. Kazdin (Eds.), *Advances in child clinical psychology,* Vol. 4. New York: Plenum, 1981.

Barkley, R. A., Copeland, A. P., & Sivage, C. A self-control classroom for hyperactive children. *Journal of Autism and Developmental Disorders,* 1980, *10,* 75–89.

Barkley, R. A., & Cunningham, C. E. Do stimulant drugs improve the academic performance of hyperkinetic children? A review of outcome studies. *Clinical Pediatrics,* 1978, *17,* 85–92.

Barkley, R. A., & Cunningham, C. E. The effects of methylphenidate on the mother-child interactions of hyperactive children. *Archives of General Psychiatry,* 1979, *36,* 201–208.

Barkley, R. A., & Jackson, T. L., Jr. Hyperkinesis, autonomic nervous system activity, and stimulant drug effects. *Journal of Child Psychology and Psychiatry,* 1977, *18,* 347–357.

Barkley, R. A., & Ullman, D. G. A comparison of objective measures of activity and distractibility in hyperactive and nonhyperactive children. *Journal of Abnormal Child Psychology,* 1975, *3,* 231–244.

Barnard, K., & Collar, B. S. Early diagnosis, interpretation, and intervention: A commentary on the nurse's role. *Annals of the New York Academy of Sciences*, 1973, *205*, 373–382.

Barrett, R. J., Leith, N. J., & Ray, O. S. Permanent facilitation of avoidance behavior by d-amphetamine and scopolamine. *Psychopharmacologia*, 1972, *25*, 321–331.

Barry, R. G. G., & O'Naullain, S. O. Cash Report: Foetal alcoholism. *Irish Journal of Medicine*, 1975, *144*, 286–287.

Barten, H. H. The expanding spectrum of the brief therapies. In H. H. Barten (Ed.), *Brief therapies*. New York: Behavioral Publications, 1971.

Battle, E. S., & Lacey, B. A context for hyperactivity in children, over time. *Child Development*, 1972, *43*, 757–773.

Bax, M. C. O. The active and the overactive school child. *Developmental Medicine and Child Neurology*, 1972, *14*, 83–86.

Bax, M. C. O. Who is hyperactive? *Developmental Medicine and Child Neurology*, 1978, *20*, 277–278.

Bax, M. C. O., & MacKeith, R. C. Minimal brain damage—a concept discarded. In R. C. MacKeith & M. C. O. Bax (Eds.), *Minimal cerebral dysfunction*. Little Club Clinics in Development Medicine, No. 10. London: Heinemann, 1963.

Baxley, G. B., Turner, P. F., & Greenwold, W. E. Hyperactive children's knowledge and attitudes concerning drug treatment. *Journal of Pediatric Psychology*, 1978, *3*, 172–176.

Bayley, N. *The Bayley scales of infant development*. New York: Psychological Corporation, 1969.

Beall, J. G. Food additives and hyperactivity in children. *U. S. Congressional Record*, S19766, October 30, 1973.

Beck, L., Langford, W. S., MacKay, M., & Sum, G. Childhood chemotherapy and later drug abuse and growth curve: A follow-up study of 30 adolescents. *American Journal of Psychiatry*, 1975, *132*, 436–438.

Beck, M. A. A follow-up study of adults who were clinically diagnosed as hyperkinetic in childhood. Unpublished doctoral dissertation, Wayne State University, 1976.

Becker, W. C., Madsen, C. H., Jr., Arnold, C. R., & Thomas, D. R. The contingent use of teacher attention and praise in reducing classroom behavior problems. *Journal of Special Education*, 1967, *1*, 287–307.

Bee, H. L. Parent–child interaction and distractibility in nine-year-old children. *Merrill–Palmer Quarterly of Behavior and Development*, 1967, *13*, 175–190.

Beiser, M. Psychiatric epidemiology. In A. M. Nicholi, Jr. (Ed.), *The Harvard guide to modern psychiatry*. Cambridge, MA: Belknap Press, 1978.

Bell, J. H. The family that fought back. *McCall's*, May 1977, pp. 26, 30, 32, 34, 36, 40.

Bell, R. Q. A reinterpretation of the direction of effects in studies of socialization. *Psychological Review*, 1968, *75*, 81–95.

Bell, R. Q. Stimulus control of parent or caretaker behavior by offspring. *Developmental Psychology*, 1971, *4*, 63–72.

Bell, R. Q., & Harper, L. V. *Child effects on adults*. Hillsdale, NJ: Erlbaum, 1977.

Bell, R. Q., Waldrop, M. F., & Weller, G. M. A rating system for assessment of hyperactive and withdrawn children in preschool samples. *American Journal of Orthopsychiatry*, 1972, *42*, 23–34.

Bellak, L. (Ed.). *Psychiatric aspects of minimal brain dysfunction in adults*. New York: Grune and Stratton, 1979.

Bellak, L., & Small, L. *Emergency psychotherapy and brief psychotherapy*, New York: Grune and Stratton, 1965.

Bender, L. Postencephalitic behavior disorders in children. In J. B. Neal (Ed.), *Encephalitis: A clinical study*. New York: Grune and Stratton, 1942.

Bender, N. N. Self-verbalization versus tutor verbalization in modifying impulsivity. *Journal of Educational Psychology*, 1976, *68*, 347–354.

Benskin v. Taft City School District C.A. No. 136795. Superior Court, Kern County, California, filed September 1975.

Bentler, P. M., & McClain, J. A multitrait-multimethod analysis of reflection-impulsivity. *Child Development*, 1976, *47*, 218–226.

Bergin, A. E., & Garfield, S. L. (Eds.). *Handbook of psychotherapy and behavior change*. New York: Wiley, 1971.

Bergin, A. E., & Suinn, R. M. Individual psychotherapy and behavior therapy. *Annual Review of Psychology*, 1975, *26*, 509–556.

Berk, R. A. The discriminative efficiency of the Bayley Scales of Infant Development. *Journal of Abnormal Child Psychology*, 1979, *7*, 113–119.

Berkowitz, B. T., & Graziano, A. M. Training parents as behavior therapists: a review. *Behavior Research and Therapy*, 1972, *10*, 297–317.

Berlin, I. Minimal brain dysfunction. Management of family distress. *Journal of the American Medical Association*, 1974, *229*, (11), 1454–1456.

Berlyne, D. E. *Conflict, arousal and curiosity*. New York: McGraw-Hill, 1960.

Berne, E. *Transactional analysis in psychotherapy*. New York: Grove, 1961.

Berne, E. *Games people play*. New York: Grove, 1964.

Bernstein, J., Page, J., & Janicki, R. Some characteristics of children with minimal brain dysfunction. In C. Conners (Ed.), *Clinical use of stimulant drugs in children*. Amsterdam: Excerpta Medica, 1974.

Berry, K., & Cook, V. J. Personality and behavior. In H. E. Rie & E. D. Rie (Eds.), *Handbook of minimal brain dysfunctions*. New York: Wiley, 1980.

Bettelheim, B. Bringing up children. *Ladies Home Journal*, 1973, *90*, 28.

Bhagavan, H. N., Coleman, M., & Coursin, D. B. The effect of pyridoxine hydrochloride on blood serotonin and pyridoxal phosphate contents in hyperactive children. *Pediatrics*, 1975, *55*, 437.

Bhatara, V., Arnold, L. E., Lorance, T., & Gupta, D. Muscle relaxation therapy in hyperkinesis: Is it effective? *Journal of Learning Disabilities*, 1979, *12*, 49–53.

Bhatara, V., Clark, D. L., Arnold, L. E., Gunsett, R., & Smeltzer, D. J. Hyperkinesis treated by vestibular stimulation: An exploratory study. *Biological Psychiatry*, 1981, *16*, 269–279.

Bierman, C. W., & Furukawa, C. T. Food additives and hyperkinesis: Are there nuts among the berries? *Pediatrics*, 1978, *61*, 932–933.

Bing, E. Effect of child rearing practices on development of differential cognitive abilities. *Child Development*, 1963, *43*, 631–648.

Birch, H. G. *Brain damage in children: The biological and social aspects*. Baltimore: Williams and Wilkins, 1964.

Birk, L. Behavior therapy and behavioral psychotherapy. In A. M. Nicholi (Ed.), *The Harvard guide to modern psychiatry*. Cambridge, MA: Belknap, 1978.

Bittinger, M. L. (Ed.). *Living with our hyperactive children*. New York: Two Continents Publishing Group, 1977.

Blacklidge, V., & Ekblad, R. The effectiveness of methylphenidate hydrochloride (Ritalin) on learning and behavior in public school educable mentally retarded children. *Pediatrics*, 1971, *47*, 923–926.

Blanchard, E. B., & Young, L. Clinical applications of biofeedback training: A review of evidence. *Archives of General Psychiatry*, 1974, *30*, 573–589.

Blau, T. H. Diagnosis of disturbed children. *American Psychologist*, 1979, *34*, 969–972.

Bloch, A. *Murphy's Law*. Los Angeles: Price/Stern/Sloan, 1977.

Block, G. H. Hyperactivity: A cultural perspective. *Journal of Learning Disabilities*, 1977, *10*, 236–240.

Block, J., Block, J. H., & Harrington, D. M. Some misgivings about the Matching Familiar Figures Test as a measure of reflection-impulsivity. *Developmental Psychology*, 1974, *10*, 611–632.

Block, J., Block, J. H., & Harrington, D. M. Comment on the Kagan–Messer reply. *Developmental Psychology*, 1975, *11*, 249–252.

Bloom, K. Social elicitation of infant vocal behavior. *Journal of Experimental Child Psychology*, 1975, *19*, 209–222.

Blouin, A. G. A., Bornstein, R., & Trites, R. Teen-age alcohol use among hyperactive children: A 5-year follow-up study. *Journal of Pediatric Psychology*, 1978, *3*, 188–194.

Blumenthal, D. S., Burke, R., & Shapiro, A. K. The validity of "identical matching placebos." *Archives of General Psychiatry*, 1974, *31*, 214–215.

Blunden, D., Spring, C., & Greenberg, L. Validation of the classroom behavior inventory. *Journal of Consulting and Clinical Psychology*, 1974, *42*, 84–88.

Boileau, R. A., Ballard, J. E., Sprague, R. L., Sleator, E. K., & Massey, B. H. Effect of methylphenidate on cardiorespiratory responses in hyperactive children. *Research Quarterly*, 1976, *47*, 590–596.

Boileau, V. K. New techniques in brief psychotherapy. *Psychological Reports*, 1958, *4*, 627–645.

Bok, S. The ethics of giving placebos. *Scientific American*, 1974, *231*, 17–23.

Bond, E. D., & Appel, K. E. *The treatment of behavior disorders following encephalitis.* New York: Commonwealth Fund, Division of Publications, 1931.

Borland, B. L. Social adaptation in men who were hyperactive: A follow-up study of hyperactive boys and their brothers. In L. Bellak (Ed.), *Psychiatric aspects of minimal brain dysfunction in adults.* New York: Grune and Stratton, 1979.

Borland, B. L., & Heckman, H. K. Hyperactive boys and their brothers: A 25-year follow-up study. *Archives of General Psychiatry*, 1976, *33*, 669–675.

Bornstein, P. H., & Quevillon, R. P. The effects of a self-instructional package on overactive preschool boys. *Journal of Applied Behavior Analysis*, 1976, *9*, 179–188.

Bosco, J. J., & Robin, S. S. The treatment of hyperkinetic children: Public policy and controversial health problems. Paper presented at the annual meeting of the American Public Health Association, New York, November 1979.

Bosco, J. J., & Robin, S. S. Hyperkinesis: Prevalence and treatment. In C. K. Whalen & B. Henker (Eds.), *Hyperactive children: The social ecology of identification and treatment.* New York: Academic Press, 1980.

Bower, G. H. Mood and memory. *American Psychologist*, 1981, *36*, 129–148.

Bradley, C. The behavior of children receiving benzedrine. *American Journal of Psychiatry*, 1937, *94*, 577–585.

Bradley, C. Characteristics and management of children with behavior problems associated with organic brain damage. *Pediatric Clinics of North America*, 1957, *4*, 1049–1060.

Braud, L. The effects of frontal EMG biofeedback and progressive relaxation upon hyperactivity and its behavioral concomitants. *Biofeedback and Self-Regulation*, 1978, *3*, 69–89.

Braud, L. W., Lupin, M. N., & Braud, W. G. The use of electromyographic biofeedback in the control of hyperactivity. *Journal of Learning Disabilities*, 1975, *3*, 420–425.

Brazelton, T. B. Psychophysiologic reaction of the neonate: I. The value of observation of the neonate. *Journal of Pediatrics*, 1961, *58*, 508–512.

Bremer, D. A., & Stern, J. A. Attention and distractibility during reading in hyperactive boys. *Journal of Abnormal Child Psychology*, 1976, *4*, 381–387.

Bremness, A. B., & Sverd, J. Methylphenidate-induced Tourette syndrome: Case report. *American Journal of Psychiatry*, 1979, *136*, 1334–1335.

Brenner, A. Trace mineral levels in hyperactive children responding to the Feingold diet. *Journal of Pediatrics*, 1979, *94*, 944–945.

Breunlin, C., & Breunlin, D. C. The family therapy approach to adolescent disturbances: A review of the literature. *Journal of Adolescence*, 1979, *2*, 153–169.

Bromwich, R. M. Focus on maternal behavior in infant intervention. *American Journal of Orthopsychiatry*, 1976, *46*, 439–446.

Bronfenbrenner, U. The origins of alienation. *Scientific American*, 1974, *231*, 53–61.

Bronfenbrenner, U. *The ecology of human development.* Cambridge, MA: Harvard University Press, 1979a.

Bronfenbrenner, U. Contexts of child rearing: Problems and prospects. *American Psychologist*, 1979b, *34*, 844–850.

Browder, J. A. Appropriate use of psychic drugs in school children. *American Journal of Diseases in Children*, 1972, *124*, 606–607.

Brown, D., Winsberg, B. G., Bialer, I., & Press, M. Imipramine therapy and seizures: Three children treated for hyperactive behavior disorders. *American Journal of Psychiatry*, 1973, *130*, 210–212.

Brown, J., Montgomery, R., & Barclay, J. An example of psychologist management of teacher reinforcement procedures in the elementary classroom. *Psychology in the Schools*, 1969, *6*, 336–340.

Bruck, C. Battle lines in the Ritalin war. *Human Behavior*, 1976, *5*, 25–33.

Brumback, R. A., & Weinberg, W. A. Relationship of hyperactivity and depression in children. *Perceptual and Motor Skills*, 1977, *45*, 247–251.

Buchan, B., Swap, S., & Swap, W. Teacher identification of hyperactive children in preschool settings. *Exceptional Children*, 1977, *43*, 314–315.

Buchsbaum, M., & Wender, P. H. Average evoked responses in normal and minimally brain dysfunctioned children treated with amphetamine: A preliminary report. *Archives of General Psychiatry*, 1973, *29*, 764–770.

Buckalew, L. W., Ross, S., & Lewis, M. J. Behavioral teratology: A formalization. *Journal of Pediatric Psychology*, 1979, *4*, 323–330.

Bugental, D. B., Whalen, C. K., & Henker, B. Causal attributions of hyperactive children and motivational assumptions of two behavior-change approaches: Evidence for an interactionist position. *Child Development*, 1977, *48*, 874–884.

Burg, C., Hart, D., Quinn, P. O., & Rapoport, J. L. Clinical evaluation of one-year-old infants: Possible predictors of risk for the "hyperactivity syndrome."*Journal of Pediatric Psychology*, 1978, *3*, 164–167.

Burg, C., Rapoport, J. L., Bartley, L. S., Quinn, P. O., & Timmins, P. Newborn minor physical anomalies and problem behavior at age three. *American Journal of Psychiatry*, 1980, *137*, 791–796.

Burns, B. J. The effect of self-directed verbal commands on arithmetic performance and activity level of urban hyperactive children. Unpublished doctoral dissertation, Boston College, 1972.

Buss, A. H., & Plomin, R. *A temperament theory of personality development.* New York: Wiley, 1975.

Butter, H. J., & Lapierre, Y. D. The effect of methylphenidate on sensory perception and integration in hyperactive children. *International Pharmacopsychiatry*, 1974, *9*, 235–244.

Butter, H. J., Lapierre, Y. D., Laprade, K., Firestone, P., Côté, A., & Pierre-Louis, F. A comparative study of the efficacy of ACTH $_{4-9}$ (Org. 2766) and methylphenidate on hyperkinetic behavior. Unpublished paper, University of Ottawa, Department of Psychiatry, 1979.

Byers, R. K., & Lord, E. E. Late effects of lead poisoning on mental development. *American Journal of Diseases of Children*, 1943, *66*, 471–494.

Cadoret, R. J., & Gath, A. Biologic correlates of hyperactivity: Evidence for a genetic factor. In S. B. Sells (Ed.), *Life history research in psychopathology*, Vol. 5. In press, 1982.

Cairns, E., & Cammock, T. Development of a more reliable version of the Matching Familiar Figures Test. *Developmental Psychology*, 1978, *14*, 555–560.

Calhoun, M. L. Teachers' causal attributions for child's hyperactivity: Race, socioeconomic status, and typicalness. *Perceptual and Motor Skills*, 1975, *41*, 195–198.

Cameron, J. R. Parental treatment, children's temperament and the risk of childhood behavioral problems: I. Relationships between parental characteristics and changes in children's temperament over time. *American Journal of Orthopsychiatry*, 1977, *47*, 568–576.

Cameron, J. R. Parental treatment, children's temperament, and the risk of childhood behavioral problems. II. Initial temperament, parental attitudes, and the incidence and form of behavioral problems. *American Journal of Orthopsychiatry*, 1978, *48*, 140–147.

Cameron, M. I., & Robinson, V. M. J. Effects of cognitive training on academic and off-task behavior of hyperactive children. *Journal of Abnormal Child Psychology*, 1980, *8*, 405–419.

Camp, J. A., Phil, M., Bialer, I., Sverd, J., & Winsberg, B. G. Clinical usefulness of the NIMH physical and neurological examination for soft signs. *American Journal of Psychiatry*, 1978, *135*, 362–364.

Campbell, E. S., & Redfering, D. L. Relationship among environmental and demographic variables and teacher-rated hyperactivity. *Journal of Abnormal Child Psychology*, 1979, *1*, 77–81.

Campbell, S. B. Mother–child interaction in reflective, impulsive, and hyperactive children. *Developmental Psychology*, 1973, *8*, 341–349.

Campbell, S. B. Mother–child interaction: A comparison of hyperactive, learning disabled, and normal boys. *American Journal of Orthopsychiatry*, 1975, *45*, 51–57.

Campbell, S. B. Hyperactivity: Course and treatment. In A. Davids (Ed.), *Child personality and psychopathology: Current topics*. Vol. 3. New York: Wiley, 1976.

Campbell, S. B. Mother–infant interaction as a function of maternal ratings of temperament. *Child Psychiatry and Human Development*, 1979a, *10*, 67–76.

Campbell, S. B. Personal communication, 1979b.

Campbell, S. B., Douglas, V. I., & Morgenstern, G. Cognitive styles in hyperactive children and the effect of methylphenidate. *Journal of Child Psychology and Psychiatry*, 1971, *12*, 55–67.

Campbell, S. B., Endman, M. W., & Bernfeld, G. A three-year follow-up of hyperactive preschoolers into elementary school. *Journal of Child Psychology and Psychiatry*, 1977, *18*, 239–249.

Campbell, S. B., & Paulauskas, S. Peer relations in hyperactive children. *Journal of Child Psychology and Psychiatry*, 1979, *20*, 233–246.

Campbell, S. B., Schleifer, M., & Weiss, G. Continuities in maternal reports and child behaviors over time in hyperactive and comparison groups. *Journal of Abnormal Child Psychology*, 1978, *6*, 33–45.

Campbell, S. B., Schleifer, M., Weiss, G., & Perlman, T. A two-year follow-up of hyperactive preschoolers. *American Journal of Orthopsychiatry*, 1977, *47*, 149–162.

Cantwell, D. P. Psychiatric illness in the families of hyperactive children. *Archives of General Psychiatry*, 1972, *27*, 414–417.

Cantwell, D. P. Early intervention with hyperactive children. *Journal of Operational Psychiatry*, 1974, *5*, 56–67.

Cantwell, D. P. The hyperactive child syndrome: Clinical aspects. In D. P. Cantwell (Ed.), *The hyperactive child*. New York: Spectrum, 1975a.

Cantwell, D. P. Genetic studies of hyperactive children. In R.R. Fieve, D. Rosenthal, & H. Brill (Eds.), *Genetic research in psychiatry*. Baltimore: John Hopkins University Press, 1975b.

Cantwell, D. P. Genetics of hyperactivity. *Journal of Child Psychology and Psychiatry*, 1975c, *16*, 261–264.

Cantwell, D. P. CNS activating drugs in the treatment of the hyperactive child. In J. P. Brady & H. K. Brodie (Eds.), *Controversy in psychiatry*. Philadelphia: Saunders, 1978a.

Cantwell, D. P. Hyperactivity and antisocial behavior. *American Academy of Child Psychiatry*, 1978b, *17*, 252–262.

Cantwell, D. P. The "hyperactive" child. *Hospital Practice*, 1979, *14*, 65–73.

Cantwell, D. P. Use of stimulant medication with psychiatrically disordered adolescents. In S. C. Feinstein & P. L. Giovacchini (Eds.), *Adolescent psychiatry: Developmental and clinical studies*, Vol. 7. New York: Basic Books, 1979a.

Cantwell, D. P. A clinician's guide to the use of stimulant medication for the psychiatric disorders of children. *Developmental and Behavioral Pediatrics*, 1980, *1*, 133–140.

Cantwell, D. P. Personal communication, 1980a.

Cantwell, D. P., & Carlson, G. A. Stimulants. In J. S. Werry (Ed.), *Pediatric Psychopharmacology*. New York: Brunner/Mazel, 1978.

Cantwell, D. P., & Satterfield, J. H. The prevalence of academic underachievement in hyperactive children. *Journal of Pediatric Psychology*, 1978, *3*, 168–171.

Cappella, B., Gentile, J. R., & Juliano, D. B. Time estimation by hyperactive and normal children. *Perceptual and Motor Skills*, 1977, *44*, 787–790.

Carey, W. B. A simplified method for measuring infant temperament. *Journal of Pediatrics*, 1970, *77*, 188–194.

Carey, W. B. Clinical applications of infant temperament measurements. *Journal of Pediatrics*, 1972, *81*, 823–828.

Carey, W. B., & McDevitt, S. C. A revision of the Infant Temperament Questionnaire. *Pediatrics*, 1978, *61*, 735–739.

Carter, E. N., & Reynolds, J. N. Imitation in the treatment of a hyperactive child. *Psychotherapy: Theory, Research & Practice*, 1976, *13*, 160–161.

Casey, P. The hyperactive child: Review and suggested management. *Texas Medicine*, 1977, *73*, 68–75.

Casey, P., Sharp, M., & Loda, F. Child-health supervision for children under two years of age: A review of its content and effectiveness. *Journal of Pediatrics*, 1979, *95*, 1–9.

Center for Disease Control. Preventing lead poisoning in young children. Atlanta, GA. 1978.

Chaiklin, H. The treadmill of lead. *American Journal of Orthopsychiatry*, 1979, *49*, 571–573.

Chamberlin, R. W. Convulsions and Ritalin? (letter). *Pediatrics*, 1974, *54*, 658–659.

Chamberlin, R. W. Authoritarian and accommodive child rearing styles: Their relationships with the behavior patterns of 2-year-old children and with other variables. *Journal of Pediatrics*, 1974, *84*, 287–293.

Chamberlin, R. W. Parental use of "positive contact" in child rearing: Its relationship to child behavior patterns and other variables. *Pediatrics*, 1975, *56*, 768–773.

Chamberlin, R. W. The use of teacher checklists to identify children at risk for later behavior and emotional problems. *American Journal of Diseases of Children*, 1976, *130*, 141–145.

Chapin, R. C. The legal rights of children with handicapping conditions and the process of mainstreaming. *Peabody Journal of Education*, 1978, *56*, 18–23.

Chedd, G. Who shall be born? *Science 81*, 1981, *2*, 32–41.

Chess, S. Diagnosis and treatment of the hyperactive child. *New York State Journal of Medicine*, 1960, *60*, 2379–2385.

Chess, S. Hyperactive children: A rational approach to medication. *Urban Review*, 1972, *5*, 33–35.

Chess, S. Development theory revisited: Findings of longitudinal study. *Canadian Journal of Psychiatry*, 1979, *24*, 101–112.

Chess, S., Thomas, A., Rutter, M., & Birch, H. G. Interaction of temperament and environment in the production of behavioral disturbances in children. *American Journal of Psychiatry*, 1963, *120*, 142–148.

Childers, A. T. Hyperactivity in children having behavior disorders. *American Journal of Orthopsychiatry*, 1935, *5*, 227–243.

Chiong, B. N. The evidence against the catecholamine hypothesis. *Psychiatric Opinion*, 1979, *16*, 10–12.

Chisolm, J. J., Jr. Current status of lead exposure and poisoning in children. *Southern Medical Journal*, 1976, *69*, 529–531.

Christensen, D. Effects of combining methylphenidate and a classroom token system in modifying hyperactive behavior. *American Journal of Mental Deficiency*, 1975, *80*, 226–276.

Clark, L. P. Psychology of essential epilepsy. *Journal of Nervous and Mental Disease*, 1926, *63*, 575–585.

Clark, M. The curse of hyperactivity. *Newsweek*, June 23, 1980, 59–60, 62.

Clarkin, J. F., Frances, A. J., & Moodie, J. L. Selection criteria for family therapy. *Family Process*, 1979, *18*, 391–403.

Clarren, S. K., & Smith, D. W. Letter to the editor. *New England Journal of Medicine*, 1978a, *298*, 556.

Clarren, S. K., & Smith, D. W. The fetal alcohol syndrome. *New England Journal of Medicine*, 1978b, *298*, 1063–1067.

Clements, S. D. *Task Force One: Minimal brain dysfunction in children*. National Institute of Neurological Diseases and Blindness, Monograph No. 3, U. S. Department of Health, Education and Welfare, 1966.

Clements, S. D., & Peters, J. E. Minimal brain dysfunctions in the school-age child. *Archives of General Psychiatry*. 1962, *6*, 185–197.

Clements, S. D., & Peters, J. E. Psychoeducational programming for children with minimal brain dysfunctions. *Annals of the New York Academy of Sciences*, 1973, *205*, 46–51.

Close, J. Scored neurological examination.*Psychopharmacology Bulletin*, National Institute of Mental Health, Washington, DC, 1973, pp. 142–150.

Cohen, M. I. Editorial comment: The reference standard. *Journal of Pediatrics*, 1975, *86*, 167–168.

Cohen, M. J. *Drugs and the special child*. New York: Gardner Press, 1979.

Cohen, N. J., Douglas, V. I., & Morgenstern, G. The effect of methylphenidate on attentive behavior and autonomic activity in hyperactive children. *Psychopharmacologia*, 1971, *22*, 282–294.

Cohen, N. J., Sullivan, S., Minde, K. K., Novak, C., & Helwig, C. Evaluation of the relative effectiveness of methylphenidate and cognitive behavior modification in the treatment of kindergarten-aged hyperactive children. *Journal of Abnormal Child Psychology*, 1981, *9*, 43–54.

Cohen, N. J., Weiss, G., & Minde, K. Cognitive styles in adolescents previously diagnosed as hyperactive. *Journal of Child Psychology and Psychiatry*, 1972, *13*, 203–209.

Cole, J. O. (Moderator). General discussion. In L. Bellak (Ed.), *Psychiatric aspects of minimal brain dysfunction in adults*. New York: Grune and Stratton, 1979, pp. 68–69.

Cole, J. O. Drug therapy of adult minimal brain dysfunction (MBD). In J. O. Cole (Ed.), *Psychopharmacology update*. Lexington, MA: Collamore Press, 1980.

Coleman, M. Serotonin levels in whole blood of hyperactive children. *Journal of Pediatrics*, 1971, *78*, 985–990.

Coleman, N., Dexheimer, P., DiMascio, A., Redman, W., & Finnerty, R. Deanol in the treatment of hyperkinetic children. *Psychosomatics*, 1976, *17*, 68–72.

Collard, R. R. Review of Bayley Scales of Infant Development (1969). In O. K. Buros (Ed.), *The seventh mental measurements yearbook*, Vol. 1. Highland Park, NJ: Gryphon Press, 1972, pp. 727–729.

Collins, B. E., Whalen, C. K., & Henker, B. Ecological and pharmacological influences on behaviors in the classroom: The hyperkinetic behavioral syndrome. In S. Salzinger, J. Antrobus, and J. Glick (Eds.), *The ecosystem of the "sick" child*. New York: Academic Press, 1980.

• Conners, C. K. A teacher rating scale for use in drug studies with children. *American Journal of Psychiatry*, 1969, *126*, 885–888.

Conners, C. K. Symptom patterns in hyperkinetic, neurotic, and normal children. *Child Development*, 1970, *41*, 667–682.

Conners, C. K. Symposium: Behavior modification by drugs. II. Psychological effects of stimulant drugs in children with minimal brain dysfunction. *Pediatrics*, 1972, *49*, 702–708.

Conners, C. K. Rating scales for use in drug studies with children. *Psychopharmacology Bulletin* (Special issue, Pharmacotherapy of Children), 1973a, 24–84.

Conners, C. K. A clinical comparison of methylphenidate and placebo in the treatment of children with minimal brain dysfunction. Paper presented at the meeting of the American Psychological Association, Montreal, August 1973b.

Conners, C. K. Deanol and behavior disorders in children: A critical review of the literature and recommended future studies for determining efficacy. *Psychopharmacology Bulletin* (Special issue: Pharmacotherapy of Children), 1973c, 188–195.

Conners, C. K. A placebo-crossover study of caffeine treatment of hyperkinetic children. *International Journal of Mental Health*, 1975a, *4*, 132–143.

Conners, C. K. Minimal brain dysfunction and psychopathology in children. In A. Davids (Ed.), *Child personality and psychopathology: Current topics*, Vol. 2. New York: Wiley, 1975b.

Conners, C. K. Methodological considerations in drug research with children. In J. M. Wiener (Ed.), *Psychopharmacology in childhood and adolescence*. New York: Basic Books, 1977.

Conners, C. K. Discussion of "Models of hyperactivity." In R. L. Trites (Ed.), *Hyperactivity in children*. Baltimore: University Park Press, 1979a.

Conners, C. K. Application of biofeedback to treatment of children. *American Academy of Child Psychiatry*, 1979b, *18*, 143–153.

Conners, C. K. The acute effects of caffeine on evoked response, vigilance, and activity level in hyperkinetic children. *Journal of Abnormal Child Psychology*, 1979c, *7*, 145–151.

Conners, C. K. *Food additives and hyperactive children*. New York: Plenum, 1980.

Conners, C. K., & Blouin, A. Hyperkinetic syndrome and psychopathology in children. In B. B. Lahey (Chair), *Is there an independent syndrome of hyperactivity in children?* Symposium presented at the meeting of the American Psychological Association, Montreal, September 1980.

Conners, C. K., Denhoff, E., Millichap, J. G., & O'Leary, S. G. Take a slow approach to hyperkinesis. *Patient Care*, June 15, 1978, *12*, 22–78.

Conners, C. K., Eisenberg, L., & Barcai, A. Effect of dextroamphetamine in children. *Archives of General Psychiatry*, 1967, *17*, 478–485.

Conners, C. K., Goyette, G. H., & Newman, E. B. Dose-time effect of artificial colors in hyperactive children. *Journal of Learning Disabilities*, 1980, *13*, 512–516.

Conners, C. K., Goyette, C. H., Southwick, D. A., Lees, J. M., & Andrulonis, P. Food additives and hyperkinesis. *Pediatrics*, 1976, *58*, 154–166.

Conners, C. K., & Rothschild, G. H. Drugs and learning in children. In J. Hellmuth (Ed.), *Learning Disorders*, Vol. 3. Seattle, WA: Special Child Publications, 1968.

Conners, C. K., & Taylor, E. Pemoline, methylphenidate, and placebo in children with minimal brain dysfunction. *Archives of General Psychiatry*, 1980, *37*, 922–930.

Conners, C. K., Taylor, E., Meo, G., Kurtz, M. A., & Fournier, M. Magnesium pemoline and dextroamphetamine: A controlled study in children with minimal brain dysfunction. *Psychopharmacologia*, 1972, *26*, 321–336.

Conners, C. K., & Wells, K. C. Method and theory for psychopharmacology with children. In R. L. Trites (Ed.), *Hyperactivity in children*. Baltimore: University Park Press, 1979.

Conners, C. K., & Werry, J. S. Pharmocotherapy of psychopathology in children. In H. Quay & J. S. Werry (Eds.), *Psychopathological disorders of childhood* (2nd ed.). New York: Wiley, 1979.

Conrad, P. The discovery of hyperkinesis: Notes on the medicalization of deviant behavior. *Social Problems*, 1975, *23*, 12–21.

Conrad, W. G., Dworkin, E. S., Shai, A., & Tobiessen, J. E. Effects of amphetamine therapy and prescriptive tutoring on the behavior and achievement of lower class hyperactive children. *Journal of Learning Disabilities*, 1971, *4*, 509–517.

Conrad, W. G., & Insel, J. Anticipating the response to amphetamine therapy in the treatment of hyperkinetic children. *Pediatrics*, 1967, *40*, 96–98.

Conway, A. An evaluation of drugs in the elementary schools: Some geographic considerations. *Journal of Psychology in the Schools*, 1976, *13*, 442–444.

Cook, P. S., & Woodhill, J. M. The Feingold dietary treatment of the hyperkinetic syndrome. *The Medical Journal of Australia*, 1976, *2*, 85–90.

Copeland, A. P. Types of private speech produced by hyperactive and nonhyperactive boys. *Journal of Abnormal Child Psychology*, 1979, *7*, 169–177.

Copeland, A. P., & Weissbrod, C. S. Effects of modeling on hyperactivity-related behavior. Paper presented at the meeting of the American Psychological Association, San Francisco, 1977.

Copeland, A. P., & Weissbrod, C. S. Behavioral correlates of the hyperactivity factor of the Conners Teacher Questionnaire. *Journal of Abnormal Child Psychology*, 1978, *6*, 339–343.

Copeland, L. Nonstop Timmy, our two-year-old terror. *Redbook Magazine*, 1971, *137*, 38–41.

Cornwall, T. P., & Freeman, D. F. The hyperactive child with primary emotional problems. *Psychiatric Opinion*, 1980, *17*, 35–38.

Cowen, E. L. Social and community interventions. *Annual Review of Psychology*, 1973, *24*, 423–472.

Cowen, E. L., Pederson, A., Babijian, H., Izzo, L., & Trost, M. A. Long-term follow-up of early detected vulnerable children. *Journal of Consulting and Clinical Psychology*, 1973, *41*, 438–446.

Cowen, E. L., Trost, M. A., Lorion, R. P., Dorr, D., Izzo, L. D., & Isaccson, R. V. *New ways in school mental health: Early detection and prevention of school maladaption*. New York: Human Science Press, 1975.

Creedon, M. P. Adolescent Parenting Program: Comprehensive prenatal and postnatal care. *Journal of Current Adolescent Medicine*, 1980, *2*, 11–22.

Cromwell, R. L., Baumeister, A., & Hawkins, W. F. Research in activity level. In N. R. Ellis (Ed.), *Handbook of mental deficiency*. New York: McGraw-Hill, 1963.

Crook, W. G. Can what a child eats make him dull, stupid, or hyperactive? *Journal of Learning Disabilities*, 1980, *13*, 53–58.

Crowe, P. B. *Aspects of body image in children with the symptoms of hyperkinesis*. Unpublished dissertation, George Washington University, 1972.

Cruickshank, W. M., Bentzen, F. A., Ratzeburg, F. H., & Tannhauser, M. T. *A teaching method of brain injured and hyperactive children*. Syracuse, NY: Syracuse University Press, 1961.

Csikszentmihalyi, M., Larson, R., & Prescott, S. The ecology of adolescent activity and experience. *Journal of Youth and Adolescence*, 1977, *6*, 281–294.

Cunningham, C. E., & Barkley, R. A. The effects of methylphenidate on the mother–child interaction of hyperactive identical twins. *Developmental Medicine and Child Neurology*, 1978a, *20*, 634–642.

Cunningham, C. E., & Barkley, R. A. The role of academic failure in hyperactive behavior. *Journal of Learning Disabilities*, 1978b, *11*, 15–21.

Cunningham, C. E., & Barkley, R. A. The interactions of normal and hyperactive children with their mothers in free play and structured tasks. *Child Development*, 1979, *50*, 217–224.

Cunningham, C. E., Siegel, L., & Offord, D. Peer relations among hyperactive children. Paper presented at the meeting of the American Psychological Association, Montreal, September 1980.

Cylert Monograph. Abbott Laboratories, Chicago, 1975.

Dalby, J. T. Environmental effects on prenatal development. *Journal of Pediatric Psychology*, 1978, *3*, 105–109.

Dalby, J. T., Kapelus, G. J., Swanson, J. M., Kinsbourne, M., & Roberts, W. An examination of the double-blind design in drug research with hyperactive children. *Progress in Neuro-Psychopharmacology*, 1978, *2*, 123–127.

Dalby, J. T., Kinsbourne, M., Swanson, J. M., & Sobol, M. P. Hyperactive children's underuse of learning time: Correction by stimulant treatment. *Child Development*, 1977, *48*, 1448–1453.

Daniels, L. K. Parental treatment of hyperactivity in a child with ulcerative colitis. *Journal of Behavior Therapy and Experimental Psychiatry*, 1973, *4*, 183–185.

David, O. J. Association between lower level lead concentrations and hyperactivity in children. *Environmental Health Perspectives*, 1974, No.7, 17–25.

David, O. J., Clark, J., & Hoffman, S. Childhood lead poisoning: A reevaluation. *Archives of Environmental Health*, 1979, *34*, 106–111.

David, O. J., Clark, J., & Voeller, K. Lead and hyperactivity. *Lancet*, 1972, *2*, 900–903.

David, O. J., Hoffman, S., & Koltun, A. Threshold levels and lead toxicity. *Psychopharmacology Bulletin*, 1978, *14*, 50–53.

David, O. J., Hoffman, S. P., Sverd, J., & Clark, J. Lead and hyperactivity: Lead levels among hyperactive children. *Journal of Abnormal Child Psychology*, 1977, *5*, 405–416.

David, O. J., Hoffman, S. P., Sverd, J., Clark, J., & Voeller, K. Lead and hyperactivity. Behavioral response to chelation: A pilot study. *American Journal of Psychiatry*, 1976, *133*, 1155–1158.

Davids, A. An objective instrument for assessing hyperkinesis in children. *Journal of Learning Disabilities*, 1971, *4*, 499–501.

DeFilippis, N. A. Source of data as a factor in assessing symptoms of hyperkinesis. *Journal of Consulting and Clinical Psychology*, 1979a, *47*, 1115–1116.

DeFilippis, N. A. The historical development of the diagnostic concept of childhood hyperkinesis. *Clinical Neuropsychology*, 1979b, *1*, 15–19.

DeFries, J. C., & Plomin, R. Behavioral genetics. *Annual Review of Psychology*, 1978, *29*, 473–515.

Delamater, A. M., Lahey, B. B., & Drake, L. Toward an empirical subclassification of "learning disabilities": A psychophysiological comparison of "hyperactive" and "nonhyperactive" subgroups. *Journal of Abnormal Child Psychology*, 1981, *9*, 65–77.

DeLong, A. R. What have we learned from psychoactive drug research on hyperactives? *American Journal of Diseases of Children*, 1972, *123*, 177–180.

Denckla, M. B., & Rudel, R. G. Anomalies of motor development in hyperactive boys. *Annals of Neurology*, 1978, *3*, 231–233.

Denhoff, E. The natural life history of children with minimal brain dysfunction. *Annals of the New York Academy of Sciences,* 1973, *205,* 188–205.

Denhoff, E., Davids, A., & Hawkins, W. F. Research in activity level: A controlled double-blind study. *Journal of Learning Disabilities,* 1971, *4,* 491–498.

Denhoff, E., Hainsworth, P. K., & Hainsworth, M. S. The child at risk for learning disorder. *Clinical Pediatrics,* 1972, *11,* 164–170.

Diagnostic and statistical manual of mental disorders (2nd ed.). Washington, D. C.: American Psychiatric Association, 1968.

Diagnostic and statistical manual of mental disorders (3rd ed.). Washington, D. C.: American Psychiatric Association, 1980.

Diamond, M. C. Uppers and downers in the air. *Psychology Today,* 1980, *14,* 128.

Diamond, M. C., Connor, J. R., Jr., Orenberg, E. K., Bissell, M., Yost, M., & Krueger, A. Environmental influences on serotonin and cyclic nucleotides in rat cerebral cortex. *Science,* 1980, *210,* 652–654.

Dickinson, L. C., Lee, J., Ringdahl, I. C., Schedewie, H. K., Kilgore, B. S., & Elders, M. J. Impaired growth in hyperkinetic children receiving pemoline. *Journal of Pediatrics,* 1979, *94,* 538–541.

Diller, L. H., & Gofman, H. F. The biopsychosocial vulnerability of the hyperactive child: A case study of a treatment approach. Unpublished manuscript, University of California, San Francisco, 1981.

Divoky, D. Behavior and food coloring: Lessons of a diet fad. *Psychology Today,* 1978, *12,* 145–148.

Doll, E. A., Phelps, W. M., & Melcher, R. T. *Mental deficiency due to birth injuries.* New York: MacMillan, 1932.

Doster, J. T. Differential base rates of hyperactive behavior in open and closed classrooms. Paper presented at the meeting of the American Psychological Association, San Francisco, August 1977.

Doubros, S. G., & Daniels, G. J. An experimental approach to the reduction of overactive behavior. *Behavior Research and Therapy,* 1966, *4,* 251–258.

Douglas, V. I. Stop, look and listen: The problem of sustained attention and impulse control in hyperactive and normal children. *Canadian Journal of Behavioural Science,* 1972, *4,* 259–282.

Douglas, V. I. Sustained attention and impulse control: Implications for the handicapped child. In J. A. Swets & L. L. Elliott (Eds.), *Psychology and the handicapped child.* Washington, D. C.: U. S. Department of Health, Education and Welfare. DHEW Pub. No. (OE) 73–05000, 1974.

Douglas, V. I. Are drugs enough? To treat or train the hyperactive child. *International Journal of Mental Health,* 1975, *4* (1–2), 199–212.

Douglas, V. I. Research on hyperactivity: Stage two. *Journal of Abnormal Child Psychology,* 1976, *4,* 307–308.

Douglas, V. I. Treatment and training approaches to hyperactivity: Establishing internal or external control. In C. K. Whalen & B. Henker (Eds.), *Hyperactive children: The social ecology' of identification and treatment.* New York: Academic Press, 1980a.

Douglas, V. I. Higher mental processes in hyperactive children: Implications for training. In R. M. Knights & D. J. Bakker (Eds.), *Rehabilitation, treatment and management of learning ι disorders.* Baltimore: University Park Press, 1980b.

Douglas, V. I., Parry, P., Marton, P., & Garson, C. Assessment of a cognitive training program for hyperactive children. *Journal of Abnormal Child Psychology,* 1976, *4,* 389–410.

Douglas, V. I., & Peters, K. G. Toward a clearer definition of the attentional deficit of hyperactive children. In G. A. Hale & M. Lewis (Eds.), *Attention and the development of cognitive skills.* New York: Plenum, 1979.

Douglas, V. I., Weiss, G., & Minde, K. Learning disabilities in hyperactive children and the effect of methylphenidate. *Canadian Psychology,* 1969, *10,* 201 (Abstract).

Dowrick, P. W., & Raeburn, J. M. Video editing and medication to produce a therapeutic self model. *Journal of Consulting and Clinical Psychology,* 1977, *45,* 1156–1158.

Drash, P. W. Treatment of hyperactivity in the two-year-old. *Pediatric Psychology,* 1975, *3,* 17–20.

Drash, P. W. Personal communication, 1981.

Drash, P. W., Stolberg, A. L., & Bostow, D. E. Hyperactivity in preschool children as non-compliance: A new conceptual basis for treatment. Arlington, VA: ERIC Document Reproduction Service, ED 13000, microfiche, 1976.

Drash, P. W., Stolberg, A. L., & Bostow, D. E. Does hyperactivity mean non-compliance? A new conceptual basis for treatment. Unpublished manuscript, 1981.

Dreger, R. A progress report on a factor analytic approach to classification in child psychiatry. In J. Jenkins & J. Cole (Eds.), *Research Report No. 18.* Washington, D. C.: American Psychiatric Association, 1964.

Dubey, D. R. Organic factors in hyperkinesis: A critical evaluation. *American Journal of Orthopsychiatry,* 1976, *46,* 353–366.

Dubey, D. R. The hyperkinetic child: Current status. *Comprehensive Therapy,* 1981, in press.

Dubey, D. R., & Kaufman, K. F. Home management of hyperkinetic children. *Journal of Pediatrics,* 1978, *93,* 141–146.

Dubey, D. R., Kaufman, K. F., & O'Leary, S. G. Behavioral and reflective parent training for hyperactive children: A comparison. Paper presented at the annual meeting of the American Psychological Association, San Francisco, 1977.

Duehn, W. D., & Mayadas, N. S. Behavioral rehearsals in group counseling with parents. *Groups: Journal of Group Dynamics and Psychotherapy,* 1976, *7,* 13–23.

Dunn, H. UBC study of low birth weight babies yields exciting results. *UBC Reports,* 1979, *10,* 4–5.

Dunn, H. Personal communication, 1980.

Durlak, J. A. Description and evaluation of a behaviorally oriented school-based preventive mental health program. *Journal of Consulting and Clinical Psychology,* 1977, *45,* 27–33.

Duva, N. A. Effects of asymptomatic lead poisoning on psychoneurological functioning of school-age urban children: A follow-up study. Unpublished doctoral dissertation, Fordham University, 1977.

Dykman, R. A., & Ackerman, P. T. Hyperactive boys as adolescents. Paper presented at the meeting of the American Psychological Association, Chicago, 1975.

Dykman, R. A., McGrew, J., & Ackerman, P. T. A double-blind clinical study of pemoline in MBD children: Comments on the psychological test results. In C. K. Conners (Ed.), *Clinical use of stimulant drugs in children.* New York: American Elsevier, 1974.

Dykman, R. A., McGrew, J., Harris, T. S., Peters, J. E., & Ackerman, P. T. Two blinded studies of the effects of stimulant drugs on children: Pemoline, methylphenidate, and placebo. In R. P. Anderson and C. G. Halcomb (Eds.), *Learning disability/minimal brain dysfunction syndrome.* Springfield, IL: Charles C. Thomas, 1976.

Dykman, R. A., Peters, J. E., & Ackerman, P. T. Experimental approaches to the study of minimal brain dysfunction. *Annals of the New York Academy of Sciences,* 1973, *205,* 93–108.

Ebaugh, F. G. Neuropsychiatric sequelae of acute epidemic encephalitis in children. *American Journal of Diseases in Children*, 1923, *25*, 89–97.

Edwards, S. A. Hyperactivity as passive behavior. *Transactional Analysis Journal*, 1979, *9*, 60–62.

Edwards, S. A. Personal communication, 1981.

Egeland, B., & Weinberg, R. A. The Matching Familiar Figures Test: A look at its psychometric credibility. *Child Development*, 1976, *47*, 483–491.

Ehrenfest, H. Birth injuries of the child. *Gynecological and Obstetrical Monographs*. New York: Appleton, 1926.

Eisenberg, L. The management of the hyperkinetic child. *Developmental Medicine and Child Neurology*, 1966, *8*, 593–632.

Eisenberg, L. The hyperkinetic child and stimulant drugs. *New England Journal of Medicine*, 1972, *287*, 249–250.

Eisenberg, L., Gilbert, A., Cytryn, L., & Molling, P. A. The effectiveness of psychotherapy alone and in conjunction with perphenazine or placebo in the treatment of neurotic and hyperkinetic children. *American Journal of Psychiatry*, 1961, *117*, 1088–1093.

Eisenberg, M. Brief psychotherapy: A viable possibility with adolescents. *Psychotherapy: Theory, Research and Practice*, 1975, *12*, 187–191.

El-Guebaly, N., & Offord, D. R. The offspring of alcoholics: A critical review. *American Journal of Psychiatry*, 1977, *134*, 357–365.

Ellis, M. J., Witt, P. A., Reynolds, R., & Sprague, R. L. Methylphenidate and the activity of hyperactives in the informal setting. *Child Development*, 1974, *45*, 217–220.

Ellis, N. R., & Pryer, R. S. Quantification of gross bodily activity in children with severe neuropathology. *American Journal of Mental Deficiency*, 1959, *63*, 1034–1037.

Engel, G. C. The need for a new medical model: A challenge for biomedicine. *Science*, 1977, *196*, 129–136.

Epstein, L. C., Lasagna, L., Conners, C. K., & Rodriguez, A. Correlation of dextroamphetamine excretion and drug response in hyperkinetic children. *Journal of Nervous and Mental Diseases*, 1968, *146*, 136–146.

Erickson, M. H. Naturalistic techniques of hypnosis. *American Journal of Clinical Hypnosis*, 1958, *1*, 3–8.

Estes, W. K. Reinforcement in human behavior. *American Scientist*, 1972, *60*, 723–729.

Etzioni, A. Caution: Too many health warnings could be counterproductive. *Psychology Today*, 1978, *12*, 20, 22.

Eyberg, S. M., & Matarazzo, R. G. Training parents as therapists: A comparison between individual parent–child interaction training and parent group didactic training. *Journal of Clinical Psychology*, 1980, *36*, 492–499.

Fay, A. *Making things better by making them worse*. New York: Hawthorne Books, 1978.

Feighner, A. C., & Feighner, J. P. Multimodality treatment of the hyperkinetic child. *American Journal of Psychiatry*, 1974, *131*, 459–463.

Feinberg, I., Hibi, S., Braun, M., Cavness, C., Westerman, G., & Small, A. Sleep amphetamine effects in MBDs and normal subjects. *Archives of General Psychiatry*, 1974, *31*, 723–731.

Feingold, B. F. *Introduction to clinical allergy*. Springfield, IL: Charles C. Thomas, 1973a.

Feingold, B. F. Food additives and child development. *Hospital Practice*, 1973b, *8*, 11–12, 17–18, 21.

Feingold, B. F. *Why your child is hyperactive*. New York: Random House, 1975a.

Feingold, B. F. Hyperkinesis and learning disabilities linked to artificial food flavors and colors. *American Journal of Nursing*, 1975b, *75*, 797–803.

Feingold, B. F. Hyperkinesis and learning disabilities (H-LD) linked to the ingestion of artificial food colors and flavors. Paper presented to the U. S. Subcommittee on Health, September 1975c.

Feingold, B. F. Hyperkinesis and learning disabilities linked to the ingestion of artificial food colors and flavors. *Journal of Learning Disabilities*, 1976a, *9*, 551–559.

Feingold, B. F. Hyperactivity—Dr. Feingold replies. *The Science Show*, No. 54, Australian Broadcasting Commission, September 4, 1976b.

Feingold, B. F., German, D. F., Brahm, R. M., & Simmers, E. Adverse reaction to food additives. Paper presented at the Annual Meeting of the American Medical Association, New York, 1973.

Feingold, H., & Feingold, B. F. *The Feingold cookbook for hyperactive children and others with problems associated with food additives and salicylates.* New York: Random House, 1979.

Ferguson, H. B., & Pappas, B. A. Evaluation of psychophysiological, neurochemical, and animal models of hyperactivity. In R. L. Trites (Ed.), *Hyperactivity in children.* Baltimore: University Park Press, 1979.

Ferguson, H. B., Rapoport, J. L., & Weingartner, H. Food dyes and impairment of performance in hyperactive children. *Science*, 1981, *211*, 410–411.

Ferguson, H. B., Simpson, S., & Trites, R. L. Psychophysiological study of methylphenidate responders and nonresponders. In R. K. Knights & D. J. Bakker (Eds.), *Neuropsychology of learning disorders.* Baltimore: University Park Press, 1976.

Ferguson, H. B., & Trites, R. L. Predicting the response of hyperactive children to Ritalin. In R. M. Knights & D. J. Bakker (Eds.), *Treatment of hyperactive and learning disordered children.* Baltimore: University Park Press, 1980.

Ferrier, P. E., Nicod, I., & Ferrier, S. Fetal alcohol syndrome. *Lancet*, 1973, *2*, 1496.

Feshbach, N. D., & Feshbach, S. (Eds.). The changing status of children: Rights, roles and responsibilities. *Journal of Social Issues*, 1978, *34*, 1–196.

Fidone, G. S. Recognizing the precursors of failure in school. *Clinical Pediatrics*, 1975, *14*, 768–778.

Field, T. Games parents play with normal and high-risk infants. *Child Psychiatry and Human Development*, 1979, *10*, 41–48.

Field, T., Hallock, N., Ting, G., Dempsey, J., Dabiri, C., & Shuman, H. H. A first-year follow-up of high risk infants: Formulating a cumulative risk index. *Child Development*, 1978, *49*, 119–131.

Firestone, P., Davey, J., Goodman, J. T., & Peters, S. The effects of caffeine and methylphenidate on hyperactive children. *Journal of Child Psychiatry*, 1978, *17*, 445–456.

Firestone, P., & Douglas, V. The effects of reward and punishment on reaction times and autonomic activity in hyperactive and normal children. *Journal of Abnormal Child Psychology*, 1975, *3*, 201–216.

Firestone, P., Lewy, F., & Douglas, V. I. Hyperactivity and physical anomalies. *Canadian Psychiatric Association Journal*, 1976, *21*, 23–26.

Firestone, P., & Martin, J. E. An analysis of the hyperactive syndrome: A comparison of hyperactive, behavior problem, asthmatic and normal children. *Journal of Abnormal Child Psychology*, 1979, *7*, 261–263.

Firestone, P., Peters, S., Rivier, M., & Knights, R. M. Minor physical anomalies in hyperactive, retarded and normal children and their families. *Journal of Child Psychology and Psychiatry*, 1978, *19*, 155–160.

Firestone, P., Poitras-Wright, H., & Douglas, V. The effects of caffeine on hyperactive children. *Journal of Learning Disabilities*, 1978, *11*, 20–28.

Fischer, K. C., & Wilson, W. P. Methylphenidate and the hyperkinetic state. *Diseases of the Nervous System*, 1971, *32*, 695–698.

Fish, B. The "one child, one drug" myth of stimulants in hyperkinesis. *Archives of General Psychiatry*, 1971, *25*, 193–203.

Fisher, M. A. Dextroamphetamine and placebo practice effects on selective attention in hyperactive children. *Journal of Abnormal Child Psychology*, 1978, *6*, 25–32.

Fleischmann, D. J. Etiological subgrouping of hyperkinetic boys. Unpublished doctoral dissertation, University of Iowa, 1977.

Flynn, N. M., & Rapoport, J. L. Hyperactivity in open and traditional classroom environments. *Journal of Special Education*, 1976, *10*, 285–290.

Forehand, R., & Baumeister, A. A. Effects of variations in auditory-visual stimulation on activity levels of severe mental retardates. *American Journal of Mental Deficiency*, 1970, *74*, 470–474.

Fouts, G. T. Effect of social reinforcement on infant activity: A pilot study. Eric Document No. ED 103 103, PS 007604. Washington, D. C.: U. S. Department of Health, Education and Welfare, National Institute of Education, 1974.

Fowlie, B. A parent's guide to amphetamine treatment of hyperkinesis. *Journal of Learning Disabilities*, 1973, *6*, 352–355.

Fox, R. E. Family therapy. In I. B. Weiner (Ed.), *Clinical methods in psychology*. New York: Wiley, 1976.

Framo, J. L. Family theory and therapy. *American Psychologist*, 1979, *34*, 988–992.

Frank, J. Therapeutic factors in psychotherapy. *American Journal of Psychotherapy*, 1971, *25*, 350–361.

Frankenburg, W. K., & Dodds, J. B. The Denver Developmental Screening Test. *Journal of Pediatrics*, 1967, *71*, 181–191.

Fras, I. Alternating caffeine and stimulants (letter). *American Journal of Psychiatry*, 1974, *131*, 228–229.

Frazier, J. R., & Schneider, H. Parental management of inappropriate hyperactivity in a young retarded child. *Journal of Behavior Therapy and Experimental Psychiatry*, 1975, *6*, 246–247.

Freed, A. M. *TA for kids*. Sacramento, CA: Jalmar, 1971.

Freed, A. M. *TA for tots*. Sacramento, CA: Jalmar, 1973.

Freedman, D. Report on the conference on the use of stimulant drugs in the treatment of behaviorally disturbed young school children. Washington, D. C.: U. S. Department of Health, Education and Welfare, 1971.

Freedman, D. G. Discussant in A. Ambrose (Ed.), *Stimulation in early infancy*. New York: Academic Press, 1969, pp. 102–103.

Freedman, J. L. *Crowding and behavior: The psychology of high-density living*. New York: Viking, 1975.

Freeman, D. F., & Cornwall, T. P. Hyperactivity and neurosis. *American Journal of Orthopsychiatry*, 1980, *50*, 704–711.

Freeman, R. D. Minimal brain dysfunction, hyperactivity and learning disorders: Epidemic or episode? *University of Chicago School Review*, 1976, *85*, 5–30.

Freibergs, V., & Douglas, V. I. Concept learning in hyperactive and normal children. *Journal of Abnormal Psychology*, 1969, *74*, 388–395.

French, G. M., & Harlow, H. F. Locomotor reaction decrement in normal and brain damaged Rhesus monkeys. *Journal of Comparative and Physiological Psychology*, 1955, *48*, 496–501.

Freudenberger, H. J. New psychotherapy approaches with teenagers in a new world. *Psychotherapy: Theory, Research and Practice*, 1971, *8*, 38–43.

Frey, A. H. Behavioral biophysics. *Psychological Bulletin*, 1965, *63*, 322–337.

Fullard, W., McDevitt, S. C., & Carey, W. B. The Toddler Temperament Scale. Unpublished manuscript, 1978.

Furman, S., & Feighner, A. Video feedback in treating hyperkinetic children: A preliminary report. *American Journal of Psychiatry*, 1973, *130*, 792–795.

Gadow, K. D. *Children on medication: A primer for school personnel.* Reston, VA: Council on Exceptional Children, 1979.

Gadow, K. D. Drug therapy for hyperactivity: Treatment procedures in natural settings. In K. D. Gadow & J. Loney (Eds.), *Psychosocial aspects of drug treatment for hyperactivity.* Boulder, CO: Westview Press, 1981.

Gadow, K. D., & Loney, J. (Eds.). *Psychosocial aspects of drug treatment for hyperactivity.* Boulder, CO: Westview Press, 1981.

Gadow, K., & Sprague, R. An anterospective follow-up study of hyperactive children into adolescence: Licit and illicit drug use. Paper presented at the meeting of the American Psychological Association, Montreal, September 1980.

Gallagher, C. E. *Federal involvement in the use of behavior modification drugs on grammar school children* (Hearing before a subcommittee of the Committee of Government Operations, House of Representatives, September 29, 1970). Washington, D. C.: U. S. Government Printing Office, 1970.

Gallagher, J. J. New educational treatment models for children with minimal brain dysfunction. In F. F. de la Cruz, B. H. Fox, & R. H. Roberts (Eds.), *Minimal brain dysfunction. Annals of the New York Academy of Sciences*, 1973, *205*, 383–389.

Gallant, D. M. General discussion of adult brain dysfunction. In L. Bellak (Ed.), *Psychiatric aspects of minimal brain dysfunction in adults.* New York: Grune and Stratton, 1979.

Gallas, H. B. Teenage parenting: Social determinants and consequences. *Journal of Social Issues*, 1980, *36*, 1–6.

Gardner, R. A. *MBD: The family book about minimal brain dysfunction.* New York: Aronson, 1973.

Gardner, R. A. The Mutual Storytelling Technique in the treatment of psychogenic problems secondary to minimal brain dysfunction. *Journal of Learning Disabilities*, 1974, *7*, 135–143.

Gardner, R. A. Psychotherapy in minimal brain dysfunction. In J. H. Masserman (Ed.), *Current Psychiatric Therapies*, Vol. 15. New York: Grune and Stratton, 1975.

Gardner, W. I., Cromwell, R. L., & Foshee, J. G. Studies in activity level: II. Effects of distal visual stimulation in organics, familials, hyperactives, and hypoactives. *American Journal of Mental Deficiency*, 1959, *63*, 1028–1033.

Garfield, S. L., & Bergin, A. E. (Eds.). *Handbook of psychotherapy and behavior change: An empirical analysis* (2nd ed.). New York: Wiley, 1978.

Garfinkel, B., Webster, C., & Sloman, L. Methylphenidate and caffeine in the treatment of children with minimal brain dysfunction. *American Journal of Psychiatry*, 1975, *132*, 723–728.

Garmezy, N. DSM III: Never mind the psychologists: Is it good for the children? *Clinical Psychologist*, 1978, *31*(1), 4–6.

Garside, R. F., Birch, H. G., Scott, D. M., Chambers, S., Kolvin, I., Tweddle, E. G., & Barber, L. M. Dimensions of temperament in infant school children. *Journal of Child Psychology and Psychiatry*, 1975, *16*, 219–231.

Garson, C. Cognitive impulsivity in children and the effects of training. Unpublished doctoral dissertation, McGill University, 1977.

Gastaut, H. Combined photic and Metrazol activation of the brain. *Electroencephalography and Clinical Neurophysiology*, 1950, *2*, 249–261.

Gelfand, C. C. The effects of an altered interpersonal environment on minimally brain-damaged children. *Dissertation Abstracts International*, 1973, *34B*, 1274–1275.

Gerz, H. O. Experience with the logotherapeutic technique of paradoxical intervention in the treatment of phobic and obsessive-compulsive patients. *American Journal of Psychiatry,* 1966, *123,* 548–553.

Gibbs, F., Gibbs, E., Spies, H., & Carpenter, P. Common types of childhood encephalitis. *Archives of Neurology,* 1964, *10,* 1–11.

Gilfillan, S. C. Lead poisoning and the fall of Rome. *Journal of Occupational Medicine,* 1965, *7,* 53–60.

Gittelman, M. Rescuing parents: Therapies for the hyperkinetic child. *Behavioral Medicine,* 1979, *6,* 33–34.

Gittelman-Klein, R. Introduction: Recent advances in child psychopharmacology. *International Journal of Mental Health,* 1975, *4,* 3–10.

Gittelman-Klein, R., Abikoff, H., Pollack, E., Klein, D. F., Katz, S., & Mattes, J. A controlled trial of behavior modification and methylphenidate in hyperactive children. In C. K. Whalen & B. Henker (Eds.), *Hyperactive children: The social ecology of identification and treatment.* New York: Academic Press, 1980.

Gittelman-Klein, R., & Klein, D. F. Are behavioral and psychometric changes related in methylphenidate-treated, hyperactive children? *International Journal of Mental Health,* 1975, *4,* 182–198.

Gittelman-Klein, R., & Klein, D. F. Methylphenidate effects in learning disabilities. Psychometric changes. *Archives of General Psychiatry,* 1976, *33,* 655–664.

Gittelman-Klein, R., Klein, D. F., Abikoff, H., Katz, S., Gloisten, C., & Kates, W. Relative efficacy of methylphenidate and behavior modification in hyperkinetic children: An interim report. *Journal of Abnormal Child Psychology,* 1976, *4,* 361–379.

Gittelman-Klein, R., Klein, D. F., Katz, S., Saraf, K., & Pollack, E. Comparative effects of methylphenidate and thioridazine in hyperkinetic children. I. Clinical results. *Archives of General Psychiatry,* 1976, *33,* 1217–1231.

Glasser, W. *Schools without failure.* New York: Harper and Row, 1968.

Glow, P. H., & Glow, R. A. Hyperkinetic impulse disorder: A developmental defect of motivation. *Genetic Psychology Monographs,* 1979, *100,* 159–231.

Glow, R. A. Cross-validity and normative data on the Conners parent and teacher rating scales. In K. D. Gadow & J. Loney (Eds.), *Psychosocial aspects of drug treatment for hyperactivity.* Boulder, CO: Westview Press, 1981.

Glow, R. A., & Glow, P. H. Peer and self-rating: Children's perception of behavior relevant to hyperkinetic impulse disorder. *Journal of Abnormal Psychology,* 1980, *8,* 471–490.

Gofman, H. F. Personal communication, 1979.

Gold, M. W. Research on the vocational habilitation of the retarded: The present, the future. In N. R. Ellis (Ed.), *International review of research in mental retardation,* Vol. 3. New York: Academic Press, 1968.

Goldberg, J. O., & Konstantareas, M. M. Vigilance in hyperactive and normal children on a self-paced operant task. *Journal of Child Psychology and Psychiatry,* 1981, *22,* 55–63.

Golden, G. S. Tourette's syndrome: The pediatric perspective. *American Journal of Diseases in Children,* 1977, *13,* 531–534.

Goldiamond, I. Toward a constructional approach to social problems. *Behaviorism.* 1974, *2,* 1–84.

Goldstein, K. *After-effects of brain injuries in war.* New York: Grune and Stratton, 1942.

Golter, M., & Michaelson, I. A. Growth, behavior, and brain catecholamines in lead-exposed neonatal rats: A reappraisal. *Science,* 1975, *187,* 359–361.

Goodman, J., & Sours, J. *The child mental status examination.* New York: Basic Books, 1967.

Goodman, L. S., & Gilman, A. *The pharmacological basis of therapeutics.* New York: Macmillan, 1970.

Goodman, L. S., & Gilman, A. (Eds.). *The pharmacological basis of therapeutics* (5th ed.). New York: Macmillan, 1975.

Goodwin, D. W., Schulsinger, F., Hermansen, L., Guze, S. B., & Winokur, G. Alcoholism and the hyperactive child syndrome. *Journal of Nervous and Mental Disease,* 1975, *160,* 349–353.

Goodwin, S. E., & Mahoney, M. J. Modification of aggression through modeling: An experimental probe. *Journal of Behavior Therapy and Experimental Psychiatry,* 1975, *6,* 200–202.

Gordon, G. G., & Lieber, C. A. The fetal alcohol syndrome: Mechanisms and models. *Hospital Practice,* 1979, *14,* 11, 15.

Gordon, M. The assessment of impulsivity and mediating behaviors in hyperactive and nonhyperactive boys. *Journal of Abnormal Child Psychology,* 1979, *7,* 317–326.

Gordon, T. *Parent effectiveness training.* New York: Wyden, 1972.

Gorenstein, E. E., & Newman, J. P. Disinhibitory psychopathology: A new perspective and a model for research. *Psychological Bulletin,* 1980, *87,* 301–315.

Gorsuch, R. L., & Butler, M. C. Initial drug abuse: A review of predisposing social psychological factors. *Psychological Bulletin,* 1976, *83,* 120–137.

Goyer, P. F., Davis, G. C., & Rapoport, J. L. Abuse of prescribed stimulant medication by a 13-year-old hyperactive boy. *Journal of the American Academy of Child Psychiatry,* 1979, *18,* 170–175.

Goyette, C. H., Conners, C. K., Petti, T. A., & Curtis, L. E. Effects of artificial colors on hyperkinetic children: A double-blind challenge study. *Psychopharmacology Bulletin,* 1978, *14,* 39–40.

Goyette, C. H., Conners, C. K., & Ulrich, R. F. Normative data on revised Conners Parent and Teacher Rating Scales. *Journal of Abnormal Child Psychology,* 1978, *6,* 221–236.

Graham, F. K., Caldwell, B. M., Ernhart, C. B., Pennoyer, M. M., & Hartmann, A. F., Sr. Anoxia as a significant perinatal experience: A critique. *Journal of Pediatrics,* 1957, *50,* 556–569.

Graham, P., Rutter, M., & George, S. Temperamental characteristics as predictors of behavior disorders of children. *American Journal of Orthopsychiatry,* 1973, *43,* 328–339.

Greenberg, L. M., McMahon, S. A., & Deem, M. A. Side effects of dextroamphetamine therapy of hyperactive children. *Western Journal of Medicine,* 1974, *120,* 105–109.

Greenberg, L. M., Yellin, A. M., Spring, C., & Metcalf, M. Clinical effects of imipramine and methylphenidate in hyperactive children. *International Journal of Mental Health,* 1975, *4,* 144–156.

Greenhill, L. L., Puig-Antich, J., Sassin, J., & Sachar, E. J. Hormone and growth response in hyperkinetic children on stimulant medication. *Psychopharmacology Bulletin,* 1977, *13,* 33–36.

Greenspan, S. I. The clinical use of operant learning approaches. Some complex issues. *American Journal of Psychiatry,* 1974, *131,* 852–857.

Greenspan, S. I. Principles of intensive psychotherapy of neurotic adults with minimal brain dysfunction. In L. Bellak (Ed.), *Psychiatric aspects of minimal brain dysfunction in adults.* New York: Grune and Stratton, 1979.

Greulich, W. W., & Pyle, S. I. *Radiographic atlas of skeletal development of hand and wrist* (2nd ed.). Stanford, CA: Stanford University Press, 1959.

Grimm, L. G. The maintenance of self- and drug-attributed behavior change: A critique. *Journal of Abnormal Psychology,* 1980, *89,* 282–285.

Grinspoon, L., & Singer, S. Amphetamine in the treatment of hyperkinetic children. *Harvard Educational Review*, 1973, *43*, 515–555.

Groover, R. V. The hyperkinetic child. *Psychiatric Annals*, 1972, *2*, 36–44.

Gross, B., & Gross, R. (Eds.). *The children's rights movement. Overcoming the oppression of young people*. Garden City, NY: Anchor, 1977.

Gross, M. B., & Wilson, W. C. *Minimal brain dysfunction*. New York: Brunner/Mazel, 1974.

Gross, M. D. Caffeine in the treatment of children with minimal brain dysfunction or hyperkinetic syndrome. *Psychosomatics*, 1975, *75*, 26–27.

Gross, M. D. Growth of hyperkinetic children taking methylphenidate, dextroamphetamine, or imipramine/desipramine. *Pediatrics*, 1976, *58*, 423–431.

Grünbaum, A. The placebo concept. *Behavior Research and Therapy*, 1981, *19*, 157–167.

Grunebaum, H., & Solomon, L. Toward a peer theory of group psychotherapy: I. On the development of significance of peers and play. *International Journal of Group Psychotherapy*, 1980, *30*, 23–49.

Gurman, A. S., & Kniskern, D. P. Research on marital and family therapy: Progress, perspective, and prospect. In S. L. Garfield & A. E. Bergin (Eds.), *Handbook of psychotherapy and behavior change: An empirical analysis*. New York: Wiley, 1978.

Gutensohn, N., & Cole, P. Childhood social environment and Hodgkin's disease. *New England Journal of Medicine*, 1981, *304*, 135–140.

Guttman, H. A contraindication for family therapy: The prepsychotic or postpsychotic young adult and his parents. *Archives of General Psychiatry*, 1973, *29*, 352–355.

Hadley, S. W., & Strupp, H. H. Contemporary views of negative effects in psychotherapy. *Archives of General Psychiatry*, 1976, *33*, 1291–1302.

Haig, J. R., Schroeder, C. S., & Schroeder, S. R. Effects of methylphenidate on hyperactive children's sleep. *Psychopharmacologia*, 1974, *37*, 185–188.

Haight, M., Jampolsky, G., & Irvine, A. The response of hyperkinesis to EMG biofeedback. *Biofeedback and Self-Regulation*, 1976, *1*, 326 (abstract).

Haith, M. M., Collins, D., & Kessen, W. Response of the human infant to level of complexity of intermittent visual movement. *Journal of Experimental Child Psychology*, 1969, *7*, 52–69.

Haley, J. *Strategies of psychotherapy*. New York: Grune and Stratton, 1963.

Haley, J. *Uncommon therapy: The psychiatric techniques of Milton H. Erickson, M.D.* New York: Norton, 1973.

Hall, R. V., & Broden, M. Behavior changes in brain-injured children through social reinforcement. *Journal of Experimental Child Psychology*, 1967, *5*, 463–479.

Hallahan, D. P., & Cruickshank, W. M. *Psychoeducational foundations of learning disabilities*. Englewood Cliffs, NJ: Prentice Hall, 1973.

Halliday, R. A., Gnauck, K., Rosenthal, J. R., McKibben, J. L., & Callaway, E. The effects of methylphenidate dosage on school and home behavior of the hyperactive child. In R. M. Knights & D. J. Bakker (Eds.), *Treatment of hyperactive and learning disordered children*. Baltimore: University Park Press, 1980.

Halliday, R. A., Rosenthal, J. H., Naylor, H., & Callaway, E. Average evoked potential predictors of clinical improvement in hyperactive children treated with methylphenidate: An initial study and replication. *Psychophysiology*, 1976, *13*, 429–440.

Halpern, W. I. The medication clinic in the spectrum of children's services. *Diseases of the Nervous System*, 1977, *38*, 687–690.

Hampstead, W. J. The effects of EMG assisted relaxation training with hyperkinetic children: An alternative to medication. Unpublished doctoral dissertation, Western Michigan University, 1977.

Hare-Mustin, R. T. Treatment of temper tantrums by a paradoxical intervention. *Family Process,* 1975, *14,* 481–485.

Hare-Mustin, R. T. Paradoxical tasks in family therapy: Who can resist? *Psychotherapy: Research, Theory and Practice,* 1976, *13,* 128–130.

Harley, J. P., Matthews, C. G., & Eichman, P. Synthetic food colors and hyperactivity in children: A double-blind challenge experiment. *Pediatrics,* 1978, *62,* 975–983.

Harley, J. P., & Matthews, C. G. Food additives and hyperactivity in children. In R. M. Knights & D. J. Bakker (Eds.), *Treatment of hyperactive and learning disordered children.* Baltimore: University Park Press, 1980.

Harley, J. P., Ray, R. S., Tomasi, L., Eichman, P. L., Matthews, C. G., Chun, R., Cleeland, C. S., & Traisman, E. Hyperkinesis and food additives: Testing the Feingold hypothesis. *Pediatrics,* 1978, *61,* 818–828.

Harrington, J., & Letemendia, F. Persistent psychiatric disorder after head injury in children. *Journal of Mental Science,* 1958, *104,* 1205–1218.

Harris, T. *I'm OK–you're OK: A practical guide to Transactional Analysis.* New York: Harper and Row, 1969.

Hartley, E. R. Radiation that's good for you. *Science Digest,* 1974, *76,* 39–45.

Hartocollis, P. The syndrome of minimal brain dysfunction in young adult patients. *Bulletin of the Menninger Clinic,* 1968, *32,* 102–114.

Hartocollis, P. Minimal brain dysfunction in young adults. In L. Bellak (Ed.), *Psychiatric aspects of minimal brain dysfunction in adults.* New York: Grune and Stratton, 1979.

Hartup, W. W. Peer interaction and the behavior development of the individual child. In E. Schopler & R. J. Reichler (Eds.), *Psychopathology and child development: Research and treatment.* New York: Plenum Press, 1976.

Hartup, W. W. The social worlds of childhood. *American Psychologist,* 1979, *10,* 944–950.

Harvey, D. P. H. Whole coffee for hyperactive children. *Modern Medicine,* 1978, *46,* 31.

Hastings, J. E., & Barkley, R. A. A review of psychophysiological research with hyperkinetic children. *Journal of Abnormal Child Psychology,* 1978, *6,* 413–447.

Hastrop, R. W., Mecklenburger, J. A., & Wilson, J. A. (Eds.). *Accountability for educational results.* Hamden, CT: Linnet Books, 1973.

Havighurst, R. J. *Developmental tasks and education* (3rd ed.). New York: McKay, 1972.

Hayes, T. A., Panitch, M. L., & Barker, E. Imipramine dosage in children: A comment on "Imipramine and electrocardiographic abnormalities in hyperactive children." *American Journal of Psychiatry,* 1975, *132,* 546–547.

Hechtman, L., Weiss, G., Finklestein, J., Wener, A., & Benn, R. Hyperactives as young adults: Preliminary report. *Canadian Medical Association Journal,* 1976, *115,* 625–630.

Hechtman, L., Weiss, G., & Perlman, T. Hyperactives as young adults: Past and current antisocial behavior (stealing, drug abuse) and moral development. Paper presented at the meeting of the American Academy of Child Psychiatry, Atlanta, October 1979.

Hechtman, L., Weiss, G., & Perlman, T. Hyperactives as young adults: Self-esteem and social skills. *Canadian Journal of Psychiatry,* 1980, *25,* 478–483.

Hechtman, L., Weiss, G., Perlman, T., & Amsel, R. Hyperactives as young adults: Adolescent predictors of adult outcome. Paper presented at the annual meeting of the American Academy of Child Psychiatry, Chicago, IL, October 1980.

Hegeman, G. A. Parental perceptions of the hyperactive child: A hyperactivity scale for the personality inventory for children. Unpublished doctoral dissertation, University of Minnesota, 1977.

Heikkila, R. E., Orlansky, H., Mytilineous, C., & Cohen, G. Amphetamine: Evaluation of d and l-isomers as releasing agents and uptake inhibitors for ^{3}H-dopamine and ^{3}H-norepinephrine in slices of rat neostriatum and cerebral cortex. *Journal of Pharmacology and Experimental Therapeutics*, 1975, *194*, 47–56.

Hein, K., Cohen, M. I., & Litt, I. F. Illicit drug use among urban adolescents. *American Journal of Diseases in Children*, 1979, *133*, 38–40.

Henderson, A. T., Dahlin, I., Partridge, C. R., & Engelsing, E. L. A hypothesis on the etiology of hyperactivity, with a pilot-study report of related non-drug therapy. *Pediatrics*, 1973, *52*, 625.

Henker, B., & Whalen, C. K. The changing faces of hyperactivity: Retrospect and prospect. In C. K. Whalen & B. Henker (Eds.), *Hyperactive children: The social ecology of identification and treatment*. New York: Academic Press, 1980a.

Henker, B., & Whalen, C. K. The many messages of medication: Hyperactive children's perceptions and attributions. In S. Salzinger, J. Antrobus, & J. Glick(Eds.), *The ecosystem of the "sick" kid*. New York: Academic Press, 1980b.

Henker, B., Whalen, C. K., Bugental, D. B., & Barker, C. Licit and illicit drug patterns in stimulant treated children and their peers. In K. D. Gadow & J. Loney, (Eds.), *Psychosocial aspects of drug treatment for hyperactivity*. Boulder, CO: Westview Press, 1981.

Henker, B., Whalen, C. K., & Collins, B. E. Double-blind and triple-blind assessments of medication and placebo responses in hyperactive children. *Journal of Abnormal Child Psychology*, 1979, *7*, 1–13.

Hentoff, N. Drug-pushing in the schools: The professionals (1). *The Village Voice*, May 25, 1972, pp. 20–22.

Herjanic, B., & Campbell, J. Differentiating psychiatrically disturbed children on the basis of a structured interview. *Journal of Abnormal Child Psychology*, 1977, *5*, 127–135.

Herjanic, B., Herjanic, M., Brown, F., & Wheatt, T. Are children reliable reporters? *Journal of Abnormal Child Psychology*, 1975, *3*, 41–48.

Herron, R. E., & Ramsden, R. W. Continuous monitoring of overt human body movement by radio telemetry: A brief review. *Perceptual and Motor Skills*, 1967, *24*, 1303–1308.

Hersher, L. Minimal brain dysfunction and otitis media. *Perceptual and Motor Skills*, 1978, *47*, 723–726.

Himwich, W. A., Hall, J. S., & MacArthur, W. F. Maternal alcohol and neonatal health. *Biological Psychiatry*, 1977, *12*, 495–505.

Hirst, I. Removal of a student on a methylphenidate (Ritalin) prescription in an open classroom condition. Paper presented at the annual meeting of the Council for Exceptional Children, Chicago, April 1976.

Hodgman, C. H., McAnarney, E. R., Myers, G. J., & Iker, H. Emotional complications of adolescent grand mal epilepsy. *Journal of Pediatrics*, 1979, *95*, 309–312.

Hoffman, S. P., Engelhardt, D. M., Margolis, R. A., Polizos, P., Waizer, J., & Rosenfeld, R. Response to methylphenidate in low socioeconomic hyperactive children. *Archives of General Psychiatry*, 1974, *30*, 354–359.

Hohman, L. B. Post-encephalitic behavior disorder in children. *Johns Hopkins Hospital Bulletin*, 1922, *33*, 372–375.

Holt, J. *How children fail*. New York: Pitman, 1964.

Horner, G. C. Hyperactive and nonhyperactive children's self-determined levels of stimulation. Unpublished doctoral dissertation, University of Missouri, 1977.

Hornstein, L., Crowe, C., & Gruppo, R. Adrenal carcinoma in a child with history of fetal alcohol syndrome. *Lancet*, 1977, *2*, 1292.

Howell, M. C., Rever, G. W., Scholl, M. L., Trowbridge, F., & Rutledge, A. Hyperactivity in children. Types, diagnosis, drug therapy, approaches to management. *Clinical Pediatrics*, 1972, *11*, 30–39.

Hoy, E., Weiss, G., Minde, K., & Cohen, N. The hyperactive child at adolescence: Emotional, social, and cognitive functioning. *Journal of Abnormal Child Psychology*, 1978, *6*, 311–324.

Huessy, H. R. Study of the prevalence and therapy of the choreatiform syndrome or hyperkinesis in rural Vermont. *Acta Paedopsychiatrica*, 1967, *34*, 130–135.

Huessy, H. R. The adult hyperkinetic (letter). *American Journal of Psychiatry*, 1974, *131*, 724–725.

Huessy, H. R. Long term treatment outcome of minimal brain dysfunction. In R. S. Lipman (Chair), *Proceedings of the National Institute of Mental Health Workshop on the hyperkinetic behavior syndrome*. N. I. M. H., Washington, D.C., 1978.

Huessy, H. R., Cohen, S. M., Blair, C. L., & Rood, P. Clinical explorations in adult minimal brain dysfunction. In L. Bellak (Ed.), *Psychiatric aspects of minimal brain dysfunction in adults*. New York: Grune and Stratton, 1979.

Huessy, H. R., & Gendron, R. Prevalence of the so-called hyperkinetic syndrome in public school children of Vermont. *Acta Paedopsychiatrica*, 1970, *37*, 243–248.

Huessy, H. R., Metoyer, M., & Townsend, M. 8–10 year follow-up of 84 children treated for behavioral disorder in rural Vermont. *Acta Paedopsychiatrica*, 1974, *40*, 230–235.

Huestis, R. D., & Arnold, L. E. Possible antagonism of amphetamine by decongestant-antihistamine compounds. *Journal of Pediatrics*, 1974, *85*, 579–580.

Huestis, R. D., Arnold, L. E., & Smeltzer, M. A. Caffeine versus methylphenidate and d-amphetamine in minimal brain dysfunction: A double-blind comparison. *American Journal of Psychiatry*, 1975, *132*, 868–870.

Hughes, H., Henry, D., & Hughes, A. The effect of frontal EMG biofeedback training on the behavior of children with activity-level problems. *Biofeedback and Self-Regulation*, 1980, *5*, 207–219.

Hughes, R., & Brewin, R. *The tranquilizing of America*. New York: Harcourt Brace Jovanovich, 1979.

Humphries, T., Kinsbourne, M., & Swanson, J. Stimulant effects on cooperation and social interaction between hyperactive children and their mothers. *Journal of Child Psychology and Psychiatry*, 1978, *19*, 13–22.

Humphries, T., Swanson, J. M., Kinsbourne, M., & Yiu, L. Stimulant effects on persistence of motor performance of hyperactive children. *Journal of Pediatric Psychology*, 1979, *4*, 55–66.

Hunsinger, S. School storm: Drugs for children. *Christian Science Monitor*, October 31, 1970, pp. 1,6.

Ingalls, T. H., & Gordon, J. E. Epidemiologic implications of developmental arrests. *American Journal of Medical Science*, 1947, *241*, 322–328.

Ingram, T. T. Soft signs. *Developmental Medicine and Child Neurology*, 1973, *15*, 527–530.

Irwin, O. C. The amount of motility of seventy-three newborn infants. *Journal of Comparative Psychology*, 1932, *14*, 415–428.

Ives, S. B. Conceptual tempo, attention, and skin conductance in Ritalin-responsive hyperkinetic boys. Unpublished doctoral dissertation, Cornell University, 1977.

Jacob, R. G., O'Leary, K. D., & Rosenblad, C. Formal and informal classroom settings: Effects on hyperactivity. *Journal of Abnormal Child Psychology*, 1978, *6*, 47–59.

Jacobson, E. *Progressive relaxation*. Chicago: University of Chicago Press, 1938.

James, M. *Born to love: Transactional analysis in the church*. Reading, MA: Addison-Wesley, 1973.

Jeffrey, T. The effects of operant conditioning and electromyographic feedback on the relaxed behavior of hyperkinetic children. Paper presented at the Ninth Annual Meeting of the Biofeedback Society of America, Albuquerque, NM, 1978.

Jessor, R., & Jessor, S. *Problem behavior and psychosocial development: A longitudinal study of youth.* New York: Academic Press, 1977.

John, E. R., Ahn, H., Prichep, L., Trepitin, M., Brown, D., & Kay, H. Developmental equations for the electroencephalogram. *Science,* 1980, *210,* 1255–1258.

Johnson, C. F., & Prinz, F. Hyperactivity is in the eye of the beholder. *Clinical Pediatrics,* 1976, *15,* 222–238.

Johnson, S., & Bolstad, O. Methodological issues in naturalistic observation: Some problems and solutions for field research. In L. Hamerlynck, L. Handy, & E. Mash (Eds.), *Behavior change: Methodology concepts in practice.* Fourth Banff International Conference on Behavior Modification. Champaign, IL: Research Press, 1973.

Johnson, W. B. An experimental study of the effect of electromyography (EMG) biofeedback on hyperactivity in children. Unpublished doctoral dissertation, University of Southern California, 1976.

Jones, K. L., Smith, D. W., Streissguth, A. P., & Myrianthopoulos, N. C. Outcome in offspring of chronic alcoholic women. *Lancet,* 1974, *1,* 1076–1078.

Jones, K. L., Smith, D. W., Ulleland, C. N., & Streissguth, A. P. Pattern of malformation in offspring of chronic alcoholic mothers. *Lancet,* 1973, *1,* 1267–1271.

Jones, N. M., Loney, J., Weissenburger, F. E., & Fleischmann, D. J. The hyperkinetic child: What do teachers know? *Psychology in the Schools,* 1975, *12,* 338–392.

Jones, R. R., Reid, J. B., & Patterson, G. R. Naturalistic observations in clinical assessment. In P. McReynolds (Ed.), *Advances in psychological assessment,* Vol. 3. San Francisco: Jossey-Bass, 1975.

Joselow, M. Environmental contrasts: Blood lead levels of children in Honolulu and Newark. *Journal of Environmental Health,* 1974, *37,* 10–12.

Kagan, J. Reflection-impulsivity: The generality and dynamics of conceptual tempo. *Journal of Abnormal Psychology,* 1966, *71,* 17–24.

Kagan, J. *Change and continuity in infancy.* New York: Wiley, 1971.

Kagan, J., & Kogan, N. Individuality and cognitive performance. In Paul H. Mussen (Ed.), *Carmichael's Manual of child psychology,* Vol. 1 (3rd ed.). New York: Wiley, 1970.

Kagan, J., & Messer, S. B. A reply to "Some misgivings about the Matching Familiar Figures Test as a measure of reflection-impulsivity." *Developmental Psychology,* 1975, *11,* 244–248.

Kagan, J., Rosman, B. L., Day, D., Albert, J., & Phillips, W. Information processing in the child: Significance of analytic and reflective attitudes. *Psychological Monographs,* 1964, *78* (1, Whole No. 578).

Kahn, E., & Cohen, L. Organic driveness: A brain stem syndrome and an experience. *New England Journal of Medicine,* 1934, *210,* 748–756.

Kalachnik, J. E., Sprague, R. L., Sleator, E. K., Cohen, M. N., & Ullman, R. K. Use of the RWT stature prediction formula in monitoring growth suppression effects in methylphenidate. Unpublished manuscript. University of Illinois, 1981.

Kalverboer, A. F., Touwen, B. C., Prechtl, H. F. Follow-up of infants at risk for minor brain dysfunction. *Annals of the New York Academy of Sciences,* 1973, *205,* 173–187.

Kandel, D. Convergences in prospective longitudinal surveys of drug use in normal populations. In D. Kandel (Ed.), *Longitudinal research on drug use: Empirical findings and methodological issues.* New York: Wiley, 1978.

Kane, J. S., & Lawler, E. E., III. Methods of peer assessment. *Psychological Bulletin,* 1978, *85,* 555–586.

Kappelman, M., Roberts, P., Rinaldi, R., & Cornblath, M. The school health team and school health physician: New role and operation. *American Journal of Diseases of Children,* 1975, *129,* 191–195.

Karasu, T. B. Psychotherapies: An overview. *American Journal of Psychiatry*, 1977, *134*, 851–863.

Kasanin, J. Personality changes in children following cerebral palsy. *Journal of Nervous and Mental Disease*, 1929, *69*, 385–408.

Kastin, A. J. Personal communication, May 1981.

Katz, S., Saraf, K., Gittelman-Klein, R., & Klein, D. F. Clinical pharmacological management of hyperkinetic children. *International Journal of Mental Health*, 1975, *4*, 157–181.

Kaufman, A. S. *Intelligence testing with the WISC-R*. New York: Wiley, 1979.

Kehne, C. W. Control of the hyperactive child via medication—at what cost to personality development: Some psychological implications and clinical interventions. *American Journal of Orthopsychiatry*, 1974, *44*, 237–238.

Kendall, P., & Finch, A., Jr. A cognitive-behavioral treatment for impulse control: A case study. *Journal of Consulting and Clinical Psychology*, 1976, *44*, 852–857.

Kendall, P. C., & Brophy, C. Activity and attentional correlates of teacher ratings of hyperactivity. *Journal of Pediatric Psychology*, in press, 1981.

Kenny, T. J. Hyperactivity. In H. E. Rie & E. D. Rie (Eds.), *Handbook of minimal brain dysfunctions: A critical view*. New York: Wiley, 1980.

Kenny, T. J., Clemmens, R. L., Hudson, B., Lentz, G. A., Jr., Cicci, R., & Nair, P. Characteristics of children referred because of hyperactivity. *Journal of Pediatrics*, 1971, *79*, 618–622.

Kent, R. N., & O'Leary, K. D. A controlled evaluation of behavior modification with conduct problem children. *Journal of Consulting and Clinical Psychology*, 1976, *44*, 586–596.

Keogh, B. K. Hyperactivity and learning problems: Implications for teachers. *Education Digest*, 1971a, *37*, 45–47.

Keogh, B. K. Hyperactivity and learning disorders: Review and speculation. *Exceptional Children*, 1971b, *38*, 101–110.

Keogh, B. K., & Barkett, C. J. Children's rights in assessment and school placement. *Journal of Social Issues*, 1978, *37*, 87–100.

Keogh, B. K., & Barkett, C. J. An educational analysis of hyperactive children's achievement problems. In C. K. Whalen & B. Henker (Eds.), *Hyperactive children: The social ecology of identification and treatment*. New York: Academic Press, 1980.

Keogh, B. K., Wetter, J., McGinty, A., & Donlon, G. Functional analysis of WISC performance of learning disordered, hyperactive, and mentally retarded boys. *Psychology in the Schools*, 1973, *10*, 178–181.

Kessler, J. W. History of minimal brain dysfunctions. In H. E. Rie & E. D. Rie (Eds.), *Handbook of minimal brain dysfunctions: A critical view*. New York: Wiley, 1980.

Kilman, G. W., & Rosenfeld, A. *Responsible parenthood: The child's psyche through the six-year pregnancy*. New York: Holt, Rinehart, and Winston, 1980.

King, C., & Young, R. D. Peer interaction in a communication task and peer popularity: A comparison of hyperactive and active boys. Unpublished manuscript. Indiana University, 1982.

Kinney, H., Faix, R., & Brazy, J. The fetal alcohol syndrome and neuroblastoma. *Pediatrics*, 1980, *66*, 130–131.

Kinsbourne, M. Minimal brain dysfunction as a neurodevelopmental lag. *Annals of the New York Academy of Science*, 1973, *205*, 263–273.

Kinsbourne, M. Discussion of "Can hyperactives be identified in infancy?" In R. L. Trites (Ed.), *Hyperactivity in children*. Baltimore: University Park Press, 1979.

Kinsbourne, M., & Swanson, J. M. Models of hyperactivity. In R. L. Trites (Ed.), *Hyperactivity in children*. Baltimore: University Park Press, 1979.

Kirk, S. P. *Educating exceptional children*. Boston: Houghton Mifflin, 1972.

Klaus, M. H., & Kennell, J. H. *Maternal-infant bonding*. St. Louis: Mosby, 1976.

Klein, A. R., & Young, R. D. Hyperactive boys in their classroom: Assessment of teacher and peer perceptions, interactions, and classroom behaviors. *Journal of Abnormal Child Psychology,* 1979, *7,* 425–442.

Klein, D. F., & Gittelman-Klein, R. Problems in the diagnosis of minimal brain dysfunction and the hyperkinetic syndrome. *International Journal of Mental Health,* 1975, *4,* 45–60.

Kløve, H. Discussion of "Method and theory for psychopharmacology." In R. L. Trites (Ed.), *Hyperactivity in children.* Baltimore: University Park Press, 1979.

Kløve, H., & Hold, K. The hyperkinetic syndrome: Criteria for diagnosis. In R. L. Trites (Ed.), *Hyperactivity in children.* Baltimore: University Park Press, 1979.

Knights, R. M., & Hinton, G. The effects of methylphenidate (Ritalin) on the motor skills and behavior of children with learning problems. *Journal of Nervous and Mental Diseases,* 1969, *148,* 643–653.

Knights, R. M., & Viets, C. A. The effects of pemoline on hyperactive boys. Unpublished paper. Carleton University, Ottawa, Canada, 1973.

Knobel, M. Psychopharmacology of the hyperkinetic child: Dynamic considerations. *Archives of General Psychiatry,* 1962, *6,* 198–202.

Knobel, M. Personal communication, 1975.

Knobel, M., Wolman, M. B., & Mason, E. Hyperkinesis and organicity in children. *Archives of General Psychiatry,* 1959, *1,* 310–321.

Knobloch, H., & Pasamanick, B. Prospective studies on the epidemiology of reproductive casualty: Methods, findings, and some implications. *Merrill-Palmer Quarterly,* 1966, *12,* 27–43.

Knopp, W., Arnold, L. E., Andras, R. L., & Smeltzer, D. J. Predicting amphetamine response in hyperkinetic children by electric pupillography. *Pharmakopsychiatrie Neuro-Psychopharmakologie,* 1973, *6,* 158–166.

Koester, L. S. Arousal and hyperactivity in open and traditional education: Test of a theory. Unpublished doctoral dissertation, University of Wisconsin, 1976.

Kornetsky, C. Psychoactive drugs in the immature organism. *Psychopharmacologia* (Berlin), 1970, *17,* 105–136.

Kovel, J. *A complete guide to therapy: From psychoanalysis to behavior modification.* New York: Pantheon, 1976.

Krager, J. M., Safer, D., & Earhart, J. Medication used to treat hyperactive children: Follow-up survey results. Paper presented at the School Health Association meeting. Detroit, Spring 1979.

Kramer, J., & Loney, J. Predicting adolescent antisocial behavior among hyperactive boys. Paper presented at the 86th Annual Convention of the American Psychological Association, Toronto, 1978.

Kramer, J., & Loney, J. Substance use among medicated and non-medicated hyperkinetic boys at adolescence. In R. Lipman (Chair), Substance abuse and childhood hyperactivity: Answers from longitudinal studies. Paper presented at the meeting of the American Psychological Association, Montreal, September 1980.

Kramer, J., & Loney, J. Childhood hyperactivity and substance abuse: A review of the literature. In K. Gadow & I. Bialer (Eds.), *Advances in learning and behavioral disabilities,* Vol. 1. Greenwich, CT: JAI Press, 1981.

Kretsinger, E. A. An experimental study of restiveness in preschool educational television audiences. *Speech Monographs,* 1959, *26,* 72–77.

Kristein, M. M., Arnold, C. B., & Wynder, E. L. Health economic and preventive care. *Science,* 1977, *195,* 457–462.

Kritzberg, N. *Structured therapeutic game method of child analytic therapy.* New York: Grune and Stratton, 1975.

Kupietz, S., Bialer, I., & Winsberg, B. G. A behavior rating scale for assessing improvement in behaviorally deviant children: A preliminary investigation. *American Journal of Psychiatry*, 1972, *128*, 116–120.

Ladd, E. T. Pills for classroom peace? *Saturday Review*, November 21, 1970, pp. 66–68; 81–83.

Lafferman, J. A., & Silbergeld, E. K. Erythrosin B inhibits dopamine transport in rat caudate synaptosomes. *Science*, 1979, *205*, 410–412.

Lahey, B. B. (Ed.). *Behavior therapy with hyperactive and learning disabled children*. New York: Oxford University Press, 1977.

Lahey, B. B., Green, K. D., & Forehand, R. On the independence of ratings of hyperactivity, conduct problems, and attention deficits in children: A multiple regression analysis. *Journal of Consulting and Clinical Psychology*, 1980, *48*, 566–574.

Lahey, B. B., Stempniak, M., Robinson, E. J. Hyperactivity and learning disabilities as independent dimensions of child behavior problems. Unpublished manuscript. University of Georgia, 1981.

Lahey, B. B., Stempniak, M., Robinson, E. J., & Tyroler, M. J. Hyperactivity and learning disabilities as independent dimensions of child behavior problems. *Journal of Abnormal Psychology*, 1978, *87*, 333–340.

Lambert, N. M. School Behavior Survey. Unpublished test. University of California, Berkeley, 1977.

Lambert, N. M. Temperament profiles of hyperactive children. *American Journal of Orthopsychiatry*, 1982, in press.

Lambert, N. M., & Hartsough (Eds.). *A process for the assessment of effective student functioning*. Monterey, CA: Publisher's Test Service, CTB/McGraw–Hill, 1979.

Lambert, N. M., & Sandoval, J. The prevalence of learning disabilities in a sample of children considered hyperactive. *Journal of Abnormal Child Psychology*, 1980, *8*, 33–50.

Lambert, N. M., Sandoval, J., & Sassone, D. Prevalence of hyperactivity in elementary school children as a function of social system definers. *American Journal of Orthopsychiatry*, 1978, *48*, 446–463.

Lambert, N. M., Windmiller, M., Sandoval, J., & Moore, B. Hyperactive children and the efficacy of psychoactive drugs as a treatment intervention. *American Journal of Orthopsychiatry*, 1976, *46*, 335–352.

Lambert, N. M., & Windmiller, M. An exploratory study of temperament traits in a population of children at risk. *Journal of Special Education*, 1977, *11*, 37–47.

Lancioni, G. E. Infant operant conditioning and its implications for early intervention. *Psychological Bulletin*, 1980, *88*, 516–534.

Langhorne, J. E. The large data set in clinical research: What would you do with it after you got it? Symposium presentation, American Psychological Association Annual Meeting, San Francisco, 1977.

Langhorne, J. E., & Loney, J. A four-fold model for subgrouping the Hyperkinetic/MBD syndrome. *Child Psychiatry and Human Development*, 1979, *9*, 153–159.

Langhorne, J. E., Loney, J., Paternite, C. E., & Bechtoldt, H. P. Childhood hyperkinesis: A return to the source. *Journal of Abnormal Psychology*, 1976, *85*, 201–209.

Langone, J., & Langone, D. D. *Women who drink*. Reading, MA: Addison-Wesley, 1980.

Lansdown, R. G., Shepherd, J., Clayton, B. E., Delves, H. T., Graham, P. J., & Turner, W. C. Blood-lead levels, behavior and intelligence: A population study. *Lancet*, 1974, *1*, 538–541.

Laufer, M. W. Cerebral dysfunction and behavior disorders in adolescents. *American Journal of Orthopsychiatry*, 1962, *32*, 501–506.

Laufer, M. W. Long-term management and some follow-up findings on the use of drugs with minimal cerebral syndromes. *Journal of Learning Disabilities*, 1971, *4*, 55–58.

Laufer, M. W., & Denhoff, E. Hyperkinetic behavior syndrome in children. *Journal of Pediatrics*, 1957, *50*, 463–474.

Laufer, M. W., Denhoff, E., & Solomons, G. Hyperkinetic impulse disorder in children's behavior problems. *Psychosomatic Medicine*, 1957, *19*, 38–49.

Lazarus, A. A. *Behavior theory and beyond.* New York: McGraw-Hill, 1971.

Leighton, A. H. *My name is legion.* New York: Basic Books, 1959.

Lemoine, P., Haronsseau, H., Borteyru, J. P., & Menuet, J. C. The children of alcoholic parents: Anomalies seen in 127 cases. *Ouest Medical*, 1968, 476.

Lerer, R. J. Do hyperactive children tend to have abnormal palmar creases? *Clinical Pediatrics*, 1977, *16*, 645–647.

Lerer, R. J., & Lerer, M. P. The effects of methylphenidate on the soft neurological signs of hyperactive children. *Pediatrics*, 1976, *57*, 521–525.

Lerer, R. J., & Lerer, M. P. Response of adolescents with minimal brain dysfunction to methylphenidate. *Journal of Learning Disabilities*, 1977, *10*, 223–228.

Lesnik-Oberstein, M., van der Vlugt, H., Hoencamp, E., Juffermans, D., & Cohen, L. Stimulus-governance and the hyperkinetic syndrome. *Journal of Abnormal Child Psychology*, 1978, *6*, 407–412.

Lessinger, L. M., & Tyler, R. W. (Eds.). *Accountability in education.* Worthington, OH: C. A. Jones, 1971.

Levine, E. M., Kozak, C., & Shaiova, C. H. Hyperactivity among white middle-class children. *Child Psychiatry and Human Development*, 1977, *7*, 156–168.

Levine, J. D., Gordon, N. C., Bornstein, J. C., & Fields, H. L. Role of pain in placebo analgesia. *Proceedings of the National Academy of Science*, 1979, *76*, 3528–3531.

Levine, M. D., & Oberklaid, F. Hyperactivity: Symptom complex or complex symptom? *American Journal of Diseases of Children*, 1980 *34*, 409–414.

Levis, D. J. Integration of behavior therapy and dynamic psychiatry techniques: A marriage with a high probability of ending in divorce. *Behavior Therapy*, 1970, *1*, 521–537.

Levitt, E. E. The results of psychotherapy with children: An evaluation. *Journal of Consulting Psychology*, 1957, *21*, 189–196.

Levitt, E. E. Psychotherapy with children: A further evaluation. *Behavior Research and Therapy*, 1963, *1*, 45–51.

Levitt, E. E. Research on psychotherapy with children. In A. E. Bergin & S. L. Garfield (Eds.), *Handbook of psychotherapy and behavior change.* New York: Wiley, 1971.

Lewis, J. A., & Lewis, B. S. Deanol in minimal brain dysfunction. *Diseases of the Nervous System*, 1977, *38*, 21–24.

Lilienfeld, A. M., Pasamanick, B., & Rogers, M. Relationship between pregnancy experience and the development of certain neuropsychiatric disorders in childhood. *American Journal of Public Health*, 1955, *45*, 637–643.

Lindsley, O. R., & Skinner, B. F. A method for the experimental analysis of behavior of psychotic patients. *American Psychologist*, 1954, *9*, 419–420.

Lindzey, G., Loehlin, J., Manosevitz, M., & Thiessen, D. Behavioral genetics. *Annual Review of Psychology*, 1971, *22*, 39–94.

Lin-Fu, J. S. Undue absorption of lead among children: A new look at an old problem. *New England Journal of Medicine*, 1972, *236*, 702–710.

Lin-Fu, J. S. Lead exposure among children: A reassessment. *New England Journal of Medicine*, 1979, *300*, 731–732.

Lipman, R. S. (Chair). *Proceedings of the National Institute of Mental Health Workshop on the Hyperkinetic Behavior Syndrome.* Washington, D.C., June 1978.

Loehlin, J. C., & Nichols, R. C. *Heredity, environment and personality.* Austin: University of Texas Press, 1976.

Logan, W. J., & Swanson, J. M. Erythrosin B inhibition of neurotransmitter accumulation by rat brain homogenate. Unpublished manuscript, University of Toronto, 1979.

London, P. The end of ideology in behavior modification. *American Psychologist,* 1972, *27,* 913–920.

Loney, J. The Teacher Approval–Disapproval Scale. University of Iowa, 1974a.

Loney, J. The intellectual functioning of hyperactive elementary school boys: A cross-sectional investigation. *American Journal of Orthopsychiatry,* 1974b, *44,* 754–762.

Loney, J. Panel on treatment. In R. S. Lipman (Chair), *Proceedings of the National Institute of Mental Health Workshop on the Hyperkinetic Behavior Syndrome.* Washington, D. C., June 1978.

Loney, J. Hyperkinesis comes of age: What do we know and where should we go? Paper presented at the annual meeting of the American Orthopsychiatric Association, New York, 1979.

Loney, J. Childhood hyperactivity. In R. H. Woody (Ed.), *Encyclopedeia of Clinical Assessment.* San Francisco: Jossey-Bass, 1980a.

Loney, J. Hyperkinesis comes of age: What do we know and where should we go? *American Journal of Orthopsychiatry,* 1980b, *50,* 28–42.

Loney, J. The Iowa theory of substance abuse among hyperactive adolescents. In D. J. Lettieri, M. Sayers, & H. W. Pearson (Eds.). Theories on drug abuse: Selected contemporary perspectives. *NIDA Research Monograph 30, March 1980c.*

Loney, J. Evaluating treatments for hyperactivity: Some methodological considerations. In K. Gadow & J. Loney (Eds.), *Psychosocial aspects of drug treatment for hyperactivity.* Boulder, CO: Westview Press, 1981.

Loney, J., Comly, H. H., & Simon, B. Parental management, self-concept, and drug response in minimal brain dysfunction. *Journal of Learning Disabilities,* 1975, *8,* 187–190.

Loney, J., Kramer, J., & Milich, R. The hyperkinetic child grows up: Predictors of symptoms, delinquency, and achievement at follow-up. In K. D. Gadow & J. Loney (Eds.), *Psychosocial aspects of drug treatment for hyperactivity.* Boulder, CO: Westview Press, 1981.

Loney, J., Langhorne, J. E., & Paternite, C. E. An empirical basis for subgrouping the Hyperkinetic/MBD syndrome. *Journal of Abnormal Psychology,* 1978, *87,* 431–441.

Loney, J., Langhorne, J. E., Paternite, C. E., Whaley-Klahn, M. A., Blair-Broeker, C. T., & Hacker, M. The Iowa HABIT: Hyperactive/aggressive boys in treatment. Paper presented at the meeting of the Society for Life History Research in Psychopathology, Fort Worth, TX, October 1976.

Loney, J., & Milich, R. Development and evaluation of a placebo for studies of operant behavioral intervention. *Journal of Behavior Therapy and Experimental Psychiatry,* 1978, *9,* 327–333.

Loney, J., & Milich, R. S. Hyperactivity, inattention, and aggression in clinical practice. In M. Wolraich & D. K. Routh (Eds.), *Advances in Behavioral Pediatrics,* Vol. 2. Greenwich, CT: JAI Press, 1981.

Loney, J., Milich, R. S., & Maurer, R. A longitudinal cluster analytic study of the hyperkinetic/MBD syndrome. Paper presented at the biennial meeting of the Society for Research in Child Development, San Francisco, 1979.

Loney, J., Prinz, R. J., Mishalow, J., & Joad, J. Hyperkinetic/aggressive boys in treatment: Predictors of clinical response to methylphenidate. *American Journal of Psychiatry,* 1978, *135,* 1487–1491.

Loney, J., Weissenburger, F. E., Woolson, R. F., & Lichty, E. C. Comparing psychological and pharmacological treatments for hyperkinetic boys and their classmates. *Journal of Abnormal Child Psychology*, 1979, *7*, 133–143.

Loney, J., Whaley-Klahn, M. A., Ponto, L. B., & Adney, K. Predictors of adolescent growth in hyperkinetic boys treated with methylphenidate. *Psychopharmacology Bulletin*, 1981 in press.

Loney, J., Whaley-Klahn, M. A., & Weissenburger, F. E. Responses of hyperactive boys to a behaviorally focused school attitude questionnaire. *Child Psychiatry and Human Development*, 1976, *6*, 123–133.

Lopez, R. E. Hyperactivity in twins. *Canadian Psychiatric Association Journal*, 1965, *10*, 421.

Lord, E. E. *Children handicapped by cerebral palsy*. New York: Commonwealth Fund, 1937.

Lovaas, O. I., & Willis, T. Behavioral control of a hyperactive child. Unpublished manuscript referred to in D. P. Cantwell (Ed.), *The hyperactive child*. New York: Spectrum, 1975, p. 134.

Lubar, J. F., & Shouse, M. N. EEG and behavioral changes in a hyperkinetic child concurrent with training of the sensorimotor rhythm. *Biofeedback and Self-Regulation*, 1976, *1*, 293–306.

Lubs, H., & Smith, S. Genetic dyslexia. Science News Report. *Science 81*, 1981, *2*, 7.

Lucas, A. R., & Weiss, M. Methylphenidate hallucinois. *Journal of the American Medical Association*, 1971, *217*, 1079–1081.

Luisada, P. V. REM deprivation and hyperactivity in children. *The Chicago Medical School Quarterly*, 1969, *28*, 97–108.

Lupin, M. N., Braud, L. W., Braud, W. G., & Duer, W. F. Children, parents and relaxation tapes. *Academic Therapy*, 1976, *12*, 105–113.

Luria, A. R. *The role of speech in the regulation of normal and abnormal behavior*. New York: Liveright, 1961.

Lyness, S. Hyperactivity and marital casualties. Paper presented at the meeting of the Michigan Association for Children with Learning Disabilities, Dearborn, MI, October 1977.

Lytton, G. J., & Knobel, M. Diagnosis and treatment of behavior disorders in children. *Diseases of the Nervous System*, 1958, *20*, 5–11.

MacIsaac, D. S. Learning and behavioral functioning of low income, black preschoolers with asymptomatic lead poisoning. Unpublished doctoral dissertation, Fordham University, 1976.

Madle, R. A., Neisworth, J. T., & Kurtz, P. D. Biasing of hyperkinetic behavior ratings by diagnostic reports: Effects of observer training and assessment method. *Journal of Learning Disabilities*, 1980, *13*, 35–38.

Madsen, C. H., & Madsen, C. K. *Teaching/discipline: A positive approach for educational development* (2nd. ed.). Boston: Allyn and Bacon, 1974.

Mainville, F., & Friedman, R. J. Peer relations of hyperactive children. *Ontario Psychologist*, 1976, *8*, 17–20.

Malone, C. A. Child psychiatry and family therapy. *American Academy of Child Psychiatry*, 1979, *18*, 4–21.

Mann, H. B., & Greenspan, S. I. The identification of treatment of adult brain dysfunction. *American Journal of Psychiatry*, 1976, *133*, 1013–1017.

Mann, J. *Time-limited psychotherapy*. Cambridge, MA: Harvard University Press, 1973.

Margolin, D. I. The hyperkinetic child syndrome and brain monoamines: Pharmacology and therapeutic implications. *Journal of Clinical Psychiatry*, 1978, *39*, 120–130.

Margules, D. L. Obesity and the hibernation response. *Psychology Today*, 1979, *13*, 136.

Marks, I. M. The current status of behavioral psychotherapy. *American Journal of Psychiatry*, 1976, *133*, 253–261.

Marmor, J., & Woods, S. *The interface between the psychodynamic and behavioral therapies.* New York: Plenum Press, 1980.

Marsden, G., & Kalter, N. Children's understanding of their emotionally disturbed peers: I. The concept of emotional disturbance. *Psychiatry,* 1976, *39,* 227–238.

Martin, G., & Zaug, P. Electrocardiographic monitoring of enuretic children receiving therapeutic doses of imipramine. *American Journal of Psychiatry,* 1975, *132,* 540–542.

Marwit, S. J., & Stenner, A. J. Hyperkinesis: Delineation of two patterns. *Exceptional Children,* 1972, *38,* 401–406.

Mash, E. J., & Dalby, J. T. Behavioral interventions for hyperactivity. In R. L. Trites (Ed.), *Hyperactivity in children.* Baltimore: University Park Press, 1979.

Mash, E. J., Handy, L. C., & Hammerlynck, L. A. *Behavior modification approaches to parenting.* New York: Brunner/Mazel, 1976.

Mash, E. J., & Johnston, C. A behavioral assessment of sibling interactions in hyperactive and normal children. Unpublished manuscript, University of Calgary, (Canada), 1981.

Mash, E. J., Terdal, L. G., & Anderson, K. A. The response-class matrix: A procedure for recording parent–child interactions. *Journal of Consulting and Clinical Psychology,* 1973, *40,* 163–164.

Masten, A. S. Family therapy as a treatment for children: A critical review of outcome research. *Family Process,* 1979, *18,* 323–335.

Mattes, J. A. The role of frontal lobe dysfunction in childhood hyperkinesis. *Comprehensive Psychiatry,* 1980, *21,* 358-369.

Mattes, J. A., & Gittelman, R. A. Effects of artificial food colorings in children with hyperactive symptoms. *Archives of General Psychiatry,* 1981, *38,* 714–718.

Mattes, J. A., & Gittelman-Klein, R. A crossover study of artificial food colorings in a hyperkinetic child. *American Journal of Psychiatry,* 1978, *135,* 987–988.

Maugh, T. H. Hair: A diagnostic tool to complement blood serum and urine. *Science,* 1978,*202,* 1271–1273.

Maurer, R., Cadoret, R. J., & Cain, C. Cluster analysis of childhood temperament data on adoptees. *American Journal of Orthopsychiatry,* 1980, *50,* 522–534.

Mausner, J. S. & Bahn, A. K. *Epidemiology.* Philadelphia: W. B. Saunders, 1974.

Maynard, R. Omaha pupils given "behavior" drugs. *Washington Post,* June 29, 1970.

Mayron, L. W. Hyperactivity from fluorescent lighting—fact or fancy: A commentary on the report by O'Leary, Rosenbaum, and Hughes. *Journal of Abnormal Child Psychology,* 1978, *6,* 291–294.

Mayron, L. W., Ott, J. N., Nations, R., & Mayron, E. L. Light, radiation, and academic behavior. *Academic Therapy,* 1974, *10,* 33–47.

McDermott, J. F., & Char, W. F. The undeclared war between child psychiatry and family therapy. *American Academy of Child Psychiatry,* 1974, *13,* 422–436.

McDermott, J. F., & Harrison, S. *Psychiatric treatment of the child.* New York: Jason Aronson, 1977.

McDevitt, S. C., & Carey, W. B. The measurement of temperament in 3–7 year old children. *Journal of Child Psychology and Psychiatry,* 1978, *19,* 245–253.

McDonald, J. E. Pharmacologic treatment and behavior therapy: Allies in the management of hyperactive children. *Psychology in the Schools,* 1978, *15,* 270–274.

McGinnis, J. M. Trends in disease prevention: Assessing the benefits of prevention. *New York Academy of Medicine Bulletin,* 1980, *56,* 38–44.

McInerny, T., & Chamberlin, R. W. Is it feasible to identify infants who are at risk for later behavioral problems? *Clinical Pediatrics,* 1978, *17,* 233–238.

McMahon, R. C. Genetic etiology in the hyperactive child syndrome. *American Journal of Orthopsychiatry,* 1980, *50,* 145–150.

McNamara, J. J. Hyperactivity in the apartment bound child. *Clinical Pediatrics*, 1972, *11*, 371–372.

McNamara, J. R. Behavior therapy in the seventies: Some changes and current issues. *Psychotherapy: Theory, Research and Practice*, 1980, *17*, 2–9.

McNutt, B. A., Ballard, J. E., Boileau, R., Sprague, R. L., & von Neumann, A. The effects of long-term stimulant medication on growth and body composition of hyperactive children. *Psychopharmacology Bulletin*, 1976, *12*, 13–15.

McNutt, B. A., Boileau, R. A., & Cohen, M. The effects of long-term stimulant medication on the growth and body composition of hyperactive children. *Psychopharmacology Bulletin*, 1977, *13*, 36–38.

Meichenbaum, D. H. *Cognitive behavior modification.* New York: Plenum Press, 1977a.

Meichenbaum, D. H. The nature and modification of impulsivity. In M. Blaw, I. Rapin, & M. Kinsbourne (Eds.), *Topics in child neurology.* Jamaica, NY: Spectrum, 1977b.

Meichenbaum, D. H. Teaching children self-control. In B. Lahey & A. Kazdin (Eds.), *Advances in child clinical psychology*, Vol. 2. New York: Plenum Press, 1978.

Meichenbaum, D. H., & Goodman, J. Training impulsive children to talk to themselves: A means of developing self-control. *Journal of Abnormal Psychology*, 1971, *77*, 115–126.

Meissner, W. W., & Nicholi, A. M., Jr. The psychotherapies: Individual, family, and group. In A. M. Nicholi, Jr., (Ed.), *The Harvard guide to modern psychiatry.* Cambridge, MA: Belknap Press, 1978.

Mendelson, J. H. The fetal alcohol syndrome. *New England Journal of Medicine*, 1978, *298*, 566.

Mendelson, W. B., Johnson, N. E., & Stewart, M. A. Hyperactive children as teenagers: A follow-up study. *Journal of Nervous and Mental Disease*, 1971, *153*, 273–279.

Mercer, J. R., & Lewis, J. F. *System of multicultural pluralistic assessment.* New York: Psychological Corporation, 1978.

Merwin, J. C. Review of the WRAT. In O. K. Buros (Ed.), *The seventh mental measurements yearbook*, Vol. 1. Highland Park, NJ: Gryphon Press, 1972, pp. 66–67.

Messer, S. B. Reflection-impulsivity: A review. *Psychological Bulletin*, 1976, *83*, 1026–1052.

Milich, R. S., & Landau, S. Socialization and peer relations in hyperactive children. In K. D. Gadow & I. Bialer (Eds.), *Advances in learning and behavior disabilities*, Vol. 1. Greenwich, CT: JAI Press, 1981, in press.

Milich, R. S., & Loney, J. The role of hyperactive and aggressive symptomatology in predicting adolescent outcome among hyperactive children. *Journal of Pediatric Psychology*, 1979a, *4*, 93–112.

Milich, R. S., & Loney, J. The factor composition of the WISC for hyperkinetic/MBD males. *Journal of Learning Disabilities*, 1979b, *12*, 491–495.

Milich, R. S., Loney, J., & Landau, S. The independent dimensions of hyperactivity and aggression: A replication and further validation. Unpublished manuscript. University of Iowa, 1981.

Milich, R. S., Roberts, M. A., Loney, J., & Caputo, J. Differentiating practice effects and statistical regression on the Conners Hyperkinesis Index. *Journal of Abnormal Child Psychology*, 1980, *8*, 549–552.

Miller, J. S. Hyperactive children: A ten-year study. *Pediatrics*, 1978a, *61*, 217–223.

Miller, L. Method factors associated with assessment of child behavior: Fact or artifact? *Journal of Abnormal Child Psychology*, 1976, *4*, 209–219.

Miller, N. E. Biofeedback and visceral learning. *Annual Review of Psychology*, 1978b, *29*, 373–404.

Miller, P. H. & Bigi, L. The development of children's understanding of attention. *Merrill–Palmer Quarterly*, 1979, *25*, 235–250.

Miller, R. G., Palkes, H. S., & Stewart, M. A. Hyperactive children in suburban elementary schools. *Child Psychiatry and Human Development*, 1973, *4*, 121–127.

Millichap, J. G. Drugs in management of minimal brain dysfunction. In F. F. de la Cruz, B. H. Fox, & R. H. Roberts (Eds.), Minimal brain dysfunction. *Annals of the New York Academy of Sciences*, 1973, *205*, 321–334.

Millichap, J. G. *The hyperactive child with minimal brain dysfunction.* Chicago: Year Book Medical Publishers, 1975.

Millman, B. S. Resources and recourses in the management of compound ("intractable") pain. *Drug Therapy*, 1978, *8*, 65–80.

Milman, D. H. Minimal brain dysfunction in childhood: Outcome in late adolescence and early adult years. *Journal of Clinical Psychiatry*, 1979, *40*, 371–380.

Minde, K. K. Hyperactivity: Where do we stand? In M. Blaw, I. Rapin, & M. Kinsbourne (Eds.), *Topics in child neurology.* Jamaica, NY: Spectrum, 1977.

Minde, K. K., & Cohen, N. J. Hyperactive children in Canada and Uganda. *Journal of Child Psychiatry*, 1978, *17*, 476–487.

Minde, K. K., Lewin, D., Weiss, G., Lavigueur, H., Douglas, V., & Sykes, E. The hyperactive child in elementary school: A 5-year controlled followup. *Exceptional Children*, 1971, *38*, 215–221.

Minde, K. K., Webb, G., & Sykes, D. Studies on the hyperactive child: VI. Prenatal and paranatal factors associated with hyperactivity. *Developmental Medicine and Child Neurology*, 1968, *10*, 355–363.

Minde, K. K., Weiss, G., & Mendelson, N. A 5-year follow-up study of 91 hyperactive school children. *Journal of the American Academy of Child Psychiatry*, 1972, *11*, 595–610.

Minerals Yearbook: United States Department of the Interior. Washington, D.C.: Government Printing Office, 1976.

Mischel, W. Continuity and change in personality. *American Psychologist*, 1969, *24*, 1012–1018.

Mnookin, R. Children's rights: Beyond kiddie libbers and child savers. *Journal of Clinical Child Psychology*, 1978, *7*, 163–167.

Mofenson, H. C., Greensher, J., & Horowitz, R. Detection of the hyperactive child (letter). *Journal of Pediatrics*, 1972, *80*, 687.

Molitch, M., & Eccles, A. K. Effect of benzedrine sulphate on intelligence scores of children. *American Journal of Psychiatry*, 1937, *94*, 587–590.

Montagu, J. D. The hyperkinetic child: A behavioural, electrodermal and EEG investigation. *Developmental Medicine and Child Neurology*, 1975, *17*, 299–305.

Moore, C. L. Behavior modification and electromyographic biofeedback as alternatives to drugs for the treatment of hyperkinesis in children. Unpublished doctoral dissertation, East Texas State University, 1977.

Moore, K., & Waite, L. Early childbearing and educational attainment. *Family Planning Perspectives*, 1977, *9*, 220–225.

Moreland, K. L. Stimulus control of hyperactivity. *Perceptual and Motor Skills*, 1977, *45*, 916.

Moreland, K. L. Personal communication, 1978.

Morrison, J. R. Diagnosis of adult psychiatric patients with childhood hyperactivity. *American Journal of Psychiatry*, 1979, *136*, 955–958.

Morrison, J. R. Adult psychiatric disorders in parents of hyperactive children. *American Journal of Psychiatry*, 1980a, *137*, 825–827.

Morrison, J. R. Childhood hyperactivity in an adult psychiatric population. *Journal of Clinical Psychiatry*, 1980b, *41*, 40–43.

Morrison, J. R., & Minkoff, K. Explosive personality as a sequel to the hyperactive-child syndrome. *Comprehensive Psychiatry*, 1975, *16*, 343–348.

Morrison, J. R., & Stewart, M. A. A family study of the hyperactive child syndrome. *Biological Psychiatry*, 1971, *3*, 189–195.

Morrison, J. R., & Stewart, M. A. Evidence for polygenetic inheritance in the hyperactive child syndrome. *American Journal of Psychiatry*, 1973a, *130*, 791–792.

Morrison, J. R., & Stewart, M. A. The psychiatric status of the legal families of adopted hyperactive children. *Archives of General Psychiatry*, 1973b, *23*, 888–891.

Morrison, J. R., & Stewart, M. A. Bilateral inheritance as evidence for polygenicity in the hyperactive child syndrome. *Journal of Nervous and Mental Diseases*, 1974, *158*, 226–228.

Munsinger, H. The identical twin transfusion syndrome: A source of error in estimating IQ resemblance and heritability. *Annals of Human Genetics*, 1977, *40*, 307–321.

Murray, M. E. Behavioral management of the hyperactive child. *Developmental and Behavioral Pediatrics*, 1980, *1*, 108–111.

Nader, P. R., Emmel, A., & Charney, E. The school health service: A new model. *Pediatrics*, 1972, *49*, 805–813.

National Advisory Committee on Hyperkinesis and Food Additives. New York, The Nutrition Foundation Inc., 1980.

Needleman, H. L. Lead poisoning in children: Neurologic implications of widespread subclinical intoxication. *Seminars in Psychiatry*, 1973, *5*, 47–53.

Needleman, H. L., Gunnoe, C., Leviton, A., Reed, R., Peresie, H., Maher, C., & Barrett, P. Deficits in psychologic and classroom performance of children with elevated dentine lead levels. *New England Journal of Medicine*, 1979, *300*, 689–695.

Neisworth, J., Kurtz, P. D., Ross, A., & Madle, R. Naturalistic assessment of neurological diagnoses and pharmacological intervention. *Journal of Learning Disabilities*, 1976, *9*, 149–152.

Nelson, W. E. *Textbook of pediatrics*. Philadelphia: Saunders, 1950.

Newell, G. R., & Henderson, B. E. Case-control study of Hodgkin's disease: I. Results of the interview questionnaire. *Journal of the National Cancer Institute*, 1973, *51*, 1437–1441.

Newlin, D. B., & Tramontana, M. G. Neuropsychological findings in a hyperactive adolescent with subcortical brain pathology. *Clinical Neuropsychology*, 1980, *2*, 178–183.

Ney, P. G. Psychosis in a child, associated with amphetamine administration. *Canadian Medical Association Journal*, 1967, *97*, 1026–1029.

Ney, P. G. Four types of hyperkinesis. *Canadian Psychiatric Association Journal*, 1974, *19*, 543–550.

Ney, P. G. Uses and abuses of operant conditioning. *Canadian Psychiatric Association Journal*, 1975, *20*, 119–132.

Nichamin, S. J. Recognizing minimal cerebral dysfunction in the infant and toddler. *Clinical Pediatrics*, 1972, *11*, 255–257.

Nicholi, A. M., Jr. The adolescent. In A. M. Nicholi, Jr. (Ed.), *The Harvard guide to modern psychiatry*. London: Belknap, 1978.

Norwood, C. *At highest risk*. New York: McGraw-Hill, 1980.

Nyquist, E. B., & Hawes, G. R. (Eds.). *Open education: A sourcebook for parents and teachers*. New York: Bantam Books, 1972.

O'Donnell, J. P., O'Neill, S., & Staley, A. Congenital correlates of distractibility. *Journal of Abnormal Child Psychology*, 1979, *7*, 465–470.

Oettinger, L. Bone age and minimal brain dysfunction (letter to the editor). *Journal of Pediatrics*, 1975, *87*, 328.

Office of Child Development. Report on the conference on the use of stimulant drugs in the treatment of behaviorally disturbed young school children, 1971. Reprinted in *The National Elementary Principal*, 1971, *50*, 53–59.

Offord, D. R., & Jones, M. B. The proband-sibling design in psychiatry with two technical notes. *Canadian Psychiatric Association Journal*, 1976, *21*, 101–107.

Offord, D. R., Sullivan, N., Allen, N., & Abrams, N. Delinquency and hyperactivity. *Journal of Nervous and Mental Diseases*, 1979, *167*, 734–741.

Okolo, C., Bartlett, S. A., & Shaw, S. F. Communication between professionals concerning medication for the hyperactive child. *Journal of Learning Disabilities*, 1978, *11*, 45–48.

Olds, S. W. Is there a tornado in the house? *Today's Health*, November 1969, *47*, 33–36.

O'Leary, K. D. Pills or skills for hyperactive children. *Journal of Applied Behavior Analysis*, 1980, *13*, 191–204.

O'Leary, K. D., & Borkovec, T. D. Conceptual, methodological, and ethical problems of placebo groups in psychotherapy research. *American Psychologist*, 1978, *33*, 821–830.

O'Leary, K. D., & Drabman, R. S. Token reinforcement programs in the classroom: A review. *Psychological Bulletin*, 1971, *75*, 379–398.

O'Leary, K. D., Pelham, W. E., Rosenbaum, A., & Price, G. H. Behavioral treatment of hyperkinetic children: An experimental evaluation of its usefulness. *Clinical Pediatrics*, 1976, *15*, 510–515.

O'Leary, K. D., Romanczyk, R. G., Kass, R. E., Dietz, A., & Santagrossi, D. Procedures for classroom observation of teachers and children. Unpublished manuscript. State University of New York at Stony Brook, 1971.

O'Leary, K. D., Rosenbaum, A., & Hughes, P. C. Fluorescent lighting: A purported source of hyperactive behavior. *Journal of Abnormal Child Psychology*, 1978a, *6*, 285–289.

O'Leary, K. D., Rosenbaum, A., & Hughes, P. C. Direct and systematic replication: A rejoinder. *Journal of Abnormal Child Psychology*, 1978b, *6*, 295–297.

Olweus, D. Personality and aggression. In J. K. Cole and D. D. Jensen (Eds.), *Nebraska symposium on motivation 1972*. Lincoln: University of Nebraska Press, 1973.

O'Malley, J. E., & Eisenberg, L. The hyperkinetic syndrome. *Seminars in Psychiatry*, 1973, *5*, 95–103.

Omenn, G. S. Genetic issues in the syndrome of minimal brain dysfunction. *Seminars in Psychiatry*, 1973, *5*, 5–17.

O'Shea, J. Sublingual immunotherapy of hyperkinetic children with food, chemical and inhalant allergens: a double-blind study. Paper presented at the Twelfth Advanced Seminar in Clinical Ecology, Key Biscayne, FL, 1979.

Oster, M. W. Cancer of the pancreas. *New England Journal of Medicine*, 1980, *302*, 232.

Ott, J. N. Responses of psychological and physiological functions to environmental radiation stress: Part II. *Journal of Learning Disabilities*, 1968, *1*, 348–354.

Ott, J. N. Influence of fluorescent lights on hyperactivity and learning disabilities. *Journal of Learning Disabilities*, 1976, *9*, 417–422.

Overton, D. A. Major theories of state dependent learning. In B. T. Ho, D. W. Richards, III, & D. L. Chute (Eds.), *Drug discrimination and state dependent learning*. New York: Academic Press, 1978.

Packer, S. Treatment of minimal brain dysfunction in a young adult. *Canadian Psychiatric Association Journal*, 1978, *23*, 501–502.

Padway, L. Federal regulation of Ritalin in the treatment of hyperactive children. *Ecology Law Quarterly*, 1978, *7*, 457–495.

Page, J. G., Bernstein, J. E., Janicki, R. S., & Michelli, F. A. A multi-clinic trial of pemoline in childhood hyperkinesis. In C. K. Conners (Ed.), *Clinical use of stimulant drugs in children*. New York: American Elsevier, 1974.

Paine, R. S., Werry, J. S., & Quay, H. C. A study of "minimal cerebral dysfunction." *Developmental Medicine and Child Neurology*, 1968, *10*, 505–520.

Palfrey, J. S., Mervis, R. C., & Butler, J. A. New directions in the evaluation and education of handicapped children. *New England Journal of Medicine*, 1978, *298*, 819–824.

Palkes, H. S., & Stewart, M. A. Intellectual ability and performance of hyperactive children. *American Journal of Orthopsychiatry*, 1972, *42*, 35–39.

Palkes, H. S., Stewart, M. A., & Freedman, J. Improvement in maze performance of hyperactive boys as a function of verbal-training procedures. *Journal of Special Education*, 1971, *5*, 337–342.

Palkes, H. S., Stewart, M. A., & Kahana, B. Porteus Maze performance of hyperactive boys after training in self-directed verbal commands. *Child Development*, 1968, *39*, 817–826.

Paradise, J. L. Otitis media in infants and children. *Pediatrics*, 1980, *65*; 917–943.

Parmelee, A. H., Sigman, M., Kopp, C. B., & Haber, A. The concept of a cumulative risk score in infants. In N. R. Ellis (Ed.), *Aberrant development in infancy: Human and animal studies.* Hillsdale, NJ: Erlbaum, 1975.

Parry, P., & Douglas, V. I. The effects of reward on the performance of hyperactive children. Cited in Douglas, V. I., Parry, P., Marton, P., & Garson, C. Assessment of a cognitive training program for hyperactive children. *Journal of Abnormal Child Psychology*, 1976, *4*, 389–410.

Pasamanick, B., Rogers, M., & Lilienfeld, A. M. Pregnancy experience and the development of behavior disorder in children. *American Journal of Psychiatry*, 1956, *112*, 613–617.

Pastor, D. L. The quality of mother–infant attachment and its relationship to toddlers' initial sociability with peers. *Developmental Psychology*, 1981, *17*, 326–335.

Paternite, C. E., & Loney, J. Childhood hyperkinesis: Relationships between symptomatology and home environment. In C. K. Whalen & B. Henker (Eds.), *Hyperactive children: The social ecology of identification and treatment.* New York: Academic Press, 1980.

Paternite, C. E., Loney, J., & Langhorne, J. E. Relationships between symptomatology and SES-related factors in hyperkinetic/MBD boys. *American Journal of Orthopsychiatry*, 1976, *46*, 291–301.

Patmon, R., & Murphy, P. Differential treatment efficacy of EEG and EMG feedback for hyperactive adolescents. Paper presented at the Ninth Annual Meeting of the Biofeedback Society of America, Albuquerque, NM, 1978.

Patterson, G. R. *Families: Applications of social learning to family life.* Champaign, IL: Research Press, 1971.

Patterson, G. R., Jones, R., Whittier, J., & Wright, M. A. A behavior modification technique for the hyperactive child. *Behavior Research and Therapy*, 1965, *2*, 217–226.

Paulauskas, S. L., & Campbell, S. B. Social perspective-taking and teacher ratings of peer interaction in hyperactive boys. *Journal of Abnormal Child Psychology*, 1979, *7*, 483–493.

Paxton, P. W. Effects of drug-induced behavior changes in hyperactive children on maternal attitude and personality. Unpublished doctoral dissertation, University of Minnesota, 1972.

Payne, D. *The assessment of learning: Cognition and affection.* Lexington, MA: Heath, 1974.

Pederson, F. A. Mother, father, and infant as an interaction system. Paper presented at the meeting of the American Psychological Association, Washington, D.C., September 1976.

Pekarik, E. G., Prinz, R. J., Liebert, D. E., Weintraub, S., & Neale, J. M. The Pupil Evaluation Inventory: A sociometric technique for assessing children's social behavior. *Journal of Abnormal Child Psychology*, 1976, *4*, 83–97.

Pelham, W. E. Withdrawal of a stimulant drug and concurrent behavioral intervention in the treatment of a hyperactive child. *Behavior Therapy*, 1977, *8*, 473–479.

Pelham, W. E. Hyperactive children. In R. P. Liberman (Ed.), Symposium on behavior therapy in psychiatry. *Psychiatric Clinics of North America*, 1978, *1*, 217–242.

Pelham, W. E. Peer relations and hyperactive children: Description and treatment effects. In R. Milich (Chair), *Peer relations among hyperactive children.* Symposium presented at the meeting of the American Psychological Association, Montreal, September 1980.

Persson-Blennow, I., & McNeil, T. F. A questionnaire for measurement of temperament in six-month-old infants: Development and standardization. *Journal of Child Psychology and Psychiatry,* 1979, *20,* 1–13.

Peters, J. E., Romine, J. S., & Dykman, R. A. A special neurological examination of children with learning disabilities. *Developmental Medicine and Child Neurology,* 1975, *17,* 63–78.

Petti, T., & Campbell, M. Imipramine and seizures. *American Journal of Psychiatry,* 1975, *32,* 538–540.

Phipps-Yonas, S. Teenage pregnancy and motherhood: A review of the literature. *American Journal of Orthopsychiatry,* 1980, *50,* 403–431.

Pihl, R. F. Conditioning procedures with hyperactive children. *Neurology,* 1967, *17,* 421–423.

Pincus, J. H., & Glaser, G. H. The syndrome of "minimal brain damage" in childhood. *New England Journal of Medicine,* 1966, *275,* 27–35.

Pletscher, A. Metabolism, transfer, and storage of 5-hydroxytrptamine in blood platelets. *British Journal of Pharmacology and Chemotherapy,* 1968, *32,* 1–16.

Plomin, R., & Foch, T. T. Hyperactivity and pediatrician diagnoses, parental ratings, specific cognitive abilities, and laboratory measures. *Journal of Abnormal Child Psychology,* 1981, *9,* 55–64.

Plotnikoff, N. Pemoline: Review of performance. *Texas Reports on Biology and Medicine,* 1971, *29,* 467–479.

Points, T. C. Testimony to Subcommittee on Government Operations, Washington, D.C., 1970.

Pope, L. Motor activity in brain-injured children. *American Journal of Orthopsychiatry,* 1970, *40,* 783–794.

Porges, S. W. Peripheral and neurochemical parallels of psychopathology: A psychophysiological model relating autonomic imbalance to hyperactivity, psychopathy, and autism. In H. W. Reese (Ed.), *Advances in child development and behavior,* Vol. 11. New York: Academic Press, 1976.

Porges, S. W. Individual differences in attention: A possible physiological substrate. *Advances in Special Education,* 1980, *2,* 111–134.

Porges, S. W., Drasgow, F., Ullman, R. K., Sleator, E. K., & Sprague, R. L. *Illinois Classroom Assessment Profile*: Development of the instrument. Unpublished manuscript. University of Illinois, 1981.

Porges, S. W., & Smith, K. M. Defining hyperactivity: Psychophysiological and behavioral strategies. In C. K. Whalen & B. Henker (Eds.), *Hyperactive children: The social ecology of identification and treatment.* New York: Academic Press, 1980.

Porges, S. W., Ullman, R. K., Drasgow, F., Sleator, E. K., & Sprague, R. L. *Illinois Classroom Assessment Profile*: A teacher rating scale. Champaign, IL: University of Illinois, 1980.

Porges, S. W., Walter, G. F., Korb, R. J., & Sprague, R. L. The influence of methylphenidate on heart rate and behavioral measures of attention in hyperactive children. *Child Development,* 1975, *46,* 727–733.

Potvin, R. H., & Lee, C. F. Multistage path models of adolescent alcohol and drug use. *Journal of Studies on Alcohol,* 1980, *41,* 531–542.

Prechtl, H. F. R. The mother–child interaction in babies with minimal brain damage: A follow-up study. In B. M. Foss (Ed.), *Determinants of infant behavior,* Vol. 2. London: Methuen, 1963.

Preis, K., & Huessy, H. R. Hyperactivity in adults. In M. J. Cohen (Ed.), *Drugs and the special child.* New York: Gardner Press, 1979a.

Preis, K., & Huessy, H. R. Hyperactive children at risk. In M. J. Cohen (Ed.), *Drugs and the special child.* New York: Gardner Press, 1979b.

Preston, M. I. Late behavioral aspects found in cases of prenatal, natal, and postnatal anoxia. *Journal of Pediatrics,* 1945, *26,* 353–366.

Prichep, L. S., Sutton, S., & Hakerem, G. Evoked potentials in hyperkinetic and normal children under certainty and uncertainty: A placebo and methylphenidate study. *Psychophysiology,* 1976, *13,* 419–428.

Prinz, R. J., Connor, P. A., & Wilson, C. C. Hyperactive and aggressive behaviors in childhood: Intertwined dimensions. *Journal of Abnormal Psychology,* 1981, *9,* 191–202.

Prinz, R. J., & Loney, J. Teacher-rated hyperactive elementary school girls: An exploratory developmental study. *Child Psychiatry and Human Development,* 1974, *4,* 246–257.

Prinz, R. J., Roberts, W. A., & Hantman, E. Dietary correlates of hyperactive behavior in children. *Journal of Consulting and Clinical Psychology,* 1980, *48,* 760–769.

Prout, H. T. Behavioral intervention with hyperactive children: A review. *Journal of Learning Disabilities,* 1977, *10,* 20–25.

Puig-Antich, J., Greenhill, L. L., Sassin, J., & Sachar, E. J. Growth hormone, prolactin, and cortisol responses and growth patterns in hyperkinetic children treated with dextroamphetamine. *American Academy of Child Psychiatry,* 1978, *17,* 457–475.

Quay, H. C. Classification. In H. C. Quay & J. S. Werry (Eds.), *Psychopathological disorders of childhood* (2nd ed.). New York: Wiley, 1979.

Quay, H. C., & Peterson, D. R. *Manual for the Behavior Problem Checklist.* Champaign, IL: Children's Research Center, University of Illinois, 1967.

Quinn, P. O., & Rapoport, J. L. One-year follow-up of hyperactive boys treated with imipramine or methylphenidate. *American Journal of Psychiatry,* 1975, *132,* 241–245.

Quinn, P. O., Renfield, M., Burg, C., & Rapoport, J. L. Minor physical anomalies: A newborn screening and 1 year follow-up. *Journal of the American Academy of Child Psychiatry,* 1977, *16,* 662–669.

Quitkin, F., & Klein, D. F. Two behavioral syndromes in young adults related to possible minimal brain dysfunction. *Journal of Psychiatric Research,* 1969, *7,* 131–142.

Rachman, S., Hodgson, R., & Marks, I. M. Treatment of chronic obsessive-compulsive neurosis. *Behavior Research and Therapy,* 1971, *9,* 237–247.

Rapoport, J. L. The "real" and "ideal" management of stimulant drug treatment for hyperactive children: Recent findings and a report from clinical practice. In C. K. Whalen & B. Henker (Eds.), *Hyperactive children: The social ecology of identification and treatment.* New York: Academic Press, 1980.

Rapoport, J. L., Abramson, A. U., Alexander, D. F., & Lott, I. T. Playroom observations of hyperactive children on medication. *Journal of the American Academy of Child Psychiatry,* 1971, *10,* 524–534.

Rapoport, J. L., & Benoit, M. The relation of direct home observations to the clinic evaluation of hyperactive school age boys. *Journal of Child Psychology and Psychiatry,* 1975, *16,* 141–147.

Rapoport, J. L., Buchsbaum, M. S., Zahn, T. P., Weingartner, H., Ludlow, C., & Mikkelsen, E. J. Dextroamphetamine: Cognitive and behavioral effects in normal prepubertal boys. *Science,* 1978, *199,* 560–563.

Rapoport, J. L., & Ferguson, H. B. Biological validation of the hyperkinetic syndrome. *Developmental Medicine and Child Neurology,* 1981, *23,* 667–682.

Rapoport, J. L., Mikkelsen, E. J., & Werry, J. S. Antidepressants. In J. S. Werry (Ed.), *Pediatric psychopharmacology: The use of behavior modifying drugs in children.* New York: Brunner/Mazel, 1978.

Rapoport, J. L., & Quinn, P. O. Minor physical anomalies and early developmental deviation. *International Journal of Mental Health*, 1975, *4*, 29–44.

Rapoport, J. L., Quinn, P. O., Bradbard, G., Riddle, D., & Brooks, E. Imipramine and methylphenidate treatments of hyperactive boys. *Archives of General Psychiatry*, 1974, *30*, 789–793.

Rapoport, J. L., Quinn, P. O., Scribanu, N., & Murphy, D. Platelet serotonin of hyperactive school-age boys. *British Journal of Psychiatry*, 1974, *125*, 138–140.

Rapoport, J. L., Quinn, P. O., Burg, C., & Bartley, L. Can hyperactives be identified in infancy? In R. L. Trites (Ed.), *Hyperactivity in children*. Baltimore: University Park Press, 1979.

Rapoport, J. L., Quinn, P. O., & Lamprecht, F. Minor physical anomalies and plasma dopamine-beta-hydroxylase activity in hyperactive boys. *American Journal of Psychiatry*, 1974, *131*, 386–390.

Rapoport, J. L., & Zametkin, A. Attention deficit disorder. *Psychiatric Clinics of North America*, 1980, *3*, 425–441.

Rapoport, R., & Repo, S. The educator as a pusher: Drug control in the classroom. *This Magazine Is About Schools*, 1971, *5*, 87–112.

Raskin, D. E., & Klein, Z. E. Losing a symptom through keeping it. *Archives of General Psychiatry*, 1976, *33*, 548–555.

Rayburn, W. F., & McKean, H. E. Maternal perception of fetal movement and perinatal outcome. *Obstetrics and Gynecology*, 1980, *56*, 161–164.

Reardon, D. M., & Bell, G. Effects of sedative and stimulative music on activity levels of severely retarded boys. *American Journal of Mental Deficiency*, 1970, *75*, 156–159.

Reichard, C. C., & Elder, S. T. The effects of caffeine on reaction time in hyperkinetic and normal children. *American Journal of Psychiatry*, 1977, *134*, 144–148.

Reisinger, J. J., Ora, J. P., & Frangia, G. W. Parents as change agents for their children: A review. *Journal of Community Psychology*, 1976, *4*, 103–123.

Renshaw, D. C. *The hyperactive child*. Chicago: Nelson Hall, 1974.

Reus, V. I., Weingartner, H., & Post, R. M. Clinical implications of state-dependent learning. *American Journal of Psychiatry*, 1979, *136*, 927–931.

Reutter, E. E., Jr., & Hamilton, R. R. *The law and education*. Mineola, NY: Foundation Press, 1976.

Richardson, N. R. Personal communication, 1978.

Rickel, A. U., Smith, R. L., & Sharp, K. C. Description and evaluation of a preventive mental health program for preschoolers. *Journal of Abnormal Child Psychology*, 1979, *7*, 101–112.

Riddle, K. D., & Rapoport, J. L. A 2-year follow-up of 72 hyperactive boys. *Journal of Nervous and Mental Disease*, 1976, *162*, 126–134.

Rie, E. D., & Rie, H. E. Recall, retention, and Ritalin. *Journal of Consulting and Clinical Psychology*, 1977, *45*, 967–972.

Rie, H. E. Hyperactivity in children. *American Journal of Diseases of Children*, 1975, *129*, 783–789.

Rie, H. E. Definitional problems. In H. E. Rie & E. D. Rie (Eds.), *Handbook of minimal brain dysfunctions: A critical view*. New York: Wiley, 1980.

Rie, H. E., & Rie, E. D. *Handbook of minimal brain dysfunctions: A critical view*. New York: Wiley, 1980.

Rie, H. E., Rie, E. D., Stewart, S., & Ambuel, J. P. Effects of methylphenidate on underachieving children. *Journal of Consulting and Clinical Psychology*, 1976a, *44*, 250–260.

Rie, H. E., Rie, E. D., Stewart, S., & Ambuel, J. P. Effects of Ritalin on underachieving children: A replication. *American Journal of Orthopsychiatry*, 1976b, *46*, 313–322.

Robertson, K. M. Personal communication, October 1978.

Robin, S. S., & Bosco, J. J. Ritalin for school children: The teachers' perspective. *Journal of School Health*, 1973, *43*, 624–628.

Robin, S. S., & Bosco, J. J. The social context of stimulant drug treatment for hyperkinetic children. *School Review*, 1976, *85*, 141–154.

Robin, S. S., & Bosco, J. J. Creating an approach for understanding the diagnosis and treatment of hyperkinetic children. Paper presented at the annual meeting of the American Educational Research Association, Boston, April 1980.

Robin, S. S., & Bosco, J. J. Parent, teacher and physician in the life of the hyperactive child: The coherence of the social environment. Unpublished manuscript, Western Michigan University, 1981.

Robins, L. N. *Deviant children grown up*. Baltimore: Williams and Wilkins, 1966.

Robins, L. N. Sturdy childhood predictors of adult outcomes: Replications from longitudinal studies. *Psychological Medicine*, 1978, *8*, 611–622.

Robinson, N. M. Personal communication, 1977.

Robinson, N. M. Mild mental retardation: Does it exist in the People's Republic of China? *Mental Retardation*, 1978, *16*, 295–298.

Robitscher, J. *The powers of psychiatry*. Boston: Houghton Mifflin, 1980.

Roche, A. F., Lipman, R. S., Overall, J. E., & Hung, W. The effects of stimulant medication on the growth of hyperkinetic children. *Pediatrics*, 1979, *63*, 847–850.

Roche, A. F., Wainer, H., & Thissen, D. Predicting adult stature for individuals. *Monographs in Pediatrics, Vol. 3*. Basel: Karger, 1975.

Rodin, E., Lucas, A., & Simson, C. A study of behavior disorders in children by means of general purpose computers. *Proceedings of the Conference on Data Acquisition and Processing in Biological Medicine*. Oxford: Pergamon, 1963.

Rosenbaum, A., O'Leary, K. D., & Jacob, R. G. Behavorial intervention with hyperactive children: Group consequences as a supplement to individual contingencies. *Behavior Therapy*, 1975, *6*, 315–323.

Rosenbaum, M. S., & Drabman, R. S. ". . . But I'd rather do it myself:" A review of self-control training in the classroom. Unpublished manuscript, 1981.

Rosenberg, J. B., & Weller, G. M. Minor physical anomalies and academic performance in young school children. *Developmental Medicine and Child Neurology*, 1973, *15*, 131–135.

Rosenberg, S., Metzig, E., & Ast, M. A methodological approach to evaluation of predictive tests for Huntington's disease. Paper presented at the 11th World Congress of Neurology, Amsterdam, September 1977.

Rosenthal, R. H., & Allen, T. W. An examination of attention, arousal, and learning dysfunctions of hyperkinetic children. *Psychological Bulletin*, 1978, *85*, 689–715.

Ross, A. O. *Psychological aspects of learning disabilities and reading disorders*. New York: McGraw-Hill, 1976.

Ross, D. C., & Klein, D. F. A comparison of analysis of covariance and the O technique as applied to illustrative psychopharmacological data. *Journal of Psychiatric Research*, 1979, *15*, 67–75.

Ross, D. M. Counterconditioning with an impulsive six-year-old boy. Unpublished manuscript, Stanford University, 1967.

Ross, D. M. Case study of a mother of a difficult, high active infant. Unpublished manuscript, University of California, San Francisco, 1973.

Ross, D. M., & Ross, S. A. Storage and utilization of previously formulated mediators in educable mentally retarded children. *Journal of Educational Psychology*, 1973, *65*, 205–210.

Ross, D. M., & Ross, S. A. *Hyperactivity: Research, theory and action*. New York: Wiley, 1976.

Ross, D. M., & Ross, S. A. A test of the generality of Bobrow and Bower's comprehension hypothesis. *American Journal of Mental Deficiency*, 1978, *82*, 453–459.

Ross, D. M., & Ross, S. A. Case study on the use of self-confrontation and imagery in a nine-year-old hyperactive boy. Unpublished manuscript, University of California, San Francisco, 1979.

Ross, D. M., Ross, S. A., & Downing, M. L. Intentional training vs. observational learning of mediational strategies in EMR children. *American Journal of Mental Deficiency*, 1973, *78*, 292–299.

Ross, R. P. Drug therapy for hyperactivity: Existing practices in physician-school communication. In M. J. Cohen (Ed.), *Drugs and the special child*. New York: Gardner Press, 1979.

Ross, S. A. Effects of intentional training in social behavior on retarded children. *American Journal of Mental Deficiency*, 1969, *73*, 912–919.

Rost, K. J., & Charles, D. C. Academic achievement of brain injured and hyperactive children in isolation. *Exceptional Children*, 1967, *34*, 125–126.

Rosvold, H. E., Mirsky, A. F., Sarason, I., Bransome, E. D., & Beck, L. H. A continuous performance test of brain damage. *Journal of Consulting Psychology*, 1956, *20*, 343–350.

Rothenberg, M. B. Reactions of children to illness and hospitalization. In D. W. Smith & R. E. Marshall (Eds.), *Introduction to clinical pediatrics*. Philadelphia: Saunders, 1972.

Rotter, J. B. *Social learning and clinical psychology*. Englewood Cliffs, NJ: Prentice-Hall, 1954.

Routh, D. K. Hyperactivity. In P. R. Magrab (Ed.), *Psychological management of pediatric problems*, Vol. 2. Baltimore: University Park Press, 1978.

Routh, D. K. Developmental and social aspects of hyperactivity. In C. K. Whalen & B. Henker (Eds.), *Hyperactive children: The social ecology of identification and treatment*. New York: Academic Press, 1980.

Routh, D. K., & Roberts, R. D. Minimal brain dysfunction in children: Failure to find evidence for a behavioral syndrome. *Psychological Reports*, 1972, *31*, 307–314.

Routh, D. K., & Schroeder, C. S. Standardized playroom measures as indices of hyperactivity. *Journal of Abnormal Child Psychology*, 1976, *4*, 199–207.

Routh, D. K., Schroeder, C. S., & O'Tuama, L. A. Development of activity level in children. *Developmental Psychology*, 1974, *10*, 163–168.

Rowe, D. C., & Plomin, R. Temperament in early childhood. *Journal of Personality Assessment*, 1977, *41*, 150–156.

Rummo, J. H., Routh, D. K., Rummo, N. J., & Brown, J. F. Behavioral and neurological effects of symptomatic and asymptomatic lead exposure in children. *Archives of Environmental Health*, 1979, *34*, 120–124.

Rutter, M. Psychological development—predictions from infancy. *Journal of Child Psychology and Psychiatry*, 1970, *11*, 49–62.

Rutter, M. Raised lead levels and impaired cognitive/behavioral functioning: A review of the evidence. *Supplement to Developmental Medicine and Child Neurology*, 1980, *22*, 1–26.

Rutter, M., & Graham, P. The reliability and validity of the psychiatric assessment of the child: 1. Interview with the child. *British Journal of Psychiatry*, 1968, *114*, 563–579.

Rutter, M., Lebovici, S., Eisenberg, L., Sneznenvskij, A. V., Sadoun, R., Brooke, E., & Lin, T-Y. A tri-axial classification of mental disorders in childhood. *Journal of Child Psychology and Psychiatry*, 1969, *10*, 41–61.

Ryor, J. 94–142—The perspective of regular education. *Learning Disability Quarterly*, 1978, *1*, 6–14.

Sabatino, D., & Cramblett, H. Behavioral sequelae of California encephalitis virus infection in children. *Developmental Medicine and Child Neurology*, 1968, *10*, 331–337.

Sachar, E. J. Growth hormone responses in hyperactive children. *Psychopharmacology Bulletin*, 1977, *13*, 55.

Safer, D. J. A familial factor in minimal brain dysfunction. *Behavior Genetics*, 1973, *3*, 175–186.

Safer, D. J., & Allen, R. P. Factors influencing the suppressant effects of two stimulant drugs on the growth of hyperactive children. *Pediatrics*, 1973, *51*, 660–667.

Safer, D. J., & Allen, R. P. Side effects from long-term use of stimulants in children. *International Journal of Mental Health*, 1975a, *4*, 105–118.

Safer, D. J., & Allen, R. P. Stimulant drug treatment of hyperactive adolescents. *Diseases of the Nervous System*, 1975b, *36*, 454–457.

Safer, D. J., & Allen, R. P. *Hyperactive children: Diagnosis and management.* Baltimore: University Park Press, 1976.

Safer, D. J., Allen, R. P., & Barr, E. Depression of growth in hyperactive children on stimulant drugs. *New England Journal of Medicine*, 1972, *287*, 217–220.

Safer, D. J., Allen, R. P., & Barr, E. Growth rebound after termination of stimulant drugs. *Journal of Pediatrics*, 1975, *86*, 113–116.

Salkind, N. J., & Poggio, J. P. The measurement of hyperactivity: Trends and issues. In M. J. Fine (Ed.), *Principles and techniques of intervention with hyperactive children.* Springfield, IL: Charles C. Thomas, 1977.

Salkind, N. J., & Wright, J. C. The development of reflection-impulsivity and cognitive efficiency: An integrated model. *Human Development*, 1977, *20*, 377–387.

Salter, A. C. Children referred and treated for hyperactivity: A descriptive and control comparison study. Unpublished doctoral dissertation, Harvard University, 1977.

Salzinger, S., Antrobus, J., & Glick, J. (Eds.), *The ecosystem of the "sick" kid.* New York: Academic Press, 1981.

Salzman, L. K. Allergy testing, psychological assessment and dietary treatment of the hyperactive child syndrome. *The Medical Journal of Australia*, 1976, *2*, 248–251.

Sameroff, A. J. Early influences on development: Fact or fancy? *Merrill-Palmer Quarterly of Behavior and Development*, 1975, *21*, 267–294.

Sameroff, A. J., & Chandler, M. J. Reproductive risk and the continuum of caretaking casualty. In F. D. Horowitz (Ed.), *Review of child development research*, Vol. 4. Chicago: University of Chicago Press, 1975.

Sanborn, D. E., Pyke, H. F., & Sanborn, C. J. Videotape playback and psychotherapy: A review. *Psychotherapy: Theory, research and practice*, 1975, *12*, 179–186.

Sandberg, S. T., Rutter, M., & Taylor, E. Hyperkinetic disorder in psychiatric clinic attenders. *Developmental Medicine and Child Neurology*, 1978, *20*, 279–299.

Sander, L. W. The longitudinal course of early mother-child interaction: Cross-case comparison in a sample of mother-child pairs. In B. M. Foss (Ed.), *Determinants of infant behavior*, Vol. 4. London: Methuen, 1969.

Sandman, C. A., George, J., Walker, B. B., & Nolan, J. D. Neuropeptide MSH/ACTH 4–10 enhances attention in the mentally retarded. *Pharmacology, Biochemistry, and Behavior*, 1976, *5*, 23–28 (Supplement 1).

Sandman, C. A., Kastin, A. J., & Schally, A. V. Neuropeptide influences on the central nervous system: A psychobiological perspective. In P. D. Hrdina & R. L. Singal (Eds.), *Neuroendocrine regulation and altered behavior.* London: Croomhelm, 1981.

Sandoval, J. The measurement of the hyperactive syndrome in children. *Review of Educational Research*, 1977, *47*, 293–318.

Sandoval, J. Format effects in two teacher rating scales of hyperactivity. *Journal of Abnormal Child Psychology*, 1981, *9*, 203–218.

Sandoval, J., Lambert, N. M., & Sassone, D. M. Parent attitudes and treatments for children identified as hyperactive. Paper presented at Hyperkinetic Behavior Syndrome Workshop, National Institutes of Mental Health, Washington, DC, June 1978.

Sandoval, J., Lambert, N. M., & Sassone, D. The identification and labeling of hyperactivity in children: An interactive model. In C. K. Whalen & B. Henker (Eds.), *Hyperactive children: The social ecology of identification and treatment.* New York: Academic Press, 1980.

Sandoval, J., Lambert, N. M., & Yandell, W. Current medical practice and hyperactive children. *American Journal of Orthopsychiatry,* 1976, *46,* 323–334.

Santostefano, S., & Paley, E. Development of cognitive controls in children. *Journal of Clinical Psychology,* 1964, *20,* 213–218.

Sapir, S. G. Educational intervention. In H. E. Rie & E. D. Rie (Eds.), *Handbook of minimal brain dysfunctions: A critical view.* New York: Wiley, 1980.

Saraf, K. R., Klein, D. F., Gittelman-Klein, R., Gootman, N., & Greenhill, P. EKG effects of imipramine treatment in children. *Journal of the American Academy of Child Psychiatry,* 1978, *17,* 60–69.

Saraf, K. R., Klein, D. F., Gittelman-Klein, R., & Groff, S. Imipramine side effects in children. *Psuchopharmacologia,* 1974, *37,* 265–274.

Sarason, S. B. *Psychological problems in mental deficiency.* New York: Harper, 1949.

Sassone, D., Lambert, N. M., & Sandoval, J. The adolescent status of boys previously identified as hyperactive. Unpublished manuscript. University of California, 1981.

Satterfield, J. H. EEG issues in children with minimal brain dysfunction. *Seminars in Psychiatry,* 1973, *5,* 35–46.

Satterfield, J. H., & Braley, B. W. Evoked potentials and brain maturation in hyperactive and normal children. *Electroencephalography and Clinical Neurophysiology,* 1977, *43,* 43–51.

Satterfield, J. H., Cantwell, D. P., Lesser, L. I., & Podosin, R. L. Physiological studies of the hyperkinetic child: I. *American Journal of Psychiatry,* 1972, *128,* 1418–1424.

Satterfield, J. H., Cantwell, D. P., & Satterfield, B. T. Pathophysiology of the hyperactive child syndrome. *Archives of General Psychiatry,* 1974, *31,* 839–844.

Satterfield, J. H., Cantwell, D. P., & Satterfield, B. T. Multimodality treatment. *Archives of General Psychiatry,* 1979, *36,* 965–974.

Satterfield, J. H., Cantwell, D. P., Saul, R. E., Lesser, L. I., & Podosin, R. L. Response to stimulant drug treatment in hyperactive children, prediction from EEG and neurological findings. *Journal of Autism and Child Schizophrenia,* 1973, *3,* 36–48.

Satterfield, J. H., Cantwell, D. P., Schell, A., & Blaschke, T. Growth of hyperactive children treated with methylphenidate. *Archives of General Psychiatry,* 1979, *36,* 212–217.

Satterfield, J. H., & Dawson, M. E. Electrodermal correlates of hyperactivity in children. *Psychophysiology,* 1971, *8,* 191–197.

Satterfield, J. H., Lesser, L. I., Saul, R. E., & Cantwell, D. P. EEG aspects in the diagnosis and treatment of minimal brain dysfunction. *Annals of the New York Academy of Sciences,* 1973, *205,* 274–282.

Satterfield, J. H., Satterfield, B. T., & Cantwell, D. P. Multimodality treatment: A two-year evaluation of 61 hyperactive boys. *Archives of General Psychiatry,* 1980, *37,* 915–918.

Satterfield, J. H., Satterfield, B. T., & Cantwell, D. P. Three-year multimodality treatment study of 100 hyperactive boys. *Journal of Pediatrics,* 1981, *98,* 650–655.

Satterfield, J. H., Schell, A. M., & Barb, S. D. Potential risk of prolonged administration of stimulant medication for hyperactive children. *Journal of Developmental and Behavioral Pediatrics,* 1980, *1,* 102–107.

Sattler, J. M. *Assessment of children's intelligence.* Philadelphia: Saunders, 1974.

Satz, P., & Fletcher, J. M. Minimal brain dysfunctions: An appraisal of research concepts and methods. In H. E. Rie & E. D. Rie (Eds.), *Handbook of minimal brain dysfunctions: A critical view*. New York: Wiley, 1980.

Sauerhoff, M. W., & Michaelson, I. A. Hyperactivity and brain catecholamines in lead-exposed developing rats. *Science*, 1973, *182*, 1022–1024.

Saxon, S. A., Magee, J. T., & Siegel, D. S. Activity level patterns in the hyperactive Ritalin responder and non-responder. *Journal of Clinical Child Psychology*, 1977, *33*, 27–29.

Scarr, S. Genetic factors in activity motivation. *Child Development*, 1966, *37*, 663–673.

Schacter, S. *The psychology of affiliation*. Stanford, CA: Stanford University Press, 1959.

Schaefer, J. W., Palkes, H. S., & Stewart, M. A. Group counseling for parents of hyperactive children. *Child Psychiatry and Human Development*, 1974, *5*, 89–94.

Schaffer, R. *Mothering*. Cambridge, MA: Harvard University Press, 1977.

Schain, R. J. Minor physical anomalies and hyperactivity (letter). *Pediatrics*, 1974, *54*, 522.

Schain, R. J., & Reynard, C. L. Effects of a central stimulant drug (methylphenidate) in children with hyperactive behavior. *Pediatrics*, 1975, *55*, 709–716.

Schlager, G., Newman, D. E., Dunn, H. G., Crichton, J. U., & Schulzer, M. Bone age in children with minimal brain dysfunction. *Developmental Medicine and Child Neurology*, 1979, *21*, 41–51.

Schleifer, M., Weiss, G., Cohen, N. J., Elman, M., Cvejic, H., & Kruger, E. Hyperactivity in preschoolers and the effect of methylphenidate. *American Journal of Orthopsychiatry*, 1975, *45*, 38–50.

Schmidt, D. E., & Keating, J. P. Human crowding and personal control: An integration of the research. *Psychological Bulletin*, 1979, *86*, 680–700.

Schmidt, K. The effect of continuous stimulation on the behavioral sleep of infants. *Merrill-Palmer Quarterly*, 1975, *21*, 77–88.

Schmitt, B. D. The minimal brain dysfunction myth. *American Journal of Diseases of Children*, 1975, *129*, 1313–1318.

Schmitt, B. D. Ten guidelines for living with a hyperactive child. *Pediatrics*, 1977, *60*, 387.

Schmitt, B. D., Martin, H. P., Nellhaus, G., Cravens, J., Camp, B. W., & Jordan, K. The hyperactive child. *Clinical Pediatrics*, 1973, *12*, 154–169.

Schneider, M. Turtle technique in the classroom. Described in M. Herbert, *Conduct disorders of childhood and adolescence*. New York: Wiley, 1978, p. 119.

Scholom, A., & Schiff, G. Relating infant temperament to learning disabilities. *Journal of Abnormal Child Psychology*, 1980, *8*, 127–132.

Scholom, A., Zucker, R. A., & Stollak, G. E. Relating early child adjustment to infant and parent temperament. *Journal of Abnormal Child Psychology*, 1979, *7*, 297–308.

Schomer, J. Family therapy. In B. Wolman, J. Egan, & A. Ross (Eds.), *Handbook of treatment of mental disorders in childhood and adolescence*. Englewood Cliffs, NJ: Prentice-Hall, 1978.

Schrag, P., & Divoky, D. *The myth of the hyperactive child*. New York: Pantheon, 1975.

Schrager, J., Lindy, J., Harrison, S., McDermott, J., & Killins, E. The hyperkinetic child: Some consensually validated behavioral correlates. *Exceptional Children*, 1966, *32*, 635–637.

Schuckit, M. A., Petrich, J., & Chiles, J. Hyperactivity: Diagnostic confusion. *Journal of Nervous and Mental Disease*, 1978, *166*, 79–87.

Schulman, J. L., & Reisman, J. M. An objective measure of hyperactivity. *American Journal of Mental Deficiency*, 1959, *64*, 455–456.

Schulman, J. L., Stevens, T. M., & Kupst, M. J. The biometometer: A new device for the measurement and remediation of hyperactivity. *Child Development*, 1977, *48*, 1152–1154.

Schulman, J. L., Stevens, T. M., Suran, B. G., Kupst, M. J., & Naughton, M. J. Modification of activity level through biofeedback and operant conditioning. *Journal of Applied Behavior Analysis*, 1978, *11*, 145–152.

Schultz, H., & Luthe, W. *Autogenic training: A psychophysiological approach to psychotherapy.* New York: Grune and Stratton, 1959.

Seeler, R., Israel, J., & Royal, J. Ganglioneuroblastoma and fetal hydantoin-alcohol syndromes. *Pediatrics*, 1979, *63*, 524–527.

Selltiz, C., Wrightsman, L., & Cook, S. *Research methods in social relations* (3rd ed.). New York: Holt, Rinehart, and Winston, 1976.

Selman, R. L., & Selman, A. P. Children's ideas about friendship: A new theory. *Psychology Today*, 1979, *13*, 70–80.

Senior, N., Towne, D., & Huessy, H. Time estimation and hyperactivity, a replication. *Perceptual and Motor Skills*, 1979, *49*, 289–290.

Shaffer, D., & Greenhill, L. A critical note on the predictive validity of "the hyperkinetic syndrome." *Journal of Child Psychology and Psychiatry*, 1979, *20*, 61–72.

Shaffer, D., McNamara, N., & Pincus, J. Controlled observations on patterns of activity, attention, and impulsivity in brain-damaged and psychiatrically disturbed boys. *Psychological Medicine*, 1974, *4*, 4–18.

Shafto, F., & Sulzbacher, S. Comparing treatment tactics with a hyperactive preschool child: Stimulant medication and programmed teacher intervention. *Journal of Applied Behavior Analysis*, 1977, *10*, 13–20.

Shapiro, A. K., Shapiro, E. S., Bruun, R. D., & Sweet, R. D. *Gilles de la Tourette's syndrome.* New York: Raven Press, 1978.

Shapiro, M. B. The single case in fundamental clinical psychological research. *British Journal of Medical Psychology*, 1961, *34*, 255–262.

Shaywitz, B. A., Cohen, D. J., & Bowers, M. B. CSF monoamine metabolites in children with minimal brain dysfunction—evidence for alteration of brain dopamine. *Journal of Pediatrics*, 1977, *90*, 67–71.

Shaywitz, B. A., Yager, R. D., & Klopper, J. H. Selective brain dopamine depletion in developing rats: An experimental model of minimal brain dysfunction. *Science*, 1976, *191*, 305–308.

Shaywitz, S. E., Cohen, D. J., & Shaywitz, B. A. The biochemical basis of minimal brain dysfunction. *Journal of Pediatrics*, 1978, *92*, 179–187.

Shelley, E. M., & Riester, A. Syndrome of minimal brain damage in young adults. *Diseases of the Nervous System*, 1972, *33*, 335–338.

Sheppard, D. S. *Interpolation in SYMAP Version 4 Contouring Program.* Boston: Harvard University, Laboratory for Computer Graphics, 1973.

Shetty, T. Photic responses in hyperkinesis of childhood. *Science*, 1971, *174*, 1356–1357.

Shetty, T., & Chase, T. N. Central monoamines and hyperkinesis of childhood. *Neurology*, 1976, *26*, 1000–1002.

Shores, R. E., & Haubrich, P. A. Effect of cubicles in educating emotionally disturbed children. *Exceptional Children*, 1969, *36*, 21–24.

Sidman, M. *Tactics of scientific research.* New York: Basic Books, 1960.

Silbergeld, E. K., & Adler, H. S. Subcellular mechanisms of lead neurotoxicity. *Brain Research*, 1978, *148*, 451–467.

Silbergeld, E. K., & Chisolm, J. J. Lead poisoning: Altered urinary catecholamine metabolites as indicators of intoxication in mice and children. *Science*, 1976, *192*, 153–154.

Silbergeld, E. K., & Goldberg, A. M. Hyperactivity: A lead-induced behavior disorder. *Life Sciences*, 1973, *13*, 1275–1283.

Silbergeld, E. K., & Goldberg, A. M. Lead-induced behavioral dysfunction: An animal model of hyperactivity. *Experimental Neurology*, 1974, *42*, 146–157.

Silberman, C. E. *Crisis in the classroom*. New York: Random House, 1970.

Simpson, R. H. The specific meanings of certain terms indicating differing degrees of frequency. *Quarterly Journal of Speech*, 1944, *30*, 328–330.

Skinner, B. F. *Science and human behavior*. New York: Macmillan, 1953.

Skinner, B. F. *Contingencies of reinforcement: A theoretical analysis*. New York: Appleton-Century-Crofts, 1969.

Skynner, A. C. R. *Systems of family and marital psychotherapy*. New York: Brunner/Mazel, 1976.

Slater, E. Expectation of abnormality on paternal and maternal sides: A computational model. *Journal of Medical Genetics*, 1966, *3*, 159–161.

Slavson, S. R. *An introduction to group therapy*. New York: International Universities Press, 1943.

Slavson, S. R., & Schiffer, M. *Group psychotherapies for children*. New York: International Universities Press, 1974.

Sleator, E. K. Deleterious effects of drugs used for hyperactivity on patients with Gilles de la Tourette's syndrome. *Clinical Pediatrics*, 1980, *19*, 453–454.

Sleator, E. K. Office diagnosis of hyperactivity by the physician. In K. D. Gadow & I. Bialer (Eds.), *Advances in learning and behavioral disabilities*. Greenwich, CT: JAI Press, 1981, in press.

Sleator, E. K., & Ullman, R. K. Can the physician diagnose hyperactivity in the office? *Pediatrics*, 1981, *67*, 13–17.

Sleator, E. K., & von Neumann, A. W. Methylphenidate in the treatment of hyperkinetic children. *Clinical Pediatrics*, 1974, *13*, 19–24.

Sleator, E. K., von Neumann, A., & Sprague, R. L. Hyperactive children: A continuous long-term placebo-controlled follow-up. *Journal of the American Medical Association*, 1974, *229*, 316–317.

Sloane, R. B., Staples, F. F., Cristal, A. H., Yorkston, N. J., & Whipple, K. *Psychotherapy versus behavior therapy*. Cambridge, MA: Harvard University Press, 1975.

Smith, A. Ambiguities in concepts and studies of "brain damage" and "organicity." *Journal of Nervous and Mental Disease*, 1962, *135*, 311–326.

Smith, D. W. The fetal alcohol syndrome. *Hospital Practice*, 1979a, *14*, 121–128.

Smith, D. W. *Mothering your unborn baby*. Philadelphia: Saunders, 1979b.

Smith, G. B. Cerebral accidents of childhood and their relationships to mental deficiency. *Welfare Magazine*, 1926, *17*, 18–33.

Smith, L. *Washington Post* description of the development of the Biofield reprinted in *San Francisco Chronicle*, July 23, 1980.

Sneed, R. C. The fetal alcohol syndrome. Is alcohol, lead, or something else the culprit? (Letter to the editor). *Journal of Pediatrics*, 1978, *92*, 324.

Sobotka, T. J. Estimates of average, 90th percentile and maximum daily intakes of FD and C artificial colors in one day's diets among two age groups of children. Memorandum of July 30, 1976, to the DHEW, Food and Drug Administration, Biochemical Toxicology Branch.

Sobotka, T. J., & Cook, M. P. Postnatal lead acetate exposure in rats: Possible relationship to minimal brain dysfunction. *American Journal of Mental Deficiency*, 1974, *79*, 5–9.

Soldin, S. J., Hill, B. M., Chan, Y. M., Swanson, J. M., & Hill, J. E. A liquid-chromatographic analysis for ritalinic acid [a-Phenyl-a-(z-piperidyl) acetic acid] in serum. *Clinical Chemistry*, 1979, *25*, 51–54.

Solomons, G. The role of methylphenidate and dextroamphetamine in children. *Drug Letter* (University of Iowa Hospitals and Clinics), 1971, *10*, 7–9.

Solomons, G. Drug therapy: Initiation and follow-up. *Annals of the New York Academy of Sciences*, 1973, *205*, 335–344.

Sorenson, C. A., Vayer, J. S., & Goldberg, C. S. Amphetamine reduction of motor activity in rats after neonatal administration of 6-hydroxydopamine. *Biological Psychiatry*, 1977, *12*, 133–137.

Spiegel, E. D. The effects of self-observation on the social behavior of hyperactive children. Unpublished doctoral dissertation, University of Southern California, 1977.

Sprague, R. L. Critical review of food additive studies. In C. G. Mathews (Chair), *Food additives and hyperkinesis*. Symposium presented at the meeting of the American Psychological Association, Washington, DC, 1976.

Sprague, R. L. Psychopharmacotherapy in children. In M. F. McMillan & S. Henao (Eds.), *Child psychiatry: Treatment and research*. New York: Brunner/Mazel, 1977.

Sprague, R. L. Principles of clinical drug trials and social, ethical and legal issues of drug use in children. In J. S. Werry (Ed.), *Pediatric psychopharmacology: The use of behavior modifying drugs in children*. New York: Brunner/Mazel, 1978.

Sprague, R. L. Assessment of intervention. In R. L. Trites (Ed.), *Hyperactivity in children*. Baltimore: University Park Press, 1979.

Sprague, R. L. Litigation, laws, and regulations regarding psychoactive drug use. In S. Breuning & A. Poling (Eds.), *Drugs and mental retardation*. Springfield, IL: Charles C. Thomas, 1981.

Sprague, R. L., Christensen, D. E., & Werry, J. S. Experimental psychology and stimulant drugs. In C. K. Conners (Ed.), *Clinical use of stimulant drugs in children*. The Hague: Excerpta Medica, 1974.

Sprague, R. L., Barnes, K., & Werry, J. S. Methylphenidate and thioridazine: Learning, reaction time, activity, and classroom behavior in disturbed children. *American Journal of Orthopsychiatry*, 1970, *40*, 615–628.

Sprague, R. L., & Berger, B. D. Drug effects on learning performance. In R. M. Knights & D. J. Bakker (Eds.), *Treatment of hyperactivity and learning disordered children*. Baltimore: University Park Press, 1980.

Sprague, R. L., Cohen, M. N., & Eichlseder, W. Are there hyperactive children in Europe and the South Pacific? Paper presented at the American Psychological Association meeting, San Francisco, 1977.

Sprague, R. L., Cohen, M., & Werry, J. S. Normative data on the Conners Teacher Rating Scale and Abbreviated Scale. Technical Report, Children's Research Center, University of Illinois, November 1974.

Sprague, R. L., & Sleator, E. K. Effects of psychopharmacologic agents on learning disorders. *Pediatric Clinics of North America*, 1973, *20*, 719–735.

Sprague, R. L., & Sleator, E. K. What is the proper dose of stimulant drugs in children? *International Journal of Mental Health*, 1975, *4*, 75–104.

Sprague, R. L., & Sleator, E. K. Drugs and dosages: Implications for learning disabilities. In R. M. Knights & D. J. Bakker (Eds.), *Neuropsychology of learning disorders: Theoretical approaches*. Baltimore: University Park Press, 1976.

Sprague, R. L., & Sleator, E. K. Methylphenidate in hyperkinetic children: Difference in dose effects on learning and social behavior. *Science*, 1977, *198*, 1274–1276.

Sprague, R. L., & Ullmann, R. Psychoactive drugs and child management. In J. M. Kaufman & D. P. Hallahan (Eds.), *Handbook of special education*. New York: Prentice-Hall, 1981.

Sprague, R. L., Ullman, R. K., & Sleator, E. K. Characteristics of subjects selected by using a cut-off point on the Conners Teacher Rating Scale. Unpublished manuscript. University of Illinois, 1981.

Sprague, R. L., & Werry, J. S. Methodology of psychopharmacological studies with the retarded. In N. R. Ellis (Ed.), *International review of research in mental retardation*, Vol. 5. New York: Academic Press, 1971.

Sprague, R. L., Werry, J. S., & Davis, K. Psychotropic drug effects on learning and activity level of children. Paper presented at the Gatlinburg Conference on Research and Theory in Mental Retardation, March 1969.

Spring, C., Blunden, D., Greenberg, L. M., & Yellin, A. M. Validity and norms of hyperactivity rating scale. *Journal of Special Education*, 1977, *11*, 313–321.

Spring, C., Greenberg, L. M., & Yellin, A. M. Agreement of mothers' and teachers' hyperactivity ratings with scores on drug-sensitive psychological tests. *Journal of Abnormal Child Psychology*, 1977, *5*, 199–204.

Spring, C., & Sandoval, J. Food additives and hyperkinesis. A critical evaluation of the evidence. *Journal of Learning Disabilities*, 1976, *9*, 560–569.

Spring, C., Yellin, A. M., & Greenberg, L. M. Effects of imipramine and methylphenidate on perceptual-motor performance of hyperactive children. *Perceptual and Motor Skills*, 1976, *43*, 459–470.

Sroufe, L. A. Drug treatment of children with behavior problems. In F. D. Horowitz (Ed.), *Review of child development research*, Vol. 4. Chicago: University of Chicago Press, 1975.

Sroufe, L. A., Sonies, B. C., West, W. D., & Wright, F. S. Anticipatory heart rate deceleration and reaction time in children with and without referral for learning disability. *Child Development*, 1973, *44*, 267–273.

Stableford, W., Butz, R., Hasazi, J., Leitenberg, H., & Peyser, J. Sequential withdrawal of stimulant drugs and use of behavior therapy with two hyperactive boys. *American Journal of Orthopsychiatry*, 1976, *46*, 302–312.

Stampfl, T. G., & Levis, D. J. Essentials of implosive therapy: A learning-theory-based psychodynamic behavioral therapy. *Journal of Abnormal Psychology*, 1967, *72*, 496–503.

Stare, F. J., Whelan, E. M., & Sheridan, M. Diet and hyperactivity: Is there a relationship? *Pediatrics*, 1980, *66*, 521–525.

Stayton, D. J., Hogan, R., & Ainsworth, M. D. S. Infant obedience and maternal behavior: The origins of socialization reconsidered. *Child Development*, 1971, *42*, 1057–1065.

Steg, J. P., & Rapoport, J. L. Minor physical anomalies in normal, neurotic, learning disabled, and severely disturbed children. *Journal of Autism and Childhood Schizophrenia*, 1975, *5*, 299–307.

Stein, T. J. Some ethical considerations of short-term workshops in the principles and methods of behavior modification. *Journal of Applied Behavior Analysis*, 1975, *8*, 113–115.

Steinberg, G. G., Troshinsky, C., & Steinberg, H. R. Dextroamphetamine-responsive behavior disorder in school children. *American Journal of Psychiatry*, 1971, *128*, 174–179.

Steinkamp, M. W. The problem of children's failure to take medication during psychotropic drug trials. Institute for Child Behavior and Development. Unpublished manuscript, University of Illinois. In press, 1981.

Stern, G. S., & Berrenberg, J. L. Biofeedback training in frontalis muscle relaxation and enhancement of belief in personal control. *Biofeedback and Self-Regulation*, 1977, *2*, 173–183.

Stevens, D. A., Stover, C. E., & Backus, J. T. The hyperkinetic child: The effect of incentives on the speed of rapid tapping. *Journal of Consulting and Clinical Psychology*, 1970, *34*, 56–59.

Stevens, T. M., Kupst, M. J., Suran, B. G., & Schulman, J. L. Activity level: A comparison between actometer scores and behavior ratings. *Journal of Abnormal Child Psychology*, 1978, *6*, 163–173.

Stewart, M. A. Genetic, perinatal, and constitutional factors in minimal brain dysfunctions. In H. E. Rie & E. D. Rie (Eds.), *Handbook of minimal brain dysfunctions*. New York: Wiley, 1980.

Stewart, M. A., deBlois, C. S., & Cummings, C. Psychiatric disorder in the parents of hyperactive boys and those with conduct disorder. *Journal of Child Psychology & Psychiatry,* 1980, *21,* 283–292.

Stewart, M. A., deBlois, C. S., & Singer, S. Alcoholism and hyperactivity revisited: A preliminary report. In M. Gallanter (Ed.), *Biomedical issues and clinical effects of alcoholism,* Vol. 5. New York: Grune and Stratton, 1979.

Stewart, M. A., Cummings, C., Singer, S., & deBlois, C. S. The overlap between hyperactive and unsocialized aggressive children. *Journal of Child Psychology and Psychiatry,* 1981, *22,* 35–45.

Stewart, M. A., & Leone, L. A family study of unsocialized aggressive boys. *Biological Psychiatry,* 1978, *13,* 107–118.

Stewart, M. A., Mendelson, W. B., & Johnson, N. E. Hyperactive children as adolescents: How they describe themselves. *Child Psychiatry and Human Development,* 1973, *4,* 3–11.

✹ Stewart, M. A., & Olds, S. W. *Raising a hyperactive child.* New York: Harper and Row, 1973.

Stewart, M. A., Pitts, F. N., Craig, A. G., & Dieruf, W. The hyperactive child syndrome. *American Journal of Orthopsychiatry,* 1966, *36,* 861–867.

Stewart, M. A., Thach, B. T., & Freidin, M. R. Accidental poisoning and the hyperactive child syndrome. *Diseases of the Nervous System,* 1970, *31,* 403–407.

Still, G. F. The Coulstonian Lectures on some abnormal physical conditions in children. *Lancet,* 1902, *1,* 1008–1012, 1077–1082, 1163–1168.

Stine, J. J. Symptom alleviation in the hyperactive child by dietary modification: A report of two cases. *American Journal of Orthopsychiatry,* 1976, *46,* 637–645.

Strain, W. H., Pories, W. J., Flynn, A., & Hill, O. A. Trace element nutriture and metabolism through head hair analysis. In D. D. H. Hemphill (Ed.), *Trace substances in environmental health.* Columbia, MO: University of Missouri Press, 1972.

Strauss, A. A., & Kephart, N. C. *Psychopathology and education of the brain-injured child.* Vol. 2, *Progress in theory and clinic.* New York: Grune and Stratton, 1955.

Strauss, A. A., & Lehtinen, L. E. *Psychopathology and education of the brain-injured child.* New York: Grune and Stratton, 1947.

Strecker, E. A., & Ebaugh, F. G. Neuropsychiatric sequelae of cerebral trauma in children. *Archives of Neurology and Psychiatry,* 1924, *12,* 443–453.

Streissguth, A. P., Herman, C. S., & Smith, D. W. Intelligence, behavior, and dysmorphogenesis in the fetal alcohol syndrome. A report on 20 patients. *Journal of Pediatrics,* 1978, *92,* 363–367.

Stroop, J. R., Studies of interference in serial verbal reactions. *Journal of Experimental Psychology,* 1935, *18,* 643–661.

Strother, C. R. Minimal cerebral dysfunction: A historical overview. *Annals of the New York Academy of Sciences,* 1973, *205,* 6–17.

Sulzbacher, S. I. The learning-disabled or hyperactive child. *Journal of the American Medical Association,* 1975, *234,* 938–941.

Surgeon General's Report on Smoking and Health. Washington, D.C.: Government Printing Office, 1979.

Surwillo, W. W. Changes in the electronecephalogram accompanying the use of stimulant drugs (methylphenidate and dextroamphetamine) in hyperactive children. *Biological Psychiatry,* 1977, *12,* 787–799.

Swanson, J. M. Personal communication, 1981.

Swanson, J. M., Eich, J., & Kinsbourne, M. State-dependent retrieval in hyperactive children. Paper presented at the annual meeting of the Psychonomic Society, San Antonio, October 1978.

Swanson, J. M., & Kinsbourne, M. Stimulant-related state-dependent learning in hyperactive children. *Science*, 1976, *192*, 1354–1357.

Swanson, J. M., & Kinsbourne, M. Should you use stimulants to treat the hyperactive child? *Modern Medicine*, 1978, *46*, 71–80.

Swanson, J. M., & Kinsbourne, M. The cognitive effects of stimulant drugs on hyperactive children. In G. A. Hale & M. Lewis (Eds.), *Attention and cognitive development*. New York: Plenum, 1979.

Swanson, J. M., & Kinsbourne, M. Artificial color and hyperactive behavior. In R. M. Knights & D. J. Bakker (Eds.), *Treatment of hyperactive and learning disordered children*. Baltimore: University Park Press, 1980a.

Swanson, J. M., & Kinsbourne, M. Food dyes impair performance of hyperactive children on a laboratory learning test. *Science*, 1980b, *207*, 1485–1487.

Swanson, J. M., & Kinsbourne, M. In rebuttal. *American Journal of Diseases of Children*, 1980c, *134*, 1124–1125.

Swanson, J. M., Kinsbourne, M., Roberts, W., & Zucker, K. Time-response analysis of the effect of stimulant medication on the learning ability of children referred for hyperactivity. *Pediatrics*, 1978, *61*, 21–29.

Sykes, D. H., Douglas, V. I., & Morgenstern, G. Sustained attention in hyperactive children. *Journal of Child Psychology and Psychiatry*, 1973, *14*, 213–220.

Tams, V., & Eyberg, S. M. A group treatment program for parents. In E. J. Mash, L. C. Handy, & L. A. Hamerlynk (Eds.), *Behavior modification approaches to parenting*. New York: Brunner/Mazel, 1976.

Tanner, J. M., Whitehouse, R. H., Takaishi, M. Standards from birth to maturity for height, weight, height velocity and weight velocity: British children, 1965, Part 1. *Archives of Disease in Childhood*, 1966, *41*, 454–471.

Tarter, R. E. Etiology of alcoholism: Interdisciplinary integration. In P. E. Nathan, G. A. Marlatt, & T. Loberg (Eds.), *Alcoholism: New directions in behavioral research and treatment*. New York: Plenum, 1979.

Tarter, R. E., McBride, N. Buonpane, N., & Schneider, D. U. Differentiation of alcoholics: Childhood history of minimal brain dysfunction, family history, and drinking pattern. *Archives of General Psychiatry*, 1977, *34*, 761–768.

Taylor, E. Annotation. Food additives, allergy and hyperkinesis. *Journal of Child Psychology and Psychiatry*, 1979, *20*, 357–363.

Taylor, J. F. *The hyperactive child and the family*. New York: Everest House, 1980.

Terestman, N. Mood quality and intensity in nursery school children as predictors of behavior disorder. *American Journal of Orthopsychiatry*, 1980, *50*, 125–138.

Terman, L. M., & Merrill, M. A. *Mental and physical traits of a thousand gifted children*. Stanford, CA: Stanford University Press, 1926.

Thelen, M. H., Fry, R. A., Fehrenbach, P. A., & Frautschi, N. M. Therapeutic videotape and film modeling: A review. *Psychological Bulletin*, 1979, *86*, 701–720.

Thomas, A., & Chess, S. *Temperament and development*. New York: Brunner/Mazel, 1977.

Thomas, A., Chess, S., & Birch, H. G. *Temperament and behavior disorders in children*. New York: New York University Press, 1968.

Thomas, A., Chess, S., Birch, H. G., & Hertzig, M. E. A longitudinal study of primary reaction patterns in children. *Comprehensive Psychiatry*, 1960, *1*, 103–112.

Thomas, A., Chess, S., Birch, H. G., Hertzig, M. E., & Korn, S. *Behavioral individuality in early childhood*. New York: New York University Press, 1963.

Thomas, A., Chess, S., Sillen, J., & Mendez, O. Cross-cultural study of behavior in children with special vulnerabilities to stress. In D. Ricks, A. Thomas, and M. Roff (Eds.), *Life history research in psychopathology*, Vol. 3. Minneapolis: University of Minnesota Press, 1974, pp. 53–67.

Thomas, H. Psychological assessment instruments for use with human infants. *Merrill-Palmer Quarterly*, 1970, *16*, 179–223.

Thompson, W. D., Kidd, J. R., & Weissman, M. M. A procedure for the efficient collection and processing of pedigree data suitable for genetic analysis. *Journal of Psychiatric Research*, 1980, *15*, 291–303.

Thorndike, R. R. Review of the WRAT. In O. K. Buros (Ed.), *The seventh mental measurements yearbook*, Vol. 1. Highland Park, NJ: Gryphon Press, 1972, pp. 67–68.

Tinklenberg, J. R. Personal communication, 1981.

Tiwary, C. M., Rosenbloom, A. L., Robertson, M. F., & Parker, J. C. Effects of thyrotropin-releasing hormone in minimal brain dysfunction. *Pediatrics*, 1975, *56*, 119–121.

Tobiessen, J., & Karowe, H. E. A role for the school in the pharmacological treatment of hyperkinetic children. *Psychology in the Schools*, 1969, *6*, 340–346.

Tonick, I., Friehling, J., & Warhit, J. Classroom observation code. Unpublished manuscript. State University of New York at Stony Brook, 1973.

Toutant, C., & Lippman, S. Fetal alcohol syndrome. *American Family Physician*, 1980, *22*, 113–117.

Touwen, B. C. L., & Sporrel, T. Soft signs and MBD. *Developmental Medicine and Child Neurology*, 1979, *21*, 528–530.

Tredgold, C. H. *Mental deficiency (amentia)*. New York: Wood, 1908.

Treegoob, M. R. A contrast of the knowledge and attitudes of special education teachers and elementary teachers about Ritalin in its use with hyperkinetic children. Unpublished doctoral dissertation, Indiana State University, 1976.

Trehub, S. E. Infant antecedents: A search for the precursors of learning disabilities. In M. Blaw, I. Rapin, & M. Kinsbourne (Eds.), *Topics in child neurology*. Jamaica, NY: Spectrum, 1977.

Trites, R. L. Prevalence of hyperactivity in Ottawa, Canada. In R. L. Trites (Ed.), *Hyperactivity in children*. Baltimore: University Park Press, 1979a.

Trites, R. L. (Ed.). *Hyperactivity in children: Etiology, measurement, and treatment implications*. Baltimore: University Park Press, 1979b.

Trites, R. L. Personal communication, 1981.

Trites, R. L., Blouin, A. G. A., Ferguson, H. B., & Lynch, G. The Conners Teacher Rating Scale: An epidemiologic, inter-rater reliability and follow-up investigation. In K. D. Gadow & J. Loney (Eds.). *Psychosocial aspects of drug treatment for hyperactivity*. Boulder, CO: Westview Press, 1981.

Trites, R. L., Tryphonas, H., & Ferguson, H. B. Diet treatment for hyperactive children with food allergies. In R. M. Knights & D. J. Bakker (Eds.), *Treatment of hyperactive and learning disordered children*. Baltimore: University Park Press, 1980.

Ullman, D. G., Barkley, R. A., & Brown, H. W. The behavioral symptoms of hyperkinetic children who successfully responded to stimulant drug treatment. *American Journal of Orthopsychiatry*, 1978, *48*, 425–437.

Ullman, R. Validity of teacher ratings. In R. L. Lipman (Chair), *Proceedings of the National Institute of Mental Health Workshop on the hyperkinetic behavior syndrome*. Washington, DC, June 15–16, 1978.

Urbain, E. S., & Kendall, P. C. Review of social-cognitive problem-solving interventions with children. *Psychological Bulletin*, 1980, *88*, 190–243.

Vandenberg, S. G. The heredity abilities study: Hereditary components in a psychological test battery. *American Journal of Human Genetics*, 1962, *14*, 220–237.

Van den Daele, L. D. Infant reactivity to redundant proprioceptive and auditory stimulation: A twin study. *Journal of Psychology*, 1971, *78*, 269–276.

Van Osdol, B. M., & Carlson, L. A study of developmental hyperactivity. *Mental Retardation*, 1972, *10*, 18–24.

Varga, J. The hyperactive child: Should we be paying more attention? *American Journal of Diseases of Children*, 1979, *133*, 413–418.

Varni, J. W. A self-regulatory approach to the treatment of the hyperactive child: Intervention with and without stimulant medication. Unpublished doctoral dissertation, University of California, Los Angeles, 1976.

Varni, J. W., Boyd, E. F., & Cataldo, M. F. Self-monitoring, external reinforcement, and time-out procedures in the control of high rate tic behaviors in a hyperactive child. *Behavior Therapy & Experimental Psychiatry*, 1978, *9*, 353–358.

Varni, J. W., & Henker, B. A self-regulation approach to the treatment of three hyperactive boys. *Child Behavior Therapy*, 1979, *1*, 171–192.

Villeneuve, C. The specific participation of the child in family therapy. *American Academy of Child Psychiatry*, 1979, *18*, 44–53.

Vincent, J. P., Williams, B. J., & Elrod, J. T. Ratings of observations of hyperactivity. Paper presented at the meeting of the American Psychological Association, San Francisco, August 1977.

Vincent, J. P., Williams, B. J., Harris, G. E., Jr., & Duval, G. C. Classroom observations of hyperactive children: A multiple validation study. In K. D. Gadow & J. Loney (Eds.), *Psychosocial aspects of drug treatment for hyperactivity*. Boulder, CO: Westview Press, 1981.

Vogel, A. V., Goodwin, J. S., & Goodwin, J. M. The therapeutics of placebo. *American Family Physician*, 1980, *22*, 105–109.

Vorhees, C. V., Brunner, R. L., & Butcher, R. E. Psychotropic drugs as behavioral teratogens. *Science*, 1979, *205*, 1220–1225.

Vygotsky, L. *Thought and language*. New York: Wiley, 1962.

Wachtel, P. L. *Psychoanalysis and behavior therapy: Toward an integration*. New York: Basic Books, 1977.

Wade, M. G., & Ellis, M. J. Measurement of free-range activity in children as modified by social and environmental complexity. *American Journal of Clinical Nutrition*, 1971, *24*, 1457–1460.

Wahler, R. G., Sperling, K. A., Thomas, M. R., Teeter, N. C., & Luper, H. L. The modification of childhood stuttering: Some response-response relationships. *Journal of Experimental Child Psychology*, 1970, *9*, 411–428.

Waizer, J., Hoffman, S. P., Polizos, P., & Engelhardt, D. M. Outpatient treatment of hyperactive school children with imipramine. *American Journal of Psychiatry*, 1974, *131*, 587–591.

Waldrop, M. F., Bell, R. Q., & Goering, J. D. Minor physical anomalies and inhibited behavior in elementary school girls. *Journal of Child Psychology and Psychiatry*, 1976, *17*, 113–122.

Waldrop, M. F., Bell, R. Q., McLaughlin, B., & Halverson, C. F. Newborn minor physical anomalies predict short attention span, peer aggression, and impulsivity at age 3. *Science*, 1978, *199*, 563–565.

Waldrop, M. F., & Goering, J. D. Hyperactivity and minor physical anomalies in elementary school children. *American Journal of Orthopsychiatry*, 1971, *41*, 602–607.

Waldrop, M. F., & Halverson, C. F. Minor physical anomalies and hyperactive behavior in young children. In J. Hellmuth (Ed.), *Exceptional infant*. New York: Brunner/Mazel, 1971.

Waldrop, M. F., Pederson, F. A., & Bell, R. Q. Minor physical anomalies and behavior in pre-school children. *Child Development,* 1968, *39,* 391–400.

Walker, B. B., & Sandman, C. A. Influences of an analog of the neuropeptide ACTH 4–9 on mentally retarded adults. *American Journal of Mental Deficiency,* 1979, *83,* 346–352.

Walker, S., III. Drugging the American child: We're too cavalier about hyperactivity. *Psychology Today,* 1974, *8,* 43–48.

Warme, G. E. In "Current issues in child psychiatry: A dialogue with John Bowlby." *Canadian Journal of Psychiatry,* 1980, *25,* 367–376.

Warren, R. J., Karduck, W. A., Bussaratid, S., Stewart, M. A., & Sly, W. S. The hyperactive child syndrome. *Archives of General Psychiatry,* 1971, *24,* 161–162.

Watson, J. B. *Psychological care of the infant and child.* New York: Norton, 1928.

Watzlawick, P., Weakland, J. H., & Fisch, R. *Change: Principles of problem formation and problem resolution.* New York: Norton, 1974.

Waxer, P. H. Short-term group psychotherapy: Some principles and techniques. *International Journal of Group Psychotherapy,* 1977, *27,* 33–42.

Weakland, J. H. The double-blind theory: Some current implications for child psychiatry. *American Academy of Child Psychiatry,* 1979, *18,* 54–66.

Weakland, J. H., & Fisch, R. Case study (personal communication), 1975.

Weakland, J. H., Fisch, R., Watzlawick, P., & Bodin, A. M. Brief therapy: Focused problem resolution. *Family Process,* 1974, *13,* 141–168.

Wechsler, D. *Wechsler Intelligence Scale for Children–Revised.* New York: Psychological Corporation, 1974.

Weintraub, S., Prinz, R. J., & Neale, J. M. Peer evaluations of the competence of children vulnerable to psychopathology. *Journal of Abnormal Child Psychology,* 1978, *6,* 461–473.

Weiss, B. In rebuttal. *American Journal of Diseases of Children,* 1980, *134,* 1126–1128.

Weiss, B., & Laties, V. Enhancement of human performance by caffeine and the amphetamines. *Pharmacological Review,* 1962, *14,* 1–36.

Weiss, B. Williams, J. H., Margen, S., Abrams, B., Caan, B., Citron, L. J., Cox, C., McKibben, J., Oga, D. & Schultz, S. Behavioral responses to artificial food colors. *Science,* 1980, *207,* 1487–1489.

Weiss, G. The natural history of hyperactivity in children and treatment with stimulant medication at different ages. *International Journal of Mental Health,* 1975, *4,* 213–226.

Weiss, G. MBD: Critical diagnostic issues. In H. E. Rie & E. D. Rie (Eds.), *Handbook of minimal brain dysfunctions: A critical view.* New York: Wiley, 1980.

Weiss, G., & Hechtman, L. The hyperactive child syndrome. *Science,* 1979, *205,* 1348–1354.

Weiss, G., Hechtman, L., & Perlman, T. Hyperactives as young adults: School, employer, and self-rating scales obtained during ten-year follow-up evaluation. *American Journal of Orthopsychiatry,* 1978, *48,* 438–445.

Weiss, G., Hechtman, L., Perlman, T., Hopkins, J., & Wener, A. Hyperactive children as young adults: A controlled prospective 10 year follow-up of the psychiatric status of 75 hyperactive children. *Archives of General Psychiatry,* 1979, *36,* 675–681.

Weiss, G., Kruger, E., Danielson, U. & Elman, M. Effects of long-term treatment of hyperactive children with methylphenidate. *Canadian Medical Association Journal,* 1975, *112,* 159–165.

Weiss, G., Minde, K., Douglas, V., Werry, J., & Sykes, D. H. Comparison of the effects of chlorpromazine, dextroamphetamine, and methylphenidate on the behaviour and intellectual functioning of hyperactive children. *Canadian Medical Association Journal,* 1971, *104,* 20–25.

Weiss, G., Minde, K., Werry, J. S., Douglas, V. I., & Nemeth, E. Studies on the hyperactive child, VIII: Five-year follow-up. *Archives of General Psychiatry,* 1971, *24,* 409–414.

Weiss, G., Werry, J. S., Minde, K., Douglas, V., & Sykes, D. Studies on the hyperactive child, V: The effects of dextroamphetamine and chlorpromazine on behavior and intellectual functioning. *Journal of Child Psychology and Psychiatry,* 1968, *9,* 145–156.

Weissenburger, F. E., & Loney, J. Hyperkinesis in the classroom: If cerebral stimulants are the last resort, what is the first resort? *Journal of Learning Disabilities,* 1977, *10,* 339–348.

Weisz, J. R., O'Neill, P., & O'Neill, P. C. Field dependence-independence on the Children's Embedded Figures Test: Cognitive style or cognitive level? *Developmental Psychology,* 1975, *11,* 539–540.

Weithorn, C. J. The relationship between hyperactivity and impulsive responsiveness in elementary school children. *Dissertation Abstracts International,* 1970, *30B,* 3899.

Weithorn, L. Drug therapy: Children's rights. In M. J. Cohen (Ed.), *Drugs and the special child.* New York: Gardner Press, 1979.

Wells, W. W. Drug control of school children: The child's right to choose. *Southern California Law Review,* 1973, *46,* 585–616.

Welner, Z., Welner, A., Stewart, M. A., Palkes, H., & Wish, E. A controlled study of siblings of hyperactive children. *Journal of Nervous and Mental Disease,* 1977, *165,* 110–117.

Welsch, E. You may not know it, but your schools probably are deeply into the potentially dangerous business of teaching with drugs. *American School Board Journal,* 1974, *161,* 41–45.

Wender, E. H. New evidence on food additives and hyperkinesis. *American Journal of Diseases of Children,* 1980, *134,* 1122–1124.

Wender, P. H. The minimal brain dysfunction syndrome. *Annual Review of Medicine,* 1975, *26,* 45–62.

Wender, P. H. The diagnosis and treatment of adult minimal brain dysfunction. In R. S. Lipman (Chair), *Proceedings of the National Institute of Mental Health Workshop on the hyperkinetic behavior syndrome.* Washington, DC, 1978.

Wender, P. H. The concept of adult minimal brain dysfunction. In L. Bellak (Ed.), *Psychiatric aspects of minimal brain dysfunction in adults.* New York: Grune and Stratton, 1979.

Wender, P. H., Epstein, R. S., Kopin, I. J., & Gordon, E. K. Urinary monoamine metabolites in children with minimal brain dysfunction. *American Journal of Psychiatry,* 1971, *127,* 1411–1415.

Wender, P. H., Reimherr, F. W., & Wood, M. D. Diagnosis and drug treatment of attentional deficit disorder (minimal brain dysfunction) in adults: A replication. *Archives of General Psychiatry,* 1981, in press.

Wender, P. H., & Wender, E. *The hyperactive child and the learning disabled child.* New York: Crown, 1978.

Werner, E. E. Environmental interaction in minimal brain dysfunctions. In H. E. Rie & E. D. Rie (Eds.), *Handbook of minimal brain dysfunctions.* New York: Wiley, 1980.

Werner, E. E., Bierman, J. M., French, F. E., Simonian, K., Connor, A., Smith, R. S., & Campbell, M. Reproductive and environmental casualties: A report on the 10-year follow-up of the children of the Kauai pregnancy study. *Pediatrics,* 1968, *42,* 112–127.

Werner, E. E., & Smith, R. S. *Kauai's children come of age.* Honolulu: University of Hawaii Press, 1977.

Werry, J.S. Developmental hyperactivity. *Pediatric Clinics of North America,* 1968, *15,* 581–599.

Werry, J. S. Food additives and hyperactivity. Guest editorial. *The Medical Journal of Australia,* 1976, *2,* 281–282.

Werry, J. S. The use of psychotropic drugs in children. *American Academy of Child Psychiatry,* 1977, *16,* 446–468.

Werry, J. S., Measures in pediatric psychopharmacology. In J. S. Werry (Ed.), *Pediatric psychopharmacology: The use of behavior modifying drugs in children.* New York: Brunner/Mazel, 1978a.

Werry, J. S. (Ed.). *Pediatric psychopharmacology: The use of behavior drugs in children.* New York: Brunner/Mazel, 1978b.

Werry, J. S. Family therapy: Behavioral approaches. *American Academy of Child Psychiatry,* 1979, *18,* 91–101.

Werry, J. S., & Aman, M. G. Methylphenidate and haloperidol in children: Effects on attention, memory, and activity. *Archives of General Psychiatry,* 1975, *32,* 790–795.

Werry, J. S., Aman, M. G., & Diamond, E. Imipramine and methylphenidate in hyperactive children. *Journal of Child Psychology and Psychiatry,* 1980, *21,* 27–35.

Werry, J. S., Aman, M. G., & Lampen, E. Haloperidol and methylphenidate in hyperactive children. *Acta Paedopsychiatrica,* 1975, *42,* 26–40.

Werry, J. S., Minde, K., Guzman, A., Weiss, G., Dogan, K., & Hoy, E. Studies on the hyperactive child: VII. Neurological status compared with neurotic and normal children. *American Journal of Orthopsychiatry,* 1972, *42,* 441–451.

Werry, J. S., & Sprague, R. L. Hyperactivity. In C. G. Costello (Ed.), *Symptoms of psychopathology.* New York: Wiley, 1970.

Werry, J. S., & Sprague, R. L. Methylphenidate in children: Effect of dosage. *Australian and New Zealand Journal of Psychiatry,* 1974, *8,* 9–19.

Werry, J. S., Sprague, R. L., & Cohen, M. M. Conners Teacher Rating Scale for use in drug studies with children—an empirical study. *Journal of Abnormal Child Psychology,* 1975, *3,* 217–230.

Werry, J. S., Weiss, G., & Douglas, V. Studies on the hyperactive child: I. Some preliminary findings. *Canadian Psychiatric Association Journal,* 1964, *9,* 120–130.

Werry, J. S., Weiss, G., Douglas, V. I., & Martin, J. Studies on the hyperactive child: III. The effect of chlorpromazine upon behavior and learning ability. *Journal of the American Academy of Child Psychiatry,* 1966, *5,* 292–312.

Whalen, C. K. Hyperactivity, learning problems, and the attention deficit disorders. In T. H. Ollendick & M. Hersen (Eds.), *Handbook of child psychopathology.* New York: Plenum Press, 1982, in press.

Whalen, C. K., Collins, B. E., Henker, B., Alkus, S. R., Adams, D., & Stapp, S. Behavior observations of hyperactive children and methylphenidate (Ritalin) effects in systematically structured classroom environments: Now you see them, now you don't. *Journal of Pediatric Psychology,* 1978, *3,* 177–184.

Whalen, C. K., Henker, B., Collins, B. E., McAulliffe, S., & Vaux, A. Peer interaction in structured communication task: Comparisons of normal and hyperactive boys and of methylphenidate (Ritalin) and placebo effects. *Child Development,* 1979, *50,* 388–401.

Whalen, C. K., & Henker, B. Psychostimulants and children: A review and analysis. *Psychological Bulletin,* 1976, 83, 1113–1130.

Whalen, C. K., & Henker, B. The pitfalls of politicization. A response to Conrad's "The discovery of hyperkinesis: Notes on the medicalization of deviant behavior." *Social Problems,* 1977, *24,* 590–595.

Whalen, C. K., & Henker, B. (Eds.). *Hyperactive children: The social ecology of identification and treatment.* New York: Academic Press, 1980a.

Whalen, C. K., & Henker, B. The social ecology of psychostimulant treatment: A model for conceptual and empirical analysis. In C. K. Whalen & B. Henker (Eds.), *Hyperactive children: The social ecology of identification and treatment.* New York: Academic Press, 1980b.

Whalen, C. K., Henker, B., Collins, B. E., Finck, D., & Dotemoto, S. A social ecology of hyperactive boys: Medication effects in systematically structured classroom environments. *Journal of Applied Behavioral Analysis,* 1979, *12,* 65–81.

Whalen, C. K., Henker, B., & Dotemoto, S. Methylphenidate and hyperactivity: Effects on teacher behaviors. *Science,* 1980, *208,* 1280–1282.

Whalen, C. K., Henker, B., & Dotemoto, S. Teacher response to the methylphenidate (Ritalin) versus placebo status of hyperactive boys in the classroom. *Child Development,* 1981, *52,* 1005–1014.

Whalen, C. K., Henker, B., & Finck, D. Medication effects in the classroom: Three naturalistic indicators. *Journal of Abnormal Child Psychology,* 1981, in press.

Whaley-Klahn, M., Loney, J., Weissenburger, F. E., & Prinz, R. Responses of boys and girls to a behaviorally focused school attitude questionnaire. *Journal of School Psychology,* 1976, *14,* 283–290.

White, J. H., & Oshanick, G. Juvenile manic-depressive illness. *American Journal of Psychiatry,* 1977, *134,* 1035–1036.

Whitehouse, D., Shah, U., & Palmer, F. B. Comparison of sustained-release and standard methylphenidate in the treatment of minimal brain dysfunction. *Journal of Clinical Psychiatry,* 1980, *41,* 283–285.

Whiting, B. B. The dependency hangup and experiments in alternative life styles. In J. M. Yinger & S. J. Cutler (Eds.), *Major social issues: A multidisciplinary view.* New York: Free Press, 1978.

Wiener, J. (Ed.). *Psychopharmacology in childhood and adolescence.* New York: Basic Books, 1977.

Wiggins, J. S., & Winder, C. L. The Peer Nomination Inventory: An empirically derived sociometric measure of adjustment in preadolescent boys. *Psychological Reports,* 1961, *9,* 643–677.

Wikler, A., Dixon, J. R., & Parker, J. B. Brain function in problem children and controls. Psychometric, neurological, and electroencephalographic comparison. *American Journal of Psychiatry,* 1970, *127,* 634–645.

Willerman, L. Activity level and hyperactivity in twins. *Child Development,* 1973, *44,* 288–293.

Williams, C. D. The elimination of tantrum behaviors by extinction procedures. *Journal of Abnormal and Social Psychology,* 1959, *59,* 269.

Williamson, G. A., Anderson, R. P., & Lundy, N. C. The ecological treatment of hyperkinesis. *Psychology in the Schools,* 1980, *17,* 249–256.

Wilson, A. Multivariate analysis: Data reduction and treatment evaluation. *British Journal of Psychiatry,* 1976, *128,* 404–407.

Wiltz, N. A., & Gordon, S. B. Parental modification of a child's behavior in an experimental residence. *Journal of Behavior Therapy and Experimental Psychiatry,* 1974, *5,* 107–109.

Winsberg, B. G., Goldstein, S., Yepes, L. E., & Perel, J. M. Imipramine and electrocardiographic abnormalities in hyperactive children. *American Journal of Psychiatry,* 1975, *132,* 542–545.

Winsberg, B. G., & Yepes, L. E. Antipsychotics (major tranquilizers, neuroleptics). In J. S. Werry (Ed.), *Pediatric psychopharmacology,* New York: Brunner/Mazel, 1978.

Winter, R. *The scientific case against smoking.* New York: Crown, 1980.

Witkin, H. A. The perception of the upright. *Scientific American,* 1959, *200,* 50–56.

Wodarski, J. S., Feldman, R. A., & Flax, N. Group therapy and antisocial children: A social learning theory perspective. *Small Group Behavior,* 1974, *5,* 182–210.

Wohlwill, J. F. The confluence of environmental and developmental psychology: Signpost to an ecology of development? *Human Development,* 1980, *23,* 354–358.

Wolberg, L. R., Aronson, M. L., & Wolberg, A. R. (Eds.) *Group therapy 1977: An overview.* New York: Stratton Intercontinental Medical Book Corporation, 1977.

Wolf, C. W. Transactional analysis and the management of hyperactivity. In M. J. Fine (Ed.), *Principles and techniques of intervention with hyperactive children.* Springfield, IL: Thomas, 1977.

Wolff, P. H. The natural history of crying and other vocalizations in early infancy. In B. M. Foss (Ed.), *Determinants of infant behavior, Vol. 4.* London: Methuen, 1969.

Wolpe, J. *Psychotherapy by reciprocal inhibition.* Stanford, CA: Stanford University Press, 1958.

Wolraich, M. L. Stimulant drug therapy in hyperactive children: Research and clinical implications. *Pediatrics,* 1977, *60,* 512–518.

Wolraich, M. L., Drummond, T., Saloman, M. K., O'Brien, M. L., & Sivage, C. Effects of methylphenidate alone and in combination with behavior modification procedures on the behavior and academic performance of hyperactive children. *Journal of Abnormal Child Psychology,* 1978, *6,* 149–161.

Wood, D. R., Reimherr, F. W., Wender, P. H., & Johnson, G. E. Diagnosis and treatment of minimal brain dysfunction in adults. *Archives of General Psychiatry,* 1976, *33,* 1453–1460.

Woollams, S., & Brown, M. *The total handbook of Transactional Analysis.* Englewood Cliffs, NJ: Prentice-Hall, 1979.

Wright, L. S., & McKenzie, C. D. A talking group therapy for hyperactive 11 year old boys. *Devereux Schools Forum,* 1973, *8,* 1–24.

Wyatt v. *Stickney,* 344 F. Supp. 387 (M. D. Ala. 1972).

Yalom, I. D. *The theory and practice of group psychotherapy* (2nd ed.). New York: Basic Books, 1975.

Yanow, M. A report on the use of behavior modification drugs on elementary school children. In M. Yanow (Ed.), *Observations from the treadmill.* New York: Viking Press, 1973.

Yellin, A. M. A standard visual stimulus for use in studies on attention-deficit disorders: Toward the development of standardized sustained and selective attention tests. *Research Communications in Psychology, Psychiatry, and Behavior,* 1980, *5,* 137–143.

Yoss, R., & Moyers, N. The pupillogram of the hyperkinetic child and the underachiever. *Abstracts of Seventh Colloquium on the Pupil,* The Mayo Clinic. Rochester, MN: 1971.

Young, J. C. (Chair.). *United States National Commission on the International Year of the Child: Report to the President.* Washington, D.C.: U. S. Government Printing Office, 1980.

Zahn, T. P., Abate, F., Little, B. C., & Wender, P. H. Minimal brain dysfunction, stimulant drugs and autonomic nervous system activity. *Archives of General Psychiatry,* 1975, *32,* 381–387.

Zara, M. M. Effects of medication on learning in hyperactive four-year-old children. *Dissertation Abstracts International,* 1973, *A34,* 2407.

Zentall, S. S. Optimal stimulation as theoretical basis of hyperactivity. *American Journal of Orthopsychiatry,* 1975, *45,* 549–563.

Zentall, S. S. An environmental stimulation model. *Exceptional Children,* 1977, *43,* 502–510.

Zentall, S. S. Behavioral comparisons of hyperactive and normally active children in natural settings. *Journal of Abnormal Child Psychology,* 1980, *8,* 93–109.

Zentall, S. S., & Barack, R. S. Rating scales for hyperactivity: Concurrent validity, reliability, and decisions to label for the Conners and Davids Abbreviated Scales. *Journal of Abnormal Child Psychology,* 1979, *7,* 179–190.

Zentall, S. S., & Lieb, S. L. Structured tasks: Effects on activity and performance of hyperactive and normal children. Unpublished paper. Eastern Kentucky University, 1981.

Zentall, S. S., & Shaw, J. H. Effects of classroom noise on performance and activity of second grade hyperactive and control children. *Journal of Educational Psychology,* in press, 1981.

Zentall, S., & Zentall, T. R. Activity and task performance of hyperactive children as a function of environmental stimulation. *Journal of Consulting and Clinical Psychology,* 1976, *44,* 693–697.

Zentall, S. S., Zentall, T. R., & Barack, R. S. Distraction as a function of within-task stimulation for hyperactive and normal children. *Journal of Learning Disabilities*, 1978, *11*, 540–548.

Zentall, S., Zentall, T. R., & Booth, M. E. Within-task stimulation: Effects on activity and spelling performance in hyperactive and normal children. *Journal of Educational Research*, 1978, *71*, 223–230.

Zeskind, P. S., Lester, B. M., & Eitzman, D. V. Cry behaviors of low and high risk infants. Paper presented at the biennial meeting of the Society for Research in Child Development, New Orleans, March 1977.

Zimmerman, F. T., & Burgemeister, B. B. Action of methylphenidylacetate (Ritalin) and reserpine in behavior disorders in children and adults. *American Journal of Psychiatry*, 1958, *115*, 323–328.

Zivin,G. How to make a boring thing more boring. *Child Development*, 1974, *45*, 232–236.

Zuckerman, B., Winsmore, G., & Alpert, J. J. A study of attitudes and support systems of inner city adolescent mothers. *Journal of Pediatrics*, 1979, *95*, 122–125.

Zukow, P. G., Zukow, A. H., & Bentler, P. M. Rating scales for the identification and treatment of hyperkinesis. *Journal of Consulting and Clinical Psychology*, 1978, *46*, 213–222.

Zupnick, S. A new approach to disturbed children: The Medical College School Program. *Psychiatric Quarterly*, 1974, *48*, 76–85.

Author Index

Subject Index

Activity level, 29, 35, 42–43, 47
  vs. hyperactivity, 69
  measures of, 126–156
  in peer interactions, 37, 39, 42, 43, 45–46
  as temperament characteristic, 152–156, 160
Adolescence:
  academic performance in, 51–52, 176
  antisocial behavior in, 52–54, 175–176
  and childhood aggression model, 22–24, 68, 175–177
  depression in, 52
  and drug abuse, 199–201
  and drug-induced growth suppression, 201–204
  emotional adjustment in, 52, 175–176
  follow-up studies in, 48–49, 175–177
  natural history of, 48–54
  and poorness of fit in, 51
  pregnancy in, early, 313–316
    education level, 315
    hospital support systems, 314
  prognosis, 47–48, 175–177
  secondary problems in, 49, 175–177
  social interaction in, 50–51, 177
  temperament in, 162
Adulthood, 54–62
  diagnosis in, opposition to, 57
  drug intervention in, 56–57, 186–187
    conference on, 227–228
    and drug abuse, 200
  hyperactivity in, evidence of, 54–56
    adolescent predictors of, 177
    and psychiatric disorders, 60–61, 67–68
  outcome in, 57–60
  time concept in, 56
Advances, major, 20–24
  childhood aggression, importance of, 22–24
  in conceptualization, 21–22
  hyperactive child, in role of, 22
Aggression in childhood:
  and adolescent outcome, 175–177
  and hyperactivity, 23–24, 61, 68

and peer relations, 35–36
as secondary symptom, 2
Assessment:
  of body lead levels, 84–85, 87
  classroom observation schedules, 147–152
  in early secondary prevention, 317–331
    of infants, 319–321
    of young children, 321–331
  electroencephalographic, 78
    developmental equations for, 78
  environmental, in management process, 361
  of mother-child adaptation, infancy, 31–33
  of peer interactions, 45–46, 47
  of primary symptoms, 119–126
  psychoeducational, in management process, 352–361
  rating scales, 126–147. *See also* Rating scales, descriptions of
  of soft signs, 79
  of temperament, 152–156
Attention:
  components of, 121
  deficit, and social skills, 50–51
  as deficit disorder, DSM III, 4, 5, 21
  in developmental delay, 103
  in directing materials, 298
  drug response as predictor of, 172, 174
  drug therapy in, 4
    caffeine, 221–222
    exaggerated control, 205
    focal, 190
    paradoxical effect, 220
    pemoline, 223–224
    tricyclic antidepressants, 225–226
  and environmental constraints, 116
  in Hyperactivity factor (Loney), 175–176
  inattention, 1, 5
    diagnostic criteria, DSM III, 5
    in preschool setting, 37
  in infancy, 322
  measures of, 121–123, 171–174
    for distractibility, 124
    Finger Twitch Test, 165

Psychology and Psychiatry in Courts and Corrections: Controversy and Change
  by Ellsworth A. Fersch, Jr.
Restricted Environmental Stimulation: Research and Clinical Applications
  by Peter Suedfeld
Personal Construct Psychology: Psychotherapy and Personality
  edited by Alvin W. Landfield and Larry M. Leitner
Mothers, Grandmothers, and Daughters: Personality and Child Care in
Three-Generation Families
  by Bertram J. Cohler and Henry U. Grunebaum
Further Explorations in Personality
  edited by A. I. Rabin, Joel Aronoff, Andrew M. Barclay, and Robert A. Zucker
Hypnosis and Relaxation: Modern Verification of an Old Equation
  by William E. Edmonston, Jr.
Handbook of Clinical Behavior Therapy
  edited by Samuel M. Turner, Karen S. Calhoun, and Henry E. Adams
Handbook of Clinical Neuropsychology
  edited by Susan B. Filskov and Thomas J. Boll
The Course of Alcoholism: Four Years After Treatment
  by J. Michael Polich, David J. Armor, and Harriet B. Braiker
Handbook of Innovative Psychotherapies
  edited by Raymond J. Corsini
The Role of the Father in Child Development (Second Edition)
  edited by Michael E. Lamb
Behavioral Medicine: Clinical Applications
  by Susan S. Pinkerton, Howard Hughes, and W. W. Wenrich
Handbook for the Practice of Pediatric Psychology
  edited by June M. Tuma
Change Through Interaction: Social Psychological Processes of Counseling and Psychotherapy
  by Stanley R. Strong and Charles D. Claiborn
Drugs and Behavior (Second Edition)
  by Fred Leavitt
Handbook of Research Methods in Clinical Psychology
  edited by Philip C. Kendall and James N. Butcher
A Social Psychology of Developing Adults
  by Thomas O. Blank
Women in the Middle Years: Current Knowledge and Directions for Research and Policy
  edited by Janet Zollinger Giele
Loneliness: A Sourcebook of Current Theory, Research and Therapy
  edited by Letitia Anne Peplau and Daniel Perlman
Hyperactivity: Current Issues, Research, and Theory (Second Edition)
  by Dorothea M. Ross and Sheila A. Ross